Advances in Thyroid Research

Advances in Thyroid Research

Editor: Dakota Marshall

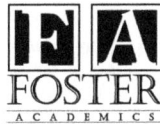

FA
FOSTER
ACADEMICS

www.fosteracademics.com

www.fosteracademics.com

FA
FOSTER
ACADEMICS

Cataloging-in-Publication Data

Advances in thyroid research / edited by Dakota Marshall.
    p. cm.
Includes bibliographical references and index.
ISBN 978-1-63242-643-7
1. Thyroid gland. 2. Thyroid gland--Diseases. I. Marshall, Dakota.
RC655 .A38 2019
61644--dc23

Foster Academics,
118-35 Queens Blvd., Suite 400,
Forest Hills, NY 11375, USA

ISBN 978-1-63242-643-7 (Hardback)

Contents

Preface

The main aim of this book is to educate learners and enhance their research focus by presenting diverse topics covering this vast field. This is an advanced book which compiles significant studies by distinguished experts in the area of analysis. This book addresses successive solutions to the challenges arising in the area of application, along with it; the book provides scope for future developments.

The thyroid is an endocrine gland, located at the front of the neck, which produces the thyroid hormones. Due to certain factors, there may arise a disruption in the normal functioning of the thyroid gland. This condition is termed as thyroid disease. When the thyroid gland does not produce sufficient thyroid hormone or produces excess hormone, it leads to the conditions called hypothyroidism and hyperthyroidism respectively. Various structural abnormalities of the thyroid gland occur such as in the case of goiter, lingual thyroid and thyroglossal duct cyst. Tumors of the thyroid can also occur and can be cancerous or non-cancerous. Side effects of medicines such as amiodarone, some types of interferon and IL-2, lithium salts, dopamine agonists, etc. can affect the thyroid gland. The diagnosis of thyroid disease is primarily determined through blood tests that measure different thyroid hormones, antithyroid antibodies, thyroidglobulin levels, calcitonin levels, etc. In some cases, ultrasound, radioiodine scanning or biopsy may be required. There are several medication pathways for the treatment of thyroid diseases. This book is compiled in such a manner, that it will provide in-depth knowledge about the study of the thyroid gland and associated disorders. The aim of this book is to present researches that have transformed the understanding of thyroid diseases. It is appropriate for students seeking detailed information in this area as well as for experts.

It was a great honour to edit this book, though there were challenges, as it involved a lot of communication and networking between me and the editorial team. However, the end result was this all-inclusive book covering diverse themes in the field.

Finally, it is important to acknowledge the efforts of the contributors for their excellent chapters, through which a wide variety of issues have been addressed. I would also like to thank my colleagues for their valuable feedback during the making of this book.

Editor

Targeted Treatment of Differentiated and Medullary Thyroid Cancer

Shannon R. Bales and Inder J. Chopra

Division of Endocrinology, Diabetes, and Hypertension, University of California, Los Angeles, CA 90095, USA

Correspondence should be addressed to Inder J. Chopra, ichopra@mednet.ucla.edu

Academic Editor: Nelson Wohllk

The incidence of thyroid cancer is increasing, with a concomitant increase in the number of patients with advanced and metastatic disease. Discoveries regarding the pathogenesis of thyroid cancer have led to the recent development of new therapeutic agents that are beginning to appear on the market. Many of these new agents are targeted kinase inhibitors primarily affecting oncogenic kinases (BRAF V600E, RET/PTC) or signaling kinases (VEGFR, PDGFR). Some of these agents report significant partial response rates, while others attain stabilization of disease as their best response. Their impact on survival is unclear. While these agents target similar pathways, a wide variety of differences exist regarding efficacy and side effect profile. Current expert opinion advises that these agents be used only in a specific subset of patients.

1. Introduction

The incidence of thyroid cancer is increasing at an alarming rate. In fact, the incidence has more than doubled in the past fifty years, and it rose approximately 6% per year from 1997 to 2006 [1]. Peak incidence is in the early fifth decade for women and the late sixth decade for men. It is two to three times more common in women than in men, though mortality rates are higher in men. Mortality rates are also higher in patients with African ethnic heritage [1].

Total thyroidectomy followed by radioactive iodine (^{131}I) ablation and thyroid hormone suppression of serum TSH are the mainstay of treatment for differentiated thyroid cancer (DTC). While cure is generally attainable in well-differentiated thyroid carcinomas (papillary and follicular subtypes), recurrence occurs in up to 40% of patients [2]. Unfortunately, in a small percentage of patients with thyroid cancer recurrence, the tumor becomes dedifferentiated. It does not concentrate iodine and thereby becomes unresponsive to (^{131}I) treatment, likely the result of mutational changes in the sodium-iodine symporter [3]. Such tumor often shows increased aggressiveness and has a tendency to metastasize [4, 5].

Patients with medullary thyroid cancer (MTC) are susceptible to early metastatic disease. Between 20 to 30% of patients with T1 tumors at the time of diagnosis already have metastasis to lymph nodes [6]. The mainstay of treatment for these patients is total thyroidectomy with aggressive lymph node dissection. For patients with a family history of MTC or multiple endocrine neoplasia 2A or 2B, prophylactic thyroidectomy is recommended as soon as possible, even in patients who are less than one-year-old [6].

Popular treatment options for advanced stages of DTC and MTC consist of radiotherapy and chemotherapy, which confer only a modest benefit on tumor burden and overall survival. Current treatment regimens for advanced thyroid cancer include bleomycin, doxorubicin, platinum-containing compounds, or a combination of these agents. For the most part, they result in minor responses, and their use is limited by their toxicities. Bleomycin is well known for its pulmonary toxicity, while doxorubicin can cause both cardiac arrhythmias and heart failure. Platinum-based therapies result in neuropathy, nausea, and renal toxicity [7].

However, recent research has shed light on the underlying molecular mechanisms of thyroid cancer and on the role of oncogenic kinases in metastatic thyroid cancer in particular

[8]. Given the high incidence of thyroid cancer and its recently elucidated molecular mechanisms, thyroid cancer has become a focus of effort for use of new targeted therapies, especially the new class of agents that inhibit kinases involved in signaling, cellular growth, and angiogenesis [8]. Most of the therapeutic agents being developed actually target both the oncogenic and the signaling pathways.

2. Overview of the Molecular Pathways of Thyroid Cancer

Comprehensive studies of mutation pathways in DTC and MTC have been undertaken in the past two decades [9–21]. The knowledge gained from these analyses may render DTC and MTC amenable to designer therapeutics. The most important findings center on the discovery of oncogenic kinases, as well as the elucidation of various signaling pathway adaptations occurring in malignant cells. Of the oncogenic kinases, BRAF V600E mutation and RET/PTC mutations are being targeted as potential pathways for therapeutic intervention. Both of these mutations have the potential to activate the mitogen-activated protein kinase (MAPK) pathway downstream. Therapeutics targeting RET/PTC are being developed particularly for use in MTC. The vascular endothelial growth factor (VEGF) and platelet-derived growth factor (PDGF) pathways, as well as the phosphatidylinositol-3-kinase-(PI3K-) phosphatase with tensin homology (PTEN) pathway are important signaling cascades being investigated for possible development of therapeutic kinase inhibitors (Figure 1).

2.1. Oncogenic Kinases.
BRAF mutations are the most commonly encountered mutation in PTC [13, 22, 23]. BRAF mutations are present in 29–83% of cases of papillary thyroid cancer (PTC) [8, 24]. Anaplastic thyroid carcinoma (ATC) also has a high frequency of BRAF mutations, with up to 50% of ATC harboring a mutation in this entity [25]. The BRAF gene is located on chromosome 7q24. Oncogenic BRAF mutations in PTC commonly (approximately 80%) are comprised of a thymidine to adenine substitution in exon 15 (T1799A) resulting in an amino acid sequence change of valine to glutamate (V600E) [22, 26]. This change destabilizes the inactive conformation of BRAF, rendering it constitutively active [14, 26, 27]. Activated oncogenic mutant BRAF has a higher affinity for MEK1 and MEK2 and increases the phosphorylation of MEK. BRAF V600E also potently activates MAPK pathway directly. BRAF can be activated by another genetic rearrangement leading to formation of a fusion protein, AKAP9-BRAF, which can activate MAPK pathways. This rearrangement is present in approximately 11% of PTC [28]. The basis of these mutations is not known. The BRAF V600E mutant does not seem related to radiation exposure. In contrast, the AKAP9-BRAF is thought to be related to irradiation [28–30].

Some authors suggest that PTCs with BRAF mutations are more aggressive and tend to present at a more advanced clinical stage and with extrathyroidal invasion [24, 31]. BRAF mutations are more frequently present in older patients with otherwise classical PTC, who are at a more advanced stage of the disease at the time of diagnosis [24, 31, 32]. This suggestion is also supported by the observation that the tall-cell variant of PTC has a high prevalence of BRAF mutations [33]. Additionally, BRAF mutation is common in aggressive microcarcinomas [34, 35]. These mutations occur rarely or not at all in follicular or medullary thyroid carcinomas, benign adenomas, or benign hyperplasias [23, 36, 37]. Many undifferentiated and anaplastic carcinomas arising from pre-existing PTC have BRAF mutations [32, 38]. Additionally, tumors with BRAF mutations tend to have decreased expression of NIS symporter, and leading the tumor to become refractory to radioiodine treatment [39–41]. Interestingly, BRAF mutation is generally present without other common mutations found in PTC, suggesting that BRAF mutation alone may be sufficient for tumorigenesis [13, 36, 37].

The oncogenic RET/PTC mutation is also commonly found in PTCs, approximately 10–50% [21]. Familial forms of medullary thyroid carcinoma (MTC) also arise from inheritable activating mutations in RET (the most studied being the C634R change) [42, 43]. RET/PTC rearrangements are very common in thyroid tissue exposed to radiation, and are also commonly noted in pediatric PTC [44, 45]. Radiation has been shown to induce this recombination in thyroid cell lines and in normal human thyroid tissue transplanted onto SCID mice [46]. Twelve forms of RET/PTC mutations have been described, with forms 1 and 3 being the most common [16]. RET/PTC1 is typically associated with classical PTC, while RET/PTC3 rearrangement is associated with solid-variant PTCs [17]. These mutations result in the linking of the promoter and N-terminus to unrelated C-terminus fragments of RET, leading to a chimeric receptor that is constitutively active. RET/PTC mutations are uncommon in poorly differentiated cancers, suggesting that this mutation may imply a favorable prognosis [18]. Curiously, RET/PTC expression in thyroid cells has been found to be associated with impaired hormonogenesis and hypothyroidism, particularly Hashimoto's thyroiditis (HT). Whether or not this predisposes an individual with HT to thyroid cancer is unclear [47–49].

2.2. Signaling Kinases.
A few of the important signaling cascades being investigated for the possible development of therapeutic kinase inhibitors are the VEGF and PDGF pathways, as well as the PI3K/PTEN pathway. VEGF is a proangiogenic factor that binds to two receptor tyrosine kinases (VEGFR-1 and VEGFR-2), of which VEGFR-2 is widely recognized to be the primary mediator of angiogenesis. PDGF-B is required for the maturation of microvasculature, while tumor-derived PDGF-A recruits angiogenic stroma to the tissue. VEGFR and PDGFR mutually support the increased activity of each other [50]. Increased VEGF expression appears to be related to worse prognosis, increased risk of recurrence, and the presence of metastasis [51, 52].

The PI3K/PTEN pathway is responsible for regulating glucose metabolism, cell survival, adhesion, and motility [20, 53, 54]. It is found in some thyroid carcinomas (particularly follicular carcinomas) as well as other types of cancers [55–60]. Epigenetic methylation leads to silencing of the negative

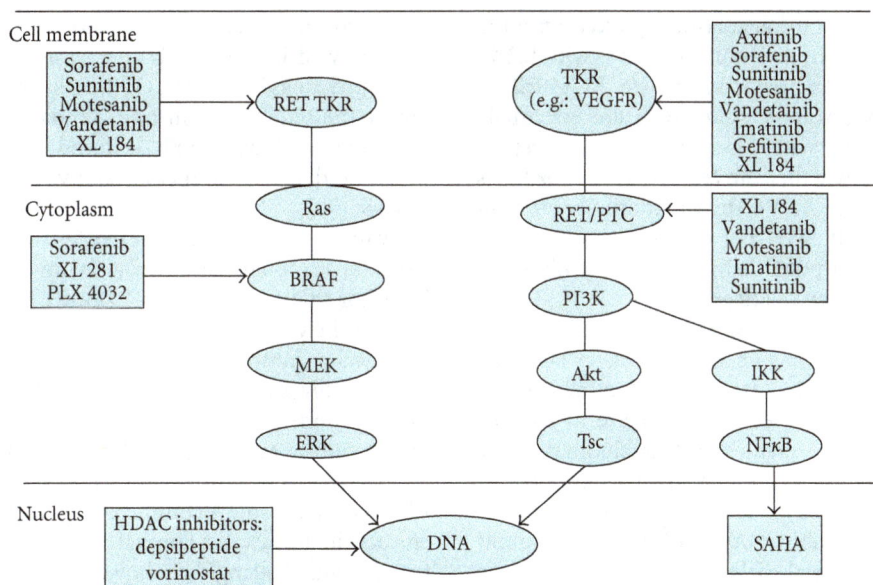

FIGURE 1: Molecular pathways of thyroid cancer and their corresponding therapeutic agents.

regulator PTEN gene, thus facilitating increased activity of the downstream PI3K/Akt pathway [61]. Changes in this pathway occurred in 31% of benign thyroid adenomas, 24% of PTCs, 55% of FTCs, and 58% of ATCs according to one study. The authors concluded that this pathway may be important in the progression from benign thyroid adenoma to follicular cancer to ATC [62]. BRAF mutations have been found along with mutations in PI3K/PTEN pathway in undifferentiated thyroid carcinoma, perhaps promoting progression from DTC to undifferentiated thyroid cancer [15].

3. New Agents for the Treatment of Thyroid Cancer

3.1. Agents Primarily Targeting Oncogenic Kinases. Given the increased frequency of BRAF mutations in PTC, a number of newer therapeutic agents have been developed that inhibit BRAF. The BRAF inhibitor studied most in thyroid cancer is sorafenib. Sorafenib (Nexavar, BAY 43-9006, Bayer) is an oral tyrosine kinase inhibitor which has been approved by the Food and Drug Administration for the treatment of advanced renal cell carcinoma and unresectable hepatocellular carcinoma. It inhibits VEGFR 2/3, RET including RET/PTC1 mutant, c-kit, PDGFR-beta, and BRAF (including the V600E mutation) [63, 64]. It is a biaryl compound that locks the mutant constitutively active kinase in an inactive state. It competitively inhibits ATP binding in the catalytic domains of both normal and mutant BRAF. This triggers G1 phase arrest.

None of the four phase 1 trials of sorafenib included subjects with thyroid cancer, but there is in vitro data in thyroid cancer cell lines that demonstrated efficacy. The phase 1 trials established the optimum dosing regimen as 400 mg twice a day [65]. A number of phase II trials

of sorafenib involved advanced or metastatic DTC. These patients' tumors demonstrated partial responses in 15–27% of participants, and stable disease in a little over 34–61% [66–68]. It should be noted that a recent retrospective review of thirteen patients with advanced DTC from MD Anderson demonstrated particular efficacy of this agent in lung metastasis, while it was less efficacious in bone metastasis [69]. Given its ability to interfere with RET and RET/PTC pathways, treatment with sorafenib was attempted in a phase II trial of MTC. Only a very small portion of patients achieved a partial response, although stable disease response rates were comparable to those seen in the DTC phase II trials [70].

While sorafenib is generally well tolerated with side effects including rash, diarrhea, hand-foot syndrome, and fatigue, treatment with sorafenib may be associated with an increased risk of cardiac toxicities, with up to 40% of patients experiencing EKG changes. Myocardial infarction has also been reported as a side effect of sorafenib in patients being treated for renal cell carcinoma [71, 72]. Increased risk for cutaneous squamous cell carcinomas has been ascribed to the entire class of BRAF inhibitors, and sorafenib is no exception [73].

PLX4032 (RG7204, a Plexxikon drug being codeveloped with Roche) is a 7-azaindole derivative that is currently in clinical trials. PLX4032 specifically inhibits BRAF V600E to a greater extent than wild-type BRAF [74, 75]. Unlike sorafenib which only binds to the inactive conformation of BRAF and keeps it inactive, PLX4032 binds to both the active form and inactive forms of BRAF. It has been shown to actively inhibit proliferation of BRAF-mutant-positive cell lines, particularly in melanoma; thus, most of the clinical trials have been focused on melanoma [76].

Notably, not all cell lines with BRAF V600E mutations respond equally to treatment with PLX4032. Although mutant BRAF V600E has been identified in ATC, PLX4032 did not lead to apoptosis of the anaplastic thyroid carcinoma cell line ARO [77]. Different melanoma cell lines with BRAF V600E demonstrate differential response to PLX4032 as well; some are highly sensitive while some are essentially unresponsive to treatment with this agent. These differences might be explained by whether the cell line is homozygous or heterozygous for the BRAF V600E mutation. Variation in the upregulation of the PI3K/PTEN pathway in response to treatment with this agent potentially mediates the observed resistance in nonresponding cell lines [78].

An early clinical trial of PLX4032 demonstrated that one out of three participants with thyroid cancer achieved a partial response [79]. Rashes are the most common side effect of this agent. Again noted is an increase in risk for development of cutaneous squamous cell carcinomas, likely owing to its anti-BRAF activity [79]. XL281 (Exelixis, Bristol-Meyers-Squibb BMS-908662) is another oral agent similar to PLX4032 in that it inhibits both wild-type and mutant BRAF kinases. Phase I clinical trials are ongoing and include subjects with thyroid carcinoma though early results are not encouraging [80].

Sunitinib (Sutent, SU11248, Pfizer) is a tyrosine kinase inhibitor affecting VEGFR 1/2/3, RET, RET/PTC1, and RET/PTC3 [81]. Of DTC and MTC patients enrolled in a phase II trial of sunitinib receiving 50 mg/day, partial response was observed in 13% of patients with DTC, while stable disease was the best response in 68% of patients with DTC. Eighty-three percent of patients with MTC achieved stable disease [82]. Additionally, there are case reports of patients with advanced MTC having a dramatic response to treatment with sunitinib with respect to both serum calcitonin levels and tumor burden [83]. Patients experience side effects primarily relating to fatigue, and diarrhea when treated with sunitinib. Another unique adverse effect of this agent is palmar-plantar erythrodesia.

Sunitinib can also cause hypothyroidism like many of the tyrosine kinase inhibitors. The mechanism is thought to be related to a destructive thyroiditis when administered for the treatment of renal cell carcinoma [84, 85]. However, this is unlikely to be the cause of hypothyroidism in thyroid cancer patients, as they have all presumably undergone total thyroidectomy. There is other evidence suggesting that increases in TSH in athyreotic patients are associated with increased type 3 deiodination and augmented peripheral thyroid hormone metabolism [86]. Interestingly, some studies suggest that development of hypothyroidism during treatment for other cancers other than thyroid cancer may actually be an encouraging prognostic factor [87, 88].

Heart failure may also be a serious adverse effect sunitinib, occurring in 2.7% of patients from a retrospective study of 600 patients at MD Anderson [69]. A different retrospective analysis including 75 patients involved in phase I and II trials with sunitinib at several centers around the United States reported an 11% cardiac event rate, and a decrease in left ventricular ejection fraction of greater than 10% in 47% of included subjects. Half of the included patients developed hypertension [89]. While the mechanism of heart failure associated with tyrosine kinase inhibitors may be related to mitochondrial damage, recent studies postulate that myocyte damage occurs secondary to a lack of target selectivity of binding to both tyrosine kinases and serine-threonine kinases [89–91]. Of the clinically available tyrosine kinase inhibitors used in one comparison study, sunitinib, sorafenib, and pazopanib induced the highest degree of myocyte damage as measured by lactate dehydrogenase leakage [90].

Vandetanib (Zactima, ZD6474, iPR Pharmaceuticals, AstraZeneca Pharmaceuticals) is an oral tyrosine kinase inhibitor that targets VEGFR 2/3, RET, and EGFR [92, 93]. It is a heteroaromatic-substituted anilinoquinazoline. It specifically inhibits RET/PTC1 and RET/PTC3 in PTC, and M918R RET mutations in MEN2B [94, 95]. Recent investigations into the mechanism of action of vandetanib in cell culture revealed that the agents ability to block both RET and EGFR simultaneously can prevent escape from RET blockade [96]. A completed phase II trial demonstrated efficacy in metastatic familial MTC [97]; 21% of patients treated with 300 mg/day showed a partial response, while 53% patients had stable disease at 24 weeks. There was a decrease in levels of calcitonin in most patients. Adverse effects were significant enough to require dose reductions in several subjects and consisted of diarrhea, severe rash, fatigue, and QTC prolongation [97].

The vandetanib safety database, which accrues data from treatment of multiple cancer types, noted a potential increase in other serious entities such as cerebrovascular accidents and interstitial lung disease [98]. Recent US Food and Drug Administration review cites concern regarding the side effect profile of this agent and propose limiting the indications to progressive symptomatic disease [98]. Another recently published study of subjects with locally advanced or metastatic hereditary MTC administered only 100 mg/day of the drug with nearly similar response rates compared to the above study, and was somewhat better tolerated regarding side effects [99]. Other phase II trials for familial MTC and DTC are underway, as are phase III trials for metastatic MTC. Based on the above mentioned trials as well as other recent data, in April 2011, the US Food and Drug Administration approved vandetanib for use in late-stage MTC. This is the first medication approved by the FDA for the treatment of MTC [100].

Imatinib Mesylate (STI571, Gleevec, Novartis) is an oral tyrosine kinase inhibitor (TKI) that suppresses c-ABL mutation, c-KIT, and inhibits RET autophosphorylation [101]. It was first utilized in the 1990s for treatment of BCR/ABL-positive leukemias. In anaplastic thyroid cancer cell lines (FRO and ARO), it caused growth inhibition, but did not inhibit growth in papillary thyroid cancer cell lines [102, 103]. Two small phase II trials of patients with MTC showed only a small percentage of subjects achieving a stable disease as their best tumor response [104, 105]. These patients were treated with 600 mg daily of imatinib. Over half of the patients were noted to have profound hypothyroidism and required significant increases in their need for thyroid hormone.

New agents are also on the horizon, particularly in RET-mutant MTC. Withaferin A (WA) is a novel compound which appears effective against MTC cell proliferation in culture. WA inhibits both activation and phosphorylation of RET as well as total RET expression. The investigators recently published evidence of its efficacy in a murine model of MTC. Treatment with WA resulted in 80% regression of tumor volume in the treated animals with a corresponding significant decrease in calcitonin levels. Additionally, all the treated animals were alive at 6 weeks, while essentially all the control animals died by this point in time [106].

3.2. Agents Primarily Targeting Signaling Kinases. Pazopanib (Votrient, GlaxoSmithKline, GW786034) is a second-generation oral small molecule kinase inhibitor that targets VEGFR-1, 2, and 3, as well as alpha and beta PDGFR [107]. There is new data from studies of breast cancer indicating that it also targets multiple forms of Raf, though it likely does not affect the common BRAF V600E mutant [108]. It is approved for use in renal cell carcinoma and is likely effective in other forms of cancer including ovarian cancer, and nonsmall cell lung carcinoma [109–111].

A phase II study completed in early 2009 of thyroid cancer patients led by the Mayo Clinic demonstrated a confirmed partial response rate by RECIST criteria in 49% of enrolled subjects (18 patients). There were no complete responses [112]. Starting dose was 800 mg per day. Patients able to tolerate maximum doses of the medication significantly decreased their tumor size as compared to those patients unable to tolerate maximum doses of the agent. Although not statistically significant, the subset of patients with FTC attained a partial response more frequently than subjects with PTC. Forty-three percent (43%) required dose reductions, owing most frequently to fatigue, skin and hair hypopigmentation, diarrhea, and nausea. Nearly 66% of patients doubled their TSH concentrations. Also of note, three patients (8%) developed grade 3 lower gastrointestinal hemorrhage, which according to the authors is similar to the rate noted in trials with Sorafenib [112].

Motesanib (AMG706, Amgen) is an oral tyrosine-kinase inhibitor that inhibits autophosphorylation of RET and also targets VEGFR 1, 2, and 3, PDGFR, and c-KIT. It demonstrates both direct antitumor and antiangiogenic properties [113]. Phase 1 trials were encouraging with 3 DTC patients registering a partial response [114]. A subsequent phase II trial administering 125 mg/day to patients with DTC demonstrated a partial response in 14% of patients, while 35% of patients had stable disease after 48 weeks [115]. A separate arm of this study examined a cohort of patients with advanced, progressive, symptomatic, or metastatic MTC. In this MTC cohort, 2% of patients showed an objective response, 81% maintained stable disease, and an overall 76% of patients showed decrease in the size of their target lesions [116]. Motesanib was generally well tolerated in both cohorts with fatigue, nausea, diarrhea, and hypertension comprising the majority of adverse side effects. As a result of treatment with motesanib, greater than 60% of patients experienced a TSH elevation out of the desired therapeutic range at some time during the study [116]. A recent study of both DTC and MTC revealed that a decrease in soluble VEGFR-2 and a concurrent increase in placental growth factor (PlGF) during the course of treatment with motesanib predicted

which patients would respond to treatment with this agent [117].

Axitinib (AG-013736) inhibits VEGFR more specifically than the agents discussed above. A phase I study included patients with thyroid cancer though none demonstrated partial responses [118]. A phase II study using a dose of 5 mg orally two times per day noted partial responses in 31% of the patients with DTC and in 18% of the patients with MTC. Side effects included fatigue, stomatitis, and hypertension [119]. Further trials are ongoing.

XL 184 (BMS-907351) inhibits VEGF 1 and 2, C-MET, RET, c-kit, fms-related tyrosine kinase 3 (FLT3), and TIE-2. A unique aspect of this agent is its activity against hepatocyte growth factor (HGF) and C-MET, both of which are overexpressed in PTC [120]. A phase 1 trial was promising; 55% of 36 patients MTC demonstrated a partial response, and 84% overall had stable disease [121]. Interestingly, patients both with and without RET mutations responded. A phase III trial exploring XL 184 in MTC is currently underway.

Other recently evaluated novel agents include pyrazolopyrimidine derivatives like CLM3 and CLM29, which also appear to be widely effective against cytoplasmic and receptor ATP competitive tyrosine kinases including RET, EGFR, VEGFR, and angiogenesis pathways. These agents are unique because they induce apoptosis and decrease tumor volume in murine models of dedifferentiated PTC, irrespective of BRAFV600E mutation [122].

4. Conclusion

Recent increased incidence of thyroid cancer is associated with a rise in the number of patients with metastatic disease and tumors that are resistant to the effect of radioiodine. Presently, there are no consensus guidelines about safe and effective methods to treat advanced-stage thyroid cancers. However, the recent elucidation of the pathogenesis of thyroid cancer has facilitated the development of new targeted agents intended to have activity against specific biochemical and oncologic pathways. Many of these newer agents being developed and tested are kinase inhibitors that show a promise for improved treatment of advanced DTC, as well as MTC.

In general, options for the chemotherapeutic treatment of advanced-stage thyroid cancers remain limited. The most promising agents display activity against VEGFR, including pazopanib, motesanib, sorafenib, sunitinib, and vandetanib. There is structural similarity between VEGFR and RET kinases, and cross-activity likely occurs perhaps increasing the efficacy of these agents. Interestingly, axitinib (a tyrosine kinase inhibitor that more specifically targets VEGFR) garnered similar promising tumor responses to the above noted multitargeted kinase inhibitors [119]. In addition, the effective targeted kinase inhibitors not only demonstrate specific activity against VEGFR, but also exhibit activity against a wide array of cellular pathways.

Perhaps owing to their wide ranging cellular targets, there are also numerous concerning side effects of these multitargeted kinase inhibitors. Several trials of the above listed agents reported a significant percentage of patients requiring a dose reduction during the study period for general tolerability. The most concerning adverse effects are increases in the incidence of cardiomyopathy and associated hypertension and stroke. Additionally, minor-to-severe bleeding (often in the form of gastrointestinal bleeding) should not be overlooked. Trials of motesanib and sunitinib noted increasing TSH values during the course of treatment, placing patients at risk for being on subtherapeutic doses of suppressive thyroid hormone for a period of time.

Other targeted kinase agents have been shown less effective than previously hoped. Imatinib does not appear to be a candidate for further study in MTC, nor does gefitinib which was not discussed in detail because a phase II trial did not demonstrate any partial responses [123]. Agents specifically targeting the BRAF pathway and BRAF V600E are in earlier stages of clinical trials; however, stable disease appears to be the best response achieved in this class of agents, including PLX4032 as well as XL281. The more specific BRAF inhibitors also have concerning side effects, including an increased incidence of squamous cell neoplasms.

Overall, options for targeted therapy of patients with advanced thyroid cancer remain limited. While these agents may improve radiographic tumor response, change in survival is unclear. Most trials have demonstrated that only small percentages of patients achieved partial responses. There has been a lack of complete responses [124]. Current expert opinion advises that these agents be used only in a specific subset of patients. They should be administered only to patients with rapidly progressive radioiodine refractory metastatic disease. Locally recurrent, unresectable cancer which is unresponsive to radiation may also be considered appropriate for treatment [125].

Other lines of research must be pursued including immunotherapy with vaccines and interferon administration, as well as efforts to induce redifferentiation of tumor cells to take up radioiodine with histone deacetylase inhibitors Romidepsin and Vorinostat, for example [126–131]. Another area that warrants further investigation is the exploration of biomarkers that may be able to predict response to a given agent, which may help tailor treatment to an individual. Additionally, both *in vivo* and *in vitro* chemosensitivity testing is becoming more common, and is currently available in several clinical trials. These tests appear to be most useful in terms of negative predictability, meaning a treatment is very likely to be unsuccessful in vivo if it is unsuccessful in vitro. Unfortunately the positive predictability of such tests is not as robust. There are many diverse challenges to be addressed before chemosensitivity becomes routine [122, 132]. Promising new studies are being performed investigating combinations of tyrosine kinase inhibitors with other conventional modalities of treatment, like radiation [133]. Much new data is required before such agents are offered routinely for the treatment of advanced or dedifferentiated thyroid cancer.

References

[1] "Surveillance, Epidemiology, and End Results (S.E.E.R. Program)," Generate custom reports from the cancer statistics review, Seer 9: 1975–2007, December 2010, http://seer.cancer.gov/.

[2] M. J. Schlumberger, "Papillary and follicular thyroid carcinoma," *New England Journal of Medicine*, vol. 338, no. 5, pp. 297–306, 1998.

[3] M. R. Castro, E. R. Bergert, J. R. Goellner, I. D. Hay, and J. C. Morris, "Immunohistochemical analysis of sodium iodide symporter expression in metastatic differentiated thyroid cancer: correlation with radioiodine uptake," *Journal of Clinical Endocrinology and Metabolism*, vol. 86, no. 11, pp. 5627–5632, 2001.

[4] L. S. Ward, P. L. Santarosa, F. Granja, L. V. M. Da Assumpção, M. Savoldi, and G. H. Goldman, "Low expression of sodium iodide symporter identifies aggressive thyroid tumors," *Cancer Letters*, vol. 200, no. 1, pp. 85–91, 2003.

[5] J. A. Fagin, "How thyroid tumors start and why it matters: kinase mutants as targets for solid cancer pharmacotherapy," *Journal of Endocrinology*, vol. 183, no. 2, pp. 249–256, 2004.

[6] C. Scollo, E. Baudin, J. P. Travagli et al., "Rationale for central and bilateral lymph node dissection in sporadic and hereditary medullary thyroid cancer," *Journal of Clinical Endocrinology and Metabolism*, vol. 88, no. 5, pp. 2070–2075, 2003.

[7] S. I. Sherman, "Cytotoxic chemotherapy for differentiated thyroid carcinoma," *Clinical Oncology*, vol. 22, no. 6, pp. 464–468, 2010.

[8] M. Xing, "BRAF mutation in thyroid cancer," *Endocrine-Related Cancer*, vol. 12, no. 2, pp. 245–262, 2005.

[9] G. Salvatore, V. De Falco, P. Salerno et al., "BRAF is a therapeutic target in aggressive thyroid carcinoma," *Clinical Cancer Research*, vol. 12, no. 5, pp. 1623–1629, 2006.

[10] B. Ouyang, J. A. Knauf, E. P. Smith et al., "Inhibitors of Raf kinase activity block growth of thyroid cancer cells with RET/PTC or BRAF mutations in vitro and in vivo," *Clinical Cancer Research*, vol. 12, no. 6, pp. 1785–1793, 2006.

[11] P. Hou, E. Bojdani, and M. Xing, "Induction of thyroid gene expression and radioiodine uptake in thyroid cancer cells by targeting major signaling pathways," *Journal of Clinical Endocrinology and Metabolism*, vol. 95, no. 2, pp. 820–828, 2010.

[12] D. J. Lim, K. H. Baek, Y. S. Lee et al., "Clinical, histopathological, and molecular characteristics of papillary thyroid microcarcinoma," *Thyroid*, vol. 17, no. 9, pp. 883–888, 2007.

[13] E. T. Kimura, M. N. Nikiforova, Z. Zhu, J. A. Knauf, Y. E. Nikiforov, and J. A. Fagin, "High prevalence of BRAF mutations in thyroid cancer: genetic evidence for constitutive activation of the RET/PTC-RAS-BRAF signaling pathway in papillary thyroid carcinoma," *Cancer Research*, vol. 63, no. 7, pp. 1454–1457, 2003.

[14] P. T. C. Wan, M. J. Garnett, S. M. Roe et al., "Mechanism of activation of the RAF-ERK signaling pathway by oncogenic mutations of B-RAF," *Cell*, vol. 116, no. 6, pp. 855–867, 2004.

[15] P. Hou, D. Liu, Y. Shan et al., "Genetic alterations and their relationship in the phosphatidylinositol 3-kinase/Akt pathway in thyroid cancer," *Clinical Cancer Research*, vol. 13, no. 4, pp. 1161–1170, 2007.

[16] M. Santoro, N. A. Dathan, M. T. Berlingieri et al., "Molecular characterization of RET/PTC3; a novel rearranged version of the RETproto-oncogene in a human thyroid papillary carcinoma," *Oncogene*, vol. 9, no. 2, pp. 509–516, 1994.

[17] Y. E. Nikiforov, J. M. Rowland, K. E. Bove, H. Monforte-Munoz, and J. A. Fagin, "Distinct pattern of ret oncogene rearrangements in morphological variants of radiation-induced and sporadic thyroid papillary carcinomas in children," *Cancer Research*, vol. 57, no. 9, pp. 1690–1694, 1997.

[18] G. Tallini, M. Santoro, M. Helie et al., "RET/PTC oncogene activation defines a subset of papillary thyroid carcinomas lacking evidence of progression to poorly differentiated or undifferentiated tumor phenotypes," *Clinical Cancer Research*, vol. 4, no. 2, pp. 287–294, 1998.

[19] M. D. Ringel, N. Hayre, J. Saito et al., "Overexpression and overactivation of Akt in thyroid carcinoma," *Cancer Research*, vol. 61, no. 16, pp. 6105–6111, 2001.

[20] H. Sun, R. Lesche, D. M. Li et al., "PTEN modulates cell cycle progression and cell survival by regulating phosphatidylinositol 3,4,5,-trisphosphate and Akt/protein kinase B signaling pathway," *Proceedings of the National Academy of Sciences of the United States of America*, vol. 96, no. 11, pp. 6199–6204, 1999.

[21] R. Ciampi and Y. E. Nikiforov, "Minireview: RET/PTC rearrangements and braf mutations in thyroid tumorigenesis," *Endocrinology*, vol. 148, no. 3, pp. 936–941, 2007.

[22] Y. Cohen, M. Xing, E. Mambo et al., "BRAF mutation in papillary thyroid carcinoma," *Journal of the National Cancer Institute*, vol. 95, no. 8, pp. 625–627, 2003.

[23] E. Puxeddu, S. Moretti, R. Elisei et al., "BRAFV599E mutation is the leading genetic event in adult sporadic papillary thyroid carcinomas," *Journal of Clinical Endocrinology and Metabolism*, vol. 89, no. 5, pp. 2414–2420, 2004.

[24] R. Elisei, C. Ugolini, D. Viola et al., "BRAFV600E mutation and outcome of patients with papillary thyroid carcinoma: a 15-year median follow-up study," *Journal of Clinical Endocrinology and Metabolism*, vol. 93, no. 10, pp. 3943–3949, 2008.

[25] A. M. Costa, A. Herrero, M. F. Fresno et al., "BRAF mutation associated with other genetic events identifies a subset of aggressive papillary thyroid carcinoma," *Clinical Endocrinology*, vol. 68, no. 4, pp. 618–634, 2008.

[26] H. Davies, G. R. Bignell, C. Cox et al., "Mutations of the BRAF gene in human cancer," *Nature*, vol. 417, no. 6892, pp. 949–954, 2002.

[27] T. Brummer, H. Naegele, M. Reth, and Y. Misawa, "Identification of novel ERK-mediated feedback phosphorylation sites at the C-terminus of B-Raf," *Oncogene*, vol. 22, no. 55, pp. 8823–8834, 2003.

[28] R. Ciampi, J. A. Knauf, R. Kerler et al., "Oncogenic AKAP9-BRAF fusion is a novel mechanism of MAPK pathway activation in thyroid cancer," *Journal of Clinical Investigation*, vol. 115, no. 1, pp. 94–101, 2005.

[29] M. N. Nikiforova, R. Ciampi, G. Salvatore et al., "Low prevalence of BRAF mutations in radiation-induced thyroid tumors in contrast to sporadic papillary carcinomas," *Cancer Letters*, vol. 209, no. 1, pp. 1–6, 2004.

[30] B. J. Collins, A. B. Schneider, R. A. Prinz, and X. Xu, "Low frequency of BRAF mutations in adult patients with papillary thyroid cancers following childhood radiation exposure," *Thyroid*, vol. 16, no. 1, pp. 61–66, 2006.

[31] M. Xing, W. H. Westra, R. P. Tufano et al., "BRAF mutation predicts a poorer clinical prognosis for papillary thyroid cancer," *Journal of Clinical Endocrinology and Metabolism*, vol. 90, no. 12, pp. 6373–6379, 2005.

[32] M. N. Nikiforova, E. T. Kimura, M. Gandhi et al., "BRAF mutations in thyroid tumors are restricted to papillary carcinomas and anaplastic or poorly differentiated carcinomas arising from papillary carcinomas," *Journal of Clinical Endocrinology and Metabolism*, vol. 88, no. 11, pp. 5399–5404, 2003.

[33] A. J. Adeniran, Z. Zhu, M. Gandhi et al., "Correlation between genetic alterations and microscopic features, clinical manifestations, and prognostic characteristics of thyroid papillary carcinomas," *American Journal of Surgical Pathology*, vol. 30, no. 2, pp. 216–222, 2006.

[34] I. Sedliarou, V. Saenko, D. Lantsov et al., "The BRAFT1796A transversion is a prevalent mutational event in human thyroid microcarcinoma," *International journal of oncology*, vol. 25, no. 6, pp. 1729–1735, 2004.

[35] X. Lee, M. Gao, Y. Ji et al., "Analysis of differential BRAFV600E mutational status in high aggressive papillary thyroid microcarcinoma," *Annals of Surgical Oncology*, vol. 16, no. 2, pp. 240–245, 2009.

[36] M. Frattini, C. Ferrario, P. Bressan et al., "Alternative mutations of BRAF, RET and NTRK1 are associated with similar but distinct gene expression patterns in papillary thyroid cancer," *Oncogene*, vol. 23, no. 44, pp. 7436–7440, 2004.

[37] P. Soares, V. Trovisco, A. S. Rocha et al., "BRAF mutations and RET/PTC rearrangements are alternative events in the etiopathogenesis of PTC," *Oncogene*, vol. 22, no. 29, pp. 4578–4580, 2003.

[38] R. M. Quiros, H. G. Ding, P. Gattuso, R. A. Prinz, and X. Xu, "Evidence that one subset of anaplastic thyroid carcinomas are derived from papillary carcinomas due to BRAF and p53 mutations," *Cancer*, vol. 103, no. 11, pp. 2261–2268, 2005.

[39] C. Durante, E. Puxeddu, E. Ferretti et al., "Brief report: BRAF mutations in papillary thyroid carcinomas inhibit genes involved in iodine metabolism," *Journal of Clinical Endocrinology and Metabolism*, vol. 92, no. 7, pp. 2840–2843, 2007.

[40] D. Liu, S. Hu, P. Hou, D. Jiang, S. Condouris, and M. Xing, "Suppression of BRAF/MEK/MAP kinase pathway restores expression of iodide-metabolizing genes in thyroid cells expressing the V600E BRAF mutant," *Clinical Cancer Research*, vol. 13, no. 4, pp. 1341–1349, 2007.

[41] G. Riesco-Eizaguirre, I. Rodríguez, A. De La Vieja et al., "The BRAFV600E oncogene induces transforming growth factor β secretion leading to sodium iodide symporter repression and increased malignancy in thyroid cancer," *Cancer Research*, vol. 69, no. 21, pp. 8317–8325, 2009.

[42] J. A. Fagin, K. Matsuo, A. Karmakar, Dan Lin Chen, S. H. Tang, and H. P. Koeffler, "High prevalence of mutations of the p53 gene in poorly differentiated human thyroid carcinomas," *Journal of Clinical Investigation*, vol. 91, no. 1, pp. 179–184, 1993.

[43] L. Ludwig, H. Kessler, M. Wagner et al., "Nuclear factor-κB is constitutively active in C-cell carcinoma and required for RET-induced transformation," *Cancer Research*, vol. 61, no. 11, pp. 4526–4535, 2001.

[44] A. Bounacer, R. Wicker, B. Caillou et al., "High prevalence of activating ret proto-oncogene rearrangements, in thyroid tumors from patients who had received external radiation," *Oncogene*, vol. 15, no. 11, pp. 1263–1273, 1997.

[45] C. L. Fenton, Y. Lukes, D. Nicholson, C. A. Dinauer, G. L. Francis, and R. M. Tuttle, "The ret/PTC mutations are common in sporadic papillary thyroid carcinoma of children and young adults," *Journal of Clinical Endocrinology and Metabolism*, vol. 85, no. 3, pp. 1170–1175, 2000.

[46] T. Mizuno, K. S. Iwamoto, S. Kyoizumi et al., "Preferential induction of RET/PTC1 rearrangement by X-ray irradiation," *Oncogene*, vol. 19, no. 3, pp. 438–443, 2000.

[47] A. Wirtschafter, R. Schmidt, D. Rosen et al., "Expression of the RET/PTC fusion gene as a marker for papillary carcinoma in Hashimoto's thyroiditis," *Laryngoscope*, vol. 107, no. 1, pp. 95–100, 1997.

[48] O. M. Sheils, J. J. O'Leary, V. Uhlmann, K. Lüttich, and E. C. Sweeney, "ret/PTC-1 activation in Hashimoto thyroiditis," *International Journal of Surgical Pathology*, vol. 8, no. 3, pp. 185–189, 2000.

[49] M. N. Nikiforova, C. M. Caudill, P. Biddinger, and Y. E. Nikiforov, "Prevalence of RET/PTC rearrangements in Hashimoto's thyroiditis and papillary thyroid carcinomas," *International Journal of Surgical Pathology*, vol. 10, no. 1, pp. 15–22, 2002.

[50] N. Ferrara and R. S. Kerbel, "Angiogenesis as a therapeutic target," *Nature*, vol. 438, no. 7070, pp. 967–974, 2005.

[51] M. Klein, J. M. Vignaud, V. Hennequin et al., "Increased expression of the vascular endothelial growth factor is a pejorative prognosis marker in papillary thyroid carcinoma," *Journal of Clinical Endocrinology and Metabolism*, vol. 86, no. 2, pp. 656–658, 2001.

[52] C. M. Lennard, A. Patel, J. Wilson et al., "Intensity of vascular endothelial growth factor expression is associated with increased risk of recurrence and decreased disease-free survival in papillary thyroid cancer," *Surgery*, vol. 129, no. 5, pp. 552–558, 2001.

[53] A. K. Ghosh, I. Grigorieva, R. Steele, R. G. Hoover, and R. B. Ray, "PTEN transcriptionally modulates c-myc gene expression in human breast carcinoma cells and is involved in cell growth regulation," *Gene*, vol. 235, no. 1-2, pp. 85–91, 1999.

[54] M. Tamura, J. Gu, E. H. J. Danen, T. Takino, S. Miyamoto, and K. M. Yamada, "PTEN interactions with focal adhesion kinase and suppression of the extracellular matrix-dependent phosphatidylinositol 3-kinase/Akt cell survival pathway," *Journal of Biological Chemistry*, vol. 274, no. 29, pp. 20693–20703, 1999.

[55] P. A. Steck, M. A. Pershouse, S. A. Jasser et al., "Identification of a candidate tumour suppressor gene, MMAC1, at chromosome 10q23.3 that is mutated in multiple advanced cancers," *Nature Genetics*, vol. 15, no. 4, pp. 356–362, 1997.

[56] D. S. Byun, K. Cho, B. K. Ryu et al., "Frequent monoallelic deletion of PTEN and its reciprocal associatioin with PIK3CA amplification in gastric carcinoma," *International Journal of Cancer*, vol. 104, no. 3, pp. 318–327, 2003.

[57] T. Kimura, A. Suzuki, Y. Fujita et al., "Conditional loss of PTEN leads to testicular teratoma and enhances embryonic germ cell production," *Development*, vol. 130, no. 8, pp. 1691–1700, 2003.

[58] S. Wang, A. J. Garcia, M. Wu, D. A. Lawson, O. N. Witte, and H. Wu, "Pten deletion leads to the expansion of a prostatic stem/progenitor cell subpopulation and tumor initiation," *Proceedings of the National Academy of Sciences of the United States of America*, vol. 103, no. 5, pp. 1480–1485, 2006.

[59] A. Yokomizo, D. J. Tindall, L. Hartmann, R. B. Jenkins, D. I. Smith, and W. Liu, "Mutation analysis of the putative tumor suppressor PTEN/MMAC1 in human ovarian cancer," *International Journal of Oncology*, vol. 13, no. 1, pp. 101–105, 1998.

[60] M. E. McMenamin, P. Soung, S. Perera, I. Kaplan, M. Loda, and W. R. Sellers, "Loss of PTEN expression in paraffin-embedded primary prostate cancer correlates with high Gleason score and advanced stage," *Cancer Research*, vol. 59, no. 17, pp. 4291–4296, 1999.

[61] P. Hou, M. Ji, and M. Xing, "Association of PTEN gene methylation with genetic alterations in the phosphatidylinositol 3-kinase/AKT signaling pathway in thyroid tumors," *Cancer*, vol. 113, no. 9, pp. 2440–2447, 2008.

[62] P. Hou, D. Liu, Y. Shan et al., "Genetic alterations and their relationship in the phosphatidylinositol 3-kinase/Akt pathway in thyroid cancer," *Clinical Cancer Research*, vol. 13, no. 4, pp. 1161–1170, 2007.

[63] S. M. Wilhelm, C. Carter, L. Tang et al., "BAY 43-9006 exhibits broad spectrum oral antitumor activity and targets the RAF/MEK/ERK pathway and receptor tyrosine kinases involved in tumor progression and angiogenesis," *Cancer Research*, vol. 64, no. 19, pp. 7099–7109, 2004.

[64] Y. C. Henderson, S. H. Ann, Y. Kang, and G. L. Clayman, "Sorafenib potently inhibits papillary thyroid carcinomas harboring RET/PTC1 rearrangement," *Clinical Cancer Research*, vol. 14, no. 15, pp. 4908–4914, 2008.

[65] D. Strumberg, J. W. Clark, A. Awada et al., "Safety, pharmacokinetics, and preliminary antitumor activity of sorafenib: a review of four phase I trials in patients with advanced refractory solid tumors," *Oncologist*, vol. 12, no. 4, pp. 426–437, 2007.

[66] V. Gupta-Abramson, A. B. Troxel, A. Nellore et al., "Phase II trial of sorafenib in advanced thyroid cancer," *Journal of Clinical Oncology*, vol. 26, no. 29, pp. 4714–4719, 2008.

[67] R. T. Kloos, M. D. Ringel, M. V. Knopp et al., "Phase II trial of sorafenib in metastatic thyroid cancer," *Journal of Clinical Oncology*, vol. 27, no. 10, pp. 1675–1684, 2009.

[68] H. Hoftijzer, K. A. Heemstra, H. Morreau et al., "Beneficial effects of sorafenib on tumor progression, but not on radioiodine uptake, in patients with differentiated thyroid carcinoma," *European Journal of Endocrinology*, vol. 161, no. 6, pp. 923–931, 2009.

[69] M. E. Cabanillas, S. G. Waguespack, Y. Bronstein et al., "Treatment with tyrosine kinase inhibitors for patients with differentiated thyroid cancer: the M. D. Anderson experience," *Journal of Clinical Endocrinology and Metabolism*, vol. 95, no. 6, pp. 2588–2595, 2010.

[70] E. T. Lam, M. D. Ringel, R. T. Kloos et al., "Phase II clinical trial of sorafenib in metastatic medullary thyroid cancer," *Journal of Clinical Oncology*, vol. 28, no. 14, pp. 2323–2330, 2010.

[71] M. Schmidinger, C. C. Zielinski, U. M. Vogl et al., "Cardiac toxicity of sunitinib and sorafenib in patients with metastatic renal cell carcinoma," *Journal of Clinical Oncology*, vol. 26, no. 32, pp. 5204–5212, 2008.

[72] Y. Arima, S. Oshima, K. Noda et al., "Sorafenib-induced acute myocardial infarction due to coronary artery spasm," *Journal of Cardiology*, vol. 54, no. 3, pp. 512–515, 2009.

[73] J. P. Arnault, J. Wechsler, B. Escudier et al., "Keratoacanthomas and squamous cell carcinomas in patients receiving sorafenib," *Journal of Clinical Oncology*, vol. 27, no. 23, pp. e59–e61, 2009.

[74] G. Bollag, P. Hirth, J. Tsai et al., "Clinical efficacy of a RAF inhibitor needs broad target blockade in BRAF-mutant melanoma," *Nature*, vol. 467, no. 7315, pp. 596–599, 2010.

[75] E. W. Joseph, C. A. Pratilas, P. I. Poulikakos et al., "The RAF inhibitor PLX4032 inhibits ERK signaling and tumor cell proliferation in a V600E BRAF-selective manner," *Proceedings of the National Academy of Sciences of the United States of America*, vol. 107, no. 33, pp. 14903–14908, 2010.

[76] P. Salerno, V. De Falco, A. Tamburrino et al., "Cytostatic activity of adenosine triphosphate-competitive kinase inhibitors in BRAF mutant thyroid carcinoma cells," *Journal of Clinical Endocrinology and Metabolism*, vol. 95, no. 1, pp. 450–455, 2010.

[77] E. Sala, L. Mologni, S. Truffa, C. Gaetano, G. E. Bollag, and C. Gambacorti-Passerini, "BRAF silencing by short hairpin RNA or chemical blockade by PLX4032 leads to different responses in melanoma and thyroid carcinoma cells," *Molecular Cancer Research*, vol. 6, no. 5, pp. 751–759, 2008.

[78] J. N. Søndergaard, R. Nazarian, Q. Wang et al., "Differential sensitivity of melanoma cell lines with BRAFV600Emutation to the specific Raf inhibitor PLX4032," *Journal of Translational Medicine*, vol. 8, article 39, 2010.

[79] K. T. Flaherty, I. Puzanov, K. B. Kim et al., "Inhibition of mutated, activated BRAF in metastatic melanoma," *New England Journal of Medicine*, vol. 363, no. 9, pp. 809–819, 2010.

[80] G. K. Schwartz, S. Robertson, A. Shen et al., "A Phase I study of XL281, a selective oral RAF kinase inhibitor, in patients with advanced solid tumors," *Journal of Clinical Oncology*, vol. 27, no. 15s, abstract 3513, 2009.

[81] D. W. Kim, Y. S. Jo, H. S. Jung et al., "An orally administered multitarget tyrosine kinase inhibitor, SU11248, is a novel potent inhibitor of thyroid oncogenic RET/papillary thyroid cancer kinases," *Journal of Clinical Endocrinology and Metabolism*, vol. 91, no. 10, pp. 4070–4076, 2006.

[82] E. E. W. Cohen, B. M. Needles, K. J. Cullen et al., "Phase II study of sunitinib in refractory thyroid cancer," *Journal of Clinical Oncology*, vol. 26, abstract 6025, 2008.

[83] M. J. Bugalho, R. Domingues, and A. Borges, "A case of advanced medullary thyroid carcinoma successfully treated with sunitinib," *Oncologist*, vol. 14, no. 11, pp. 1083–1087, 2009.

[84] D. Mannavola, P. Coco, G. Vannucchi et al., "A novel tyrosine-kinase selective inhibitor, sunitinib, induces transient hypothyroidism by blocking iodine uptake," *Journal of Clinical Endocrinology and Metabolism*, vol. 92, no. 9, pp. 3531–3534, 2007.

[85] E. Wong, L. S. Rosen, M. Mulay et al., "Sunitinib induces hypothyroidism in advanced cancer patients and may inhibit thyroid peroxidase activity," *Thyroid*, vol. 17, no. 4, pp. 351–355, 2007.

[86] M. B. Bass, S. I. Sherman, M. J. Schlumberger et al., "Biomarkers as predictors of response to treatment with motesanib in patients with progressive advanced thyroid cancer," *Journal of Clinical Endocrinology and Metabolism*, vol. 95, no. 11, pp. 5018–5027, 2010.

[87] V. Baldazzi, R. Tassi, A. Lapini, C. Santomaggio, M. Carini, and R. Mazzanti, "The impact of sunitinib-induced hypothyroidism on progression-free survival of metastatic renal cancer patients: a prospective single-center study," *Urologic Oncology: Seminars and Original Investigations*. In press.

[88] M. Schmidinger, U. M. Vogl, M. Bojic et al., "Hypothyroidism in patients with renal cell carcinoma: blessing or curse?" *Cancer*, vol. 117, no. 3, pp. 534–544, 2011.

[89] T. F. Chu, M. A. Rupnick, R. Kerkela et al., "Cardiotoxicity associated with tyrosine kinase inhibitor sunitinib," *Lancet*, vol. 370, no. 9604, pp. 2011–2019, 2007.

[90] B. B. Hasinoff and D. Patel, "The lack of target specificity of small molecule anticancer kinase inhibitors is correlated with their ability to damage myocytes in vitro," *Toxicology and Applied Pharmacology*, vol. 249, no. 2, pp. 132–139, 2010.

[91] M. H. Chen, R. Kerkelä, and T. Force, "Mechanisms of cardiac dysfunction associated with tyrosine kinase inhibitor cancer therapeutics," *Circulation*, vol. 118, no. 1, pp. 84–95, 2008.

[92] S. R. Wedge, D. J. Ogilvie, M. Dukes et al., "ZD6474 inhibits vascular endothelial growth factor signaling, angiogenesis, and tumor growth following oral administration," *Cancer Research*, vol. 62, no. 16, pp. 4645–4655, 2002.

[93] F. Ciardiello, R. Caputo, V. Damiano et al., "Antitumor effects of ZD6474, a small molecule vascular endothelial growth factor receptor tyrosine kinase inhibitor, with additional activity against epidermal growth factor receptor tyrosine kinase," *Clinical Cancer Research*, vol. 9, no. 4, pp. 1546–1556, 2003.

[94] R. S. Herbst, J. V. Heymach, M. S. O'Reilly, A. Onn, and A. J. Ryan, "Vandetanib (ZD6474): an orally available receptor tyrosine kinase inhibitor that selectively targets pathways critical for tumor growth and angiogenesis," *Expert Opinion on Investigational Drugs*, vol. 16, no. 2, pp. 239–249, 2007.

[95] F. Carlomagno, D. Vitagliano, T. Guida et al., "ZD6474, an orally available inhibitor of KDR tyrosine kinase activity, efficiently blocks oncogenic RET kinases," *Cancer Research*, vol. 62, no. 24, pp. 7284–7290, 2002.

[96] D. Vitagliano, V. De Falco, A. Tamburrino et al., "The tyrosine kinase inhibitor ZD6474 blocks proliferation of RET mutant medullary thyroid carcinoma cells," *Endocrine-Related Cancer*, vol. 18, no. 1, pp. 1–11, 2011.

[97] S. A. Wells Jr., J. E. Gosnell, R. F. Gagel et al., "Vandetanib for the treatment of patients with locally advanced or metastatic hereditary medullary thyroid cancer," *Journal of Clinical Oncology*, vol. 28, no. 5, pp. 767–772, 2010.

[98] "FDA Briefing Document Oncologic Drugs Advisory Committee Meeting," December 2010, http://www.fda.gov/downloads/AdvisoryCommittees/CommitteesMeetingMaterials/Drugs/OncologicDrugsAdvisoryCommittee/UCM235086.pdf.

[99] B. G. Robinson, L. Paz-Ares, A. Krebs, J. Vasselli, and R. Haddad, "Vandetanib (100 mg) in patients with locally advanced or metastatic hereditary medullary thyroid cancer," *Journal of Clinical Endocrinology and Metabolism*, vol. 95, no. 6, pp. 2664–2671, 2010.

[100] United States Food and Drug Administration Press Release, "FDA approves new treatment for rare form of thyroid cancer," April 2011, http://www.fda.gov/NewsEvents/Newsroom/PressAnnouncements/ucm250168.htm.

[101] M. Carroll, S. Ohno-Jones, S. Tamura et al., "CGP 57148, a tyrosine kinase inhibitor, inhibits the growth of cells expressing BCR-ABL, TEL-ABL, and TEL-PDGFR fusion proteins," *Blood*, vol. 90, no. 12, pp. 4947–4952, 1997.

[102] A. Podtcheko, A. Ohtsuru, S. Tsuda et al., "The selective tyrosine kinase inhibitor, STI571, inhibits growth of anaplastic thyroid cancer cells," *Journal of Clinical Endocrinology and Metabolism*, vol. 88, no. 4, pp. 1889–1896, 2003.

[103] J. M. Dziba and K. B. Ain, "Imatinib mesylate (Gleevec; STI571) monotherapy is ineffective in suppressing human anaplastic thyroid carcinoma cell growth in vitro," *Journal of Clinical Endocrinology and Metabolism*, vol. 89, no. 5, pp. 2127–2135, 2004.

[104] J. W. B. De Groot, B. A. Zonnenberg, P. Q. Van Ufford-Mannesse et al., "A phase II trial of imatinib therapy for metastatic medullary thyroid carcinoma," *Journal of Clinical Endocrinology and Metabolism*, vol. 92, no. 9, pp. 3466–3469, 2007.

[105] K. Frank-Raue, M. Fabel, S. Delorme, U. Haberkorn, and F. Raue, "Efficacy of imatinib mesylate in advanced medullary thyroid carcinoma," *European Journal of Endocrinology*, vol. 157, no. 2, pp. 215–220, 2007.

[106] A. K. Samadi, R. Mukerji, A. Shah, B. N. Timmermann, and M. S. Cohen, "A novel RET inhibitor with potent efficacy against medullary thyroid cancer in vivo," *Surgery*, vol. 148, no. 6, pp. 1228–1236, 2010.

[107] R. Kumar, V. B. Knick, S. K. Rudolph et al., "Pharmacokinetic-pharmacodynamic correlation from mouse to human with pazopanib, a multikinase angiogenesis inhibitor with potent antitumor and antiangiogenic activity," *Molecular Cancer Therapeutics*, vol. 6, no. 7, pp. 2012–2021, 2007.

[108] B. Gril, D. Palmieri, Y. Qian et al., "Pazopanib reveals a role for tumor cell B-Raf in the prevention of HER2+ breast cancer brain metastasis," *Clinical Cancer Research*, vol. 17, no. 1, pp. 142–153, 2011.

[109] M. Friedlander, K. C. Hancock, D. Rischin et al., "A Phase II, open-label study evaluating pazopanib in patients with recurrent ovarian cancer," *Gynecologic Oncology*, vol. 119, no. 1, pp. 32–37, 2010.

[110] N. Altorki, M. E. Lane, T. Bauer et al., "Phase II proof-of-concept study of pazopanib monotherapy in treatment-naive patients with stage I/II resectable non-small-cell lung cancer," *Journal of Clinical Oncology*, vol. 28, no. 19, pp. 3131–3137, 2010.

[111] J. E. Ward and W. M. Stadler, "Pazopanib in renal cell carcinoma," *Clinical Cancer Research*, vol. 16, no. 24, pp. 5923–5927, 2010.

[112] K. C. Bible, V. J. Suman, J. R. Molina et al., "Efficacy of pazopanib in progressive, radioiodine-refractory, metastatic differentiated thyroid cancers: results of a phase 2 consortium study," *The Lancet Oncology*, vol. 11, no. 10, pp. 962–972, 2010.

[113] A. Polverino, A. Coxon, C. Starnes et al., "AMG 706, an oral, multikinase inhibitor that selectively targets vascular endothelial growth factor, platelet-derived growth factor, and kit receptors, potently inhibits angiogenesis and induces regression in tumor xenografts," *Cancer Research*, vol. 66, no. 17, pp. 8715–8721, 2006.

[114] L. S. Rosen, R. Kurzrock, M. Mulay et al., "Safety, pharmacokinetics, and efficacy of AMG 706, an oral multikinase inhibitor, in patients with advanced solid tumors," *Journal of Clinical Oncology*, vol. 25, no. 17, pp. 2369–2376, 2007.

[115] S. I. Sherman, L. J. Wirth, J. P. Droz et al., "Motesanib diphosphate in progressive differentiated thyroid cancer," *New England Journal of Medicine*, vol. 359, no. 1, pp. 31–42, 2008.

[116] M. J. Schlumberger, R. Elisei, L. Bastholt et al., "Phase II study of safety and efficacy of motesanib in patients with progressive or symptomatic, advanced or metastatic medullary thyroid cancer," *Journal of Clinical Oncology*, vol. 27, no. 23, pp. 3794–3801, 2009.

[117] M. B. Bass, S. I. Sherman, M. J. Schlumberger et al., "Biomarkers as predictors of response to treatment with motesanib in patients with progressive advanced thyroid cancer," *Journal of Clinical Endocrinology and Metabolism*, vol. 95, no. 11, pp. 5018–5027, 2010.

[118] H. S. Rugo, R. S. Herbst, G. Liu et al., "Phase I trial of the oral antiangiogenesis agent AG-013736 in patients with advanced solid tumors: pharmacokinetic and clinical results," *Journal of Clinical Oncology*, vol. 23, no. 24, pp. 5474–5483, 2005.

[119] E. E. W. Cohen, L. S. Rosen, E. E. Vokes et al., "Axitinib is an active treatment for all histologic subtypes of advanced thyroid cancer: results from a phase II study," *Journal of Clinical Oncology*, vol. 26, no. 29, pp. 4708–4713, 2008.

[120] R. Mineo, A. Costantino, F. Frasca et al., "Activation of the Hepatocyte Growth Factor (HGF)-Met system in papillary thyroid cancer: biological effects of HGF in thyroid cancer cells depend on Met expression levels," *Endocrinology*, vol. 145, no. 9, pp. 4355–4365, 2004.

[121] R. Kurzrock, S. Sherman, D. Hong et al., "A Phase I study of XL184, a MET, VEGFR2, and RET kinase inhibitor, administered orally to patients with advanced malignancies, including a subgroup of patients with medullary thyroid carcinoma," in *the EORTC-NCI-AACR International Conference on Molecular Targets and Cancer Therapeutics*, Geneva, Switzerland, October 2008, poster number 379.

[122] A. Antonelli, G. Bocci, C. La Motta et al., "Novel pyrazolopyrimidine derivatives as tyrosine kinase inhibitors with antitumoral activity in vitro and in vivo in papillary dedifferentiated thyroid cancer," *Journal of Clinical Endocrinology and Metabolism*, vol. 96, no. 2, pp. E288–E296, 2011.

[123] N. A. Pennell, G. H. Daniels, R. I. Haddad et al., "A phase II study of gefitinib in patients with advanced thyroid cancer," *Thyroid*, vol. 18, no. 3, pp. 317–323, 2008.

[124] S. I. Sherman, "Targeted therapy of thyroid cancer," *Biochemical Pharmacology*, vol. 80, no. 5, pp. 592–601, 2010.

[125] J. A. Fagin, R. M. Tuttle, and D. G. Pfister, "Harvesting the low-hanging fruit: kinase inhibitors for therapy of advanced medullary and nonmedullary thyroid cancer," *Journal of Clinical Endocrinology and Metabolism*, vol. 95, no. 6, pp. 2621–2624, 2010.

[126] F. Furuya, H. Shimura, H. Suzuki et al., "Histone deacetylase inhibitors restore radioiodide uptake and retention in poorly differentiated and anaplastic thyroid cancer cells by expression of the sodium/iodide symporter thyroperoxidase and thyroglobulin," *Endocrinology*, vol. 145, no. 6, pp. 2865–2875, 2004.

[127] J. A. Woyach, R. T. Kloos, M. D. Ringel et al., "Lack of therapeutic effect of the histone deacetylase inhibitor vorinostat in patients with metastatic radioiodine-refractory thyroid carcinoma," *Journal of Clinical Endocrinology and Metabolism*, vol. 94, no. 1, pp. 164–170, 2009.

[128] F. Furuya, H. Shimura, H. Suzuki et al., "Histone deacetylase inhibitors restore radioiodide uptake and retention in poorly differentiated and anaplastic thyroid cancer cells by expression of the sodium/iodide symporter thyroperoxidase and thyroglobulin," *Endocrinology*, vol. 145, no. 6, pp. 2865–2875, 2004.

[129] P. Hou, E. Bojdani, and M. Xing, "Induction of thyroid gene expression and radioiodine uptake in thyroid cancer cells by targeting major signaling pathways," *Journal of Clinical Endocrinology and Metabolism*, vol. 95, no. 2, pp. 820–828, 2010.

[130] G. Vitale, P. Tagliaferri, M. Caraglia et al., "Slow release lanreotide in combination with interferon-α2b in the treatment of symptomatic advanced medullary thyroid carcinoma," *Journal of Clinical Endocrinology and Metabolism*, vol. 85, no. 3, pp. 983–988, 2000.

[131] T. Bachleitner-Hofmann, J. Friedl, M. Hassler et al., "Pilot trial of autologous dendritic cells loaded with tumor lysate(s) from allogeneic tumor cell lines in patients with metastatic medullary thyroid carcinoma," *Oncology Reports*, vol. 21, no. 6, pp. 1585–1592, 2009.

[132] R. D. Blumenthal and D. M. Goldenberg, "Methods and goals for the use of in vitro and in vivo chemosensitivity testing," *Molecular Biotechnology*, vol. 35, no. 2, pp. 185–197, 2007.

2

The Morbidity of Reoperative Surgery for Recurrent Benign Nodular Goitre: Impact of Previous Unilateral Thyroid Lobectomy versus Subtotal Thyroidectomy

Navin Rudolph, Claudia Dominguez, Anthony Beaulieu, Pierre De Wailly, and Jean-Louis Kraimps

Department of Endocrine Surgery, University Hospital of Poitiers, 86021 Poitiers, France

Correspondence should be addressed to Navin Rudolph; navin.rudolph@gmail.com

Academic Editor: Thomas J. Fahey

Background. Subtotal thyroidectomy (STT) was previously considered the gold standard in the surgical management of multinodular goitre despite its propensity for recurrence. Our aim was to assess whether prior STT or unilateral lobectomy was associated with increased reoperative morbidity. *Methods.* A retrospective analysis was conducted extracting data from our endocrine surgical database for the period from January 1991 to June 2006. Two patient groups were defined: Group 1 consisted of patients with previous unilateral thyroid lobectomy; Group 2 had undergone previous STT. Specific outcomes investigated were transient and permanent recurrent laryngeal nerve (RLN) injury and hypoparathyroidism. *Results.* 494 reoperative cases were performed which consisted of 259 patients with previous unilateral lobectomy (Group 1) and 235 patients with previous subtotal thyroidectomy (Group 2). A statistically significant increase relating to previous STT was demonstrated in both permanent RLN injury (0.77% versus 3.4%, RR 4.38, $P = 0.038$) and permanent hypoparathyroidism (1.5% versus 5.1%, RR 3.14, $P = 0.041$). Transient nerve injury and hypocalcaemia incidence was comparable. *Conclusions.* Reoperative surgery following subtotal thyroidectomy is associated with a significantly increased risk of permanent recurrent laryngeal nerve injury and hypoparathyroidism when compared with previous unilateral thyroidectomy. Subtotal thyroidectomy should therefore no longer be recommended in the management of multinodular goitre.

1. Background

Subtotal thyroidectomy (STT) was for many years the accepted standard of management for benign multinodular goitre. Although its role has significantly diminished with the recognition of the safety of total thyroidectomy, it continues to be practised in several centres worldwide both in locations endemic and nonendemic for this disease. The purported benefits of the subtotal approach include a reduced morbidity profile with respect to recurrent laryngeal (RLN) injury and hypoparathyroidism as well as a reduced need for thyroid hormone replacement therapy. The exact deployment of the surgical technique has varied amongst institutions with regard to the size and location of the thyroid remnant and whether it has been performed unilaterally or bilaterally. This marked potential for heterogeneity has hampered reliable scientific appraisal of the technique's efficacy.

Despite these methodological encumbrances, several concerns regarding STT have emerged that challenge its legitimacy within the surgical armamentarium of the thyroid surgeon. First, recurrent disease, often manifesting many years following the initial surgery, is identified in a significant number of patients [1]. Moreover, thyroid insufficiency and consequent need for thyroid hormone replacement therapy are only infrequently eradicated [2]. The presence of a thyroid remnant is problematic if an incidental malignancy is discovered. Finally, the identification of recurrent disease heralds technically demanding reoperative surgery fraught with potential for significant morbidity.

Alongside this, total thyroidectomy (TT) has been demonstrated to be a safe and efficacious procedure. Technological advancements in haemostatic vessel sealing devices have hastened the operative technique significantly and more recently nerve monitoring has been widely adopted to further combat the low rates of RLN paralysis already demonstrated. Other benefits relate to its superiority in cases of malignancy by removing all gross thyroid and potentially malignant tissue, facilitating radioactive iodine (RAI) ablation therapy and facilitating surveillance with ultrasound imaging of the thyroid bed and thyroglobulin (Tg) monitoring.

Our unit is a high volume tertiary endocrine surgery centre performing over 500 thyroid procedures per year. Having previously practiced STT for many years we have a vast experience with recurrent benign thyroid goitre following this procedure. In addition, a large number of patients who underwent unilateral thyroid lobectomy for unilateral benign nodular disease have subsequently required completion totalization thyroidectomy for contralateral recurrent disease. Our unique study approach endeavoured to assess whether reoperative surgery in these two settings conferred any difference in morbidity specifically with regard to RLN injury and hypoparathyroidism.

2. Materials and Methods

A retrospective analysis was conducted utilizing our endocrine surgical database for the period from January 1991 to June 2006. There were 494 patients that required reoperation for recurrent benign goitre and were thus selected for this study. The indications for the reoperative surgery included enlarging neck lump, pressure symptoms, and imaging suspicious for malignancy. The patients were divided into two groups on the basis of the previous surgery: group 1 consisted of patients who had previous unilateral thyroid lobectomy; group 2 included patients who had undergone prior subtotal thyroidectomy. In all cases both the initial and reoperative procedure had been performed at our own institution.

The technique of unilateral extracapsular thyroidectomy at our institution has been well documented previously [3]. Our subtotal thyroidectomy procedure performed during this period is detailed here to avoid potential ambiguity. Careful preoperative study of the thyroid ultrasound was paramount in order to appreciate the location of the nodules within each thyroid lobe. A small (less than 5 grams) homogeneous remnant was left unilaterally at either the superior pole or posteriorly depending on the location of the sonographically or intraoperatively detected nodules. This combination of unilateral lobectomy and unilateral subtotal resection has been labelled elsewhere as the Dunhill procedure [4]. The operations were all performed by or under the direct supervision of a senior endocrine surgeon (JLK) following a highly standardized procedure. Postoperative nonsuppressive thyroxine therapy was employed for restoration of euthyroidism as dictated by thyroid function tests (thyroid-stimulating hormone (TSH); free T4 and T3).

Prior to reoperative surgery all patients underwent imaging by ultrasound; computed tomography scans and technetium thyroid uptake scans were performed on an individualized basis depending on the extent of the recurrence. Intraoperative nerve monitoring was used in all reoperative cases. Fibreoptic flexible laryngoscopy was routinely performed in

TABLE 1: Group demographics and timing and indication for reoperation.

	Group 1 $n = 259$	Group 2 $n = 235$
Sex		
Male	21 (8%)	20 (9%)
Female	238 (92%)	215 (91%)
Age		
Age at first operation	38.0 years	40.0 years
Age at reoperation	53.2 years	53.9 years
Interval between initial and reoperative surgery	15.2 years	13.9 years
Indication for reoperation		
Isolated nodule	38 (14.7%)	36 (15.3%)
Multinodular goitre	221 (85.3%)	199 (84.7%)

all patients both preoperatively and on the first postoperative day permitting an accurate calculation of our temporary RLN injury rate. Patients with any detected abnormalities at this examination underwent a further laryngoscopy at 6 months postoperatively; vocal cord dysfunction at this stage was defined as permanent RLN injury. Calcium levels were obtained on the first and second postoperative days and at a 6-month followup appointment. Hypocalcaemia was defined as less than 2.00 mmol/L and permanent if requiring ongoing oral calcium supplementation beyond 3 months. Morbidity arising from the initial operation was not the intended focus of this study and was excluded from the analysis; only new morbidity events specifically relating to the reoperative surgery were included. Descriptive statistics were obtained and data subjected to analysis by Fisher's exact test and chi-square test to examine the relative risk of reoperative morbidity for group 1 and group 2. Statistical significance was accepted at $P < 0.05$.

3. Results

During the study period our unit performed thyroid surgery on 6780 patients. There were 494 patients that required reoperation for recurrent benign goitre, which constituted 7.3% of the unit's thyroid surgery throughput during this period.

Group 1 comprised 259 patients with previous thyroid lobectomy and group 2 comprised 235 patients with previous subtotal thyroidectomy (Table 1). The groups displayed demographic parity with respect to mean age (group 1, 38 years; group 2, 40 years) and female predominance (92% and 91%, resp.).

The mean interval between initial surgery and reoperation was 15.2 years in group 1 and 13.9 years in group 2. The indication for reoperation in groups 1 and 2 was also comparable: isolated nodules in 14.7% and 15.3% and multinodular goitre in 85.3% and 84.7%, respectively.

The impact of the initial surgery on the morbidity related to the reoperative case was statistically significant for both permanent RLN injury and permanent hypocalcaemia.

TABLE 2: Incidence of RLN injury following reoperative surgery.

	Group 1 (lobectomy) n = 259	Group 2 (subtotal) n = 235	P value	Relative risk
Normal laryngoscopy	241 (83.9%)	214 (83.4%)		
Transient RLN paralysis	16 (6.18%)	13 (5.53%)	0.85	0.92
Permanent RLN paralysis	2 (0.77%)	8 (3.4%)	0.038	4.38

TABLE 3: Incidence of hypocalcaemia following reoperative surgery.

	Group 1 (lobectomy) n = 259	Group 2 (subtotal) n = 235	P value	Relative risk
Normocalcaemia	220 (84.9%)	202 (85.9%)		
Temporary hypocalcaemia	35 (13.5%)	21 (8.93%)	0.15	0.69
Permanent hypocalcaemia	4 (1.54%)	12 (5.1%)	0.041	3.14

Permanent RLN palsy was observed in only 2 from group 1 and 8 from group 2 (Table 2). This correlates with a statistically significant detrimental effect of initial subtotal thyroidectomy on long-term RLN function ($P < 0.038$). This indicates a relative risk increase of 4.38 in patients who underwent initial subtotal thyroidectomy (CI_{95} 0.94–20.4). Transient paralysis was observed in both groups (group 1, 6.18%; group 2, 5.53%). The majority of patients in both groups, however, have no disturbance in postoperative RLN function (group 1, 83.9%; group 2, 83.4%).

Permanent hypocalcaemia was observed in 1.54% of group 1 patients and 5.11% of group 2 patients (Table 3). Again, this reflected a statistically significant detrimental effect of initial subtotal thyroidectomy on the development of permanent hypocalcaemia following reoperative surgery ($P < 0.041$) and correlates with an relative risk increase of 3.14 (CI_{95} 1.09–9.59). No association was determined for temporary hypocalcaemia and the nature of prior surgery (RR 0.69, CI_{95} 0.41–1.14). Of note, postoperative normocalcaemia was evident in 84.9% and 85.9% of patients from group 1 and group 2, respectively.

Incidental malignancy within the reoperative specimen was determined in 21 patients (4.22%). There was an equitable distribution within the two groups, with 11 cases in group 1 and 10 cases in group 2.

4. Discussion

The optimum extent of initial surgery in the management of benign thyroid goitre continues to generate considerable controversy. The debate between the safety and efficacy of a total versus a less than total thyroidectomy has successfully accomplished the widespread adoption of total thyroidectomy although not fully extinguishing the practice of subtotal thyroidectomy in several centres worldwide. Our study, drawing on a vast experience with reoperative surgery in benign thyroid disease, approaches the debate from a different angle. Rather than focussing on the morbidity of an initial subtotal thyroidectomy versus an extracapsular technique, our study represents the first direct comparison on the morbidity relating to the reoperative surgery in the setting of

previous subtotal and unilateral thyroid resections. Although the results may appear intuitive, the study did expose some interesting and important facets of reoperative surgery in these circumstances.

Reoperative thyroid surgery is inherently difficult on account of the distortion of central neck area anatomy and fibrotic encasement of important structures such as the recurrent laryngeal nerve [5]. This has led to the recommendation by several authors to avoid reoperations by performing definitive initial treatment [6]. Despite these difficulties Levin et al. demonstrated that reoperations could still be performed with minimal morbidity [7]. In their series, a low permanent RLN injury rate of less than 1% and permanent hypoparathyroidism rate of 3.8% was attained—the authors consequently stressed that, for patients manifesting with recurrent disease, reoperative surgery should not be withheld for fear of generating the aforementioned complications. Our rates of permanent RLN palsy (2%) and hypoparathyroidism (3.2%) from the two groups combined likewise demonstrate that satisfactory outcomes are achievable within specialized centres. Other authors have published series of reoperative cases with permanent RLN rates of 0–1.5% and highlighted that, although being hardly an innocuous procedure, reoperative surgery is safe in the hands of experienced surgeons; however, a complete initial procedure should obviate the exposure to this unnecessary additional risk [8, 9].

A different scenario exists when a patient requires secondary thyroid surgery for recurrent benign disease with a background of unilateral hemithyroidectomy. In this situation, where the contralateral side is completely untouched, no increased risk is conferred as shown by Chao et al. and confirmed in our study with rates of permanent RLN injury and permanent hypoparathyroidism rates of 0.77% and 1.54%, respectively [10]. However, previous STT, in which both sides have been dissected, is associated with an up to fivefold increase in complications with reoperative surgery [11, 12]. Despite the scar tissue and degenerative changes cited by Katz and Bronson as the principle culprit factors relating to reoperative morbidity [13], Bron and O'Brien found no significant correlation between complication rate and previous surgery [14]. Transient hypoparathyroidism was seen in 13.5% of group 1 patients in our study representing a nonstatistically significant difference from the previous STT group. Germane to this finding, Barczyński et al. remark that transient hypoparathyroidism following TT in an era where parathyroid autotransplantation is common should be viewed as a sequel rather than a complication [15].

The technique of reoperative thyroid surgery is clearly important when analysing complications. Farrag and colleagues have recently promulgated an algorithm for safe and effective thyroid bed surgery for malignancy although many aspects can be readily extrapolated to the benign sphere as well [5]. The principle tenets of the algorithm include preoperative high-resolution ultrasound examination, preoperative vocal fold examination by fibreoptic laryngoscopy, and routine nerve identification that should be facilitated by the use of intraoperative nerve monitoring (IONM). Several of these attributes are endorsed by international thyroid surgery guidelines [16]. Additionally, Menegaux et al. recommend a lateral approach to the thyroid bed with division of the infrahyoid musculature in an effort to avoid fibrous tissue surrounding the thyroid remnant [17].

TT emerged as an alternative to STT initially in the malignant domain. Clark embraced the technique for management of well-differentiated thyroid cancer and demonstrated the safety of the technique and low complication rate [18]. It is recommended as the operation of choice in all current treatment guidelines for thyroid cancer [19]. The purported benefits of a total gland resection in thyroid cancer include the removal of the primary tumour, elimination of any potential contralateral disease and facilitation of postoperative RAI ablation, Tg surveillance, and ultrasound scanning of the thyroid bed [20]. These benefits are not present when dealing with benign disease. Proponents of a subtotal resection claim a reduced rate of RLN injury and hypoparathyroidism and assert that the majority of thyroid malignancies detected fortuitously on final histopathology are of limited clinical significance. Furthermore, if recurrences do occur they can be managed surgically when indicated with less morbidity than if total thyroidectomy was performed on all cases of thyroid malignancy at the outset [20].

Numerous publications have since established the low morbidity of the extracapsular TT procedure. Mishra et al. demonstrated an 0.8% permanent RLN rate and 1.6% permanent hypoparathyroidism rate whilst Müller et al. found a 0.9% rate for both morbidities [21, 22]. Many other studies confirmed similar findings [23–25]. Serpell and Phan found a permanent RLN palsy rate of 0.3% and hypoparathyroidism rate of 1.8% and concluded that TT can be performed safely in a standard endocrine surgical unit with low complication rates matching world centres of excellence [26]. Documented high rates of incidental thyroid malignancy fortified the growing argument in favour of total thyroidectomy. Our present study revealed an incidental papillary microcarcinoma rate of 4.22% that was equally distributed within the two groups. We have previously published a 3% rate of occult carcinoma, somewhat lower than other subsequently published series from Bron and O'Brien (4.6%) [14], Colak et al. (7.4%) [27], and Levin et al. (22%) [7]. Menegaux et al. determined that thyroid cancer might be found in

approximately 10% of reoperative cases for recurrent goitre even though the preceding operation was performed for benign disease [28]. By the same token, Tezelman et al. found that within a cohort of patients diagnosed with thyroid cancer following a subtotal thyroidectomy, completion resection of the thyroid remnants yielded papillary microcarcinoma in 5.26% [1].

Recurrence of goitre and failure to prevent hypothyroidism have further weakened the validity of subtotal thyroidectomy as a surgical strategy for benign thyroid disease. Goitre recurrence rates associated with STT range from 7.1% to 43% [1, 12]. The incidence of recurrence appears directly related to the length of surveillance [29, 30]—although our study and others have found that a peak incidence of recurrence occurs at approximately 13 to 15 years from the primary operation [31], a 43% recurrence rate may be observed with up to 30 years of followup [12]. Many have noted the failure of thyroxine suppression to prevent recurrence with a 14.5% recurrence rate demonstrated in the study by Pappalardo et al. in spite of drug prophylaxis [24]. Conversely, thyroxine replacement is not obviated in 36.6–47.8% of subtotal thyroidectomy procedures and hence should not be used to justify practice of the procedure [32].

The fundamental difficulty with STT is allotting a tissue remnant unaffected by the nodular process. Colak et al. highlighted the predicament of leaving healthy tissue intact in patients with huge goitres where the nodular disease often reaches the dorsal capsule [27]. There is generally an increasing recognition that the nodular transformations in multinodular goitre inherently encompass the entire gland; hence, although STT permits a reduction in the bulk of disease, it is not an optimal treatment [33]. Moreover, the remnant posterolateral tissue often extends into the retrotracheal and retrooesophageal areas where recurrence portends early pressure symptoms that may require technically demanding reoperative surgery [34]. We have previously shown that multinodular goitre is a highly significant risk factor for recurrence in benign thyroid disease where a less than total thyroidectomy has been performed [35]. Recently, a novel study by Tekin et al. demonstrated that Ki-67 proliferation marker levels in remnant STT thyroid tissue were significantly higher than in normal thyroid tissue [36]. They found that despite the relatively small size of remnant micronodules the high Ki-67 levels reflect high cellular mitotic activity and ensuing significant goitrogenic potential of remnant tissue. Furthermore, the existence of micronodules in the remnant specimens harbouring similar proliferation index values as the main thyroid specimen establishes the homogeneous nature of the parenchymal alteration in multinodular goitre. Gerard et al. postulate that recurrent goitres resistant to thyroxine suppression may arise due to the polyclonal nature of nodule formation involving goitrogenic insulin-like growth factors and their binding proteins. These may occur separate to iodine deficiency related mechanisms of goitre development based on TSH and vascular-endothelial growth factor (VEGF) angiogenesis [37].

Finally, the often-overlooked denominator and perhaps most crucial determinant of morbidity is surgical technique.

Thomusch et al. commented on the importance of "well-trained surgeons using an appropriate intraoperative technique" in the performance of total thyroidectomy [38]. The ability to perform a safe total thyroidectomy is clearly a direct derivative of one's surgical training and experience [39]. The evolution of more dedicated endocrine surgery training programmes and specialized units combined with technological refinements such as IONM is likely to further enhance the safe implementation of TT for both malignant and benign thyroid disease alike [40].

5. Conclusion

Reoperative surgery for recurrent benign thyroid disease is associated with increased morbidity when preceded by initial subtotal thyroidectomy. Associated high levels of recurrence and increased permanent RLN injury and hypoparathyroidism rates seen in this setting call for the abandonment of this procedure in favour of total thyroidectomy. It should be noted however that successful reoperative thyroid surgery performed by experienced, well-trained surgeons may be accomplished with low overall rates of morbidity.

References

[1] S. Tezelman, I. Borucu, Y. Senyurek, F. Tunca, and T. Terzioglu, "The change in surgical practice from subtotal to near-total or total thyroidectomy in the treatment of patients with benign multinodular goiter," World Journal of Surgery, vol. 33, no. 3, pp. 400–405, 2009.

[2] A. Koyuncu, H. S. Dökmetaş, M. Turan et al., "Comparison of different thyroidectomy techniques for benign thyroid disease," Endocrine Journal, vol. 50, no. 6, pp. 723–727, 2003.

[3] "Technique of thyroidectomy," in Endocrine Surgery: Principles and Practice, H. Gibelin, T. Desurmont, J. L. Kraimps, and J. G. H. Hubbard, Eds., Springer Specialist Surgery Series, chapter 12, pp. 163–171, Springer, London, UK, 1st edition, 2009.

[4] M. Barczyński, A. Konturek, A. Hubalewska-Dydejczyk, F. Golkowski, S. Cichoń, and W. Nowak, "Five-year follow-up of a randomized clinical trial of total thyroidectomy versus dunhill operation versus bilateral subtotal thyroidectomy for multinodular nontoxic goiter," World Journal of Surgery, vol. 34, no. 6, pp. 1203–1213, 2010.

[5] T. Y. Farrag, N. Agrawal, S. Sheth et al., "Algorithm for safe and effective reoperative thyroid bed surgery for recurrent/persistent papillary thyroid carcinoma," Head and Neck, vol. 29, no. 12, pp. 1069–1074, 2007.

[6] D. B. Wilson, E. D. Staren, and R. A. Prinz, "Thyroid reoperations: indications and risks," The American Surgeon, vol. 64, no. 7, pp. 674–679, 1998.

[7] K. E. Levin, A. H. Clark, Q. Duh, M. Demeure, A. E. Siperstein, and O. H. Clark, "Reoperative thyroid surgery," Surgery, vol. 111, no. 6, pp. 604–609, 1992.

[8] D. J. Terris, S. S. Khichi, S. K. Anderson, and M. W. Seybt, "Reoperative thyroidectomy for benign thyroid disease: the case for phasing out subtotal thyroidectomy," Laryngoscope, vol. 119, no. 1, p. S89, 2009.

[9] J. H. Lefevre, C. Tresallet, L. Leenhardt, C. Jublanc, J. Chigot, and F. Menegaux, "Reoperative surgery for thyroid disease," Langenbeck's Archives of Surgery, vol. 392, no. 6, pp. 685–691, 2007.

[10] T. Chao, L. Jeng, J. Lin, and M. Chen, "Reoperative thyroid surgery," World Journal of Surgery, vol. 21, no. 6, pp. 644–647, 1997.

[11] T. S. Reeve, L. Delbridge, P. Brady, P. Crummer, and C. Smyth, "Secondary thyroidectomy: a twenty-year experience," World Journal of Surgery, vol. 12, no. 4, pp. 449–453, 1988.

[12] J. Rojdmark and J. Jarhult, "High long term recurrence rate after subtotal thyroidectomy for nodular goitre," European Journal of Surgery, vol. 161, no. 10, pp. 725–727, 1995.

[13] A. D. Katz and D. Bronson, "Total thyroidectomy. The indications and results of 630 cases," The American Journal of Surgery, vol. 136, no. 4, pp. 450–454, 1978.

[14] L. P. Bron and C. J. O'Brien, "Total thyroidectomy for clinically benign disease of the thyroid gland," The British Journal of Surgery, vol. 91, no. 5, pp. 569–574, 2004.

[15] M. Barczyński, A. Konturek, A. Hubalewska-Dydejczyk, F. Golkowski, S. Cichoń, and W. Nowak, "Five-year follow-up of a randomized clinical trial of total thyroidectomy versus dunhill operation versus bilateral subtotal thyroidectomy for multinodular nontoxic goiter," World Journal of Surgery, vol. 34, no. 6, pp. 1203–1213, 2010.

[16] "British Thyroid Association Guidelines for the management of thyroid cancer in adults," 2012, http://www.british-thyroid-association.org/Guidelines/.

[17] F. Menegaux, G. Turpin, M. Dahman et al., "Secondary thyroidectomy in patients with prior thyroid surgery for benign disease: a study of 203 cases," Surgery, vol. 126, no. 3, pp. 479–483, 1999.

[18] O. H. Clark, "Total thyroidectomy. The treatment of choice for patients with differentiated thyroid cancer," Annals of Surgery, vol. 196, no. 3, pp. 361–370, 1982.

[19] D. S. Cooper, G. M. Doherty, B. R. Haugen et al., "Revised American thyroid association management guidelines for patients with thyroid nodules and differentiated thyroid cancer," Thyroid, vol. 19, no. 11, pp. 1167–1214, 2009.

[20] M. Friedman and H. Ibrahim, "Total versus subtotal thyroidectomy: arguments, approaches, and recommendations," Operative Techniques in Otolaryngology, vol. 13, no. 3, pp. 196–202, 2002.

[21] P. Müller, S. Kabus, E. Robens, and F. Spelsberg, "Indications, risks, and acceptance of total thyroidectomy for multinodular benign goiter," Surgery Today, vol. 31, no. 11, pp. 958–962, 2001.

[22] A. Mishra, A. Agarwal, G. Agarwal, and S. K. Mishra, "Total thyroidectomy for benign thyroid disorders in an endemic region," World Journal of Surgery, vol. 25, no. 3, pp. 307–310, 2001.

[23] N. Korun, C. Aşci, T. Yilmazlar et al., "Total thyroidectomy or lobectomy in benign nodular disease of the thyroid: changing trends in surgery," International Surgery, vol. 82, no. 4, pp. 417–419, 1997.

[24] G. Pappalardo, A. Guadalaxara, F. M. Frattaroli, G. Illomei, and P. Falaschi, "Total compared with subtotal thyroidectomy in benign nodular disease: personal series and review of published reports," European Journal of Surgery, vol. 164, no. 7, pp. 501–506, 1998.

[25] D. B. de Roy van Zuidewijn, I. Songun, J. Kievit, and C. J. van de Velde, "Complications of thyroid surgery," *Annals of Surgical Oncology*, vol. 2, no. 1, pp. 56–60, 1995.

[26] J. W. Serpell and D. Phan, "Safety of total thyroidectomy," *Australian and New Zealand Journal of Surgery*, vol. 77, no. 1-2, pp. 15–19, 2007.

[27] T. Colak, T. Akca, A. Kanik, D. Yapici, and S. Aydin, "Total versus subtotal thyroidectomy for the management of benign multinodular goiter in an endemic region," *Australian and New Zealand Journal of Surgery*, vol. 74, no. 11, pp. 974–978, 2004.

[28] F. Menegaux, G. Turpin, M. Dahman et al., "Secondary thyroidectomy in patients with prior thyroid surgery for benign disease: a study of 203 cases," *Surgery*, vol. 126, no. 3, pp. 479–483, 1999.

[29] P. E. Anderson, P. R. Hurley, and P. Rosswick, "Conservative treatment and long term prophylactic thyroxine in the prevention of recurrence of multinodular goiter," *Surgery Gynecology and Obstetrics*, vol. 171, no. 4, pp. 309–314, 1990.

[30] J. L. Kraimps, R. Marechaud, D. Gineste et al., "Analysis and prevention of recurrent goiter," *Surgery Gynecology and Obstetrics*, vol. 176, no. 4, pp. 319–322, 1993.

[31] L. Delbridge, A. I. Guinea, and T. S. Reeve, "Total thyroidectomy for bilateral benign multinodular goiter: effect of changing practice," *Archives of Surgery*, vol. 134, no. 12, pp. 1389–1393, 1999.

[32] A. Koyuncu, H. S. Dökmetaş, M. Turan et al., "Comparison of different thyroidectomy techniques for benign thyroid disease," *Endocrine Journal*, vol. 50, no. 6, pp. 723–727, 2003.

[33] T. S. Reeve, L. Delbridge, A. Cohen, and P. Crummer, "Total thyroidectomy. The preferred option for multinodular goiter," *Annals of Surgery*, vol. 206, no. 6, pp. 782–786, 1987.

[34] T. Colak, T. Akca, A. Kanik, D. Yapici, and S. Aydin, "Total versus subtotal thyroidectomy for the management of benign multinodular goiter in an endemic region," *Australian and New Zealand Journal of Surgery*, vol. 74, no. 11, pp. 974–978, 2004.

[35] H. Gibelin, M. Sierra, D. Mothes et al., "Risk factors for recurrent nodular goiter after thyroidectomy for benign disease: case-control study of 244 patients," *World Journal of Surgery*, vol. 28, no. 11, pp. 1079–1082, 2004.

[36] K. Tekin, S. Yilmaz, N. Yalçin et al., "What would be left behind if subtotal thyroidectomy were preferred instead of total thyroidectomy?" *The American Journal of Surgery*, vol. 199, no. 6, pp. 765–769, 2010.

[37] A. Gerard, S. Poncin, B. Caetano et al., "Iodine deficiency induces a thyroid stimulating hormone-independent early phase of microvascular reshaping in the thyroid," *The American Journal of Pathology*, vol. 172, no. 3, pp. 748–760, 2008.

[38] O. Thomusch, C. Sekulla, and H. Dralle, "Is primary total thyroidectomy justified in benign multinodular goiter? Results of a prospective quality assurance study of 45 hospitals offering different levels of care," *Chirurg*, vol. 74, no. 5, pp. 437–443, 2003.

[39] J. K. Harness, C. H. Organ Jr., and N. W. Thompson, "Operative experience of U.S. general surgery residents in thyroid and parathyroid disease," *Surgery*, vol. 118, no. 6, pp. 1063–1070, 1995.

[40] H. Dralle, C. Sekulla, K. Lorenz, M. Brauckhoff, and A. Machens, "Intraoperative monitoring of the recurrent laryngeal nerve in thyroid surgery," *World Journal of Surgery*, vol. 32, no. 7, pp. 1358–1366, 2008.

3

There Is No Elevation of Immunoglobulin E Levels in Albanian Patients with Autoimmune Thyroid Diseases

Hatixhe Latifi-Pupovci, Besa Gacaferri-Lumezi, and Violeta Lokaj-Berisha

Department of Physiology and Immunology, Faculty of Medicine, University of Prishtina, Deshmoret e Kombit Street,
10000 Prishtina, Kosovo

Correspondence should be addressed to Hatixhe Latifi-Pupovci; hatixhe.pupovci@uni-pr.edu

Academic Editor: C. Marcocci

Background. Studies in several ethnic groups reported high incidence of elevated levels of immunoglobulin E (IgE) in patients with autoimmune thyroid diseases (ATD), especially in patients with Graves' disease. *Objective.* To study association between serum levels of IgE and thyroid stimulating hormone receptor antibodies (TRAb) in Albanian patients with ATD. *Material and Methods.* Study was performed in 40 patients with Graves' disease, 15 patients with Hashimoto's thyroiditis, and 14 subjects in the control group. The IgE levels were measured by immunoradiometric assay, whereas the TRAb levels were measured by radioreceptor assay. *Results.* In all groups of subjects the IgE levels were within reference values (<200 kIU/L). Significant difference in mean concentration of IgE was found between two groups of Graves' disease patients, and those with normal and elevated TRAb levels (22.57 versus 45.03, $P < 0.05$). Positive correlation was found between TRAb and IgE only in Graves' disease patients ($r = 0.43$, $P = 0.006$). *Conclusion.* In Albanian patients with ATD there is no elevation of IgE levels. This could be the result of low prevalence of allergic diseases in Albanian population determined by genetic and environmental factors.

1. Introduction

The master switch in the regulation of the thyroid gland is the thyroid-stimulating hormone (TSH) receptor (TSHR) [1]. Autoantibodies against thyroid-stimulating hormone receptor (TRAb) are directly involved in the pathogenesis of Graves' disease and autoimmune hypothyroidism [2]. Although the immunoglobulin E (IgE) is the main regulator of allergic reactions, there is evidence which suggests a relationship between autoimmune thyroid diseases (AITD) and allergic diseases. It has been noted that allergic sensitization is more frequent in Graves' disease and allergic seasonality may explain the fluctuation in the onset of Graves' disease [3]; seasonal allergic rhinitis aggravates the clinical course of Graves' disease [4–6]; the serum levels of IgE are significantly elevated in one-third of patients with Graves' disease and lesser reduction in TRAb exists in patients with elevated IgE levels than in patients with normal IgE [7]. Studies in several ethnic groups reported high incidence of elevated levels of IgE in patients with autoimmune thyroid diseases, especially in

Graves' diseases [7–13]. Therefore, we conducted ambulatory-based study to investigate whether IgE levels were elevated in Albanian patients with autoimmune thyroid diseases and evaluated potential relationship between IgE and TRAb in patients with Graves' disease and Hashimoto's thyroiditis.

2. Material and Methods

2.1. Patients. This prospective study included 40 patients with Graves' disease (36 females and 4 males, ages 11–69 yr), 15 patients with Hashimoto's thyroiditis (11 females and 4 males, ages 26–69 yr), and 14 individuals in control group (10 females and 4 males, ages 29–53 yr). Patients included in this study were diagnosed at the Department of Endocrinology, whereas laboratory measurements were done at the Department of Physiology, University Clinical Center, Prishtina, Kosovo. This research was approved by the Faculty of Medicine, Teaching-Science Council, and was conformed to the provisions of the Declaration of Helsinki (paragraphs 11, 13, 15, 16,

TABLE 1: Patients' characteristics and thyroid parameters in various thyroid diseases.

Subject group	Number of patients	Sex (%) F	Sex (%) M	Age (yr)	T3 (nM)	T4 (nM)	TSH (IU/L)
Graves' disease	40	90	10	41 ± 15	4.85 ± 1.81	258.15 ± 108.9	0.49 ± 0.64
Hashimoto's thyroiditis	15	73	27	46 ± 11	0.89 ± 0.34	36.18 ± 22.97	37.15 ± 46.58
Control group	14	71	29	39 ± 6	2.07 ± 0.50	111.82 ± 18.53	1.11 ± 0.64

TABLE 2: Prevalence of positive TRAb levels and elevated IgE levels in various thyroid diseases.

Subject group	TgAb levels (%)	TgAb (U/mL)	TPOAb levels (%)	TPOAb (U/mL)	TRAb levels (%)	TRAb (IU/L)	IgE (kU/L)
Graves' disease	35	135.92 ± 269.4	77.5	1492.97 ± 2413.9	85	50.32 ± 30.9	41.65 ± 26.36
Hashimoto's thyroiditis	93.3	1178.04 ± 1206.5	100	2124.24 ± 1847.6	40	3.63 ± 3.63	33.72 ± 25.79
Control group	7.4	34.35 ± 16.12	21.4	45.92 ± 35.93	21.4	1.15 ± 0.53	37.24 ± 30.63

20). Informed written consent was obtained from all subjects before inclusion in the study.

The subjects included in this study were untreated patients. Disease diagnosis was based on clinical status, laboratory data—TSH, T3 and T4 levels, and ultrasonographic and histopathologic findings. Basic precondition for inclusion of patients in the study was disease diagnosis based on clinical status and, at least, two of above-mentioned parameters. Patients included in the study were without prescribed therapy for thyroid diseases.

Blood was obtained at their first visit and serum thyroid hormones and TSH were measured at that time. In this study serum concentrations of T3 were measured by total T3 RIA test (reference range: 1.2–2.8 nM) (Immunotech Co., Marseille, France) and T4 was measured by total T4 RIA test (reference range: 60–160 nM) (Immunotech Co., Marseille, France). TSH was measured by total TSH IRMA test (reference range: 60–160 mIU/L) (Immunotech Co., Marseille, France).

2.2. Measurement of Autoantibodies and IgE. Sera for measuring autoantibodies and IgE were collected and stored in −20°C until assay. The TRAb concentration was measured by radioreceptor assay (RRA) with DYNOtest TRAK human (B.R.A.H.M.S. Diagnostica, Berlin, Germany). In this study, and as the manufacturer recommends, TRAK human values below 1.0 IU/L were defined as negative and values above 1.5 IU/L as positive. Thyroglobulin autoantibodies (TgAb) concentration was measured by radioimmunoassay (RIA) with DYNOtest anti-Tg$_n$, (B.R.A.H.M.S. Diagnostica GmbH, Germany). With this method, levels above 60 U/mL were considered positive. Thyroperoxidase antibodies (TPOAb) were determined by radioimmunoassay (RIA) with DYNOtest anti-TPO$_n$, (B.R.A.H.M.S. Diagnostica GmbH, Germany). Levels of TPOAb above 60 U/mL were considered positive. The IgE concentration was measured by immunoradiometric assay with total IgE IRMA (reference range: 2–200 kIU/L) (Immunotech Co., Marseille, France).

2.3. Statistical Analyses. Statistical analyses were performed using two-tailed unpaired Student's *t*-test. $P < 0.05$ was considered statistically significant. Correlation analysis was performed with Pearson's correlation. For statistical analysis the GraphPad Prism 5 software version 5.01 was used.

3. Results

3.1. Prevalence of Positive TRAb Levels and Mean TRAb Levels in Thyroid Diseases. As stated in materials and methods, sera from 40 patients with Graves' disease, 15 patients with Hashimoto's thyroiditis, and 14 individuals in control group were used for this research. The clinical and laboratory data of patients are shown in Table 1.

In Table 1, data are shown as mean ± SD. In this study, significant difference in prevalence of positive TRAb levels was found between Graves' patients and control group ($P < 0.001$). But prevalence of positive TRAb levels in Hashimoto's thyroiditis did not show significant difference compared to control group ($P = 0.3$). The highest levels of mean TRAb values were found in Graves' patients (mean = 50.32, SD = 30.91) showing significant difference compared to other groups of subjects: Graves' disease versus Hashimoto's thyroiditis and Graves' disease versus control group ($P < 0.001$) (Table 2).

In Table 2, data are shown as mean ± SD. Statistical analyses were performed with Student's *t*-test, $P < 0.05$. Prevalence of positive TRAb levels in Graves' disease is significantly greater than that of control group ($P < 0.001$) but the prevalence of positive TRAb levels is not significant in Hashimoto's thyroiditis compared to control group ($P = 0.3$). The mean TRAb levels are significantly greater in Graves' disease versus Hashimoto's thyroiditis and control group ($P < 0.001$).

3.2. Relationship between TRAb Levels and IgE Levels. In this study, the IgE levels were within reference values in all groups of subjects (Table 2).

Although IgE levels were within reference values, we analyzed if there is any relationship between TRAb levels and IgE levels. First, we grouped all patients in two categories depending on the TRAb levels: patients with normal TRAb levels (negative) and those with elevated TRAb levels (positive). Then we compared mean concentration of IgE among

TABLE 3: Mean serum IgE levels among patients with normal (NEG.) and elevated levels (POZ.) of TRAb.

		TRAb (IU/L)	IgE (kIU/L)
Graves' disease			
TRAb	NEG.	0.9 ± 0.00	22.57 ± 15.86
TRAb	POZ.	59.04 ± 24.64	45.03 ± 26.56
Hashimoto's thyroiditis			
TRAb	NEG.	0.96 ± 0.05	5.4 ± 3.11
TRAb	POZ.	7.63 ± 2.13	38.08 ± 24.92
Control group			
TRAb	NEG.	1.08 ± 0.47	36.38 ± 31.71

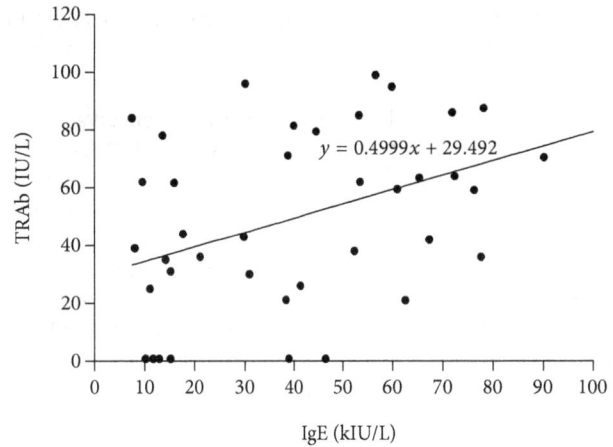

FIGURE 1: Correlation between TRAb and IgE in Graves' disease patients. Positive correlation between TRAb and IgE in Graves' disease patients and Pearson's correlation coefficient, $r = 0.43$ ($P = 0.006$), with regression line $y = 0.4999x + 29.492$.

two categories of patients within each group of subjects. Significant difference in mean concentration of IgE was found between two categories of patients with Graves' disease and those with normal and elevated TRAb levels (22.57 versus 45.03, $P < 0.05$). On the other hand, no significant difference in mean concentration of IgE was found among two categories of patients with Hashimoto's thyroiditis and the control group (Table 3).

In Table 3, data are shown as mean ± SD. Data are shown as mean ± SD. Statistical analyses were performed with Student's t-test, $P < 0.05$. Significant difference in mean concentration of IgE was found among two categories of patients with Graves' disease and those with normal and elevated TRAb levels (22.57 versus 45.03, $P < 0.05$). No significant difference in mean concentration of IgE was found among two categories of patients with Hashimoto's and the control group.

3.3. Correlation between TRAb and IgE. Among all groups of patients studied, we found a positive correlation between levels of TRAb and IgE only in Graves' disease patients ($r = 0.43$, $P = 0.006$). From the determination coefficient ($r^2 = 0.18$) 18% of changes in TRAb level are due to changes in IgE level (Figure 1).

4. Discussion

In this study, as expected, the highest prevalence of positive TRAb and the highest mean TRAb levels were found in patients with Graves' disease and our findings support other reports [14–16]. But, in this study, the prevalence of positive TRAb levels was very high in Hashimoto's patients and in the control group. The same implies for TPOAb and TgAb in the control group (Table 2). There are other publications showing positive TgAb and TPOAb in healthy subjects, although being in lower levels [17–19]. Hasse-Lazar et al. found that positive TRAb levels were present in 12.5% of patients with Hashimoto's disease and 4.8% of subjects in control group [15]. According to Trbojevic, the TRAb levels are positive in 50% of patients with Hashimoto's thyroiditis which have TSH levels higher than 5 IU/L [20]. The author Robert Volpe

explains this with the fact that the elevated levels of TSH in Hashimotos' thyroiditis could raise the expression of HLA-DR antigens and thyroid antigens which in turn stimulate TRAb elevation [18]. Although the prevalence of TRAb in Hashimoto's patients and healthy subjects was higher than reported by other authors, in this study, mean concentration of these autoantibodies was very low.

In our study, the serum IgE levels in all groups of subjects were within the reference values. Unlike our findings, research carried out on other ethnic groups (Japanese, Chinese, and Korean) showed high prevalence of elevated levels of IgE in two main thyroid autoimmune diseases, particularly Graves' disease [7, 13, 20]. Yamada et al. suggested that an underlying state of autoimmune thyroid diseases may be a permissive factor for IgE elevation [8]. So, given the fact that certain percentage of hyperthyroid Graves' and Hashimoto's thyroiditis patients have allergen sensitization [3] and atopic allergies [8] suggests that allergic states could have an underlying effect which is permissive for thyroid autoimmunity. This could be explained with IL-13 stimulation of B cells to secrete TBII, TSAb, and IgE in Graves' disease patients [13]. Genetic studies in Japanese, Chinese, and Caucasian populations found different data regarding IgE levels in GD [9, 11, 21]. The discrepancy between studies of Caucasian and Japanese populations with regard to IgE synthesis suggests that different genetic factors influence IgE synthesis in different ethnic groups [11].

The absence of elevated level of IgE in Albanian patients with thyroid diseases could be explained with the low prevalence of allergic diseases in Albanian population based on the publications from the International Study on Asthma and Allergy in Childhood (ISAAC) [22–25]. Despite the fact that the above mentioned studies were carried out in Albania, it should be noted that our study was carried out in Kosovo which is inhabited with genetically the same population [26]. Also, environmental factors that influence prevalence of allergic diseases are the same because of geographic proximity and similar social status of ethnic Albanians in Kosovo and Albania.

Although the IgE levels were within reference values in all three groups of subjects, in order to examine if there is any relationship between TRAb and IgE, we grouped patients in two categories: patients with normal TRAb levels and those with positive TRAb. In that case, surprisingly, although being within normal IgE values, we found significant difference in mean concentration of IgE between Graves' disease patients with normal TRAb levels and patients with positive TRAb. Also, there was a positive correlation between TRAb and IgE only in patients with Graves' disease. This suggests that mechanisms for TRAb and IgE synthesis could be linked somewhat in TRAb positive Graves' disease patients. Although there is an association between IgE levels and TRAb, the exact mechanism remains to be determined.

The most striking finding in this study is the absence of elevated IgE levels in Albanian patients with thyroid diseases in Kosovo, which could be a result of genetic and environmental factors associated with allergic diseases, prevalence of which is low in Albanian population. But a small sample may be a limitation for this study. Our data needs to be confirmed with further investigations, such as a study replication on another sample and genetic analyses, to increase confidence in our findings.

Acknowledgment

The authors are indebted to Prof. Hysri Tafarshiku for his help in diagnosing the patients at the University Clinic for Internal Diseases, who passed away before the paper was ready for submission.

References

[1] T. F. Davies, T. Ando, R.-Y. Lin, Y. Tomer, and R. Latif, "Thyrotropin receptor-associated diseases: from adenomata to Graves disease," *The Journal of Clinical Investigation*, vol. 115, no. 8, pp. 1972–1983, 2005.

[2] B. Y. Cho, "Clinical applications of TSH receptor antibodies in thyroid diseases," *Journal of Korean medical science*, vol. 17, no. 3, pp. 293–301, 2002.

[3] I. Molnár, "What is the role of allergic sensitization in Graves'disease?" *Orvosi Hetilap*, vol. 148, no. 29, pp. 1347–1352, 2007.

[4] Y. Hidaka, N. Amino, Y. Iwatani, E. Itoh, M. Matsunaga, and H. Tamaki, "Recurrence of thyrotoxicosis after attack of allergic rhinitis in patients with Graves' disease," *Journal of Clinical Endocrinology and Metabolism*, vol. 77, no. 6, pp. 1667–1670, 1993.

[5] Y. Hidaka, T. Masai, H. Sumizaki, K. Takeoka, H. Tada, and N. Amino, "Onset of Graves' thyrotoxicosis after an attack of allergic rhinitis," *Thyroid*, vol. 6, no. 4, pp. 349–351, 1996.

[6] K. Takeoka, Y. Hidaka, H. Hanada et al., "Increase in serum levels of autoantibodies after attack of seasonal allergic rhinitis in patients with graves' disease," *International Archives of Allergy and Immunology*, vol. 132, no. 3, pp. 268–276, 2003.

[7] A. Sato, Y. Takemura, T. Yamada et al., "A possible role of immunoglobulin E in patients with hyperthyroid Graves' disease," *Journal of Clinical Endocrinology and Metabolism*, vol. 84, no. 10, pp. 3602–3605, 1999.

[8] T. Yamada, A. Sato, I. Komiya et al., "An elevation of serum immunoglobulin E provides a new aspect of hyperthyroid Graves' disease," *Journal of Clinical Endocrinology and Metabolism*, vol. 85, no. 8, pp. 2775–2778, 2000.

[9] K. K. L. Chong, S. W. Y. Chiang, G. W. K. Wong et al., "Association of CTLA-4 and IL-13 gene polymorphisms with Graves' disease and ophthalmopathy in Chinese children," *Investigative Ophthalmology and Visual Science*, vol. 49, no. 6, pp. 2409–2415, 2008.

[10] T. Yamada, I. Komiya, Y. Miyahara et al., "Effect of methimazole treatment for 2 years on circulating IL-4, IgE, TBII, and TSAb in patients with hyperthyroid Graves' disease," *Endocrine Journal*, vol. 53, no. 6, pp. 783–788, 2006.

[11] Y. Hiromatsu, T. Fukutani, M. Ichimura et al., "Interleukin-13 gene polymorphisms confer the susceptibility of Japanese populations to Graves' disease," *Journal of Clinical Endocrinology and Metabolism*, vol. 90, no. 1, pp. 296–301, 2005.

[12] H. Y. Kim, K. R. Park, S. H. Kim et al., "The relationship between Graves' disease and serum immunoglobulin-E," *Journal of Korean Society of Pediatric Endocrinology*, vol. 17, no. 5, pp. 640–648, 2002.

[13] I. Komiya, T. Yamada, A. Sato, T. Kouki, T. Nishimori, and N. Takasu, "Remission and recurrence of hyperthyroid Graves' disease during and after methimazole treatment when assessed by IgE and interleukin 13," *Journal of Clinical Endocrinology and Metabolism*, vol. 86, no. 8, pp. 3540–3544, 2001.

[14] M. R. Sérgio, C. Godinho, L. Guerra, A. Agapito, F. Fonseca, and C. Costa, "TSH anti-receptor antibodies in Graves' disease," *Acta Médica Portuguesa*, vol. 9, no. 7–9, pp. 229–231.

[15] K. Hasse-Lazar, B. Jarzab, A. Podwiński et al., "TSH-receptor antibodies in thyroid diseases," *Polish Archives of Internal Medicine*, vol. 97, no. 3, pp. 239–251, 1997.

[16] L. Giovanella, L. Ceriani, and S. Garancini, "Clinical applications of the 2nd generation assay for anti-TSH receptor antibodies in Graves' disease. Evaluation in patients with negative 1st generation test," *Clinical Chemistry and Laboratory Medicine*, vol. 39, no. 1, pp. 25–28, 2001.

[17] H. Nakamura, Y. Mikami, Y. Aono et al., "Measurement of anti-microsomal and anti-thyroglobulin antibodies by radioimmunoassay," *Rinsho byori. The Japanese journal of clinical pathology*, vol. 39, no. 4, pp. 373–378, 1991.

[18] R. Volpe, *Autoimmune Endocrinopathies*, Humana Press, New Jersey, NJ, USA, 1999.

[19] K. Yabiku, M. Hayashi, I. Komiya et al., "Polymorphisms of interleukin (IL)-4 receptor alpha and signal transducer and activator of transcription-6 (Stat6) are associated with increased IL-4Rα-Stat6 signalling in lymphocytes and elevated serum IgE in patients with Graves' disease," *Clinical and Experimental Immunology*, vol. 148, no. 3, pp. 425–431, 2007.

[20] B. Trbojević, *TIroIdna Žlezda—PatofIzIološke Osnove I klInIčkI prIstup, Drugo Izmenjeno Izdanje*, Zavod Za Udžbenike I Nastavna Sredstva, Beograd, Serbia, 1998.

[21] P. E. Graves, M. Kabesch, M. Halonen et al., "A cluster of seven tightly linked polymorphisms in the IL-13 gene is associated

with total serum IgE levels in three populations of white children," *Journal of Allergy and Clinical Immunology*, vol. 105, no. 3, pp. 506–513, 2000.

[22] G. Weinmayr, S. K. Weiland, B. Björkstén et al., "Atopic sensitization and the international variation of asthma symptom prevalence in children," *American Journal of Respiratory and Critical Care Medicine*, vol. 176, no. 6, pp. 565–574, 2007.

[23] G. Weinmayr, F. Forastiere, S. K. Weiland et al., "International variation in prevalence of rhinitis and its relationship with sensitisation to perennial and seasonal allergens," *European Respiratory Journal*, vol. 32, no. 5, pp. 1250–1261, 2008.

[24] N. Pearce, N. Aït-Khaled, R. Beasley et al., "Worldwide trends in the prevalence of asthma symptoms: phase III of the International Study of Asthma and Allergies in Childhood (ISAAC)," *Thorax*, vol. 62, no. 9, pp. 757–765, 2007.

[25] J. Bousquet, N. Khaltaev, A. A. Cruz et al., "Allergic Rhinitis and its Impact on Asthma (ARIA) 2008," *Allergy: European Journal of Allergy and Clinical Immunology*, vol. 63, no. 86, pp. 8–160, 2008.

[26] G. Sulcebe, M. Cuenod, A. Sanchez-Mazas et al., "Human leukocyte antigen-A, -B, -C, -DRB1 and -DQB1 allele and haplotype frequencies in an Albanian population from Kosovo," *International Journal of Immunogenetics*, vol. 40, no. 2, pp. 104–107, 2013.

4

Is the Use of a Drain for Thyroid Surgery Realistic? A Prospective Randomized Interventional Study

Ugur Deveci,[1] Fatih Altintoprak,[2] Mahmut Sertan Kapakli,[1] Manuk Norayk Manukyan,[1] Rahmi Cubuk,[3] Nese Yener,[4] and Abut Kebudi[1]

[1] General Surgery Department, School of Medicine, Maltepe University, 34843 Istanbul, Turkey
[2] General Surgery Department, School of Medicine, Sakarya University, 54100 Sakarya, Turkey
[3] Radiology Department, School of Medicine, Maltepe University, 34843 Istanbul, Turkey
[4] Pathology Department, School of Medicine, Maltepe University, 34843 Istanbul, Turkey

Correspondence should be addressed to Ugur Deveci; opdrdeveci@yahoo.com

Academic Editor: C. Marcocci

Background. The use of a suction drain in thyroid surgery is common practice in order to avoid hematomas or seromas. The aim of this study was to determine the efficacy of routine drainage after thyroid surgery. *Methods.* In this prospective randomized trial, 400 patients who underwent either a total thyroidectomy or lobectomy for thyroid disorders were randomly allocated to either the nondrainage (group 1) or the drainage (group 2) group. The volume of fluid collection in the operative bed, postoperative pain, complications, and length of hospital stay were then recorded. *Results.* Both groups were homogeneous according to age, gender, thyroid volume, type of procedure performed, and histopathological diagnosis. After assessment by USG, no significant difference was found between the groups in the fluid collection of the thyroid bed ($P = 0.117$), but the length of hospital stay was significantly reduced in group 1 ($P = 0.004$). *Conclusions.* In our experience, the use of drain for thyroid surgery is not a routine procedure. However, it should be used in the presence of extensive dead space, particularly when there is retrosternal or intrathoracic extension, or when the patient is on anticoagulant treatment. This trial was registered with Clinical Trials.gov NCT01771523.

1. Introduction

It is believed that many surgeons use a drain following thyroid surgery to obliterate the dead space and evacuate collected blood and serum. This is further reinforced by the fact that postoperative drains usually yield fluid. Hemorrhage can be life threatening, thus necessitating an immediate reoperation. This fear prompts surgeons to use a routine drain after any type of thyroid surgery. Although the rate of bleeding might increase in a subtotal thyroidectomy due to vascularized remnant tissue, postoperative bleeding is actually quite rare and occurs in only 0.3–1% of patients after a thyroidectomy [1, 2]. Many studies have suggested that drains may be blocked with clotted blood; therefore, the surgeon is not alerted even if major bleeding occurs [1–4]. In addition, numerous studies have also failed to show any benefits of drainage in thyroid surgery [3–5]. Hence, the goal of this prospective study was to evaluate the necessity of drainage after thyroid surgery.

2. Patients and Methods

This interventional, randomized, double-blind, prospective study was approved by the local ethics committee at the Turkish Ministry of Health, and informed consent was obtained from all the patients. The subjects were 400 patients who underwent thyroid surgery between January 2010 and January 2012. These patients were randomized via a computer-generated random number table into two groups according to whether or not drains were inserted at the time of surgery. Group 1 consisted of 200 patients without drains and group 2 consisted of 200 patients with drains. The indications for surgery, procedures performed, local complications (infection, seroma, bleeding, hematoma, laryngeal nerve palsy, and hypoparathyroidism), necessity for reoperation, and length of hospital stay were recorded for all of the participants. Those with substernal goiter or malignant disease requiring lymphatic dissection were excluded from

Is the Use of a Drain for Thyroid Surgery Realistic? A Prospective Randomized Interventional Study

23

the study. In addition, nondifferentiated cancer patients and those undergoing anticoagulant therapy were also not included.

Depending on the thyroid disorder, either a total thyroidectomy or a lobectomy plus an isthmectomy was performed. The duration of the operation was defined as the time from the first incision to the last suture placement. Wound closure was done via subcutaneous 4/0 absorbable sutures (Figure 1). Additionally a closed suction drain with negative pressure (Hemovac evacuator, Zimmer Inc., Warsaw, IN, USA) was inserted through a separate wound in the patients in group 2. An ultrasound of the neck using the B mode with a linear frequency of 7.5 MHz was performed on both groups at the postoperative 24th hour of surgery by the same radiologist. The volume of fluid collection in the operative bed was calculated by measuring the maximum diameter in three dimensions, and the fluid which collected in the drain was measured separately. The drains were removed from all of the patients after 24 hours since less than 100 cc had been collected.

Postoperative pain was assessed according to a visual analogue scale (VAS) with scores ranging from 0 (no pain) to 10 (worst pain imaginable) at the postoperative sixth hour and postoperative first day. A standard analgesic protocol comprised of diclofenac sodium (75 mg intramuscularly) and oral paracetamol (500 mg twice a day) was then given to the patients. Differences in the pain scores were analyzed using the Mann-Whitney U test. Thyroid gland volumes were calculated according to the ultrasound measurements of all the patients, and the correlation between thyroid volume and volume of fluid was evaluated in the thyroid bed. The differences between the two groups were analyzed with Student's t-test, and a value of $P < 0.05$ was accepted as being significant.

3. Results

Between January 2010 and January 2012, we performed 400 thyroidectomies in our clinic and analyzed 403 surgical interventions in these patients (mean age 46.8 ± 12.9 years; range 17–82). The male to female ratio was $1 : 7.51$, and there was equal distribution in both groups based on the type of surgery and size of the nodule. The patients' characteristics are presented in Table 1, and there were no significant differences with regard to gender, age, hormonal status, or histopathological results between the two groups ($P = 0.39$, $P = 0.45$, $P = 0.24$, and $P = 0.32$, resp.).

Similar average operating times occurred in group 1 (86.45 (50–120) ± 18.93 min) and in group 2 (88.80 (45–120) ± 21.33 min) ($P = 0.19$). However, the mean VAS score was significantly lower in group 1 than in group 2 at the postoperative sixth hour (3.64 (2–7) ± 1.06 and 4.95 (2–8) ± 1.05, resp.) ($P = 0.002$) and at the postoperative first day (2.08 (1–5) ± 0.74 and 3.09 (1–5) ± 0.77, resp.) ($P = 0.001$) (Table 2). An intramuscular analgesic was requried for all of the patients in group 2, whereas 162 (81%) of the patients in group 1 needed this medication.

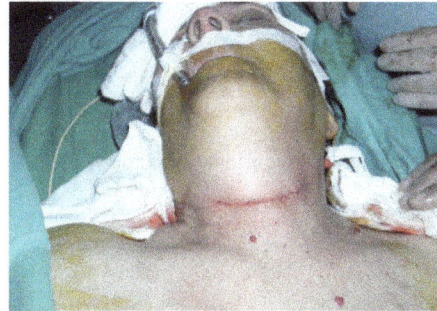

FIGURE 1: Postoperative patient in group 1.

The amount of fluid collection in the thyroid bed was assessed by USG for both groups at the postoperative 24th hour, and the results are shown in Table 3. Student's t-test was applied to detect any difference in the means of fluid collection between the groups, but there was no statistically significant difference in the volume of fluid collection ($P = 0.117$). In group 2, the amount of fluid collected in the suction drain was noted over a 24-hour period, with an average finding of 53.32 mL (range 30–90 mL/day). The mean volume of the thyroid gland was 54.31 (17.3–116.4) ± 22.48 mL and 53.72 (16.8–120.4) ± 21.61 mL in groups 1 and 2, respectively. A linear regression analysis was performed, and no significant statistical difference was seen in the amount of collection according to the volume of the thyroid gland in groups 1 and 2 ($P = 0.73$ and $P = 0.16$, resp.). The groups were also divided into toxic and nontoxic subgroups, and there was no significant difference in the volume of fluid collection ($P = 0.192$). This data is shown in Table 3.

The complications that we observed are shown in Table 4, and the complication rates were similar between the groups ($P = 0.43$). Two cases of hematoma (1%), four cases of seroma (2%), one case of transient recurrent laryngeal nerve palsy (0.5%), one case of reaction to the silk sutures (0.5%), and eight cases of transient hypoparathyroidism (4%) occurred in group 1, whereas three cases of hematoma (1.5%), three cases of seroma (2%), two cases of wound infections (1%), one case of persistent single-side recurrent laryngeal nerve injury (0.5%), two cases of reaction to the silk sutures (1%), and six cases of transient hypoparathyroidism (3%) were present in group 2 ($P = 0.56$). Two of patients in group 1 and three in group 2 required single aspiration due to seroma. In addition, one patient in group 1 and two more in group 2 needed surgical intervention for postoperative bleeding and hematoma. The alerting symptom was the sudden increase in neck volume with dyspnea. In the second intervention, a suction drain was inserted and then removed at the postoperative 24th hour.

The average length of hospital stay was 1.10 (1–3) ± 0.33 days for group 1 and 1.53 (1–6) ± 0.80 days for group 2, and there was a statistically significant difference noted after conducting an analysis with a two-sample t-test ($P = 0.004$). The mean follow-up period was 23.60 (12–36) ± 7.51 months. In the end, we concluded that the presence or absence of

TABLE 1: Patient characteristics.

	Group 1	Group 2
Age	46.80 (17–82) ± 12.90	44.33 (20–79) ± 12.01
Gender (male/female)	21/179	26/174
Type of surgery (total thyroidectomy/lobectomy)	164/36	172/28
Diagnosis		
Benign	178 (89%)	184 (92%)
Malign	22 (11%)	16 (8%)
Toxic	24 (12%)	28 (14%)
Non-toxic	176 (88%)	172 (86%)

TABLE 2: Operative and postoperative values of the patients.

	Group 1	Group 2	P
*Operating time (min)	86.45 (50–120) ± 18.93	88.80 (45–120) ± 21.33	0.19
*Thyroid volume (mL)	54.31 (17.3–116.4) ± 22.48	53.72 (16.8–120.4) ± 21.61	0.80
**Postoperative sixth hour VAS	3.64 (2–7) ± 1.06	4.95 (2–8) ± 1.05	0.002
**Postoperative first day VAS	2.08 (1–5) ± 0.74	3.09 (1–5) ± 0.77	0.001
*Hospital stay (day)	1.10 (1–3) ± 0.33	1.53 (1–6) ± 0.80	0.04

VAS: visual analog scale. The data is presented as mean (min–max) ± SD. *Student's t-test was used for assessment. **The Mann-Whitney U test was used for assessment.

the drain did not contribute significantly to the postoperative complications.

4. Discussion

Drains have been traditionally used in most of the surgical procedures involving the thyroid, and there is limited evidence to suggest that they provide any benefit [4–7]. Our study failed to show any advantage in the routine use of the drain after thyroid surgery. Arterial bleeding near the trachea leads to decreased space, which subsequently compresses the airway and produces significant edema in the soft tissues of the larynx and pharynx. All this causes in the syndrome known as suffocating hematoma, and immediate treatment and surgical revision in the operating theater are then required. This complication appears very infrequently, with figures ranging from 0.3 to 2.5%; however, when it does exist, it presents a big challenge for both the surgeon and the anesthesiologist [8–10]. The risk is greater in patients with intrathoracic goiter and those with Graves' disease [10]. Suffocating hematoma tends to appear between two and six hours after surgery, and most patients report coughing, vomiting, or nausea prior to the hemorrhage. Possible causes for this complication include displacement of an improperly applied suture, the opening of a vessel in which diathermia was used for coagulation, or "drooling" of an area that has been improperly cauterized [10].

In our series, postoperative bleeding occurred in three patients (two in group 1 and one in group 2) two hours after surgery. These patients presented with dyspnea and neck swelling, although the drain was clean. Surgical drains neither prevent this complication from occurring nor contribute to early detection [3–6, 10]. In fact, hemorrhage can appear, and the container may be empty because the blood has clotted inside the drain. Bandages do not reduce the risk of hemorrhage either. They keep blood from collecting in the subcutaneous plane, but the blood may dissect the deep plane to the prethyroid musculature in the paratracheal region, leading to compression of the airway at that level [10].

Two large nonrandomized studies of 250 and 400 patients have also documented that the use of drains after thyroid surgery produces no benefits [8, 11]. In our study, there was an absence of fluid in the thyroid bed on USG, but it was present in the suction drain. This could be caused by the drain itself, since by virtue of the inflammation caused by their presence, they may actually increase the drainage. In addition, the vacuum created by the negative suction of the drain may prevent the lymphatics from sealing off, thus causing an increase in seroma formation and drainage [4, 12]. Furthermore, a possible relationship between drain insertion and infective complications has been observed in some studies [1, 11, 13]. However, we found no relationship between wound infection and drain usage in our study (Table 4). Two studies also investigated the relationship between drain insertion and postoperative pain [1, 14], and the authors noted an approximate 50% reduction in the VAS score in the group in which no drains were used. We obtained similar results in our study. These results indicate that drain insertion might be directly associated with higher levels of postoperative discomfort due to increased pain. This would be reflected by patient satisfaction and early discharge independent of any complications. Morrissey et al. demonstrated that thyroid surgery without the use of a drain decreases the length of hospital stay while producing no increase in patient morbidity [15]. We also observed that performing a thyroidectomy without the use of drain decreased the length of hospital stay.

TABLE 3: Volume of fluid collection in the groups as assessed by USG.

Group 1 ($N = 200$)		Group 2 ($N = 200$)	
4.09 (0–25) ± 6.08 mL		3.64 (0–30) ± 5.07 mL	
	$P = 0.11$		
Group 1		Group 2	
Toxic ($N = 24$)	Nontoxic ($N = 176$)	Toxic ($N = 28$)	Nontoxic ($N = 172$)
4.37 (0–18.4) ± 4.24	4.39 (0–25) ± 5.97	3.81 (0–18.3) ± 5.41	3.83 (0–30) ± 5.05
$P = 0.19$		$P = 0.16$	

The data is presented as mean (min–max) ± SD. Student's t-test was used for assessment.

TABLE 4: Postoperative complications ($P > 0.05^{*}$).

	Group 1	Group 2
Hematoma	2 (1%)	3 (1.5%)
Seroma	4 (2%)	3 (1.5%)
Wound infection	0 (0%)	1 (0.5%)
Suture reaction	1 (0.5%)	2 (1%)
Transient recurrent nerve praxy	1 (0.5%)	0 (0%)
Persistant recurrent nerve injury	0 (0%)	1 (0.5%)
Transient hypoparathyroidism	8 (4%)	6 (3%)
Persistant hypoparathyroidism	0 (0%)	0 (0%)

The data is presented as the number of patients with percentiles in parenthesis. A chi-square test was used for all of the complications. $^{*}P$ value is presented for the total number of complications.

Meticulous hemostasis and an adequate surgical technique are the keys for avoiding hemorrhage and hematoma formation. Herranz and Latorre suggested using a drain in cases in which there is extensive dead space or retrosternal goiters and also noted that routine drainage of the thyroidectomy bed is not effective in decreasing the rate of postoperative complications after thyroid surgery [10]. In a meta-analysis, Corsten et al. concluded that the use of suction drains in thyroid surgery to prevent postoperative hematoma is not evidence based [16]. Furthermore, Khanna et al. reported no significant differences between patients with drains and those without in the collection of the thyroid bed when this was assessed by postoperative USG [5]. In this study, we also demonstrated that the use of a drain for thyroid surgery was not effective for decreasing the rate of complications associated with toxic thyroid disorders. Additionally, a total thyroidectomy performed without a drain is safe and effective for patients with Graves' disease or toxic goiter.

Most studies have revealed that drainage is unnecessary after routine thyroid surgery [1, 3–5, 13, 14]. However, many of these studies had a small number of patients and a retrospective design. This prospective study contains the largest number of patients on this topic in the literature. We do not routinely use drains in our department for thyroid surgery. We only recommend that they should be used in thyroidectomies for patients with substernal goiter and nondifferentiated cancer along with those who are undergoing anticoagulant therapy or require lymphatic dissection. We believe that thyroidectomies without drains are safe for differentiated thyroid cancer, Graves' disease, and other toxic goiters.

5. Conclusion

Our randomized prospective study verified that routine drain placement after thyroid surgery is not necessary nor is it effective in decreasing the rate of postoperative complications. Meticulous hemostasis and attention to finer details during surgery are more important for achieving this goal. Thyroid surgery without the drain decreases the length of hospital stay without increasing patient morbidity. Hence, we found no positive evidence that the use of drains improves patient outcomes.

Authors' Contribution

The study presented here was carried out in collaboration with all authors. U. Deveci, M. N. Manukyan, and A. Kebudi performed surgical interventions. U. Deveci and F. Altintoprak codesigned the research and methods. F. Altintoprak analyzed the data and interpreted the results. Pathological and radiological assessments were performed by N. Yener and R. Cubuk. Discussed analyses, interpretations, and presentation were codesigned by all authors. U. Deveci wrote the paper. All authors have read and approved the paper and take full responsibility for its content.

References

[1] T. Colak, T. Akca, O. Turkmenoglu et al., "Drainage after total thyroidectomy or lobectomy for benign thyroidal disorders," *Journal of Zhejiang University: Science B*, vol. 9, no. 4, pp. 319–323, 2008.

[2] D. Bergqvist and S. Kallero, "Reoperation for postoperative haemorrhagic complications. Analysis of a 10-year series," *Acta Chirurgica Scandinavica*, vol. 151, no. 1, pp. 17–22, 1985.

[3] L. M. Hurtado-López, S. López-Romero, C. Rizzo-Fuentes, F. R. Zaldívar-Ramirez, and C. Cervantes-Sánchez, "Selective use of drains in thyroid surgery," *Head & Neck*, vol. 23, no. 3, pp. 189–193, 2001.

[4] N. Suslu, S. Vural, M. Oncel et al., "Is the insertion of drains after uncomplicated thyroid surgery always necessary?" *Surgery Today*, vol. 36, no. 3, pp. 215–218, 2006.

[5] J. Khanna, R. S. Mohil, Chintamani et al., "Is the routine drainage after surgery for thyroid necessary? A prospective randomized clinical study [ISRCTN63623153]," *BMC Surgery*, vol. 5, article 11, 2005.

[6] R. T. Lewis, R. G. Goodall, B. Marien, M. Park, W. Lloyd-Smith, and F. M. Wiegand, "Simple elective cholecystectomy: to drain or not," *American Journal of Surgery*, vol. 159, no. 2, pp. 241–245, 1990.

[7] J. Hoffmann, M. H. Shokouh-Amiri, P. Damm, and R. Jensen, "A prospective, controlled study of prophylactic drainage after colonic anastomoses," *Diseases of the Colon and Rectum*, vol. 30, no. 6, pp. 449–452, 1987.

[8] A. R. Shaha and B. M. Jaffe, "Practical management of post-thyroidectomy hematoma," *Journal of Surgical Oncology*, vol. 57, no. 4, pp. 235–238, 1994.

[9] S. H. Burkey, J. A. Van Heerden, G. B. Thompson, C. S. Grant, C. D. Schleck, and D. R. Farley, "Reexploration for symptomatic hematomas after cervical exploration," *Surgery*, vol. 130, no. 6, pp. 914–920, 2001.

[10] J. Herranz and J. Latorre, "Drainage in thyroid and parathyroid surgery," *Acta Otorrinolaringologica Espanola*, vol. 58, no. 1, pp. 7–9, 2007.

[11] D. G. Ariyanayagam, V. Naraynsingh, D. Busby, K. Sieunarine, G. Raju, and N. Jankey, "Thyroid surgery without drainage: 15 years of clinical experience," *Journal of the Royal College of Surgeons of Edinburgh*, vol. 38, no. 2, pp. 69–70, 1993.

[12] C. Debry, G. Renou, and A. Fingerhut, "Drainage after thyroid surgery: a prospective randomized study," *Journal of Laryngology and Otology*, vol. 113, no. 1, pp. 49–51, 1999.

[13] A. Kristoffersson, B. Sandzen, and J. Jarhult, "Drainage in uncomplicated thyroid and parathyroid surgery," *British Journal of Surgery*, vol. 73, no. 2, pp. 121–122, 1986.

[14] G. Schoretsanitis, J. Melissas, E. Sanidas, M. Christodoulakis, J. G. Vlachonikolis, and D. D. Tsiftsis, "Does draining the neck affect morbidity following thyroid surgery?" *American Surgeon*, vol. 64, no. 8, pp. 778–780, 1998.

[15] A. T. Morrissey, J. Chau, W. K. Yunker, B. Mechor, H. Seikaly, and J. R. Harris, "Comparison of drain versus no drain thyroidectomy: randomized prospective clinical trial," *Journal of Otolaryngology*, vol. 37, no. 1, pp. 43–47, 2008.

[16] M. Corsten, S. Johnson, and A. Alberabi, "Is suction drainage an effective means of preventing hematoma in thyroid surgery? A meta-analysis," *Journal of Otolaryngology*, vol. 34, no. 6, pp. 415–417, 2005.

5

The Central Effects of Thyroid Hormones on Appetite

Anjali Amin, Waljit S. Dhillo, and Kevin G. Murphy

Section of Investigative Medicine, Faculty of Medicine, Imperial College London, 6th Floor, Commonwealth Building, Hammersmith Hospital, Du Cane Road, London W12 0NN, UK

Correspondence should be addressed to Kevin G. Murphy, k.g.murphy@imperial.ac.uk

Academic Editor: Carmen C. Solorzano

Obesity is a major public health issue worldwide. Current pharmacological treatments are largely unsuccessful. Determining the complex pathways that regulate food intake may aid the development of new treatments. The hypothalamic-pituitary-thyroid (HPT) axis has well-known effects on energy expenditure, but its role in the regulation of food intake is less well characterised. Evidence suggests that the HPT axis can directly influence food intake. Thyroid dysfunction can have clinically significant consequences on appetite and body weight. Classically, these effects were thought to be mediated by the peripheral effects of thyroid hormone. However, more recently, local regulation of thyroid hormone in the central nervous system (CNS) is thought to play an important role in physiologically regulating appetite. This paper focuses on the role of the HPT and thyroid hormone in appetite and provides evidence for potential new targets for anti-obesity agents.

1. Introduction

Obesity, its complications, and the associated mortality are major public health issues worldwide. The major central nervous system (CNS) areas important in the regulation of appetite are the hypothalamus and brainstem. The hypothalamus interprets and integrates afferent signals from the periphery and brainstem to modulate efferent signals that regulate food intake and energy expenditure. Neural and hormonalperipheral signals communicate information including acute nutritional states and energy stores. The hypothalamus is subdivided into a number of interconnecting nuclei, including the paraventricular nucleus (PVN), the ventromedial nucleus (VMN), and the arcuate nucleus (ARC), which are particularly important in regulating energy homeostasis. The ARC is located near the median eminence, where the blood-brain barrier is incomplete, and is thus well positioned to respond to circulating factors involved in appetite and food intake [1]. Recent evidence suggests that thyroid hormones may access the ARC and other regions of the hypothalamus to regulate appetite (Figure 1).

It is well established that the hypothalamic-pituitary-thyroid (HPT) axis regulates body weight. Thyroid hormones are known to effect metabolic rate. Thyroid dysfunction can have clinically significant consequences on appetite and body weight. Hypothyroidism classically causes reduced basal energy expenditure [2] with weight gain [3, 4]. Conversely, hyperthyroidism increases energy expenditure and reduces body weight [5–7]. Traditionally, it has been assumed that it is this reduced body weight that drives the hyperphagia that can be a presenting feature in hyperthyroidism. However, recent evidence suggests that the HPT axis may play a direct role in the hypothalamic regulation of appetite, independent of effects on energy expenditure. Classically, hypothalamic thyrotropin-releasing hormone (TRH) stimulates thyroid-stimulating hormone (TSH) release from the anterior pituitary gland, which then stimulates the release of both thyroid hormones, triiodothyronine (T3) and thyroxine (T4). Reports suggest that all of these signalling molecules can directly influence food intake [8–11]. Improved understanding of the role of the HPT axis and thyroid hormone in appetite may identify new targets for antiobesity agents.

2. Effects of Thyroid Hormones on Food Intake (Table 1)

There are well-characterised effects of fasting on hypothalamic TRH expression. This is primarily thought to downregulate the HPT axis in periods of limited food availability,

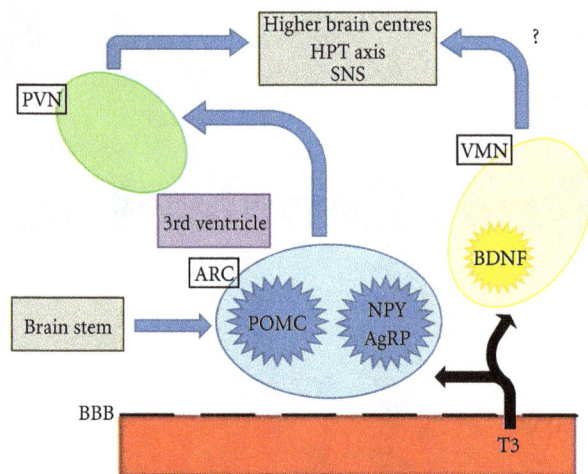

FIGURE 1: Schematic diagram of central appetite regulation. T3 can access the hypothalamus and brainstem via the incomplete blood brain barrier. PVN: paraventricular nucleus; ARC: arcuate nucleus; VMN: ventromedial nucleus; BBB: blood-brain barrier; T3: triiodothyronine; POMC: Pro-opiomelanocortin; NPY: neuropeptide Y; AgRP: agouti-related protein; BDNF: brain-derived neurotrophic factor; HPT: hypothalamic-pituitary thyroid; SNS: sympathetic nervous system.

TABLE 1: Effect of TRH, TSH, and T3 on food intake. Central administration of TRH and TSH in rodents causes a reduction in food intake [8, 12, 13]; similar effects on food intake are seen following peripheral administration of TRH [14]. Central and peripheral administration of T3 increases food intake [9–11]. TRH: thyrotropin releasing hormone; TSH: thyroid-stimulating hormone; T3: triiodothyronine.

Hormone	Effect on food intake
TRH	↓
TSH	↓
T3	↑

thus reducing food intake. However, TRH has been reported to have direct anorectic effects, suggesting it may regulate food intake independent of effects on the HPT axis. In rodents, central administration of TRH reduces food intake [8, 12, 13]; similar effects on food intake are seen following peripheral administration [14].

TSH has also been shown to reduce food intake when injected centrally into rats [8]. There is evidence that TSH from the pars tuberalis is involved in the photoperiodic response in birds and rodents, and it is thus possible that TSH is involved with the seasonal alterations in food intake and body weight that occur in some species [15–17].

The hyperphagia associated with hyperthyroidism may be a result of thyroid hormones acting directly on CNS appetite circuits. T3 directly stimulates food intake at the level of the hypothalamus. In rodent models, peripheral and central hypothalamic administration of T3 increases food intake [9–11].

There are several mechanisms postulated to mediate the orexigenic effects of thyroid hormones. The ARC contains two distinct energy homeostasis-regulating neuronal populations. One subpopulation expresses the pro-opiomelanocortin (POMC) gene which codes for the anorectic neuropeptide alpha-melanocyte-stimulating hormone (α-MSH). The other expresses the orexigenic factors neuropeptide Y (NPY) and agouti-related protein (AgRP). It has been reported that peripheral administration of T3 increases hypothalamic NPY mRNA and that intracerebroventricular (ICV) administration of a NPY Y1 receptor antagonist blunts T3 induced hyperphagia, suggesting that T3 may increase appetite via NPY [10]. T3 administration was also reported toalso reduce hypothalamic POMC expression [10]. Another study did not detect changes in hypothalamic neuropeptide

expression in response to peripheral administration of T3 though this may reflect the different doses of T3 administered [9].

However, the effects of thyroid hormones on food intake may not be mediated directly by the ARC. Direct administration of T3 into the VMN but not the ARC increases food intake in rats [9]. As appetite regulating circuits in the ARC are known to be altered by changes in the HPT, there may be an indirect effect of the ARC via the VMN allowing intra-VMN T3 to increase food intake. In keeping with this, there are excitatory inputs into POMC neurons that originate in the VMN [18].

The effects of T3 in the VMN may be mediated by glutamate [19] and/or brain-derived neurotrophic factor (BDNF) neurons [20]. The VMN is likely to be the source of glutamatergic neurons that modulate ARC POMC neurons. It has not been investigated whether T3, for example, inhibits glutamate synthesis and/or release to disrupt excitatory input into POMC neurons. However, it is interesting to note that there is evidence from other tissues that HPT activity can regulate glutamatergic neuronal machinery. For example, hypothyroidism increases expression of the vesicular glutamate transporter vGLUT-2 in the anterior pituitary [21]. BDNF is a protein belonging to the neurotrophin family of growth factors, which regulate growth, differentiation and survival of neurons. BDNF is highly expressed in the VMN and is reduced by 60% with fasting chronic ICV administration of BDNF significantly reduces food intake in rats [22]. BDNF is thought to act via the tyrosine kinase receptor TrkB. In accord with this, rodents with reduced TrkB expression develop hyperphagia and obesity [23]. In vitro data suggest that T3 reduces BDNF gene expression when applied to hypothalamic explants [20]. However, VMN BDNF may not be physiologically important in the regulation of food intake. Steroidogenic factor-1 (SF1) is a transcription factor which is expressed in of the VMN and which is often used as a molecular marker for the VMN. Leptin depolarizes and increases the firing rate of VMN SF1 neurons, suggesting they are involved in the regulation of energy homeostasis. Mice specifically lacking BDNF in SF1 neurons do not develop the obese phenotype observed in other BDNF-deficient models, suggesting that VMN BDNF may not play an important role in food intake [24]. Further work is required to determine the role of BDNF in mediating the effects of T3 on appetite.

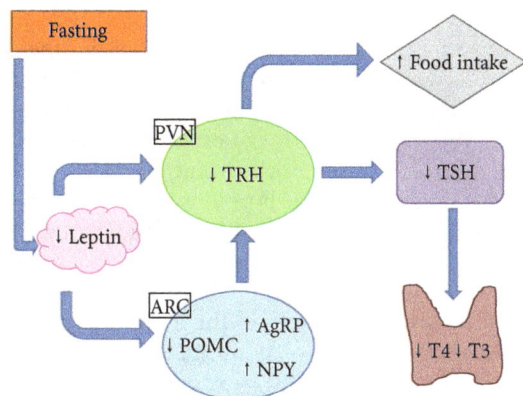

FIGURE 2: Effect of fasting on the hypothalamo-pituitary-thyroid axis. PVN: paraventricular nucleus; ARC: arcuate nucleus; TRH: thyrotropin releasing hormone; TSH: Thyroid-stimulating hormone; T3: triiodothyronine; T4: thyroxine; POMC: Pro-opiomelanocortin; NPY: neuropeptide Y; AgRP: agouti-related protein.

The enzyme 5′ adenosine monophosphate-activated protein kinase (AMPK) is thought to act as a sensor which regulates cellular energy homeostasis. AMPK is activated by phosphorylation, and AMPK activation in the ARC increases food intake [25]. Peripherally administered T3 increases hypothalamic AMPK phosphorylation, which thus may mediate the orexigenic effects of T3 [11].

Thyroid hormone derivatives have also been implicated in the regulation of appetite. G protein-coupled trace amine-associated receptor 1 (TAAR1) is expressed in the rat hypothalamus and is associated with the regulation of energy homeostasis. Thyroid hormone derivative 3-iodothyronamine (T1AM), an endogenous biogenic amine, is a potent agonist of TAAR1. Rodent studies show that T1AM significantly increases food intake in rats, when administered intraperitoneally, ICV, or directly into the ARC [26]. However, the physiological relevance of these effects remains unknown.

The thyroid hormone receptor (TR) or receptors that mediate the effects of thyroid hormones on appetite are unknown. There are two main types of thyroid hormone receptors—thyroid hormone receptor α (THRA) and thyroid hormone receptor β (THRB), each coded by a distinct gene. These genes are alternately spliced to generate three major highly homologous nuclear receptor isoforms (TRα1, TRβ1, and TRβ2) with specific tissue distributions [27]. The three main isoforms bind T3 with high affinity, and regulate thyroid hormone-mediated transcription. TRα is the main isoform regulating T3 activity in the heart, skeletal muscle, bone and brain; TRβ is the main isoform regulating T3 activity in the liver. Adipose tissue expresses both TRα and TRβ. TRβ1 is expressed in most tissues, whilst TRβ2 is expressed solely in the hypothalamus, pituitary, cochlea, and retina [28, 29]. All three isoforms are expressed in the human hypothalamus in a number of nuclei, including the infundibular nucleus, the human equivalent of the ARC, and the supraoptic and paraventricular nuclei.

Although thyroid hormones can directly increase food intake in the hypothalamus, selectively targeting TR subtypes have been shown to have beneficial metabolic effects. Activation of the TRβ receptor reduces body weight in obese rats [30], which may be a result of an increase in metabolic rate. Hence, TRβ agonists have been proposed as treatments for obesity. Targeting the TR with a TRβ-selective agonist may determine whether these agents address the metabolic effects of thyroid hormone, without effects on the TRα-expressing tissues such as the heart [30]. Peripheral administration of a TRβ-selective agonist to rats during feeding with a high-fat diet prevents the expected increases in fat mass, glucose intolerance, and hypertriglyceridaemia [31]. These effects may reflect the increased energy expenditure observed in rodents treated with a TRβ-selective agonist rather than the effects of thyroid hormones on appetite [32]. Further work is required to identify the receptor responsible for the orexigenic effects of T3 in the hypothalamus.

3. Effects of Nutritional State on Thyroid Hormones

Reduction in TRH in response to fasting may be important as TRH is seen to have a direct anorectic effect when injected into the hypothalamus [13]. It is possible there are distinct TRH neuronal populations regulating the HPT axis and regulating appetite.

In periods of limited food availability, there is central downregulation of the HPT axis. Serum T4 and T3 levels fall during fasting in humans [33] and rodents [34, 35]. As the majority of T3 in rodents comes from the thyroid gland, it is thought food deprivation may result in a fall in the release of T4 and T3. This is likely secondary to a reduction in hypothalamic TRH expression, an effect that may be mediated by the adipose hormone leptin (Figure 2).

Leptin is an adipocytokine that circulates in proportion to white adipose tissue and communicates information regarding body fat stores to the CNS. Administration of leptin can reverse starvation induced changes of the HPT axis [34, 36, 37]. Leptin administration partially prevents the reduction in total T4 clearly observed in fasted mice [34]. Humans and mice with mutations of leptin receptor or leptin itself exhibit central hypothyroidism [38, 39], which is ameliorated in leptin-deficient humans by the administration of leptin [40]. Leptin may directly regulate TRH expression in the PVN and may indirectly regulate TRH via effects in the ARC. Leptin increases α-MSH release and decreasesAgRP release, which results in a downregulation of TRH expression. There is also emerging evidence of the existence of a melanocortin-independent pathway by which leptin can influence the HPT axis; cotreatment with a potent melanocortin 4 receptor (MC4R) antagonist diminishes but does not fully block leptin action in restoring total T4 in a rodent model [41].

However, the changes in the HPT axis and peripheral thyroid hormone levels are at odds with the reported effects of thyroid hormones on appetite. If thyroid hormones physiologically increase appetite, they would be predicted to increase, rather than decrease in starvation. Evidence

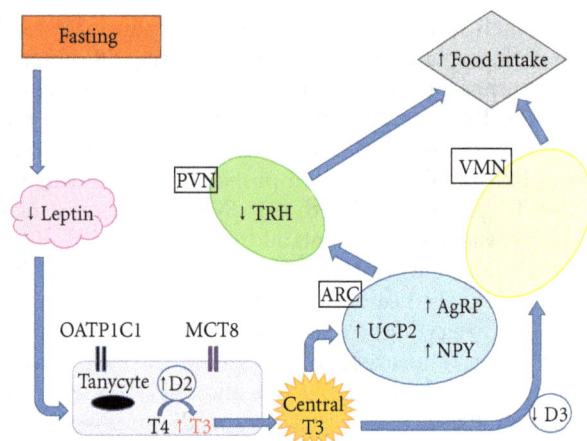

FIGURE 3: Effect and consequences of fasting on central T3 levels, mediated by D2 and D3. PVN: paraventricular nucleus; ARC: arcuate nucleus; VMN: ventromedial nucleus; TRH: thyrotropin releasing hormone; T4: thyroxine; T3: triiodothyronine; OATP1C1: Organic anion transporting polypeptide 1c1; MCT8: monocarboxylate transporter 8; D2: Deiodinase 2; D3: deiodinase 3; NPY: Neuropeptide Y; AgRP: agouti-related protein; UCP2: uncoupling protein 2.

suggests that rather than systemic thyroid hormone levels, it is local CNS concentrations of thyroid hormones that are important in the regulation of appetite.

4. Central Changes in T3 Levels Mediated by D2 and D3

A group of enzymes known as the deiodinases (thioredoxin fold enzymes) regulates the activation and inactivation of T3 and T4. These enzymes are responsible for regulating centralthyroid hormone levels. There are three types of deiodinase, each with an active site containing the amino acid selenocysteine, which is critical for the deiodination reaction catalysed by these enzymes. Deiodinases act by selectively removing of iodine from T4 and its derivatives. Iodine may be removed from the inner (tyrosyl) or outer (phenolic) ring. Deiodinase 1 (D1) is expressed predominantly in the liver, kidney, and thyroid in humans and rodents. However, Deiodinase 2 (D2) and Deiodinase 3 (D3) are highly expressed within the CNS, with some peripheral expression. The expression of each enzyme is regulated individually by thyroid hormone. Within the hypothalamus, expression and activity of D2 and D3 depend on nutritional circumstances, leading to tissue specific changes in hypothalamic T3 availability that may be important in the regulation of food intake and energy expenditure (Figure 3).

D2 catalyses the conversion of T4 to T3 to generate intracellular T3 [42]. It is particularly important in the brain. D2 plays an important part in thyroid hormone-mediated feedback regulation of TRH production. Dio2 knockout mice have higher levels of serum T4 and TSH; however, administration of T3, but not T4, suppresses TSH, suggesting central T4 resistance [43]. Hence the activity of

D2 is crucial in the feedback regulation of TSH secretion. T3-driven suppression of TRH expression in the PVN [44] can be prevented by infusion of the D2 inhibitor iopanoic acid [45]. D2 is not expressed in hypophysiotropic neurons [46] but is highly expressed in tanycytes [47], specialised endothelial cells which line the third ventricle. Tanycytes express two thyroid hormone specific transporters: monocarboxylate transporter 8 (MCT8) and organic anion transporting polypeptide 1C1 (OATP1C1) in rodent models [48]. D2 mediates the conversion of T4 to T3 within these tanycytes, allowing T3 to access the TRH neurons of the PVN. MCT8 is thought to modulate neuronal uptake of thyroid hormone in mice [49], ensuring that TRH production is regulated by peripheral T4 concentration, under basal conditions. Expression of Dio2 and D2 activity are increased in hypothyroidism [50] and fall with the administration of T4, protecting tissues from the adverse effects of extremes of thyroid dysfunction [51].

Hypothalamic D2 expression is not just regulated by thyroid status. In rodents, fasting also increases hypothalamic D2 expression and activity [9, 37], and this effect is not reversed by systemic administration of T4 [45]. It can, however, be reversed by leptin administration [37], suggesting it is more important in energy homeostasis than the HPT axis. Leptin restores the hypothalamic and pituitary components of the HPT axis during fasting, but directly blunts the response of the thyroidgland, resulting in low plasma T4 and T3 [37]. Hence, normalization of thyroid hormone may depend on changes in deiodinase activities and the long-term thyroid stimulation by TSH to oppose these direct inhibitory effects of leptin on the thyroid.

D2 activity is particularly high in the ARC and median eminence [52], where it is expressed within astrocytes and tanycytes. The processes of the D2 containing tanycytes are in direct contact with NPY/AgRP neurons of the ARC which also express UCP2 [53]. Uncoupling protein 1 (UCP1) is thought to be integral to the process of brown-fat-associated nonshivering thermogenesis, as it dissipates energy in the form of heat [54]. The role of inner mitochondrial membrane uncoupling protein 2 (UCP2) is less well defined and tissue specific, but it is subject to regulation by T3 [55].

T3 is thought to access CNS target neurons via a number of different mechanisms. One is through a direct crossing of the blood-brain barrier (BBB). Alternatively T3 may cross the BBB via astrocytes encircling endothelial cells, following 5′ deiodination of T4 taken up from the blood. Astrocytes in the ARC are of particular importance as they express leptin receptors [56, 57]. Another postulated mechanism of T3 transport to target neurons is hypothalamic thyroid hormone uptake from the CSF, with thyroid hormone being taken up from the CSF in the third ventricle and transported by tanycytes to neurons in the ARC that project to TRH cells in the PVN [58]. Upregulation of ARC D2 activity during food deprivation causes increased local bioavailability of T3 in the ARC, leading to increased UCP2 activity and mitochondrial proliferation within the NPY/AgRP neurons [53]. In Dio2 null mice, food deprivation does not result in the characteristic increase in hypothalamic NPY expression [53], suggesting that D2-driven T3 production is crucial to maintain the normal hypothalamic response to fasting. TSH from the pars tuberalis induces Dio2 expression in the mouse hypothalamus as part of the photoperiodic response, and this may thus increase hypothalamic T3 levels [16]. However, it is currently unknown whether these changes are responsible for photoperiodic changes in food intake.

D3 is responsible for the inactivation of T4 to rT3 and T3 to 3′,3′-diiodothyronine (T2) by inner-ring deiodination [59]. D3 preferentially uses T3 as a substrate rather than T4. D3 is predominantly expressed in the adult CNS [60] but is also expressed in the placenta, pregnant uterus, and fetal tissues. D3 mRNA is expressed in the rat hypothalamus and other CNS regions [61]. In the CNS, D3 activity is mediated by levels of thyroid hormone, with higher levels in hyperthyroidism and lower levels in hypothyroidism [61]. Expression of D3 in peripheral tissues is relatively low, but it can be induced in the liver and skeletal muscle of critically ill patients and has been postulated to be responsible for the characteristic changes of reduced levels of TSH and thyroid hormone seen in the sick euthyroid syndrome [62]. D3 may also play a role in the regulation of food intake. Hibernating Siberian hamsters show significant changes in food intake and energy expenditure depending on photoperiod. During short photoperiod days, which would naturally occur during winter months they have reduced food intake and body weight and their core body temperature falls [63]. Expression and activity of hypothalamic D3 is increased in these animals during the same period, causing a reduction in local bioavailability of T3. The reductions in food intake and body weight can be reversed by the implantation of a T3 pellet into the dorsomedial hypothalamus, suggesting that it may be the changes in hypothalamic D3 that is responsible for these effects on energy homeostasis [64].

5. Summary

Local regulation of thyroid hormones in the CNS may physiologically regulate appetite. Switching between the induction of D2 and D3 expression may finely control hypothalamic thyroid hormone concentrations. Further work is now required in order to characterise the pathways by which thyroid hormones regulate food intake. Determining the mechanisms by which thyroid hormones regulate energy homeostasis may aid the development of therapies for the management of obesity.

Abbreviations

T2: 3′,3′-diiodothyronine
AMPK: 5′ adenosine monophosphate-activated protein kinase
AgRP: Agouti-related protein
α-MSH: Alpha-melanocyte-stimulating hormone
ARC: Arcuate nucleus
BBB: Blood-brain barrier
BDNF: Brain-derived neurotrophic factor
CNS: Central nervous system
D1: Deiodinase 1

Dio1: Deiodinase 1 gene
D2: Deiodinase 2
Dio2: Deiodinase 2 gene
D3: Deiodinase 3
Dio3: Deiodinase 3 gene
HPT: Hypothalamic-pituitary-thyroid
ICV: Intracerebroventricular
IP: Intraperitoneal
MC4R: Melanocortin 4 receptor
MCT8: Monocarboxylate transporter 8
NPY: Neuropeptide Y
OATP1C1: Organic anion transporting polypeptide 1c1
PVN: Paraventricular nucleus
POMC: Pro-opiomelanocortin
rT3: Reverse T3
SF1: Steroidogenic factor-1
TR: Thyroid hormone receptor
TSH: Thyroid-stimulating hormone
TRH: Thyrotropin Releasing Hormone
T4: Thyroxine
T3: Tri-iodothyronine
UCP1: Uncoupling protein 1
UCP2: Uncoupling protein 2
VMN: Ventromedial nucleus.

Acknowledgments

A. Amin is supported by the National Institute for Health Research (NIHR) Biomedical Research Centre Funding Scheme. W. S. Dhillo is funded by a National Institute for Health Research Clinician Scientist Award and a Wellcome Trust Value in People Award. K. G. Murphy receives funding from the Biotechnology and Biological Sciences Research Council (BBSRC). The Department is funded by the National NIHR Biomedical Research Centre Funding Scheme, the BBSRC and under FP7-HEALTH-2009-241592 (European Union) EurOCHIP.

References

[1] M. Fry and A. V. Ferguson, "The sensory circumventricular organs: brain targets for circulating signals controlling ingestive behavior," *Physiology and Behavior*, vol. 91, no. 4, pp. 413–423, 2007.

[2] M. Wolf, A. Weigert, and G. Kreymann, "Body composition and energy expenditure in thyroidectomized patients during short-term hypothyroidism and thyrotropin-suppressive thyroxine therapy," *European Journal of Endocrinology*, vol. 134, no. 2, pp. 168–173, 1996.

[3] N. Manji, K. Boelaert, M. C. Sheppard, R. L. Holder, S. C. Gough, and J. A. Franklyn, "Lack of association between serum TSH or free T4 and body mass index in euthyroid subjects," *Clinical Endocrinology*, vol. 64, no. 2, pp. 125–128, 2006.

[4] S. Iossa, L. Lionetti, M. P. Mollica, A. Barletta, and G. Liverini, "Thermic effect of food in hypothyroid rats," *Journal of Endocrinology*, vol. 148, no. 1, pp. 167–174, 1996.

[5] S. Alton and B. P. O'Malley, "Dietary intake in thyrotoxicosis before and after adequate carbimazole therapy; The impact of dietary advice," *Clinical Endocrinology*, vol. 23, no. 5, pp. 517–520, 1985.

[6] H. Pijl, P. H. E. M. De Meijer, J. Langius et al., "Food choice in hyperthyroidism: potential influence of the autonomic nervous system and brain serotonin precursor availability," *Journal of Clinical Endocrinology and Metabolism*, vol. 86, no. 12, pp. 5848–5853, 2001.

[7] L. P. Klieverik, C. P. Coomans, E. Endert et al., "Thyroid hormone effects on whole-body energy homeostasis and tissue-specific fatty acid uptake in vivo," *Endocrinology*, vol. 150, no. 12, pp. 5639–5648, 2009.

[8] M. T. Lin, P. C. Chu, and S. Y. Leu, "Effects of TSH, TRH, LH and LHRH on thermoregulation and food and water intake in the rat," *Neuroendocrinology*, vol. 37, no. 3, pp. 206–211, 1983.

[9] W. M. Kong, N. M. Martin, K. L. Smith et al., "Triiodothyronine stimulates food intake via the hypothalamic ventromedial nucleus independent of changes in energy expenditure," *Endocrinology*, vol. 145, no. 11, pp. 5252–5258, 2004.

[10] S. Ishii, J. Kamegai, H. Tamura, T. Shimizu, H. Sugihara, and S. Oikawa, "Hypothalamic neuropeptide Y/Y1 receptor pathway activated by a reduction in circulating leptin, but not by an increase in circulating ghrelin, contributes to hyperphagia associated with triiodothyronine-induced thyrotoxicosis," *Neuroendocrinology*, vol. 78, no. 6, pp. 321–330, 2003.

[11] S. Ishii, J. Kamegai, H. Tamura, T. Shimizu, H. Sugihara, and S. Oikawa, "Triiodothyronine (T3) stimulates food intake via enhanced hypothalamic AMP-activated kinase activity," *Regulatory Peptides*, vol. 151, no. 1–3, pp. 164–169, 2008.

[12] E. Vijayan and S. M. McCann, "Suppression of feeding and drinking activity in rats following intraventricular injection of thyrotropin releasing hormone (TRH)," *Endocrinology*, vol. 100, no. 6, pp. 1727–1729, 1977.

[13] T. Suzuki, H. Kohno, T. Sakurada, T. Tadano, and K. Kisara, "Intracranial injection of thyrotropin releasing hormone (TRH) suppresses starvation-induced feeding and drinking in rats," *Pharmacology Biochemistry and Behavior*, vol. 17, no. 2, pp. 249–253, 1982.

[14] Y. H. Choi, D. Hartzell, M. J. Azain, and C. A. Baile, "TRH decreases food intake and increases water intake and body temperature in rats," *Physiology and Behavior*, vol. 77, no. 1, pp. 1–4, 2002.

[15] L. C. Drickamer, "Seasonal variation in litter size, bodyweight and sexual maturation in juvenile female house mice (Mus musculus)," *Laboratory Animals*, vol. 11, no. 3, pp. 159–162, 1977.

[16] H. Ono, Y. Hoshino, S. Yasuo et al., "Involvement of thyrotropin in photoperiodic signal transduction in mice," *Proceedings of the National Academy of Sciences of the United States of America*, vol. 105, no. 47, pp. 18238–18242, 2008.

[17] N. Nakao, H. Ono, T. Yamamura et al., "Thyrotrophin in the pars tuberalis triggers photoperiodic response," *Nature*, vol. 452, no. 7185, pp. 317–322, 2008.

[18] S. M. Sternson, G. M. G. Shepherd, and J. M. Friedman, "Topographic mapping of VMH → arcuate nucleus microcircuits and their reorganization by fasting," *Nature Neuroscience*, vol. 8, no. 10, pp. 1356–1363, 2005.

[19] D. R. Ziegler, W. E. Cullinan, and J. P. Herman, "Distribution of vesicular glutamate transporter mRNA in rat hypothalamus," *Journal of Comparative Neurology*, vol. 448, no. 3, pp. 217–229, 2002.

[20] M. S. Byerly, J. Simon, E. Lebihan-Duval, M. J. Duclos, L. A. Cogburn, and T. E. Porter, "Effects of BDNF, T, and corticosterone on expression of the hypothalamic obesity gene network in vivo and in vitro," *American Journal of Physiology*, vol. 296, no. 4, pp. R1180–R1189, 2009.

[21] E. Hrabovszky, I. Kalló, G. F. Turi et al., "Expression of vesicular glutamate transporter-2 in gonadotrope and thyrotrope cells of the rat pituitary. Regulation by estrogen and thyroid hormone status," *Endocrinology*, vol. 147, no. 8, pp. 3818–3825, 2006.

[22] P. A. Lapchak and F. Hefti, "BDNF and NGF treatment in lesioned rats: effects on cholinergic function and weight gain," *NeuroReport*, vol. 3, no. 5, pp. 405–408, 1992.

[23] S. G. Kernie, D. J. Liebl, and L. F. Parada, "BDNF regulates eating behavior and locomotor activity in mice," *EMBO Journal*, vol. 19, no. 6, pp. 1290–1300, 2000.

[24] H. Dhillon, J. M. Zigman, C. Ye et al., "Leptin directly activates SF1 neurons in the VMH, and this action by leptin is required for normal body-weight homeostasis," *Neuron*, vol. 49, no. 2, pp. 191–203, 2006.

[25] Y. Minokoshi, T. Shiuchi, S. Lee, A. Suzuki, and S. Okamoto, "Role of hypothalamic AMP-kinase in food intake regulation," *Nutrition*, vol. 24, no. 9, pp. 786–790, 2008.

[26] W. S. Dhillo, G. A. Bewick, N. E. White et al., "The thyroid hormone derivative 3-iodothyronamine increases food intake in rodents," *Diabetes, Obesity and Metabolism*, vol. 11, no. 3, pp. 251–260, 2009.

[27] M. A. Lazar, "Thyroid hormone receptors: multiple forms, multiple possibilities," *Endocrine Reviews*, vol. 14, no. 2, pp. 184–193, 1993.

[28] M. Sjoberg, B. Vennstrom, and D. Forrest, "Thyroid hormone receptors in chick retinal development: differential expression of mRNAs for α and N-terminal variant β receptors," *Development*, vol. 114, no. 1, pp. 39–47, 1992.

[29] R. A. Hodin, M. A. Lazar, and W. W. Chin, "Differential and tissue-specific regulation of the multiple rat c-erbA messenger RNA species by thyroid hormone," *Journal of Clinical Investigation*, vol. 85, no. 1, pp. 101–105, 1990.

[30] G. Bryzgalova, S. Effendic, A. Khan et al., "Anti-obesity, anti-diabetic, and lipid lowering effects of the thyroid receptor β subtype selective agonist KB-141," *Journal of Steroid Biochemistry and Molecular Biology*, vol. 111, no. 3–5, pp. 262–267, 2008.

[31] B. S. Amorim, C. B. Ueta, B. C. G. Freitas et al., "A TRβ-selective agonist confers resistance to diet-induced obesity," *Journal of Endocrinology*, vol. 203, no. 2, pp. 291–299, 2009.

[32] C. M. Villicev, F. R. S. Freitas, M. S. Aoki et al., "Thyroid hormone receptor β-specific agonist GC-1 increases energy expenditure and prevents fat-mass accumulation in rats," *Journal of Endocrinology*, vol. 193, no. 1, pp. 21–29, 2007.

[33] J. L. Chan, K. Heist, A. M. DePaoli, J. D. Veldhuis, and C. S. Mantzoros, "The role of falling leptin levels in the neuroendocrine and metabolic adaptation to short-term starvation in healthy men," *Journal of Clinical Investigation*, vol. 111, no. 9, pp. 1409–1421, 2003.

[34] R. S. Ahlma, D. Prabakaran, C. Mantzoros et al., "Role of leptin in the neuroendocrine response to fasting," *Nature*, vol. 382, no. 6588, pp. 250–252, 1996.

[35] G. Légràdi, C. H. Emerson, R. S. Ahima, J. S. Flier, and R. M. Lechan, "Leptin prevents fasting-induced suppression of prothyrotropin-releasing hormone messenger ribonucleic acid in neurons of the hypothalamic paraventricular nucleus," *Endocrinology*, vol. 138, no. 6, pp. 2569–2576, 1997.

[36] M. Rosenbaum, E. M. Murphy, S. B. Heymsfield, D. E. Matthews, and R. L. Leibel, "Low dose leptin administration reverses effects of sustained weight-reduction on energy expenditure and circulating concentrations of thyroid hormones," *Journal of Clinical Endocrinology and Metabolism*, vol. 87, no. 5, pp. 2391–2394, 2002.

[37] R. L. Araujo, B. M. Andrade, M. L. Da Silva, A. C. F. Ferreira, and D. P. Carvalho, "Tissue-specific deiodinase regulation during food restriction and low replacement dose of leptin in rats," *American Journal of Physiology*, vol. 296, no. 5, pp. E1157–E1163, 2009.

[38] M. Ohtake, G. A. Bray, and M. Azukizawa, "Studies on hypothermia and thyroid function in the obese (ob/ob) mouse," *American Journal of Physiology*, vol. 2, no. 2, pp. 110–115, 1977.

[39] K. Clément, C. Vaisse, N. Lahlou et al., "A mutation in the human leptin receptor gene causes obesity and pituitary dysfunction," *Nature*, vol. 392, no. 6674, pp. 398–401, 1998.

[40] I. Sadaf Farooqi, G. Matarese, G. M. Lord et al., "Beneficial effects of leptin on obesity, T cell hyporesponsiveness, and neuroendocrine/metabolic dysfunction of human congenital leptin deficiency," *Journal of Clinical Investigation*, vol. 110, no. 8, pp. 1093–1103, 2002.

[41] M. Ghamari-Langroudi, K. R. Vella, D. Srisai, M. L. Sugrue, A. N. Hollenberg, and R. D. Cone, "Regulation of thyrotropin-releasing hormone-expressing neurons in paraventricular nucleus of the hypothalamus by signals of adiposity," *Molecular Endocrinology*, vol. 24, no. 12, pp. 2366–2381, 2010.

[42] T. J. Visser, J. L. Leonard, M. M. Kaplan, and P. R. Larsen, "Kinetic evidence suggesting two mechanisms for iodothyronine 5'-deiodination in rat cerebral cortex," *Proceedings of the National Academy of Sciences of the United States of America*, vol. 79, no. 16, pp. 5080–5084, 1982.

[43] M. J. Schneider, S. N. Fiering, S. E. Pallud, A. F. Parlow, D. L. ST. Germain, and V. A. Galton, "Targeted disruption of the type 2 selenodeiodinase gene (Dio2) results in a phenotype of pituitary resistance to T," *Molecular Endocrinology*, vol. 15, no. 12, pp. 2137–2148, 2001.

[44] G. A. C. Van Haasteren, E. Linkels, W. Klootwijk et al., "Starvation-induced changes in the hypothalamic content of prothyrotrophin-releasing hormone (proTRH) mRNA and the hypothalamic release of proTRH-derived peptides: role of the adrenal gland," *Journal of Endocrinology*, vol. 145, no. 1, pp. 143–153, 1995.

[45] S. Diano, F. Naftolin, F. Goglia, and T. L. Horvath, "Fasting-induced increase in type II iodothyronine deiodinase activity and messenger ribonucleic acid levels is not reversed by thyroxine in the rat hypothalamus," *Endocrinology*, vol. 139, no. 6, pp. 2879–2884, 1998.

[46] H. M. Tu, S. W. Kim, D. Salvatore et al., "Regional distribution of type 2 thyroxine deiodinase messenger ribonucleic acid in rat hypothalamus and pituitary and its regulation by thyroid hormone," *Endocrinology*, vol. 138, no. 8, pp. 3359–3368, 1997.

[47] A. Guadaño-Ferraz, M. J. Obregón, D. L. Germain, and J. Bernal, "The type 2 iodothyronine deiodinase is expressed primarily in glial cells in the neonatal rat brain," *Proceedings of the National Academy of Sciences of the United States of America*, vol. 94, no. 19, pp. 10391–10396, 1997.

[48] L. M. Roberts, K. Woodford, M. Zhou et al., "Expression of the thyroid hormone transporters monocarboxylate transporter-8 (SLC16A2) and organic ion transporter-14 (SLCO1C1) at the blood-brain barrier," *Endocrinology*, vol. 149, no. 12, pp. 6251–6261, 2008.

[49] H. Heuer, M. K. Maier, S. Iden et al., "The monocarboxylate transporter 8 linked to human psychomotor retardation is highly expressed in thyroid hormone-sensitive neuron populations," *Endocrinology*, vol. 146, no. 4, pp. 1701–1706, 2005.

[50] J. E. Silva, M. B. Gordon, and F. R. Crantz, "Qualitative and quantitative differences in the pathways of extrathyroidal triiodothyronine generation between euthyroid and hypothyroid rats," *Journal of Clinical Investigation*, vol. 73, no. 4, pp. 898–907, 1984.

[51] B. Gereben, A. M. Zavacki, S. Ribich et al., "Cellular and molecular basis of deiodinase-regulated thyroid hormone signaling," *Endocrine Reviews*, vol. 29, no. 7, pp. 898–938, 2008.

[52] P. N. Riskind, J. M. Kolodny, and P. R. Larsen, "The regional hypothalamic distribution of type II 5'-monodeiodinase in euthyroid and hypothyroid rats," *Brain Research*, vol. 420, no. 1, pp. 194–198, 1987.

[53] A. Coppola, Z. W. Liu, Z. B. Andrews et al., "A central thermogenic-like mechanism in feeding regulation: an interplay between arcuate nucleus T3 and UCP2," *Cell Metabolism*, vol. 5, no. 1, pp. 21–33, 2007.

[54] D. Ricquier, "Respiration uncoupling and metabolism in the control of energy expenditure," *Proceedings of the Nutrition Society*, vol. 64, no. 1, pp. 47–52, 2005.

[55] M. L. Reitman, Y. He, and D.-W. Gong, "Thyroid hormone and other regulators of uncoupling proteins," *International Journal of Obesity*, vol. 23, pp. S56–S59, 1999.

[56] J. K. Young, "Anatomical relationship between specialized astrocytes and leptin-sensitive neurones," *Journal of Anatomy*, vol. 201, no. 1, pp. 85–90, 2002.

[57] H. Hsuchou, Y. He, A. J. Kastin et al., "Obesity induces functional astrocytic leptin receptors in hypothalamus," *Brain*, vol. 132, no. 4, pp. 889–902, 2009.

[58] A. Alkemade, E. C. Friesema, U. A. Unmehopa et al., "Neuroanatomical pathways for thyroid hormone feedback in the human hypothalamus," *Journal of Clinical Endocrinology and Metabolism*, vol. 90, no. 7, pp. 4322–4334, 2005.

[59] A. C. Bianco, D. Salvatore, B. Gereben, M. J. Berry, and P. R. Larsen, "Biochemistry, cellular and molecular biology, and physiological roles of the iodothyronine selenodeiodinases," *Endocrine Reviews*, vol. 23, no. 1, pp. 38–89, 2002.

[60] A. Campos-barros, T. Hoell, A. Musa et al., "Phenolic and tyrosyl ring iodothyronine deiodination and thyroid hormone concentrations in the human central nervous system," *Journal of Clinical Endocrinology and Metabolism*, vol. 81, no. 6, pp. 2179–2185, 1996.

[61] H. M. Tu, G. Legradi, T. Bartha, D. Salvatore, R. M. Lechan, and P. R. Larsen, "Regional expression of the type 3 iodothyronine deiodinase messenger ribonucleic acid in the rat central nervous system and its regulation by thyroid hormone," *Endocrinology*, vol. 140, no. 2, pp. 784–790, 1999.

[62] R. P. Peeters, P. J. Wouters, E. Kaptein, H. Van Toor, T. J. Visser, and G. Van Den Berghe, "Reduced activation and increased inactivation of thyroid hormone in tissues of critically ill patients," *Journal of Clinical Endocrinology and Metabolism*, vol. 88, no. 7, pp. 3202–3211, 2003.

[63] F. J. P. Ebling and P. Barrett, "The regulation of seasonal changes in food intake and body weight," *Journal of Neuroendocrinology*, vol. 20, no. 6, pp. 827–833, 2008.

[64] P. Barrett, F. J. P. Ebling, S. Schuhler et al., "Hypothalamic thyroid hormone catabolism acts as a gatekeeper for the seasonal control of body weight and reproduction," *Endocrinology*, vol. 148, no. 8, pp. 3608–3617, 2007.

6

Serum Resistin and Insulin-Like Growth Factor-1 Levels in Patients with Hypothyroidism and Hyperthyroidism

Ceren Eke Koyuncu,[1] Sembol Turkmen Yildirmak,[1] Mustafa Temizel,[2] Tevfik Ozpacaci,[3] Pinar Gunel,[4] Mustafa Cakmak,[5] and Yüksel Gülen Ozbanazi[1]

[1] Department of Clinical Biochemistry, Ministry of Health Okmeydani Educational and Research Hospital, Okmeydani, Istanbul 34384, Turkey
[2] Department of Internal Medicine, Ministry of Health Okmeydani Educational and Research Hospital, Okmeydani, Istanbul 34384, Turkey
[3] Department of Nuclear Medicine, Ministry of Health Okmeydani Educational and Research Hospital, Okmeydani, Istanbul 34384, Turkey
[4] Department of Biostatistics, Uludag University Medical Faculty, Bursa 16059, Turkey
[5] Department of Clinical Chemistry, Gulkent State Hospital, Isparta 32100, Turkey

Correspondence should be addressed to Sembol Turkmen Yildirmak; yildirmaksembol@gmail.com

Academic Editor: Jack R. Wall

Introduction. The aim of this study was to evaluate the serum levels of resistin and insulin-like growth factor-1 (IGF-1) and and also the potential relationship between thyroid function and levels of resistin and IGF-1 in hypothyroid and hyperthyroid patients. *Methods.* Fifteen cases of hypothyroid (HT), 16 of subclinically hypothyroid (SCHT), 15 of hyperthyroid (HrT), 15 of subclinically hyperthyroid (SCHrT), and 17 healthy individuals have been included in the study. Serum resistin levels were measured using enzyme-linked immunosorbent assay and IGF-1 and thyroid stimulating hormone (TSH) levels by chemiluminescence method. *Results.* Resistin levels in total HT group were significantly higher than in controls (12.66 ± 6.04 and 8.45 ± 2.90 ng/mL, resp.). In SCHrT subgroup resistin levels were significantly higher than those of controls (14.88 ± 7.73 and 8.45 ± 2.90 ng/mL, resp.). IGF-1 levels were significantly lower in total HT than in total HrT and control groups (117.22 ± 52.03, 155.17 ± 51.67, and 184.00 ± 49.73 ng/mL, resp.). Furthermore IGF-1 levels in HT subgroup were significantly lower compared to controls (123.70 ± 44.03 and 184 ± 49.73 ng/mL, resp.). In SCHT subgroup IGF-1 levels were significantly lower than those of control and SCHrT groups (111.11 ± 59.35, 184.00 ± 49.73, and 166.60 ± 47.87 ng/mL, resp.). There were significant correlations between IGF-1 and TSH in HT subgroup and between resistin and TSH in total HrT group. *Conclusion.* It was concluded that increased resistin levels are directly related to thyroid dysfunction, and GH/IGF-1 axis is influenced in clinically or subclinically hypothyroidism patients.

1. Introduction

Thyroxine (T4) and triiodothyronine (T3) hormones regulate heat production and energy utilization, and they are very important for normal growth and development. They also play important roles in regulating various homeostatic mechanisms [1]. Thyroid abnormalities are accompanied by changes in intermediary metabolism including alterations in body weight, insulin resistance, and lipid profile [2].

It has been understood that adipose tissue is not only a passive energy reservoir, it is but also an active endocrine tissue. Resistin is an adipocytokine which is considered to have an important role in energy metabolism and is secreted from adipocytes and macrophages. Resistin antagonizes insulin effect and causes insulin resistance especially in obese patients. Resistin is also playing a role in inflammation and is a potential biomarker in cardiovascular and many other diseases [3, 4].

IGF-1 is a growth factor which is secreted from liver as a response to growth hormone (GH). IGF-1 has many receptors in various tissues and manifests insulin-like effect as well; it functions in many metabolic pathways including energy metabolism [5]. There are very few studies concerning resistin and IGF-1 concentrations in patients with thyroid dysfunction, and they present conflicting results [4, 6–9]. Furthermore there is no study in the literature related to correlation between resistin and IGF-1 in thyroid dysfunction.

The aims of the present study were (1) to determine serum resistin, IGF-1, TSH, fT4, lipid, and transaminase levels together in untreated patients with hyper-and hypothyroidism and control groups for the first time and (2) to investigate potential relationship between thyroid function and serum levels of resistin and IGF-1 in HT and HrT patients.

2. Materials and Methods

The study consisted of 15 HT patients with ages 20–76, 16 SCHT patients with ages 26–71, 15 HrT patients with ages 22–79, 15 SCHrT patients with ages 26–70, and control group consisting of 17 individuals who were detected as healthy by physical examination and laboratory findings. The total number of volunteers was 78.

The individuals having TSH levels over 5.6 μIU/mL and serum free T4 (fT4) levels below 0.58 ng/dL were classified as HT; the individuals having TSH levels over 5.6 μIU/mL and serum fT4 levels 0.58–1.64 ng/dL were classified as SCHT.

The individuals having TSH levels below 0.34 μIU/mL and serum fT4 levels over 1.64 ng/dL were classified as HrT; the individuals having TSH levels below 0.34 μIU/mL and serum fT4 levels 0.58–1.64 ng/dL were classified as SCHrT. The patients who have TSH levels over 5.6 μIU/mL were classified as total HT, and the patients who have TSH levels below 0.34 μIU/mL were classified as total HrT.

In patient groups there was no individual who had any systemic disease. None of the patients had treatment concerning thyroid dysfunction.

Detailed histories of individuals included in the study were obtained; follow-up forms were prepared. All of the tests and clinical meanings of the tests performed were explained to the individuals, and their written consents were obtained. The ethical approval of study was given by the Okmeydani Educational and Research Hospital Ethics Committee.

10 mL of blood samples into plain vacuum tubes with gel were obtained after 12 hour fasting. They were centrifuged for 10 min at 2000 ×g. T-Chol, HDL-Chol, AST, ALT, TSH, and fT4 were analyzed on the same day. Undiluted serum samples were seperated into two tubes, and they were stored at −80°C for maximum 6 months. Repetative freezing and thawing were not performed.

Serum T-Chol, HDL-Chol, AST, and ALT levels were determined photometrically in Beckman Coulter AU2700 auto-analyzer (Beckman Coulter Inc., CA, USA); TSH ve fT4 levels were determined in Beckman Coulter UniCel DxI 800 autoanalyzer (Beckman Coulter Inc., CA, USA) by using access high sensitive TSH 3rd generation and access

fT4 successively by chemiluminescence method. LDL-Chol levels were calculated by the Friedewald formula. AdipoGen Human Resistin ELISA kit (AdipoGen Inc., Incheon, Korea) was used to determine resistin levels. IGF-1 levels were determined in Siemens Immulite 2000 analyzer (Siemens Healthcare Diagnostics, Deerfield, IL, USA) by solid phase enzyme marked chemiluminescence method.

In order to analyze data SPSS 17.0 ve GraphPad InStat 3.05 packet programs were used. Standart deviations (SD) and means of the Gaussian parameters included in the study were given in terms of groups. Both mean and min-max values and mean ± SD values were presented for the nonGaussian parameters. In comparison of more than two groups that were independent of each other (3 groups and 5 groups), Kruskal-Wallis and one way ANOVA tests were used. The groups which were determined to be different from one another in terms of parameters were compared again in binary groups. The correlation between resistin, IGF-I, and TSH was presented via Spearman's correlation coefficient. The results were evaluated in 95% confidence and significance in $P < 0.05$.

3. Results

Of the individuals included in the study were 17 (22%) males and 61 (78%) females. Laboratory findings and demographic properties of total HT, total HrT, and healthy control groups and HT, SCHT, HrT, and SCHrT subgroups were showed in Tables 1 and 2, respectively. A significant positive correlation between resistin and TSH in total HrT group was detected ($r = 0.463$, $P = 0.010$) (Table 3). There was a statistically significant negative correlation between IGF-1 and TSH in HT subgroup ($r = -0.704$, $P = 0.003$) (Table 3). Within and between assay variations of resistin and IGF-1 measurements were shown at Table 4.

4. Discussion

Significantly higher T-Chol and LDL-Chol levels in total HT group were observed in comparison to total HrT and control groups. Significantly higher T-Chol and LDL-Chol levels in HT subgroup were observed in comparison to HrT, SCHrT, and control groups. These parameters were also significantly higher in SCHT in comparison to HrT subgroup. These findings support the possible correlation between thyroid function and lipid metabolism.

Serum AST levels in total HT and HT groups were detected as significantly higher in comparison to control group. Hepatocellular damage due to fatty liver caused by hypercholesterolemia in hypothyroid patients causes high AST levels. Our findings are consistent with this situation.

Thyroid gland and adipose tissue functions are closely correlated with each other. Recently by the discovery of endocrine functions of adipose tissue, it has been considered that adipose tissue not only has storage function but also has active regulatory functions in energy metabolism [10]. Resistin which is one of the hormones secreted from adipose

TABLE 1: Comparisons of laboratory findings and demographic characteristics of total HT, total HrT, and healthy control groups.

Parameters	Reference ranges	Total hypothyroid group ($n = 31$) Mean ± SD Median (min-max)	Total hyperthyroid group ($n = 30$) Mean ± SD Median (min-max)	Control group ($n = 17$) Mean ± SD Median (min-max)
Age (year)	(—)	47.84 ± 13.31*	43.43 ± 15.66 39.5 (22–79)	37 ± 12.53 34 (22–72)
T-Chol (mg/dL)	120–200	235.13 ± 56.99*†	162.57 ± 42.04	178.41 ± 31.64
HDL-Chol (mg/dL)	35–70	56.61 ± 13.39	52.17 ± 11.61	59.65 ± 14.11
LDL-Kol (mg/dL)	<130	144.19 ± 48.6*†	89.9 ± 32.32	100.24 ± 26.88
AST (U/L)	0–50	41.58 ± 46.12‡ 24 (16–213)	23.43 ± 7.72	19.06 ± 4.46 18 (15–34)
ALT (U/L)	0–50	43.68 ± 58.49 21 (5–265)	24.47 ± 10.18	19.12 ± 9.76 17 (7–50)
TSH (μIU/mL)	0.34–5.6	50.85 ± 75.03*† 15.74 (5.63–306.3)	0.089 ± 0.090$^\alpha$ 0.04 (0.015–0.279)	2.10 ± 1.26
fT4 (ng/dL)	0.58–1.64	0.53 ± 0.23*	2.08 ± 1.20$^{\dagger\alpha}$ 1.68 (0.68–4.85)	0.83 ± 0.10 0.81 (0.73–1.03)
Resistin (ng/mL)	(—)	12.66 ± 6.04$^{\infty}$ 11.98 (5.28–30.32)	12.19 ± 7.13 11.1 (3.84–33.5)	8.45 ± 2.90
IGF-I (ng/mL)	64–345	117.22 ± 52.03†* 104 (58.8–241)	155.17 ± 51.67	184 ± 49.73

$P < 0.05$; *: hypothyroid and control; †: hypothyroid and hyperthyroid; $^\alpha$: hyperthyroid and control.
‡$P = 0.002$ (hypothyroid and control); $^{\infty}P = 0.025$ (hypothyroid and control).

tissue is responsible for insulin resistance, and it is a candidate marker for insulin resistance. However the correlations between resistin and thyroid hormones which are among the major regulators in energy metabolism could not be clearly established.

Changes in thyroid hormone levels have been clearly known to affect insulin secretion and sensitivity. Correlation between resistin and thyroid functions have been investigated by both human and animal studies. Syed et al. [11] reported they observed significant improvement in insulin resistance in obese rats after exogenous thyroid hormone treatment. Nogueiras et al. [6] observed resistin mRNA levels increased in adipose tissue in hypothyroid rats, whereas it decreased to almost undetectable levels in hyperthyroid rats.

In order to enlighten functions of resistin in human it is neccessary to accomplish detailed studies. There is very little information about relationship between thyroid functions and resistin. Furthermore existing studies present conflicting results [4, 6–9].

Significantly higher resistin levels in total HT and total patient group were observed in comparison to control group. It was also observed serum resistin level of total HrT group was higher in comparison to control group. But that elevation was not statistically significant. Serum resistin levels of SCHrT subgroup were significantly higher than those of control group. Although they are not statistically significant, the means of resistin levels in HT, SCHT, and HrT subgroups were higher than those of control group.

The study of Yaturu et al. [10] consisted of 69 Graves' patients as hyperthyroid group and 32 of them taking radioactive iodine as hypothyroid group. Resistin levels of patients who are in hyperthyroid status were determined higher, when compared to the ones who are in hypothyroid status, and it was positively correlated to fT4 and fT3 and negatively correlated to TSH.

In the study of Krassas et al. [12] hyperthyroid group consisting of 43 patients was compared with both 23 healthy controls and 36 treated euthyroid patients who were previously hyperthyroid. Serum resistin levels of hyperthyroid patient group were higher than those of control group. However after normalization of thyroid hormones in hyperthyroid patients, they decreased, and it was correlated with control group.

In another study consisting of 53 hypothyroid patients and 30 controls, Krassas et al. [9] also did not observe any difference between control and patient groups in terms of resistin. After a 4-5-month treatment, normalization of thyroid hormone levels did not result in a signficant change in resistin levels. Furthermore, after treatment, there was no difference in terms of resistin levels in euthyroid individuals. Resistin levels, thyroid hormones, TSH, thyroid antibodies, insulin levels, HOMA-IR index, and age, before treatment and after treatment, did not manifest correlation [9].

In their study consisting of 20 hypothyroid patients and 20 healthy controls, Iglesias et al. [7] observed similar resistin levels in pretreament and posttreatment period in hypothyroid patients, whereas those levels were significantly lower in hypothyroid patients than euthyroid control group [7]. Same research group in their study consisting of 20 hyperthyroid and 20 controls observed lower resistin levels in hyperthyroid patient group in comparison to control group. After normalization of thyroid function in hyperthyroid

TABLE 2: Comparisons of laboratory findings and demographic characteristics of 4 subgroups of patients and healthy control groups.

Parameters	Hypothyroid ($n = 15$) Mean ± SD Median (min-max)	Subclinically hypothyroid ($n = 16$) Mean ± SD Median (min-max)	Hyperthyroid ($n = 15$) Mean ± SD Median (min-max)	Subclinically hyperthyroid ($n = 15$) Mean ± SD Median (min-max)	Control group ($n = 17$) Mean ± SD Median (min-max)
Age (year)	46.53 ± 13.98	49.06 ± 12.98	40.40 ± 17.36 36 (22–79)	46.47 ± 13.66	37 ± 12.53 34 (22–72)
T-Chol (mg/dL)	254.27 ± 63.78$^{\alpha*}$	217.19 ± 44.6$^{£}$	146.47 ± 33.69	178.67 ± 44.4$^{\$}$	178.41 ± 31.64
HDL-Chol (mg/dL)	56.53 ± 11.75	56.69 ± 15.16	51.53 ± 14.0	52.8 ± 9.06	59.65 ± 14.11
LDL-Chol (mg/dL)	163.9 ± 53.91$^{\alpha\$*}$	125.69 ± 35.42$^{£}$	78.27 ± 22.37	101.53 ± 37.06	100.24 ± 26.88
AST (U/L)	51.6 ± 58.31* 26 (16–213)	32.19 ± 29.76 22.5 (16–136)	23.2 ± 7.8	23.67 ± 7.9 20 (16–40)	19.06 ± 4.46 18 (15–34)
ALT (U/L)	46.47 ± 56.83 22 (5–204)	41.06 ± 61.75 21 (9–265)	26.9 ± 9.6	22.0 ± 10.46	19.12 ± 9.76 17 (7–50)
TSH (μIU/mL)	94.4 ± 89.97$^{\alpha\$*}$ 65.19 (9.410–306.3)	10.02 ± 5.31$^{£}$ 7.67 (5.63–24.96)	0.05 ± 0.06$^{\neq}$ 0.02 (0.015–0.22)	0.13 ± 0.10$^{€}$ 0.1 (0.015–0.270)	2.10 ± 1.26
fT4 (ng/dL)	0.33 ± 0.14$^{\alpha\$*}$	0.73 ± 0.08$^{£}$	3.08 ± 0.88$^{\neq}$	1.07 ± 0.28	0.83 ± 0.10 0.81 (0.73–1.03)
Resistin (ng/mL)	13.6 ± 6.25	11.76 ± 5.89 11.35 (5.72–30.32)	9.51 ± 5.48 8.66 (4.1–24.76)	14.88 ± 7.73$^{\#}$	8.45 ± 2.90
IGF-I (ng/mL)	123.7 ± 44.03*†	111.11 ± 59.35$^{€}$ 85.95 (58.8–241)	143.73 ± 54.39	166.6 ± 47.87 148 (114–243)	184 ± 49.73

$P < 0.05$; $^{\#}$: subclinically hyperthyroid and control; *: hypothyroid and control; $^{€}$: subclinically hyperthyroid and subclinically hypothyroid; †: subclinically hypothyroid and control; $^{\alpha}$: hyperthyroid and hypothyroid; $^{£}$: hyperthyroid and subclinically hypothyroid; $^{\$}$: hypothyroid and subclinically hyperthyroid; $^{\neq}$: hyperthyroid and control.

TABLE 3: Correlations between resistin, IGF-1, and TSH in total HT and total HrT groups and HT-HrT subgroups.

		IGF-1	TSH
Total hyperthyroid group ($n = 30$)	Resistin	$r = 0.007$ $P = 0.971$	$r = \mathbf{0.463}$ $P = \mathbf{0.010}$
	IGF-I	— —	$r = -0.069$ $P = 0.718$
Total hypothyroid group ($n = 31$)	Resistin	$r = -0.026$ $P = 0.889$	$r = 0.182$ $P = 0.328$
	IGF-1	— —	$r = 0.081$ $P = 0.663$
Hypothyroid subgroup ($n = 15$)	Resistin	$r = -0.439$ $P = 0.101$	$r = 0.332$ $P = 0.226$
	IGF-I	— —	$r = \mathbf{-0.704}$ $P = \mathbf{0.003}$
Hyperthyroid subgroup ($n = 15$)	Resistin	$r = -0.086$ $P = 0.761$	$r = 0.466$ $P = 0.080$
	IGF-I	— —	$r = -0.131$ $P = 0.641$
Subclinically hypothyroid subgroup	Resistin	$r = 0.276$ $P = 0.300$	$r = 0.265$ $P = 0.322$
	IGF-I	— —	$r = 0.165$ $P = 0.542$
Subclinically hyperthyroid subgroup	Resistin	$r = -0.154$ $P = 0.583$	$r = 0.034$ $P = 0.904$
	IGF-I	— —	$r = -0.085$ $P = 0.764$

TABLE 4: Within and between assay variations of resistin and IGF-1 measurements.

	Concentration	SD	CV
Resistin (ng/mL)			
Within assay	12.57	0.47	3.73
Between assay	15.32	1.07	6.97
IGF-1 (ng/mL)			
Within assay	169	6.5	3.8
Between assay	169	9.1	5.4

patients, they did not observe any significant change in resistin levels [7].

In this study higher resistin levels in total hypothyroid group conflict in comparison to control group with study of Krassas et al. [9] in which they did not observe any difference and with study of Iglesias et al. [7] in which they observed lower resistin levels. This contradiction may be as a result of inequal demographic characteristics and therapeutic variations of patient group. Although observed higher resistin levels were in total HT group in comparison to control group, no correlation between resistin and TSH in total HT group was found. This finding is consistent with that of Krassas et al. [9]. There were no proportional correlations between resistin levels and severity of hypothyroidism, whereas the total HrT group showed positive correlation between resistin and TSH levels. This finding conflicts with study of Yaturu et al. [10] in which they observed negative correlation. In this study, resistin levels were found higher in SCHrT subgroup than in controls. This finding is consistent with study of Krassas et al. [12] in which serum resistin levels of HrT patient group were higher than those of control group and conflict with Iglesias et al. [7] in which serum resistin levels of HrT patient group were lower than those of control group.

Consequently, when limited number of studies about resistin examined, it was observed that resistin levels are variable in thyroid dysfunctions [9, 10, 12]. Higher resistin levels in both hypothyroidism and hyperthyroidism were observed compared to controls. These findings refer to a relationship between thyroid dysfunction and serum resistin levels. Conflicting results may be related to secretion of resistin by macrophages in addition to adipose tissue in humans. Differences in inflammation status of selected individuals may cause different results. In this study, individuals were classified according to their serum levels of TSH, and fT4 and it was not known what was underlying the disease of hypo-and hyperthyroid patients. This is the limitation of this study.

Before now, the correlation between growth hormone excess, insulin resistance, and carbohydrate intolerance has been presented by some studies [13–16]. It has been considered that the correlation between insulin resistances is due to both growth hormone's insulin-like effect and its structural similarity to insulin causing activation of IGF-1 by binding weakly to insulin receptors. In acromegalic patients there is excess of growth hormone and consequently IGF-1 excess, and this results in glucose intolerance and type II diabetes. Besides, in a study performed by Silha et al., similar resistin

levels in control subjects and acromegalic patients having high IGF-1 levels were observed [13]. They reported that insulin resistance in acromegaly may be due to other reasons than resistin [13]. In a study performed with transgenic GH-suppressed rats, Chiba et al. noted that low IGF-1 levels decrease resistin gene expression in white adipose tissue and plasma resistin levels, and insulin efficiency increases in dwarf rats [17]. Chen et al. reported IGF-1 decreases resistin gene expression and protein secretion in vitro [18]. Willemsen et al. performed a 2-year study with infants having low birth weight and short stature according to gestational age [19]. During this period they determined resistin levels in children having high IGF-1 levels and taking GH treatment. They observed resistin levels did not decrease after treatment, but levels of resistin were lower in children with high IGF-1 in comparison to control group. However they also observed that resistin levels increased spontaneously in children taking no treatment after 2 years, and there was a correlation between high IGF-1 levels and low resistin levels [19].

In another study performed with children having GH deficiency, Nozue et al. investigated effect of GH treatment on serum resistin levels [20]. In contrast to the study performed by Willemsen et al. [19], they reported that IGF-1 and resistin levels increased significantly after treatment with GH [20]. Schmid et al. detected that T4 replacement increased IGF-1 level in primary and central hypothyroid patients [21]. They reported that administration of thyroid hormone to the patients with GH deficiency increased IGF-1 level [21]. Völzke et al. detected high IGF-1 levels were correlated with goitre in males with presence of thyroid nodules and in females with low TSH levels [22]. Kursunluoglu et al. reported IGF-1 polymorphism can be a risk factor for hypothyroidism [23]. Akin et al. observed significantly lower serum IGF-1 levels in subclinically hypothyroid patients in comparison to control group, whereas they observed similar IGF-1 levels in subclinically hyperthyroid patients with control group [24]. They reported GH/IGF-1 axis was influenced in subclinically hypothyroid patients, but it was not influenced in subclinical hyperthyroid patients. They also reported LT4 treatment in subclinically hypothyroid patients could prevent abnormalities involving GH/IGF-1 axis.

In this study significantly lower serum IGF-1 levels were detected in total HT group in comparison to total HrT and control groups. Serum IGF-1 levels in HT subgroup were significantly lower in comparison to control group; serum IGF-1 levels in SCHT subgroup were significantly lower in comparison to control group and SCHrT subgroup. A negative correlation between TSH and IGF-1were also observed in HT subgroup. These results were compatible with that of Akin et al. [24], Schmid et al. [21] l, and Kursunluoglu et al. [23]

In this study, no correlation between resistin and IGF-1 levels was found. The reason may be limited number and age diversity of individuals in study groups. A comparement can not be made about that result because there is no study about correlation between resistin and IGF-1 in thyroid dysfunction in the literature.

In conclusion, increased resistin levels are directly related to thyroid dysfunction, and changes in levels of thyroid hormones may affect synthesis and/or secretion of resistin in adipose tissue and/or macrophages. In addition, serum IGF-1 levels decrease in hypothyroid status and correlate negatively with TSH levels. GH/IGF-1 axis may be influenced in clinical or subclinically hypothyroid patients. However, it was concluded that demographic characteristics, therapeutic variations and underlying reasons of thyroid dysfunction should be taken into consideration while interpreting the resistin and IGF-1 levels in thyroid dysfunction.

References

[1] V. Kumar, A. K. Abbas, and Nelson, *Robbins and Cotran. Pathologic Basis of Disease*, 7th edition, 2005.

[2] E. Pucci, L. Chiovato, and A. Pinchera, "Thyroid and lipid metabolism," *International Journal of Obesity*, vol. 24, no. 2, pp. S109–S112, 2000.

[3] B. Antuna-Puente, B. Feve, S. Fellahi, and J. P. Bastard, "Adipokines: the missing link between insulin resistance and obesity," *Diabetes and Metabolism*, vol. 34, no. 1, pp. 2–11, 2008.

[4] N. Pontikides and G. E. Krassas, "Basic endocrine products of adipose tissue in states of thyroid dysfunction," *Thyroid*, vol. 17, no. 5, pp. 421–431, 2007.

[5] W. F. Ganong, *Ganong Medical Physiology*, 16th edition, 2002.

[6] R. Nogueiras, O. Gualillo, J. E. Caminos, F. F. Casanueva, and C. Diéguez, "Regulation of resistin by gonadal, thyroid hormone, and nutritional status," *Obesity Research*, vol. 11, no. 3, pp. 408–414, 2003.

[7] P. Iglesias, P. Alvarez Fidalgo, R. Codoceo, and J. J. Díez, "Serum concentrations of adipocytokines in patients with hyperthyroidism and hypothyroidism before and after control of thyroid function," *Clinical Endocrinology*, vol. 59, no. 5, pp. 621–629, 2003.

[8] J. I. Botella-Carretero, F. Alvarez-Blasco, J. Sancho, and H. F. Escobar-Morreale, "Effects of thyroid hormones on serum levels of adipokines as studied in patients with differentiated thyroid carcinoma during thyroxine withdrawal," *Thyroid*, vol. 16, no. 4, pp. 397–402, 2006.

[9] G. E. Krassas, N. Pontikides, K. Loustis, G. Koliakos, T. Constantinidis, and T. Kaltsas, "Resistin levels are normal in hypothyroidism and remain unchanged after attainment of euthyroidism: relationship with insulin levels and anthropometric parameters," *Journal of Endocrinological Investigation*, vol. 29, no. 7, pp. 606–612, 2006.

[10] S. Yaturu, S. Prado, and S. R. Grimes, "Changes in adipocyte hormones leptin, resistin, and adiponectin in thyroid dysfunction," *Journal of Cellular Biochemistry*, vol. 93, no. 3, pp. 491–496, 2004.

[11] M. A. Syed, M. P. Thompson, J. Pachucki, and L. A. Burmeister, "The effect of thyroid hormone on size of fat depots accounts for most of the changes in leptin mRNA and serum levels in the rat," *Thyroid*, vol. 9, no. 5, pp. 503–512, 1999.

[12] G. E. Krassas, N. Pontikides, K. Loustis, G. Koliakos, T. Constantinidis, and D. Panidis, "Resistin levels in hyperthyroid patients before and after restoration of thyroid function: relationship with body weight and body composition," *European Journal of Endocrinology*, vol. 153, no. 2, pp. 217–221, 2005.

[13] J. V. Silha, M. Krsek, V. Hana et al., "Perturbations in adiponectin, leptin and resistin levels in acromegaly: lack of correlation with insulin resistance," *Clinical Endocrinology*, vol. 58, no. 6, pp. 736–742, 2003.

[14] S. Melmed, "Acromegaly," *The New England Journal of Medicine*, vol. 322, no. 14, pp. 966–977, 1990.

[15] P. H. Sönksen, F. C. Greenwood, J. P. Ellis, C. Lowy, A. Rutherford, and J. D. N. Nabarro, "Changes of carbohydrate tolerance in acromegaly with progress of the disease and in response to treatment," *The Journal of Clinical Endocrinology and Metabolism*, vol. 27, no. 10, pp. 1418–1430, 1967.

[16] T. Wasada, K. Aoki, A. Sato et al., "Assessment of insulin resistance in acromegaly associated with diabetes mellitus before and after transsphenoidal adenomectomy," *Endocrine Journal*, vol. 44, no. 4, pp. 617–620, 1997.

[17] T. Chiba, H. Yamaza, T. Komatsu et al., "Pituitary growth hormone suppression reduces resistin expression and enhances insulin effectiveness. Relationship with caloric restriction," *Experimental Gerontology*, vol. 43, no. 6, pp. 595–600, 2008.

[18] Y. H. Chen, P. F. Hung, and Y. H. Kao, "IGF-I downregulates resistin gene expression and protein secretion," *American Journal of Physiology*, vol. 288, no. 5, pp. E1019–E1027, 2005.

[19] R. H. Willemsen, M. Dijk, Y. B. Rijke, A. W. Toorenenbergen, P. G. Mulder, and A. C. Hokken-Koelega, "Effect of growth hormone therapy on serum adiponectin and resistin levels in short, small-for-gestational-age children and associations with cardiovascular risk parameters," *Journal of Clinical Endocrinology and Metabolism*, vol. 92, no. 1, pp. 117–123, 2007.

[20] H. Nozue, T. Kamoda, and A. Matsui, "Serum resistin concentrations in growth hormone-deficient children during growth hormone replacement therapy," *Metabolism*, vol. 56, no. 11, pp. 1514–1517, 2007.

[21] C. Schmid, C. Zwimpfer, M. Brändle, P. A. Krayenbühl, J. Zapf, and P. Wiesli, "Effect of thyroxine replacement on serum IGF-I, IGFBP-3 and the acid-labile subunit in patients with hypothyroidism and hypopituitarism," *Clinical Endocrinology*, vol. 65, no. 6, pp. 706–711, 2006.

[22] H. Völzke, N. Friedrich, S. Schipf et al., "Association between serum insulin-like growth factor-I levels and thyroid disorders in a population-based study," *Journal of Clinical Endocrinology and Metabolism*, vol. 92, no. 10, pp. 4039–4045, 2007.

[23] R. Kursunluoglu, S. Turgut, F. Akin et al., "Insulin-like growth factor-I gene and insulin-like growth factor binding protein-3 polymorphism in patients with thyroid dysfunction," *Archives of Medical Research*, vol. 40, no. 1, pp. 42–47, 2009.

[24] F. Akin, G. F. Yaylali, S. Turgut, and B. Kaptanoglu, "Growth hormone/insulin-like growth factor axis in patients with subclinical thyroid dysfunction," *Growth Hormone and IGF Research*, vol. 19, no. 3, pp. 252–255, 2009.

7

Thyroid Hormone and Tissue Repair: New Tricks for an Old Hormone?

Iordanis Mourouzis, Efstathia Politi, and Constantinos Pantos

Department of Pharmacology, University of Athens, 75 Mikras Asias Avenue, Goudi, 11527 Athens, Greece

Correspondence should be addressed to Constantinos Pantos; cpantos@med.uoa.gr

Academic Editor: Giorgio Iervasi

Although the role of thyroid hormone during embryonic development has long been recognized, its role later in adult life remains largely unknown. However, several lines of evidence show that thyroid hormone is crucial to the response to stress and to poststress recovery and repair. Along this line, TH administration in almost every tissue resulted in tissue repair after various injuries including ischemia, chemical insults, induction of inflammation, or exposure to radiation. This novel action may be of therapeutic relevance, and thyroid hormone may constitute a paradigm for pharmacologic-induced tissue repair/regeneration.

1. Introduction

Although the role of thyroid hormone (TH) during development has long been recognized, its role later in adult life remains largely unknown [1]. A growing body of evidence reveals that thyroid hormone may be a major player for the response to stress and its presence crucial to poststress adaptation and recovery. Thus, thyroid hormone is now thought to have a reparative action later in adult life, and this has been recently documented in several studies; see Table 1.

2. Adaptation to Environmental Stress and Species Evolution: The Critical Role of Thyroid Hormone

The most important challenge that living organisms faced during species evolution was the ability to adapt to the transition from the aquatic environment, a condition of low oxygen, to the ground, an oxygen-rich state. This required a gene programming that would enable organ protection and remodeling during this transition. Interestingly, studies on amphibians revealed that thyroid-hormone-regulated gene programming is critical for the metamorphosis of tadpoles into juvenile frogs [2]. Several studies have shown that the morphological and functional changes of metamorphosis are the result of alterations in the transcription of specific sets

of genes induced by TH and TH alterations can lead to developmental failures [3–6].

3. Thyroid Hormone and Stress Response: An Evolutionary Conserved Mechanism

The potential role of thyroid hormone in stress response has been, until now, underestimated. However, thyroid hormone signaling is altered during various stressful stimuli and thyroid hormone is crucial to poststress recovery and injury repair [7–9]. Interestingly, the importance of thyroid hormone for stress response has been documented in several species ranging from fish to humans [10]. Thus, exposure of air-breathing perch to water-born kerosene resulted in low T3 and unfavorable metabolic changes, while the administration of TH reversed this response [11]. Along this line, cold stunning Kemp's ridley sea turtles had undetectable levels of thyroid hormone, and recovery was observed only in those who recovered thyroid hormone levels in blood [12]. Interestingly, a similar response is also observed in humans. In fact, after an index event, such as myocardial infarction, T3 levels significantly drop and lower levels of T3 are associated with high mortality [13, 14]. Furthermore, T3 levels are strongly correlated to early and late recovery of cardiac function, with T3 levels at 6 months to be an independent predictor of the recovery of the myocardium [15]. In fact, patients

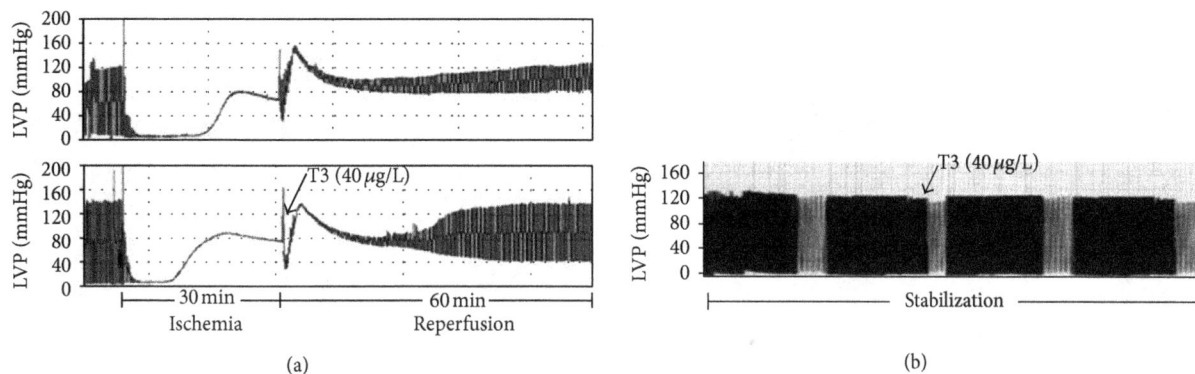

FIGURE 1: Langendorff recordings of left ventricular pressure (LVP) from isolated rat hearts subjected to zero-flow global ischemia followed by reperfusion (a) and hearts subjected only to stabilization (b). Triiodothyronine (T3) administration at reperfusion improves postischemic recovery of function, whereas T3 during stabilization does not affect contractile function.

who spontaneously recover T3 levels in plasma after myocardial infarction are those with markedly improved cardiac functional recovery [15]. These observations provide clear evidence that thyroid-hormone-regulated mechanisms may be evolutionary conserved and are crucial to the response to stress and poststress recovery and tissue repair [11]. Along this line, several studies have demonstrated the reparative action of thyroid hormone. We have recently shown that T3 at a dose which had no effect on noninjured myocardium significantly limited apoptosis in the ischemic myocardium and improved postischemic function in an isolated rat heart model of ischemia-reperfusion. This effect was due to the suppression of the ischemia-reperfusion-induced activation of the proapoptotic p38 MAPK [16, 17] as shown in, Figure 1.

4. Thyroid Hormone: The "Black Box of Repair?"

Accumulating experimental evidence shows that thyroid hormone may play a critical role in the repair after injury in almost every tissue and organ as shown in Table 1. This probably implies that organisms may have a common mechanism of repair which may be regulated by thyroid hormone and has been established during evolution. Thus, thyroid hormone was shown to control DNA repair after irradiation-induced damage in mouse intestine [38]. A single dose of T3 in rats significantly diminished hepatocellular injury induced by ischemia-reperfusion (I/R) when given 48 h before the I/R protocol. This effect was mediated by a T3 transient oxidative stress, and thus, it was abrogated by the administration of antioxidant N-acetyl-cysteine [23]. Thyroxine was cytoprotective in toxic and ischemic injury in kidney [24, 26]. Thus, T3 administration 24 h prior to renal ischemia could precondition against ischemia-reperfusion (I/R) injury. This was evident by a marked decrease in I/R-induced proteinuria. T3 treatment also improved lipid peroxidation biomarkers and increased antioxidant enzymes [24]. In another study, T4 administration immediately or 24 h after ischemia resulted in higher Inulin clearance and preserved cellular integrity [26]. In accordance with these observations

in animal models, T4 was shown to be cytoprotective, in a cellular model of reoxygenation injury in isolated proximal tubule cells [25]. Such evidence may provide an explanation to the clinical observation that low T3 has been associated with increased mortality in hemodialyzed patients [39]. T3 treatment prevented streptozocin-induced toxic injury in pancreatic cells. This effect was associated with an increased activation of the prosurvival Akt signaling [27]. Similarly, T3 was shown to improve function and survival of rat pancreatic islets in in vitro cell cultures [40]. Moreover, T3 was found to preserve ovarian granulose cells exposed to paclitaxel. In fact, T3 significantly reduced the paclitaxel-induced cell injury via downregulation of caspase3 and Bax and upregulation of Bcl2 [28]. T3 pretreatment in rats instilled with an isosmolar 5% albumin solution resulted in the upregulation of alveolar epithelial fluid clearance [41]. T3 was also shown not only to stimulate alveolar fluid clearance in normal but also in hypoxia-injured lungs [29]. The administration of T3 attenuated neointimal formation after balloon injury of carotid artery [35]. Thyroid hormone enhanced transected axonal regeneration and muscle reinnervation following rat sciatic nerve injury [22] and improved recovery of sensory function [21]. Similarly, thyroid hormone was shown to be essential for muscle regeneration after injury [33, 34]. Thyroid hormone promoted the survival of injured neurons [18] and enhanced remyelination in demyelinating inflammatory disease [20]. Thyroid hormone has also been shown to accelerate wound healing in mice and guinea pigs [36, 37].

5. Conclusions

Thyroid hormone appears to be a common player for the organ development and response to stress. Thyroid hormone was crucial for species evolution, and thyroid-hormone-regulated mechanisms have been evolutionary conserved and play an important role early during development. However, recent research has revealed that thyroid hormone has a reparative role later in adult life. This novel action may be of therapeutic relevance, and thyroid hormone may constitute a paradigm for pharmacologic induced tissue repair/regeneration.

TABLE 1: Accumulating experimental evidence shows that thyroid hormone may play a critical role for the repair after injury in several tissues and organs.

Study	Type of treatment	Tissue	Type of injury	Outcome
Shulga et al. 2009 [18]	Treatment with T4 after injury	Mouse hippocambal slices	Mechanical injury	Increased number of neurons, reduced caspase-3 activation, and increased axonal regeneration
Hiroi et al. 2006 [19]	Treatment with T4 after ischemia	Mouse central nervous system	Transient focal ischemia	Reduced cerebral infarct volume, and improved neurological deficit score
Fernandez et al. 2004 [20]	Treatment with T4 after injury	Rat nervous system	Chronic demyelinating inflammatory disease	Enhancement of remyelination
Papakostas et al. 2009 [21]	Treatment with T3 after injury	Rat sciatic nerve	Nerve transection	Increased recovery of sensory function
Panaite and Barackat-Walter 2010 [22]	Treatment with T3 after injury	Rat sciatic nerve	Nerve transection	Increased number of regenerated axons, improved muscle reinnervation
Fernández et al. 2007 [23]	Pretreatment with T3	Rat Liver	Ischemia-reperfusion	Reduced injury (serum AST and ALT levels)
Ferreyra et al. 2009 [24]	Pretreatment with T3	Rat kidney	Ischemia-reperfusion	Reduced proteinuria
Erkan et al. 2003 [25]	Pretreatment with T4	Rabbit proximal tubule cells	Anoxia reoxygenation	Better preservation of cellular structure
Sutter et al. 1988 [26]	Treatment with T4 after ischemia	Rat kidney	Ischemia-reperfusion	Improved kidney function, preserved cellular morphology
Verga Falzacappa et al. 2011 [27]	Contemporary T3 treatment	Mouse pancreas	Streptozocin-induced toxicity	Increased number, shape, and dimension of islets, increased insulin and glucagon levels
Verga Falzacappa et al. 2012 [28]	Contemporary T3 treatment	Rat ovarian granulosa cells	Chemotherapy induced toxicity	Increased number of survived cells, reduced apoptosis
Bhargava et al. 2008 [29]	Pretreatment with T3	Rat lung	Hyperoxia injury	Increased alveolar fluid clearance
Pantos et al. 2011 [16]	Treatment with T3 after ischemia	Rat heart	Ischemia-reperfusion	Increased recovery of function, reduced injury and apoptosis
Pantos et al. 2009 [17]	Treatment with T3 after ischemia	Rat heart	Ischemia-reperfusion	Increased recovery of function, reduced injury
Pantos et al. 2002 [30]	Pretreatment with T4	Rat heart	Ischemia-reperfusion	Increased recovery of function
Kuzman et al. 2005 [31]	Pretreatment with T3	Neonatal rat cardiomyocytes	Serum starvation	Increased cell viability, reduced apoptosis
Chen et al. 2008 [32]	Treatment with T3 after infarction	Rat heart	Acute myocardial infarction	Improved LV function, reduced apoptosis
Dentice et al. 2010 [33]	Treatment with T3 after injury	Mouse skeletal muscle	Mechanical injury	Improved muscle regeneration
Marsili et al. 2011 [34]	Induction of D2-increased T3	Mouse skeletal muscle	Skeletal muscle injury	Improved muscle regeneration
Fukuyama et al. 2006 [35]	Treatment with T3 after injury	Rat carotid artery	Mechanical injury	Attenuation of VSMC proliferation and neointimal formation
Safer et al. 2004 [36]	Treatment with T3 after injury	Mouse skin	Wound	Accelerated wound healing, increased keratinocyte proliferation
Kassem et al. 2012 [37]	Local T3 treatment	Guinea pig skin	Wound	Reduction in the wound surface area

References

[1] C. Pantos, I. Mourouzis, and D. V. Cokkinos, "Thyroid hormone and cardiac repair/regeneration: from Prometheus myth to reality?" *Canadian Journal of Physiology and Pharmacology*, vol. 90, no. 8, pp. 977–987, 2012.

[2] J. F. Gudernatsch, "Feeding Experiments on tadpoles - I. The influence of specific organs given as food on growth and differentiation. A contribution to the knowledge of organs with internal secretion," *Archiv für Entwicklungsmechanik der Organismen*, vol. 35, no. 3, pp. 457–483, 1912.

[3] D. L. Berry, C. S. Rose, B. F. Remo, and D. D. Brown, "The expression pattern of thyroid hormone response genes in remodeling tadpole tissues defines distinct growth and resorption gene expression programs," *Developmental Biology*, vol. 203, no. 1, pp. 24–35, 1998.

[4] J. D. Furlow and E. S. Neff, "A developmental switch induced by thyroid hormone: xenopus laevis metamorphosis," *Trends in Endocrinology and Metabolism*, vol. 17, no. 2, pp. 40–47, 2006.

[5] J. D. Furlow, H. Y. Yang, M. Hsu et al., "Induction of Larval tissue resorption in Xenopus laevis tadpoles by the thyroid hormone receptor agonist GC-1," *The Journal of Biological Chemistry*, vol. 279, no. 25, pp. 26555–26562, 2004.

[6] Y. B. Shi, L. Fu, S. C. V. Hsia, A. Tomita, and D. Buchholz, "Thyroid hormone regulation of apoptotic tissue remodeling during anuran metamorphosis," *Cell Research*, vol. 11, no. 4, pp. 245–252, 2001.

[7] C. Pantos, I. Mourouzis, and D. V. Cokkinos, "New insights into the role of thyroid hormone in cardiac remodeling: time to reconsider?" *Heart Failure Reviews*, vol. 16, no. 1, pp. 79–96, 2011.

[8] C. Pantos, I. Mourouzis, and D. V. Cokkinos, "Rebuilding the post-infarcted myocardium by activating "physiologic" hypertrophic signaling pathways: the thyroid hormone paradigm," *Heart Failure Reviews*, vol. 15, no. 2, pp. 143–154, 2010.

[9] C. Pantos, I. Mourouzis, G. Galanopoulos et al., "Thyroid hormone receptor 1 downregulation in postischemic heart failure progression: the potential role of tissue hypothyroidism," *Hormone and Metabolic Research*, vol. 42, no. 10, pp. 718–724, 2010.

[10] V. S. Peter and M. C. Peter, "The interruption of thyroid and interrenal and the inter-hormonal interference in fish: does it promote physiologic adaptation or maladaptation?" *General and Comparative Endocrinology*, vol. 174, no. 3, pp. 249–258, 2012.

[11] V. S. Peter, E. K. Joshua, S. E. Wendelaar Bonga, and M. C. S. Peter, "Metabolic and thyroidal response in air-breathing perch (Anabas testudineus) to water-borne kerosene," *General and Comparative Endocrinology*, vol. 152, no. 2-3, pp. 198–205, 2007.

[12] K. E. Hunt, C. Innis, and R. M. Rolland, "Corticosterone and thyroxine in cold-stunned Kemp's ridley sea turtles (Lepidochelys kempii)," *Journal of Zoo and Wildlife Medicine*, vol. 43, no. 3, pp. 479–493, 2012.

[13] B. Eber, M. Schumacher, W. Langsteger et al., "Changes in thyroid hormone parameters after acute myocardial infarction," *Cardiology*, vol. 86, no. 2, pp. 152–156, 1995.

[14] L. Friberg, S. Werner, G. Eggertsen, and S. Ahnve, "Rapid downregulation of thyroid hormones in acute myocardial infarction: is it cardioprotective in patients with angina?" *Archives of Internal Medicine*, vol. 162, no. 12, pp. 1388–1394, 2002.

[15] I. Lymvaios, I. Mourouzis, D. V. Cokkinos, M. A. Dimopoulos, S. T. Toumanidis, and C. Pantos, "Thyroid hormone and recovery of cardiac function in patients with acute myocardial infarction: a strong association?" *European Journal of Endocrinology*, vol. 165, no. 1, pp. 107–114, 2011.

[16] C. Pantos, I. Mourouzis, T. Saranteas et al., "Acute T3 treatment protects the heart against ischemia-reperfusion injury via TRα1 receptor," *Molecular and Cellular Biochemistry*, vol. 353, no. 1-2, pp. 235–241, 2011.

[17] C. Pantos, I. Mourouzis, T. Saranteas et al., "Thyroid hormone improves postischaemic recovery of function while limiting apoptosis: a new therapeutic approach to support hemodynamics in the setting of ischaemia-reperfusion?" *Basic Research in Cardiology*, vol. 104, no. 1, pp. 69–77, 2009.

[18] A. Shulga, A. Blaesse, K. Kysenius et al., "Thyroxin regulates BDNF expression to promote survival of injured neurons," *Molecular and Cellular Neuroscience*, vol. 42, no. 4, pp. 408–418, 2009.

[19] Y. Hiroi, H. H. Kim, H. Ying et al., "Rapid nongenomic actions of thyroid hormone," *Proceedings of the National Academy of Sciences of the United States of America*, vol. 103, no. 38, pp. 14104–14109, 2006.

[20] M. Fernandez, A. Giuliani, S. Pirondi et al., "Thyroid hormone administration enhances remyelination in chronic demyelinating inflammatory disease," *Proceedings of the National Academy of Sciences of the United States of America*, vol. 101, no. 46, pp. 16363–16368, 2004.

[21] I. Papakostas, I. Mourouzis, K. Mourouzis, G. Macheras, E. Boviatsis, and C. Pantos, "Functional effects of local thyroid hormone administration after sciatic nerve injury in rats," *Microsurgery*, vol. 29, no. 1, pp. 35–41, 2009.

[22] P. A. Panaite and I. Barakat-Walter, "Thyroid hormone enhances transected axonal regeneration and muscle reinnervation following rat sciatic nerve injury," *Journal of Neuroscience Research*, vol. 88, no. 8, pp. 1751–1763, 2010.

[23] V. Fernández, I. Castillo, G. Tapia et al., "Thyroid hormone preconditioning: protection against ischemia-reperfusion liver injury in the rat," *Hepatology*, vol. 45, no. 1, pp. 170–177, 2007.

[24] C. Ferreyra, F. O'Valle, J. M. Osorio et al., "Effect of preconditioning with triiodothyronine on renal ischemia/reperfusion injury and poly(ADP-ribose) polymerase expression in rats," *Transplantation Proceedings*, vol. 41, no. 6, pp. 2073–2075, 2009.

[25] E. Erkan, A. Sakarcan, G. Haklar, and S. Yalcin, "Thyroxine prevents reoxygenation injury in isolated proximal tubule cells," *Pediatric Nephrology*, vol. 18, no. 7, pp. 636–643, 2003.

[26] P. M. Sutter, G. Thulin, M. Stromski et al., "Beneficial effect of thyroxin in the treatment of ischemic acute renal failure," *Pediatric Nephrology*, vol. 2, no. 1, pp. 1–7, 1988.

[27] C. Verga Falzacappa, C. Mangialardo, L. Madaro et al., "Thyroid hormone T3 counteracts STZ induced diabetes in mouse," *PLoS One*, vol. 6, no. 5, Article ID e19839, 2011.

[28] C. Verga Falzacappa, E. Timperi, B. Bucci et al., "T₃ preserves ovarian granulosa cells from chemotherapy induced apoptosis," *Journal of Endocrinology*, vol. 215, pp. 281–289, 2012.

[29] M. Bhargava, M. R. Runyon, D. Smirnov et al., "Triiodo-L-thyronine rapidly stimulates alveolar fluid clearance in normal and hyperoxia-injured lungs," *American Journal of Respiratory and Critical Care Medicine*, vol. 178, no. 5, pp. 506–512, 2008.

[30] C. I. Pantos, V. A. Malliopoulou, I. S. Mourouzis et al., "Long-term thyroxine administration protects the heart in a pattern similar to ischemic preconditioning," *Thyroid*, vol. 12, no. 4, pp. 325–329, 2002.

[31] J. A. Kuzman, A. M. Gerdes, S. Kobayashi, and Q. Liang, "Thyroid hormone activates Akt and prevents serum starvation-induced cell death in neonatal rat cardiomyocytes," *Journal of Molecular and Cellular Cardiology*, vol. 39, no. 5, pp. 841–844, 2005.

[32] Y. F. Chen, S. Kobayashi, J. Chen et al., "Short term triiodo-l-thyronine treatment inhibits cardiac myocyte apoptosis in border area after myocardial infarction in rats," *Journal of Molecular and Cellular Cardiology*, vol. 44, no. 1, pp. 180–187, 2008.

[33] M. Dentice, A. Marsili, R. Ambrosio et al., "The FoxO$_3$/type 2 deiodinase pathway is required for normal mouse myogenesis and muscle regeneration," *The Journal of Clinical Investigation*, vol. 120, no. 11, pp. 4021–4030, 2010.

[34] A. Marsili, D. Tang, J. W. Harney et al., "Type II iodothyronine deiodinase provides intracellular 3, 5, 3′-triiodothyronine to normal and regenerating mouse skeletal muscle," *American Journal of Physiology*, vol. 301, no. 5, pp. 818–824, 2011.

[35] K. Fukuyama, T. Ichiki, I. Imayama et al., "Thyroid hormone inhibits vascular remodeling through suppression of cAMP response element binding protein activity," *Arteriosclerosis, Thrombosis, and Vascular Biology*, vol. 26, no. 9, pp. 2049–2055, 2006.

[36] J. D. Safer, T. M. Crawford, and M. F. Holick, "A role for thyroid hormone in wound healing through keratin gene expression," *Endocrinology*, vol. 145, no. 5, pp. 2357–2361, 2004.

[37] R. Kassem, Z. Liberty, M. Babaev et al., "Harnessing the skin-thyroid connection for wound healing: a prospective controlled trial in guinea pigs," *Journal of Clinical & Experimental Dermatology*, vol. 37, no. 8, pp. 850–856, 2012.

[38] E. Kress, A. Rezza, J. Nadjar, J. Samarut, and M. Plateroti, "The thyroid hormone receptor-α (TRα) gene encoding TRα1 controls deoxyribonucleic acid damage-induced tissue repair," *Molecular Endocrinology*, vol. 22, no. 1, pp. 47–55, 2008.

[39] J. Horacek, S. Dusilova Sulkova, M. Kubisova et al., "Thyroid hormone abnormalities in haemodialyzed patients: low triiodothyronine as well as high reverse triiodothyronine are associated with increased mortality," *Physiological Research*, vol. 61, no. 5, pp. 495–501, 2012.

[40] C. V. Falzacappa, C. Mangialardo, S. Raffa et al., "The thyroid hormone T3 improves function and survival of rat pancreatic islets during in vitro culture," *Islets*, vol. 2, no. 2, pp. 96–103, 2010.

[41] H. G. Folkesson, A. Norlin, Y. Wang, P. Abedinpour, and M. A. Matthay, "Dexamethasone and thyroid hormone pretreatment upregulate alveolar epithelial fluid clearance in adult rats," *Journal of Applied Physiology*, vol. 88, no. 2, pp. 416–424, 2000.

8

Determination of *RET* Sequence Variation in an MEN2 Unaffected Cohort Using Multiple-Sample Pooling and Next-Generation Sequencing

R. L. Margraf,[1] J. D. Durtschi,[1] J. E. Stephens,[1] M. Perez,[1] and K. V. Voelkerding[1,2]

[1] *Research & Development, ARUP Institute for Clinical and Experimental Pathology, 500 Chipeta Way, Salt Lake City, UT 84108, USA*
[2] *Department of Pathology, University of Utah School of Medicine, Salt Lake City, UT 84112, USA*

Correspondence should be addressed to R. L. Margraf, rebecca.margraf@aruplab.com

Academic Editor: Gary L. Francis

Multisample, nonindexed pooling combined with next-generation sequencing (NGS) was used to discover *RET* proto-oncogene sequence variation within a cohort known to be unaffected by multiple endocrine neoplasia type 2 (MEN2). DNA samples (113 Caucasians, 23 persons of other ethnicities) were amplified for *RET* intron 9 to intron 16 and then divided into 5 pools of <30 samples each before library prep and NGS. Two controls were included in this study, a single sample and a pool of 50 samples that had been previously sequenced by the same NGS methods. All 59 variants previously detected in the 50-pool control were present. Of the 61 variants detected in the unaffected cohort, 20 variants were novel changes. Several variants were validated by high-resolution melting analysis and Sanger sequencing, and their allelic frequencies correlated well with those determined by NGS. The results from this unaffected cohort will be added to the *RET* MEN2 database.

1. Introduction

Multiple endocrine neoplasia type 2 (MEN2) is a rare autosomal dominant inherited disorder with a high lifetime risk of medullary thyroid carcinoma (MTC) [1, 2]. MEN2 consists of three syndromes: familial medullary thyroid carcinoma (FMTC), MEN2A, and MEN2B [1, 3]. FMTC families have only MTC. MEN2A families have MTC, with at least one individual developing pheochromocytomas, parathyroid hyperplasia, or both. MEN2B patients have MTC (with or without pheochromocytoma) and other characteristic clinical features: mucosal ganglioneuromas, GI ganglioneuromas, eye abnormalities, and skeletal abnormalities including marfanoid body habitus [4–7]. MEN2 is caused by pathogenic mutations found exclusively within the *RET* proto-oncogene (REarranged during Transfection). These are gain-of-function dominant mutations which are commonly heterozygous missense mutations found at specific codons within *RET* exons 10, 11, and 13–16 and rarely found within exons 5 and 8 [1, 8–10]. The medical management for the patient and potentially their family

members is based on the familial *RET* variation, which is usually determined by Sanger sequencing [1]. Discovery of a known MEN2 pathogenic *RET* mutation within a family leads to screening for MTC, pheochromocytomas, or parathyroid hyperplasia, and potentially prophylactic thyroidectomy to increase survival rate for the intractable, aggressive MTC. Approximately 75–80% of MTC patients have the sporadic form of MTC (i.e., isolated, nonfamilial MTC), not MEN2 [6]. Patients with apparent sporadic MTC are always tested for an *RET* germline mutation, in case they actually have MEN2 and require different medical management. Although there are many well-known pathogenic *RET* mutations causative of MEN2, it may be difficult to know if a rare or novel germline *RET* variant is a pathogenic mutation (patient has MEN2) or nonpathogenic polymorphism (patient has sporadic MTC).

Interpretation of rare and novel variants will increase in importance as more people are sequenced at the exome, whole genome, or targeted gene levels. Many new changes will be found with unknown clinical significance and their presence and allele frequency within the general population is of importance to help determine pathogenicity status of a variant. Consortiums like the 1000 genome and other large sequencing projects are making great progress in understanding population sequence variation. Yet more direct studies on single genes or gene panels can yield higher sequencing read coverage and more cost-effective sequencing over a smaller genetic area. Also, a particular chosen cohort can be sequenced for a particular locus, such as in the case of this study, where a cohort that was self-reported to have no personal or family history of MEN2 or MTC was sequenced for a section of the *RET* protooncogene where most pathogenic MEN2 causative mutations are located. *RET* sequence variation detected in this MEN2 unaffected population can then be added to the MEN2 *RET* database [8]. This data could be used for several reasons: (1) to help interpret the pathogenicity of clinically detected *RET* sequence variation; (2) as a reference for any future MEN2 case studies (variant was not found in those unaffected by MEN2 disease); (3) for improved genetic test design, to avoid or minimize designing probes or primers over known *RET* sequence variation.

To further reduce costs of sequencing large numbers of individuals, multiple samples can be pooled (without indexing) before next-generation sequencing (NGS). This was the focus of several studies that analyzed the ability to detect true variants within nonindexed pooled sample sets [11–16]. Thirty samples (60 alleles) were the maximum pooling number indicated by our prior studies and in other reports [12, 14, 17, 18], for reproducible and accurate singleton allele detection within the pool (a singleton is a unique allele within the pool). A pool of this size was expected to a have a singleton allele read frequency of 1.67%, and with consideration of sequencing error rates and potential variance in NGS determined variant read frequencies, singleton variants are expected to be detected above a cutoff of >1% variant reads [17, 18].

In this study, 136 individuals of an MEN2 unaffected cohort were sequenced on the illumina genome analyzer utilizing laboratory and bioinformatics protocols from our previous studies for nonindexed, multiple sample pooling. The pool size was limited to less than 30, which is the previously determined optimal pooling size for accurate singleton variant detection [12, 14, 17, 18]. In total, 61 variants were detected within the MEN2 unaffected cohort, which included 20 novel variants.

2. Materials and Method

2.1. Samples. Peripheral blood samples from 136 adult volunteers (113 Caucasian and 23 non-Caucasians for ethnic diversity) were collected and deidentified using University of Utah IRB protocol no. 7740. The donors for this unaffected cohort were self-described as not having a personal or family history of neither medullary thyroid carcinoma nor multiple endocrine neoplasia type 2 (MEN2). The 51 samples used as controls were deidentified according to IRB no.7275 and were Sanger sequenced for *RET* exons 10, 11, and 13–16, including exon/intron boundaries. The "single-sample

control" did not have *RET* mutations causative of MEN2, while the "50 pool" control contained many samples with known MEN2 causative *RET* mutations. The 50 pool control was sequenced on the illumina genome analyzer several times previously [17, 18].

2.2. PCR, Library Prep, and NGS. DNA samples were amplified from *RET* intron 9 to intron 16 using long-range PCR technology. Amplicons were normalized by SequalPrep (Invitrogen Corp, Carlsbad, CA), quantified using Quant-iT Picogreen dsDNA kit (Invitrogen Corp), and equimolar pooled before Illumina Library Prep, utilizing previously described protocols [18]. Between 27 and 29 Caucasian samples' amplicons were combined into four separate pools (P1, P2, P3, and P4) before Illumina Library Prep and NGS. The non-Caucasian cohort's 23 samples were sequenced in a separate pool (ethnic pool). The PCR-amplified *RET* positions 1–9180 are positions 43608691–43617870 in reference sequence NC_000010.10 (Table 1). Two controls were also included in this study, a single sample and also a pool of 50 samples. Each pool and each control were sequenced in a separate flow cell lane on the illumina genome analyzer, using single-end read chemistry.

2.3. Data Analysis. Sequencing image files were processed and reads aligned to the *RET* reference sequence with SeqMan NGen version 2.1 software (DNAstar, Madison, WI), as described previously [17, 18]. Reads used were of 67 base lengths since the 3′ end read positions of longer reads can have an increase in sequencing background errors, as shown in previous studies [17, 19, 20]. As previously described, several base quality score screening thresholds (Q-threshold) evaluated for read coverage, errors (especially for outlier errors, which could be mistaken for false positives in a pool), variant read percentage, and base quality score statistics to determine the 30 Q-threshold should be used for analysis of all data sets, which minimized errors while maintaining adequate target read coverage (data not shown) [17, 18].

Excluded from analysis was a region of repeats and homopolymers that caused misalignment errors in all data sets (designated "repeat region," amplicon positions 7686 to 7720). Changes from the reference sequence were designated variants, and the variant read percentage is the NGS-determined allele frequency. The previously developed subtractive correction method of variant detection was applied wherein the control's variant read percentages (at every position and possible variant change) are subtracted from the pooled data's variant read percentages, to yield a pooled data set without background sequencing error [17, 18].

2.4. Variant Validation. A subset of the NGS-detected *RET* sequence variants were validated by either high-resolution melting analysis (HRM) and/or Sanger sequencing. The HRM analysis PCR primers for *RET* exons 13 and 15 were described previously [21]. *RET* intron 9 used HRM analysis primers (5′ to 3′): forward ACA CTG CAA TGT GCG GGT CA and reverse GTC CCC CAA CAA TGC TGC CC.

TABLE 1: Variants detected in the pooled data sets and their NGS percent variant read values[a].

RET amplicon position	Chr 10 positions	RET gene location	Genotype	dbSNP	dbSNP allele frequency	Found only in which pool	Ethnic % variant reads	Caucasian combined pop freq	P1 % variant reads	P2 % variant reads	P3 % variant reads	P4 % variant reads	Control % variant reads
117	43,608,807	Intron 9	c.1760−197G>T	112675631	8.0%		6.20%	6.19%	5.62%	8.05%	7.77%	2.90%	0.00%
156	43,608,846	Intron 9	c.1760−158C>G	Novel		Caucasian	0.01%	0.88%	0.01%	1.12%	0.00%	1.49%	0.00%
174	43,608,864	Intron 9	c.1760−140C>G	3026758		Ethnic	6.66%	0.00%	0.00%	0.00%	0.00%	0.00%	0.00%
819	43,609,509	Intron 10	c.1880−419G>A	Novel		Caucasian	0.05%	0.44%	0.06%	1.85%	0.05%	0.05%	0.06%
1429	43,610,119	exon 11	c.2071G>A	1799939	14.7%		12.79%	18.14%	15.00%	15.33%	17.30%	24.78%	0.07%
1645	43,610,335	Intron 11	c.2136+151G>A	Novel		Caucasian	0.10%	0.44%	1.92%	0.10%	0.10%	0.10%	0.12%
1676	43,610,366	Intron 11	c.2136+182G>A	1864400	75.2%		68.62%	75.66%	79.53%	76.35%	68.79%	79.64%	0.02%
1765	43,610,455	Intron 11	c.2136+271T>C	1864399	73.2%		63.96%	69.47%	72.74%	67.72%	62.75%	75.90%	0.10%
1766	43,610,456	Intron 11	c.2136+272G>A	Novel		Caucasian	0.03%	0.44%	1.79%	0.04%	0.03%	0.03%	0.02%
1868	43,610,558	Intron 11	c.2136+374C>T	2742233	72.3%		61.79%	69.47%	73.34%	67.78%	61.11%	76.34%	0.07%
1931	43,610,621	Intron 11	c.2136+437T>C	Novel		Caucasian	0.16%	0.44%	0.15%	0.14%	2.15%	0.17%	0.13%
1981	43,610,671	Intron 11	c.2136+487G>T	3026762	6.2%		6.09%	9.29%	8.80%	3.32%	10.17%	13.42%	0.01%
2003	43,610,693	Intron 11	c.2136+509G>T	Novel		Caucasian	0.01%	0.44%	1.75%	0.00%	0.01%	0.01%	0.00%
2096	43,610,786	Intron 11	c.2136+602T>C	Novel		Caucasian	0.08%	0.88%	1.59%	1.61%	0.06%	0.07%	0.06%
2207	43,610,897	Intron 11	c.2136+713C>T	Novel		Caucasian	0.04%	0.44%	0.04%	1.84%	0.03%	0.03%	0.03%
2598	43,611,288	Intron 11	c.2137−744A>G	50 pool		Caucasian	0.23%	1.33%	1.94%	1.89%	0.22%	1.68%	0.24%
2618	43,611,308	Intron 11	c.2137−724G>A	Novel		Caucasian	0.07%	0.44%	1.92%	0.06%	0.07%	0.06%	0.05%
2958	43,611,648	Intron 11	c.2137−384C>T	50 pool			1.92%	0.44%	0.08%	1.69%	0.09%	0.09%	0.12%
3018	43,611,708	Intron 11	c.2137−324A>G	741968	76.0%		68.18%	76.11%	78.72%	76.37%	68.79%	81.20%	0.04%
3089	43,611,779	Intron 11	c.2137−253C>T	74135468	6.9%	Ethnic	1.54%	0.00%	0.03%	0.03%	0.04%	0.04%	0.04%
3175	43,611,865	Intron 11	c.2137−167T>C	2256550	47.2%		46.33%	45.58%	51.81%	45.88%	39.24%	45.15%	0.22%
3535	43,612,225	Intron 12	c.2284+46G>C	Novel		Ethnic	1.85%	0.00%	0.00%	0.00%	0.00%	0.01%	0.00%
3536	43,612,226	Intron 12	c.2284+47C>T	760466	14.5%		10.07%	17.26%	18.80%	15.39%	14.88%	20.45%	0.05%
3919	43,612,609	Intron 12	c.2284+430C>T	2742234	70.1%		62.23%	69.91%	73.95%	68.56%	60.98%	76.51%	0.04%
4382	43,613,072	Intron 12	c.2285−749C>T	3026765	2.2%	Caucasian	0.04%	4.87%	5.61%	6.82%	3.42%	3.62%	0.05%
4418	43,613,108	Intron 12	c.2285−713G>A	79045327	0.4%		1.97%	0.44%	0.06%	1.71%	0.06%	0.05%	0.07%
4503	43,613,193	Intron 12	c.2285−628T>C	Novel		Caucasian	0.23%	0.44%	1.99%	0.23%	0.23%	0.24%	0.25%
4710	43,613,400	Intron 12	c.2285−421G>A	114921735	2.9%	Ethnic	1.86%	0.00%	0.11%	0.08%	0.09%	0.08%	0.11%
4750	43,613,440	Intron 12	c.2285−381G>A	Novel		Ethnic	2.15%	0.00%	0.09%	0.08%	0.07%	0.09%	0.10%
5153	43,613,843	Exon 13	c.2307G>T	1800861	72.3%		62.24%	70.35%	74.10%	68.58%	61.27%	76.98%	0.01%
5397	43,614,087	Intron 13	c.2392+159G>A	3026767	1.6%	Caucasian	0.03%	3.54%	3.37%	1.71%	4.93%	3.68%	0.02%
5540	43,614,230	Intron 13	c.2392+302G>A	2075910	72.2%		62.45%	70.35%	74.57%	68.59%	61.28%	76.56%	0.04%
5630	43,614,320	Intron 13	c.2392+392G>A	Novel		Caucasian	0.04%	0.44%	0.03%	0.03%	0.02%	1.60%	0.03%

TABLE 1: Continued.

RET amplicon position	Chr 10 positions	RET gene location	Genotype	dbSNP	dbSNP allele frequency	Found only in which pool	Ethnic % variant reads	Caucasian combined pop freq	P1 % variant reads	P2 % variant reads	P3 % variant reads	P4 % variant reads	Control % variant reads
5752	43,614,442	Intron 13	c.2392+514G>A	50 pool		Caucasian	0.06%	0.88%	0.06%	1.76%	1.93%	0.06%	0.07%
5770	43,614,460	Intron 13	c.2393–519G>A	2075911	14.7%		12.43%	18.14%	14.55%	14.88%	17.04%	24.21%	0.04%
5820	43,614,510	Intron 13	c.2393–469C>A	Novel		Caucasian	0.02%	0.44%	1.82%	0.01%	0.01%	0.01%	0.01%
6004	43,614,694	Intron 13	c.2393–285G>A	78453984	5.4%	Caucasian	0.03%	0.44%	0.03%	0.02%	0.03%	1.52%	0.03%
6195	43,614,885	Intron 13	c.2393–94C>T	111264957	4.2%		5.77%	6.19%	5.22%	7.80%	7.37%	3.01%	0.09%
6221	43,614,911	Intron 13	c.2393–68A>G	Novel		Ethnic	2.19%	0.00%	0.18%	0.15%	0.15%	0.15%	0.12%
6404	43,615,094	exon 14	c.2508C>T	1800862	4.1%		5.86%	5.75%	5.13%	7.67%	7.39%	2.98%	0.04%
6639	43,615,329	Intron 14	c.2607+136A>G	50 pool			2.06%	0.44%	0.16%	1.90%	0.15%	0.17%	0.14%
6692	43,615,382	Intron 14	c.2608–147C>T	11238441	14.8%		12.78%	18.58%	14.55%	15.09%	17.30%	25.23%	0.06%
6696	43,615,386	Intron 14	c.2608–143C>G	Novel		Ethnic	1.90%	0.00%	0.00%	0.00%	0.00%	0.00%	0.00%
6715	43,615,405	Intron 14	c.2608–124G>A	111306965	8.9%	Ethnic	1.93%	0.00%	0.04%	0.06%	0.04%	0.05%	0.06%
6815	43,615,505	Intron 14	c.2608–24G>A	2472737	16.0%		19.84%	17.26%	21.52%	18.75%	14.39%	13.81%	0.04%
6943	43,615,633	Exon 15	c.2712C>G	1800863	14.9%		11.74%	16.37%	13.17%	13.92%	16.24%	22.34%	0.00%
7190	43,615,880	Intron 15	c.2730+229T>C	3026768	5.1%		6.07%	6.64%	5.40%	8.07%	7.75%	4.57%	0.21%
7218	43,615,908	Intron 15	c.2730+257C>T	2435353	14.4%		19.91%	17.26%	21.81%	18.89%	14.51%	14.19%	0.08%
7283	43,615,973	Intron 15	c.2730+322C>T	3026769	4.3%		1.79%	1.33%	0.07%	1.66%	1.68%	1.37%	0.06%
7392	43,616,082	Intron 15	c.2730+431G>A	Novel		Ethnic	1.93%	0.00%	0.17%	0.13%	0.17%	0.17%	0.18%
7491	43,616,181	Intron 15	c.2730+530A>G	79094522	11.1%	Caucasian	0.21%	0.44%	0.25%	0.23%	0.20%	1.66%	0.22%
7635	43,616,325	Intron 15	c.2730+674A>G	2742235	76.0%		68.78%	76.99%	79.66%	77.02%	71.18%	79.24%	0.18%
7844	43,616,534	Intron 15	c.2731–860G>A	Novel		Ethnic	1.94%	0.00%	0.02%	0.03%	0.02%	0.03%	0.02%
8061	43,616,751	Intron 15	c.2731–643C>A	715106	76.7%		68.41%	77.43%	79.60%	77.02%	70.90%	80.13%	0.01%
8179	43,616,869	Intron 15	c.2731–525G>A	Novel		Caucasian	0.04%	0.44%	1.80%	0.03%	0.03%	0.04%	0.03%
8181	43,616,871	Intron 15	c.2731–523T>G	Novel		Caucasian	0.01%	0.88%	0.00%	0.00%	0.01%	0.00%	0.00%
8328	43,617,018	Intron 15	c.2731–376A>G	3026770	1.0%	Caucasian	0.17%	0.88%	0.17%	0.17%	1.81%	1.47%	0.15%
8414	43,617,104	Intron 15	c.2731–290A>G	2565202	47.6%		47.17%	52.21%	58.83%	52.76%	45.68%	50.20%	0.05%
8477	43,617,167	Intron 15	c.2731–227C>G	3026771	4.5%		5.82%	6.19%	5.09%	7.64%	7.36%	4.31%	0.00%
8828	43,617,518	intron 16	c.2801+54A>T	3026772	0.5%	Caucasian	0.01%	0.44%	0.00%	0.00%	0.00%	1.66%	0.00%
9017	43,617,707	intron 16	c.2801+243G>C	3026774	2.1%	Caucasian	0.02%	5.75%	5.21%	6.66%	6.77%	3.63%	0.00%

[a]Table headings. RET amplicon position and Chr 10: amplicon positions 1–9180 correlate to Chr 10 positions 43608691–43617870 in reference sequence NC_000010.10. Genotype: nomenclature (cDNA) for known variants is from the MEN2 RET database—http://www.arup.utah.edu/database/MEN2/MEN2_welcome.php, which uses the Human Genome Variation Society sequence variation nomenclature and RET reference sequence NC_000010.10. dbSNP column lists rs number; "50 pool" (if novel from dbSNP, but was found in 50 pool data set), or "novel" change. Found only in which pool: variation was found only within the ethnic or Caucasian pools. % variant reads: NGS determined variant read percentage for each variant found within each pool. Ethnic: data was from 23 pooled non-Caucasian samples. Caucasian combined pop freq: it combines all the data from the 4 Caucasian pools (P1, P2, P3, and P4), for comparison to the ethnic pool as well as the NCBI dbSNP 132 stated allele frequencies. Control: this single-sample control matched the reference sequence exactly, so no variations were detected and the values in this control column are only background sequencing error rates (0% to 0.25% variant read values).

Sample DNA (~5 to 15 ng/uL final concentration) was amplified and analyzed as described previously [21], except the LightScanner 32 instrument (Idaho Technology, Inc., Salt Lake City, UT) which was used for both PCR and HRM analysis. The LightScanner parameters included Uracil-DNA glycosylase step (50°C for 10 min); polymerase activation (95°C for 10 min); 40 PCR cycles (denaturation at 95°C for 1 s, annealing at 62°C for 1 s, extension at 72°C for 4 s); formation of amplicon heteroduplexes (95°C for 1 s, then cool rapidly to 40°C for 10 s with ramp rate of 20°C/s); high-resolution melting protocol (70 to 96°C with ramp rate of 0.3°C/s) [21]. In order to detect samples with a homozygous *RET* variant that could not be distinguished from homozygous wild-type samples during HRM analysis, the same procedure was performed, except wild-type DNA (~5 ng/uL final concentration) which was spiked into the PCR reaction [22]. If needed, Sanger sequencing was used to confirm HRM determined variant results.

3. Results

3.1. Next-Generation Sequencing (NGS) of the 50-Pool and Single-Sample Controls.
The sequence of the single-sample control used in this study exactly matched the reference sequence and therefore had no true variant changes from the reference sequence, only background sequencing error (Table 1). This sample was an ideal control for error rates since any variant reads from the *RET* reference at each sequence position reflects the background NGS error rates, and also illumina genome analyzer sequencing has demonstrated reproducible, nonuniform, sequence-specific background error rates, read coverage, and base quality scores between lanes and runs using the same version chemistry [11, 12, 17–20, 23, 24]. This single sample controls for the sequence-specific error rates within the pooled data sets by using the subtractive correction method, as described in our previous studies [17, 18]. For subtractive correction, the single-sample control's variant reads at every possible sequence position, and change from the reference sequence is subtracted from the pool's variant read percentages. This yields an estimation of the pooled data without background sequencing error rates contributing to the variant read percentages (examples in Figure 1). The single-sample control and 50-pool data were also used for selection of the 30 Q-threshold used for quality screening of the data before analysis (data not shown) [17, 18].

The 50-pool control demonstrated sensitivity to detect known variants with low read percentages for this NGS run and for using the subtractive correction method (as shown in Figure 1). The 50-pool contained 100 alleles and had an expected 1% singleton variant read frequency (singleton is unique within the pool). All 59 variants previously detected in the 50-pool were present at >0.5% variant reads and at similar percentage variant read values as determined in a previous NGS run with the same library ($R^2 = 0.9991$, Figure 1(a)). The 50-pool data had some potential false positives around the cutoff of 0.5% variant reads but after subtractive correction with the single-sample control

data, and all true variants were readily detected from the background error (Figure 1(b)).

3.2. NGS of MEN2 Unaffected Cohort.
Based on our previous work and other studies, sample pools were restricted to 30 or less samples within each pool to result in a variant read percentage above 1%, the chosen cutoff for the most accurate singleton variant detection [12, 14, 17]. The 113 Caucasian samples were divided into 4 pools with less than 30 samples. Caucasian pool P1 had 27 samples, P2 had 29, P3 had 28, and P4 had 29 samples, with an expected 1.85%, 1.72%, 1.77%, and 1.72% singleton variant read frequency, respectively. All pool data sets were evaluated with and without subtractive correction of sequencing background error rates using the single-sample control (Figure 1(c) and data not shown). A total of 51 variants were detected in the Caucasian MEN2 unaffected cohort with >1% variant read values, of which 23 were not found in the non-Caucasian MEN2 unaffected cohort (ethnic pool) (Table 1). The lowest singleton variant in the Caucasian data sets was in P2 with 1.12% variant read frequency. The 23 non-Caucasian samples were in one pool (ethnic pool), with an expected 2.17% singleton allele read frequency. A total of 38 variants were detected in this ethnically diverse MEN2 unaffected cohort with >1% variant read values, of which 10 were not found in the Caucasian data sets. The lowest singleton variant in the ethnic pool had 1.79% variant read frequency. The variant read percentages for each detected variant is shown in Table 1 per pool and also summarized for the four Caucasian pools. For comparison, the NCBI dbSNP allele frequency values for detected variants are also shown. All variants detected were intronic changes, except the expected common polymorphisms found in exons 11, 13, 14, and 15. Of the total 61 variants found in the MEN2 unaffected cohort, 20 variants were novel changes, not seen in the 50-pool control or in NCBI dbSNP132.

3.3. Validation of NGS-Detected Variations.
Since the 136 unaffected cohort samples had not been sequenced previously by either Sanger or NGS methods, several variant locations within three pools (total of 79 samples) were chosen for validation. The high-resolution melting (HRM) analysis method, which is a rapid, closed-tube mutation scanning assay, was chosen to genotype each individual sample for validation of NGS variant detection and the NGS determined variant allele frequency (Table 2). High-resolution melting analysis detects sequence variation within the PCR amplicon using a saturating dsDNA dye and in many cases can uniquely identify each variant based on differential melting profiles (Figure 2(a)) [25–28]. HRM assay states 100% specificity and sensitivity for detection of heterozygous variants within small amplicons (<300 bp) [29]. HRM analysis was used to detect sequence variations within a section of *RET* intron 9 and exons 13 and 15 (Figure 2 and data not shown). *RET* exons 13 and 15 were chosen since they each contain a common polymorphism present in all pools that could be detected using the previously developed HRM

(a)

(b)

(c)

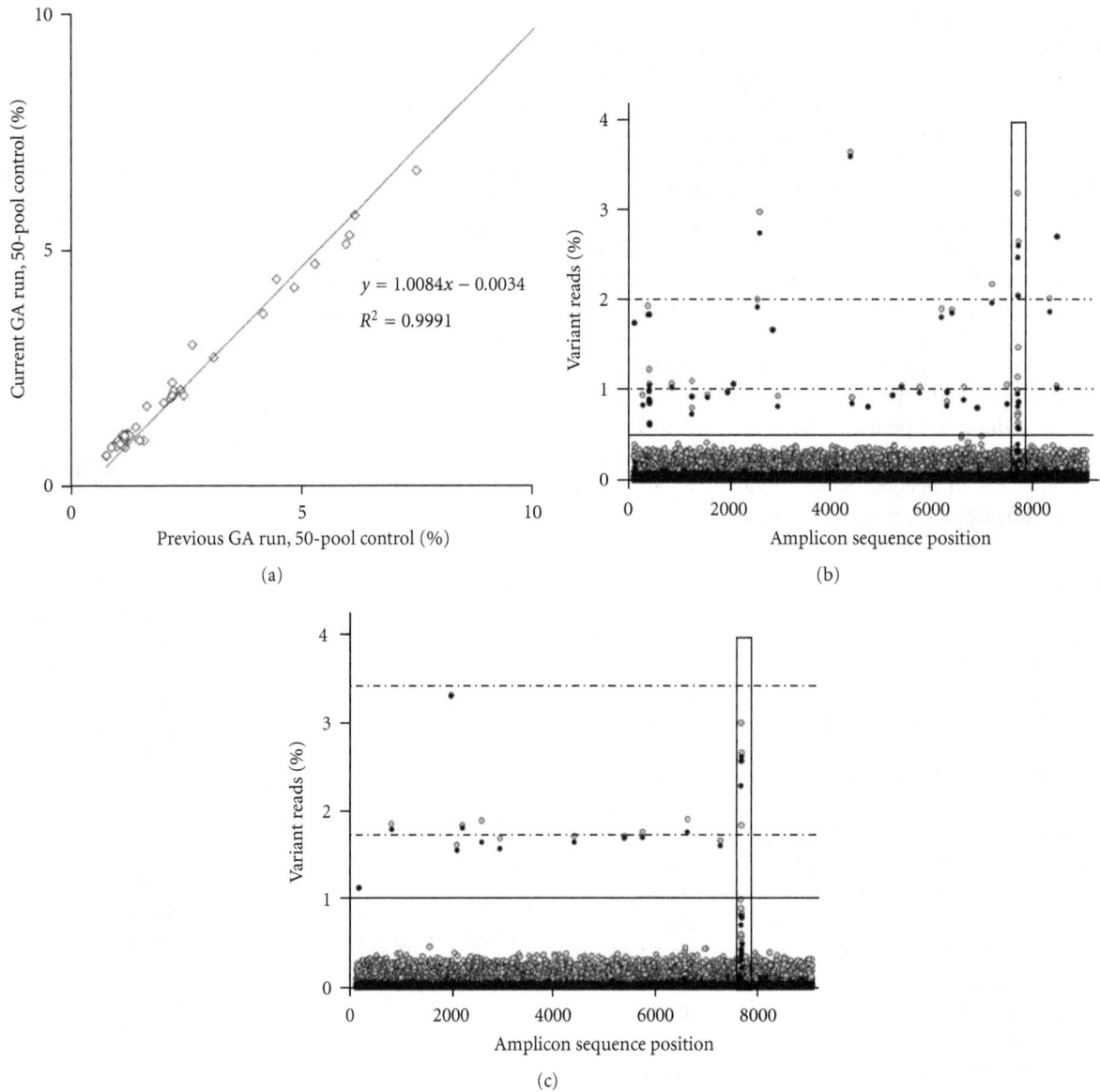

FIGURE 1: Variant identification in the 50-pool control and Caucasian P2 pool. (a) Variant read percentages for variants detected in the 50-pool control below 10% variant reads are shown. The variants detected in the 50-pool data for the current NGS run (Y-axis) is compared to the same library sequenced previously in a different NGS run (X-axis) with trendline and R^2 value shown on chart. (b and c) Variant read percentages for the pool data (gray circles) and the variant read percentages for the pool data after the subtractive correction with the single-sample control data (black circles) are shown together in each panel. The "repeat region" is boxed in black line. (b) 50-pool control data. Variant detection read cutoff value of 0.5% is the solid horizontal black line. The horizontal dotted lines mark the singleton and doubleton alleles' expected variant read percentages of 1% and 2%, respectively. (c) Caucasian pool P2 data. Variant detection read cutoff value of 1% is the solid horizontal black line. The horizontal dotted lines mark the singleton and doubleton alleles' expected variant read percentages of 1.7% and 3.4%, respectively.

assay [21]. Exon 13 contains c.2307G>T variant and exon 15 contains c.2712C>G variant (RET amplicon positions 5153 and 6943, respectively, Tables 1 and 2). Intron 9 was chosen since it contains three NGS-detected variants in close proximity at RET amplicon positions 117, 156, and 174 (c.1760−197G>T, c.1760−158C>G, and c.1760−140C>G, resp.), and also to verify the novel c.1760−158C>G variant detected in Caucasian pool P2 which had the lowest variant read percentage of 1.12% (expected 1.72% singleton read

frequency within that pool of 29 samples). Since some homozygous variants can have similar melting profiles as the wild-type sample [22], a technique that spikes wild-type DNA into the PCR reaction to allow distinction of homozygous variants was performed on any sample that appeared wild-type after testing in the first HRM assay. This technique identified four homozygous variants in RET exon 15 and one homozygous variant in RET intron 9 (Figure 2(b) and data not shown). The HRM determined allele frequency

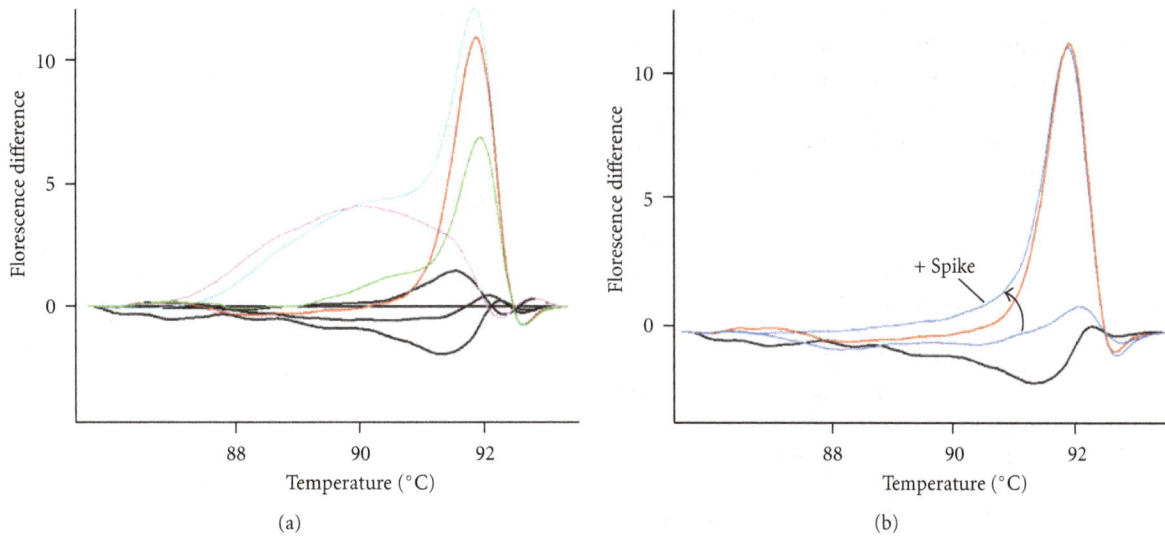

(a)   (b)

FIGURE 2: Variant validation within *RET* intron 9 by high-resolution melting analysis. The fluorescence difference plot (fluorescence difference versus temperature) of the melting curve data is shown in each panel. (a) *RET* intron 9. The black lines are samples of homozygous wild-type sequence. Data from four samples with unique variants within intron 9 are shown: heterozygous at amplicon position 156 (green trace, c.1760−158C>G), heterozygous at 174 (red trace, c.1760−140C>G), heterozygous at 117 (pink trace, c.1760−197G>T), and a sample heterozygous at both positions 117 and 174 (light blue). (b) Intron 9 with wild-type DNA spiked into the PCR reaction to help differentiate homozygous variants. One sample with a homozygous variant at position 174 with ("+spike") and without wild-type DNA spiked in is shown (blue traces) compared to a 174 heterozygous (red trace) and wild-type sample (black trace).

TABLE 2: Validation of several variants and comparison of NGS and HRM determined variant allele frequencies.

Pool	No. of samples[a]	117[b] in intron 9		156 in intron 9		174 in intron 9		5153 in exon 13		6943 in exon 15	
		NGS[c]	HRM[c]	NGS	HRM	NGS	HRM	NGS	HRM	NGS	HRM
Ethnic	23	6.2%	6.5%	0.01%	0.00%	6.7%	8.7%	62%	63%	12%	13%
P1	27	5.6%	5.6%	0.01%	0.00%	0.0%	0.0%	74%	74%	13%	19%
P2	29	8.1%	8.6%	1.12%[d]	1.70%	0.0%	0.0%	69%	72%	14%	16%

[a] A total of 79 samples were individually tested for variants by HRM analysis for three regions of the *RET* gene (which analyzed the 5 NGS-detected variant positions shown in this table).
[b] *RET* amplicon position shown, see Table 1 for more information on each variant change.
[c] NGS: illumina genome analyzer determined allele frequency (variant read percentage) from a pooled sample set. HRM: high-resolution melting analysis determined allele frequency, where each individual in the pool was tested separately for variation.
[d] Lowest NGS variant read percentage for all pools. This suspected variant was verified as a singleton allele within Caucasian pool P2 by HRM and Sanger sequencing.

correlated well with the NGS variant read percentage for each variant in each pool (Table 2). The variant with the lowest read percentage (position 156 in P2, 1.12%) was verified as present and heterozygous in one sample within Caucasian pool P2.

4. Discussion

This paper describes *RET* proto-oncogene sequence variation detected in an MEN2 unaffected cohort of 136 individuals. The previous genome analyzer sequenced 50-pool library [17, 18] was used to control for the detection of variations with low read frequency, and all known variants were detected >0.5% variant reads. With similar error rates between genome analyzer lanes of the same run [11, 12, 17, 19, 20, 23, 24], the singleton variants in a less than or equal to 30-sample pool should be accurately detected above

background error using our previously determined cutoff value of >1% variant read frequency. The single sample controlled for background sequencing error rates across each *RET* sequence position and was used for the subtractive correction method of variant detection for pools [17, 18].

The majority of the MEN2 unaffected cohort were of Caucasian ethnicity, while 23 samples were non-Caucasian (ethnic pool) and were used to identify *RET* variants within a more ethnically diverse sample set. The 136 samples were distributed into five nonindexed pools and were sequenced in five separate flow cell lanes. Using previously described protocols for bioinformatics, subtractive correction, and variant read cutoff value of >1% [17, 18], a total of 61 *RET* variants were detected within the MEN2 unaffected cohort. Twenty of these variants were novel, not in NCBI dbSNP 132 (which includes 1000 Genome data) or found in our previous sample pooling studies on the *RET* proto oncogene

[17, 18]. Many of these novel changes were specific to either the Caucasian or ethnic samples and were of low variant read frequency, so they were likely to be singleton or doubleton variants within the pools. Several variants were verified by HRM and Sanger sequencing, including the novel change (c.1760−158C>G) with the lowest variant read percentage (1.12%).

The *RET* MEN2 database developed by the author so far has 147 entries, of which 74 are known pathogenic mutations and 62 are variants of uncertain significance. This database has been used as a model for predictions of phenotypic severity of variants of unknown clinical significance within the *RET* proto oncogene [30]. *RET* sequence variation data for these MEN2 unaffected cohorts will be added to the MEN2 *RET* database [8]. This variant data will help in medical interpretation of variations found in this *RET* proto-oncogene region using methods such as Sanger sequencing or NGS (targeted to the *RET* gene, the whole exome, or whole genome sequencing). Any *RET* sequence change detected in individuals with a family history of MEN2 symptoms or where MEN2 is suspected (patient with apparent sporadic MTC or Pheochromocytoma) can be compared to the available *RET* MEN2 database, and also to the benign *RET* sequence variation present in the large cohort of unaffected individuals that was generated in this paper. This highlights the importance of clinically relevant databases with not only known pathogenic changes, but also the inclusion of known benign changes for clinical test interpretation. The MEN2 unaffected cohort's variant results can also be used in comparison to variants detected in suspected MEN2 patients for case reports. A potential problem for genetic test design is unknown variants present in the location of the PCR primers, Sanger sequencing primers, or melting analysis probes. Results from this unaffected population will help with genetic test design, so that primers, and probes will not be designed over the known *RET* sequence changes.

This paper presents sequence variation detection methods that could be used for other genes and analysis for specific cohorts (unaffected versus affected, by different ethnicities, or those with specific symptoms of disease). The resulting data can be added to locus-specific databases to help interpret the pathogenicity of clinically detected sequence variation. These validated methods can also apply to other pooled samples (such as genetic locations for GWAS followup or for testing-specific populations) and natural pools (such as mitochondrial heteroplasmy or mixed tumor populations).

Abbreviations

MEN2:	Multiple endocrine neoplasia type 2
RET:	REarranged during transfection
MTC:	Medullary thyroid carcinoma
FMTC:	Familial medullary thyroid carcinoma
PCR:	Polymerase chain reaction
Q-threshold:	Base quality score screening threshold
NGS:	Next generation sequencing.

Acknowledgments

The authors thank Brian Dalley and David Nix of the Huntsman Cancer Institute for running our sample libraries on the illumina genome analyzer.

References

[1] R. T. Kloos, C. Eng, D. B. Evans et al., "Medullary thyroid cancer: management guidelines of the American thyroid association," *Thyroid*, vol. 19, no. 6, pp. 565–612, 2009.

[2] M. A. Kouvaraki, S. E. Shapiro, N. D. Perrier et al., "RET proto-oncogene: a review and update of genotype-phenotype correlations in hereditary medullary thyroid cancer and associated endocrine tumors," *Thyroid*, vol. 15, no. 6, pp. 531–544, 2005.

[3] C. Eng, D. Clayton, I. Schuffenecker et al., "The relationship between specific ret proto-oncogene mutations and disease phenotype in multiple endocrine neoplasia type 2: international RET mutation consortium analysis," *Journal of the American Medical Association*, vol. 276, no. 19, pp. 1575–1579, 1996.

[4] J. W. de Groot, T. P. Links, J. T. Plukker, C. J. Lips, and R. M. Hofstra, "RET as a diagnostic and therapeutic target in sporadic and hereditary endocrine tumors," *Endocrine Reviews*, vol. 27, no. 5, pp. 535–560, 2006.

[5] P. J. Morrison and N. C. Nevin, "Multiple endocrine neoplasia type 2B (mucosal neuroma syndrome, Wagenmann-Froboese syndrome)," *Journal of Medical Genetics*, vol. 33, no. 9, pp. 779–782, 1996.

[6] G. Wiesner and K. Snow-Bailey, "GeneReviews: Multiple Endocrine Neoplasia Type 2," 2005, http://www.geneclinics.org/servlet/access?db=geneclinics&site=gt&id=8888892&key=2paoNNdpDmi-r&gry=&fcn=y&fw=ZVFB&filename=/profiles/men2/indexhtml.

[7] C. J. Wray, T. A. Rich, S. G. Waguespack, J. E. Lee, N. D. Perrier, and D. B. Evans, "Failure to recognize multiple endocrine neoplasia 2B: more common than we think?" *Annals of Surgical Oncology*, vol. 15, no. 1, pp. 293–301, 2008.

[8] R. L. Margraf, D. K. Crockett, P. M. Krautscheid et al., "Multiple endocrine neoplasia type 2 RET protooncogene database: repository of MEN2-associated RET sequence variation and reference for genotype/phenotype correlations," *Human Mutation*, vol. 30, no. 4, pp. 548–556, 2009.

[9] C. Eng, D. Clayton, I. Schuffenecker et al., "The relationship between specific ret proto-oncogene mutations and disease phenotype in multiple endocrine neoplasia type 2: international RET mutation consortium analysis," *Journal of the American Medical Association*, vol. 276, no. 19, pp. 1575–1579, 1996.

[10] A. Z. Lai, T. S. Gujral, L. M. Mulligan et al., "RET signaling in endocrine tumors: delving deeper into molecular mechanisms," *Endocrine Pathology*, vol. 18, no. 2, pp. 57–67, 2007.

[11] V. Bansal, O. Harismendy, R. Tewhey et al., "Accurate detection and genotyping of SNPs utilizing population sequencing data," *Genome Research*, vol. 20, no. 4, pp. 537–545, 2010.

[12] T. E. Druley, F. L. Vallania, D. J. Wegner et al., "Quantification of rare allelic variants from pooled genomic DNA," *Nature Methods*, vol. 6, no. 4, pp. 263–265, 2009.

[13] D. C. Koboldt, K. Chen, T. Wylie et al., "VarScan: variant detection in massively parallel sequencing of individual and pooled samples," *Bioinformatics*, vol. 25, no. 17, pp. 2283–2285, 2009.

[14] A. A. Out, I. J. van Minderhout, J. J. Goeman et al., "Deep sequencing to reveal new variants in pooled DNA samples," *Human Mutation*, vol. 30, no. 12, pp. 1703–1712, 2009.

[15] S. E. Calvo, E. J. Tucker, A. G. Compton et al., "High-throughput, pooled sequencing identifies mutations in NUBPL and FOXRED1 in human complex i deficiency," *Nature Genetics*, vol. 42, no. 10, pp. 851–858, 2010.

[16] V. Bansal, "A statistical method for the detection of variants from next-generation resequencing of DNA pools," *Bioinformatics*, vol. 26, no. 12, pp. i318–i324, 2010.

[17] R. L. Margraf, J. D. Durtschi, S. Dames et al., "Multi-sample pooling and illumina genome analyzer sequencing methods to determine gene sequence variation for database development," *Journal of Biomolecular Techniques*, vol. 21, no. 3, pp. 126–140, 2010.

[18] R. L. Margraf, J. D. Durtschi, S. Dames, D. C. Pattison, J. E. Stephens, and K. V. Voelkerding, "Variant identification in multi-sample pools by illumina genome analyzer sequencing," *Journal of Biomolecular Techniques*, vol. 22, no. 2, pp. 74–84, 2011.

[19] J. C. Dohm, C. Lottaz, T. Borodina, and H. Himmelbauer, "Substantial biases in ultra-short read data sets from high-throughput DNA sequencing," *Nucleic Acids Research*, vol. 36, no. 16, article e105, 2008.

[20] R. Li, Y. Li, X. Fang et al., "SNP detection for massively parallel whole-genome resequencing," *Genome Research*, vol. 19, no. 6, pp. 1124–1132, 2009.

[21] R. L. Margraf, R. Mao, W. E. Highsmith, L. M. Holtegaard, and C. T. Wittwer, "Mutation scanning of the RET protooncogene using high-resolution melting analysis," *Clinical Chemistry*, vol. 52, no. 1, pp. 138–141, 2006.

[22] R. A. Palais, M. A. Liew, and C. T. Wittwer, "Quantitative heteroduplex analysis for single nucleotide polymorphism genotyping," *Analytical Biochemistry*, vol. 346, no. 1, pp. 167–175, 2005.

[23] D. W. Craig, J. V. Pearson, S. Szelinger et al., "Identification of genetic variants using bar-coded multiplexed sequencing," *Nature Methods*, vol. 5, no. 10, pp. 887–893, 2008.

[24] O. Harismendy, P. C. Ng, R. L. Strausberg et al., "Evaluation of next generation sequencing platforms for population targeted sequencing studies," *Genome Biology*, vol. 10, no. 3, article R32, 2009.

[25] C. T. Wittwer, G. H. Reed, C. N. Gundry, J. G. Vandersteen, and R. J. Pryor, "High-resolution genotyping by amplicon melting analysis using LCGreen," *Clinical Chemistry*, vol. 49, no. 6, part 1, pp. 853–860, 2003.

[26] M. Liew, R. Pryor, R. Palais et al., "Genotyping of single-nucleotide polymorphisms by high-resolution melting of small amplicons," *Clinical Chemistry*, vol. 50, no. 7, pp. 1156–1164, 2004.

[27] S. F. Dobrowolski, J. T. McKinney, C. A. di San Filippo, G. S. Keow, B. Wilcken, and N. Longo, "Validation of dye-binding/high-resolution thermal denaturation for the identification of mutations in the *SLC22A5* gene," *Human Mutation*, vol. 25, no. 3, pp. 306–313, 2005.

[28] C. Willmore, J. A. Holden, L. Zhou, S. Tripp, C. T. Wittwer, and L. J. Layfield, "Detection of c-kit-activating mutations in gastrointestinal stromal tumors by high-resolution amplicon melting analysis," *American Journal of Clinical Pathology*, vol. 122, no. 2, pp. 206–216, 2004.

[29] G. H. Reed and C. T. Wittwer, "Sensitivity and specificity of single-nucleotide polymorphism scanning by high-resolution melting analysis," *Clinical Chemistry*, vol. 50, no. 10, pp. 1748–1754, 2004.

[30] D. K. Crockett, S. R. Piccolo, P. G. Ridge et al., "Predicting phenotypic severity of uncertain gene variants in the RET proto-oncogene," *Plos ONE*, vol. 6, no. 3, 2011.

9

Iodine Status Has No Impact on Thyroid Function in Early Healthy Pregnancy

F. Brucker-Davis,[1] **P. Ferrari,**[2] **J. Gal,**[3] **F. Berthier,**[3] **P. Fenichel,**[1] **and S. Hieronimus**[1]

[1] Department of Endocrinology, Diabetology and Reproductive Medicine, l'Archet Hospital, CHU de Nice,
  151 route de Saint-Antoine, 06200 Nice, France
[2] Department of Biochemistry, CHU de Nice, 151 route de Saint-Antoine, 06200 Nice, France
[3] Department of Biostatistics, CHU de Nice, 151 route de Saint-Antoine, 06200 Nice, France

Correspondence should be addressed to F. Brucker-Davis, brucker-davis.f@chu-nice.fr

Academic Editor: Noriyuki Koibuchi

Aim. To assess the impact of iodine status in early pregnancy on thyroid function. *Methods*. Women >18 years old seen at their first prenatal consult before 12 weeks of amenorrhea and without personal thyroid history were proposed thyroid screening and were eligible if they had strictly normal thyroid tests (fT4 > 10th percentile, TSH < 2.5 mUI/L, negative anti-TPO antibodies). Evaluation included thyroid ultrasound, extensive thyroid tests, and ioduria (UIE). *Results*. 110 women (27.5 y, 8 weeks of amenorrhea, smoking status: 28% current smokers) were enrolled. Results are expressed as medians. UIE was 116 μg/L. 66.3% of women had iodine deficiency (ID) defined as UIE < 150. FT4 was 14.35 pmol/L; TSH 1.18 mUI/L; fT3 5 pmol/L; thyroglobulin 17.4 ng/mL; rT3 0.27 ng/mL; thyroid volume: 9.4 ml. UIE did not correlate with any thyroid tests, but correlated negatively with thyroid volume. UIE and all thyroid tests, except fT3, correlated strongly with βhCG. Smoking correlated with higher thyroid volume and thyroglobulin and with lower rT3. *Conclusions*. In pregnant women selected for normal thyroid function, mild ID is present in 66% during the 1st trimester. The absence of correlation between UIE and thyroid tests at that stage contrasts with the impact of βhCG and, to a lesser degree, maternal smoking.

1. Introduction

Mild iodine deficiency (ID) is still common in western Europe, despite government programs aiming at its eradication, usually based on salt iodination. Diagnosis of ID still rests on spot ioduria (UIE) at the population level, though this tool is imperfect [1]. We have previously shown in a cross-sectional study that the prevalence of ID in pregnant women of our area was present during the 3d trimester in more than three-quarter of cases [2].

While severe ID is associated with dramatic impairment of neurocognitive development of the offspring, the deleterious developmental impact of mild to moderate ID is less documented [3, 4]. It could be mediated by fetal ID per se or via maternal hypothyroxinemia or hypothyroidism that may develop in predisposed women during pregnancy [5–7]. The changes of thyroid economy throughout pregnancy include a drop in fT4 after an early phase of thyroid stimulation

[8]. However, the definition of maternal hypothyroxinemia is debated [5, 9]. The benefit of iodine supplementation is documented for women selected for thyroid hyperstimulation in early pregnancy and their offspring, based on fetal thyroglobulin (Tg) [10], or in case of severe to moderate ID based on neurodevelopmental evaluation [3, 11, 12]. However, there is no definitive evidence of a benefit both in terms of maternal thyroid function and of neurocognitive development of her offspring in healthy pregnant women with normal thyroid function at the beginning of pregnancy [13].

We report here results assessing the impact of iodine status on thyroid function during the first trimester of pregnancy in healthy women.

2. Patients and Methods

2.1. Patients. In order to select pregnant women with normal thyroid tests, we proposed a thyroid screen to all women who age > 18 years, without personal history of thyroid disease consulting at the obstetric clinic of our hospital before 12 weeks of amenorrhea (WA) with a singleton pregnancy between July 2007 and July 2008. The screening evaluation included free T4, TSH, and antithyroperoxidase (TPO) antibodies. For this study, we specifically recruited women who were not taking iodine supplementation. A spot urine sample was also collected to allow UIE measurement in case of participation to the study. We included 110 TPO-negative women with strict criteria of normal thyroid tests who agreed to participate and signed a consent form. Ranges for normal thyroid tests in our laboratory for the first trimester are (2.5–97.5 percentile of TPO negative women) fT4: 11.47–19.3 pmol/L; TSH: 0.053–3.23 mUL/L. We selected women with fT4 > 10th percentile (12 pmol/L) and TSH < 2.5 mUL/mL, as that threshold is currently recommended for pregnant women [14].

Maternal smoking was assessed qualitatively by self-reported statement: never smoked, current smokers, and former smokers (regroup women who quit smoking before pregnancy or when diagnosed as pregnant).

Thyroid ultrasound was performed by two of us (F. Barker Davis and S. Hieronimus) who concerted and agreed before the study about thyroid volume measurement criteria using an En Visor scanner (Philips Medical System) equipped with a commercially available from 5 to 12 MHz linear transducer (50 mm length). Volume was calculated in mL for each lobe according to the formula $0.52 \times$ height $\times$ width $\times$ thickness in centimeters. Total thyroid volume was the sum of each lobe's volume, the isthmus was not taken into account in volume calculation.

2.2. Assays. Spot UIE was measured by mass spectrometry ICP/MS (Pasteur-Cerba Laboratory, Cergy Pontoise, France, detection threshold 15 μg/L; intra- and interseries CV < 10%). Free T4 (fT4), free T3 (fT3), total T4 (TT4), TSH, βhCG, and anti-TPO and anti-Tg antibodies were measured by chemiluminescence (ADVIA Centaur, Siemens Healthcare Diagnostics, France). Tg was measured by immunoradiometric assay (Thyroglobulin IRMA, Cis bio International, Gif sur Yvette, France). Thyroxin binding globulin (TBG) and reverse T3 (rT3) were measured by radio-immunoassay (RIA): RIA-gnost TBG (Cis bio International, Gif sur Yvette, France) and RIA rT3 (Pasteur Cerba Laboratory, Cergy Pontoise, France). Reference ranges outside pregnancy, intra- and intercoefficients of variation were as the following: fT4 9–23 pmol/L (intra-assay coefficient of variation (CV) 2.31%; interassay CV 1.95%); fT3 3–7 pmol/L (intra-assay CV 2.35); TT4 during pregnancy 82.6–138 nmol/L (intra-assay CV 1.77%; interassay CV 2.9%); TSH 0.1–4 mUI/L (intra-assay CV 2.67%; interassay CV 3.97%); βhCG < 10 UI/L (intra-assay CV 2.8%; interassay CV 4.3%); TPO antibodies < 100 UI/mL (intra-assay CV 4.1%, interassay CV 8.0%); Tg antibodies < 60 UI/mL (intra-assay CV 5.5%; interassay CV 1.8%); Tg 5–50 ng/mL (intra-assay CV 2.4%; interassay CV 4.5%); rT3 0.14–0.54 nmol/L (intra-assay CV 8.54% interassay CV 6.21%); reference range for TBG for the first trimester 20.5 ± 4.8 μg/mL (interassay CV 4.4%).

2.3. Statistics. Quantitative variables are expressed as means and standard deviation, medians, and range. Qualitative variables are expressed as counts and percentages. Student's *t* test or Mann-Whitney's *U* test were used to compare continuous variables. Chi-2 test or Fisher's exact test were used for categorical variables. The correlations between variables were determined using the Pearson's test or Spearman's rank test. The nonparametric Kruskal-Wallis test was used to examine associations between maternal smoking and thyroid function tests.

Statistical analyses were performed using the software SAS version 9.1. Values were considered significant when $P < 0.05$. All tests were two-sided.

3. Results

3.1. Clinical Characteristics of the 110 Included Women. Their median age was 27.5 y (18–40), their body mass index (BMI) was 22.4 (16–45.3), with a weight at inclusion of 61.5 kg (43–128 kg), and they were nulliparous in 44.5%. 53% had never smoked, 18% were former smokers, and 28% were current smokers. 15% had a family history of thyroid disease; 82% were born in France (including 56% in our area). Thyroid ultrasound allowed the detection of 16 nodules (14.6%), including six women with nodules >1 cm. Global thyroid volume was 9.4 mL (4.5–17.9 mL); thus, no patient had thyroid hyperplasia or goiter.

3.2. UIE and Thyroid Tests (Table 1). Median ioduria was 116 μg/L. The repartition of the population according to WHO criteria during pregnancy (WHO) for iodine status (15) is shown in Figure 1: 1% (n = 1) with severe ID <20 μg/L; 18% (n = 17) with moderate iodine deficiency, UIE between 20 and 50 μg/L; 47% (n = 45) with mild ID, UIE between 50 and 149 μg/L; 19% (n = 18) with adequate iodine intake, UIE between 150–250 μg/L; 15% (n = 14) with more than adequate iodine intake. With a threshold of UIE at 150 μg/L, 66% of pregnant women seen early were considered iodine deficient. There was no seasonal variation in UIE (data not shown). Women with ID based on UIE < 150 μg/L tended to have higher thyroid volumes (n = 61, median 10 mL) compared to women with UIE between 150 and 250 μg/L (n = 19, median 8.9 mL), while women with UIE > 250 mcg/L had intermediate volume (n = 14, median 9.4 mL).

Table 1 summarizes all thyroid tests. Among those women with normal thyroid tests, seven had a Tg > 50 ng/L (upper limit of normal for nonpregnant women). Those seven women had higher TSH (1.73 versus 1.15 mUI/L, P = 0.04), less homogenous thyroid on ultrasound (four out of seven, versus nine out of 103, P < 0.0001) and were more often smokers (five out of seven, versus 24 out of 103, P = 0.0006). Last, women who later had a miscarriage (n = 7) had lower βhCG (9930 versus 66704 UI/L, P = 0.005) and lower TT4 (94.9 versus 111.6 pmol/L, P = 0.04).

3.3. Correlations (Table 2). UIE did not correlate with any of the thyroid tests. However, it correlated negatively with

TABLE 1: Ioduria and thyroid tests performed at 8 weeks of amenorrhea (5–12) in the 110 included women.

	Median	Mean ± SD	Min	Max
Ioduria μg/L	116	139 ± 98	<15	399
fT4 pmol/L	14.35	14.57 ± 1.65	12.0	19.16
TSH mUI/L	1.18	1.24 ± 0.58	0.13	2.47
fT3 pmol/L	5.0	5.1 ± 0.5	3.8	6.7
TT4 nmol/L	110.7	111.1 ± 23	50.7	167.4
TBG μg/mL	26.7	28.1 ± 7.2	12.8	50
Tg ng/mL	17.4	22.3 ± 17.2	1.3	100
βhCG UI/L	62724	65289 ± 47845	1025	220731
rT3 nmol/L	0.27	0.27 ± 0.07	0.13	0.51

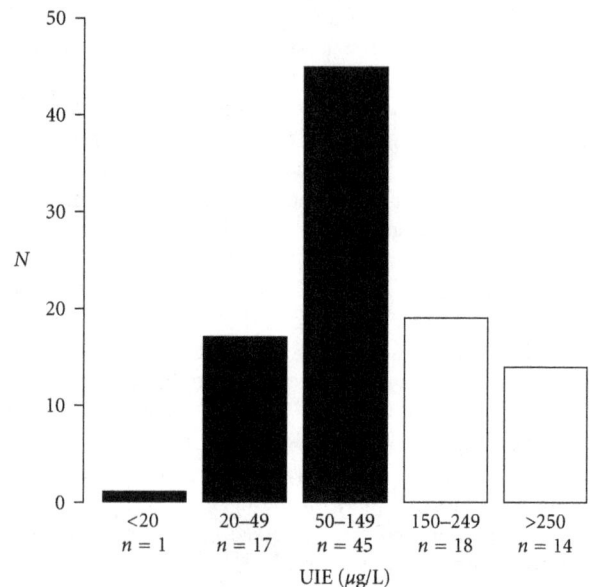

FIGURE 1: Distribution of ioduria (UIE) in healthy euthyroid pregnant women. Solid black histograms represent women (n = 63 of 95) with UIE reflecting ID according to the latest WHO guidelines (UIE < 150 μg/L).

thyroid volume and maternal age, but not with parity nor gravidity. It correlated positively with βHCG.

Thyroid tests correlated strongly with term (data not shown) and even more with βhCG: βhCG correlated negatively with TSH and positively with TT4, rT3, and TBG, and marginally with fT4. Maternal weight tended to correlate negatively with fT4 and positively with TSH. There was no correlation of thyroid volume with thyroid tests, including Tg (data not shown).

Maternal smoking was associated with higher thyroid volume (smokers 10.6 mL versus 9.3 mL in nonsmokers, P = 0.04) and higher Tg (smokers 30.6 versus nonsmokers 14.8 ng/mL, P = 0.0005), and with lower rT3 (smokers 0.2 versus nonsmokers 0.3 nmol/L, P = 0.01).

4. Discussion

We have selected women with strictly normal thyroid function, in choosing stringent criteria (above 10th percentile of our trimester specific reference range for fT4 and <2.5 mUI/L for TSH). There was no goiter nor thyroid hypertrophy as assessed by ultrasound. Thyroid volume in our population was smaller than the volume observed by Glinoer et al. (14.3 mL) in his population with "stimulated" thyroid [10]. The rate of thyroid incidentaloma was similar to the rate observed in the general population [15].

The median UIE in our population with no iodine supplementation was 116 μg/L, which is below the currently recommended threshold in pregnancy (150 μg/L), in the range of mild iodine deficiency [16]. While spot ioduria is useless to establish the diagnosis of ID at an individual level, given its variation from day to day [1], so far it remains the gold standard at the population level [17]. There is a wide range of published UIE values in pregnancy, depending in part on national public health policies to tackle iodine deficiency. Another important variation factor is gestational age, with a steady decline from the first trimester to the end of pregnancy [18]. Indeed, the apparent better iodine status in early pregnancy may be instead due to the increase of glomerular filtration during first trimester causing an increased UIE [19] and, thus, an increased loss of iodine. Two previous studies in France, including one from our Department, have shown lower UIE values at the end of pregnancy: 54 μg/L [20] and 64 μg/L [2]. When focusing on the

first trimester, in other Mediterranean countries, figures were similar or lower in Spain 95 μg/L [21] and 125 μg/L [22], and in Italy (115 in long-term supplementation versus 63 μg/L in short-term supplementation [23]). However, UIE was higher in Switzerland (267 μg/L) where an active program of supplementation exists [24, 25]. On the other hand, in Belgium, UIE was very low (36 μg/L) in a selected population of women with excessive thyroid stimulation [10]. Based on UIE, in our study of selected women with normal thyroid function in early pregnancy, ID was present in 66% of cases, using a threshold of 150 μg/L. This prevalence was similar to those many studies worldwide performed at the same gestational age, except for Brander in Switzerland [24].

UIE did not correlate with any parameters of maternal thyroid function at this stage of pregnancy in our selected healthy population. We had already reported this lack of correlation in our previous study performed during the third trimester [2]. This has also been reported by Fuse et al. [26] in a large population in an area of sufficient iodine intake, though women with excessive intake (UIE > 1 mg/L) had higher TSH [26]. In a population with moderate-to-severe iodine deficiency, it is usually reported a relative hypothyroxinemia, with or without elevation of TSH, particularly in women with predisposition to thyroid disease [8]. On the other hand, Orito et al. had shown in early pregnancy a positive correlation of UIE with TSH and a negative correlation with fT4 and fT3 in an area of excess iodine intake [27]. This suggests a U-shape curve with higher TSH observed in case of iodine deficiency and in areas of iodine excess. To some degree, this is true with thyroid volume as well. UIE in our patients correlated negatively with thyroid volume as measured by ultrasound, the smaller volume of thyroid being noted in women with

TABLE 2: Main significant correlations.

Ioduria			
Negatively	Maternal age	$r = -0.2$	$P = 0.05$
	Thyroid volume	$r = -0.22$	$P = 0.03$
Positively	βHCG	$r = 0.27$	$P < 0.01$
TSH			
Negatively	fT4	$r = -0.27$	$P < 0.005$
	rT3	$r = -0.24$	$P = 0.01$
	βhCG	$r = -0.36$	$P < 0.0001$
Positively	Maternal weight	$r = 0.19$	$P = 0.06$
fT4			
Negatively	Maternal weight	$r = -0.2$	$P = 0.05$
Positively	TT4	$r = 0.44$	$P < 0.0001$
	rT3	$r = 0.44$	$P < 0.0001$
	β hCG	$r = 0.18$	$P = 0.058$
fT3			
Positively	Tg	$r = 0.22$	$P = 0.02$
rT3			
Negatively	Smoking		$P = 0.001$
Positively	βhCG	$r = 0.4$	$P < 0.0001$
	fT4	$r = 0.44$	$P < 0.0001$
	TT4	$r = 0.5$	$P < 0.0001$
	TBG	$r = 0.33$	$P = 0.0005$
Tg			
Positively	fT3	$r = 0.22$	$P = 0.02$
	Smoking		$P = 0.0001$
βhCG			
Negatively	TSH	$r = -0.36$	$P < 0.0001$
Positively	Ioduria	$r = 0.27$	$P < 0.01$
	TT4	$r = 0.3$	$P < 0.005$
	fT4	$r = 0.18$	$P = 0.058$
	rT3	$r = 0.4$	$P < 0.0001$
	TBG	$r = 0.40$	$P < 0.0001$
Thyroid volume			
Negatively	Ioduria	$r = -0.22$	$P = 0.05$
Positively	Smoking		$P = 0.02$

adequate iodine intake. An inverse relationship between UIE and thyroid volume has also been well documented in schoolchildren in Europe, including France [28].

In contrast with UIE, βhCG correlated strongly with thyroid tests. As expected, we found a negative correlation of βhCG and TSH, reflecting the classical TSH-like activity of βhCG [8]. βHCG correlated positively with all the tested parameters, including rT3, except for fT3. Thus, βhCG appears as the main driver of thyroid function at this stage of pregnancy, as also suggested by Haddow [29]. We report here a correlation of βHCG with rT3. Interestingly, Asakura et al. have reported a correlation of rT3 with the severity of hyperemesis gravidarum [30], a condition generally associated with high βhCG levels. This could suggest a shift in deiodinase activity in that condition.

Of note, we report a strong correlation of βhCG with UIE. One physiological explanation could be that βhCG stimulates relaxin secretion by the corpus luteum, which plays an important physiologic role in the maternal renal adaptation to pregnancy [31]. We speculate that this could contribute to gestational increased UIE during the first trimester.

Maternal smoking is recognized as a stress on the thyroid [32]. The higher thyroid volume and higher thyroglobulin levels we report here in smokers illustrate the deleterious impact of tobacco on the thyroid. We found no correlation between maternal smoking and UIE, though median UIE was slightly lower in smokers (data not shown). Importantly, there was no correlation as well between Tg and UIE. This shows that Tg is more likely a marker of maternal smoking than iodine deficiency at this stage of pregnancy in an area of mild iodine deficiency. However, later in pregnancy, maternal smoking has a significant impact on CB Tg only, but not on maternal Tg [33]. The strong negative correlation of smoking with rT3 has not been reported before and could suggest an effect of tobacco on deiodinase activity. In contrast, we found no correlation of maternal smoking with other thyroid parameters. Shields et al. had found correlations during the first trimester with TSH (lower), and fT3 (higher), and no correlation with fT4 [34]. There was no information on Tg nor thyroid volume, nor rT3. On the other hand, Pearce et al. found that fT4 was lower in women smoking during pregnancy. They did not find association of TSH with smoking or the use of iodine containing vitamins [35]. The impact of other toxics, such as known endocrine disruptors (e.g., PCBs) could also play a role in pregnancy [36, 37].

5. Conclusion

In pregnant women of our area selected for a strictly normal thyroid function, ID is present in two-third of women during the 1st trimester, though usually mild. The absence of correlation between UIE and thyroid tests at that stage of pregnancy contrasts with the impact of βHCG that appears as the main driver of maternal thyroid function in early pregnancy, possibly overriding ID. In addition, our study illustrates the impact of maternal smoking on thyroid volume, Tg, and rT3.

Abbreviations

BMI: Body mass index
CV: Coefficient of variation
fT3: Free T3
fT4: Free T4
ID: Iodine deficiency
rT3: Reverse T3
RIA: Radio-immunoassay
TBG: Thyroxin Binding Globulin
Tg: Thyroglobulin
UIE: Urinary iodine excretion
WA: Weeks of amenorrhea.

Acknowledgments

The authors wish to thank the women who participated in this study, André Bongain, the Head of the Obstetrics ward, for his support, Laurie Zabeo, the midwife in charge of the screening, and Eva Baez, our data manager. This work was funded by a grant from the French Ministry of Health and was promoted by the Direction of Clinical Research of Nice University Hospital.

References

[1] O. P. Soldin, "Controversies in urinary iodine determinations," *Clinical Biochemistry*, vol. 35, no. 8, pp. 575–579, 2002.

[2] S. Hiéronimus, M. Bec-Roche, P. Ferrari, N. Chevalier, P. Fénichel, and F. Brucker-Davis, "Iodine status and thyroid function of 330 pregnant women from Nice area assessed during the second part of pregnancy," *Annales d'Endocrinologie*, vol. 70, no. 4, pp. 218–224, 2009.

[3] F. Delange, "Iodine deficiency as a cause of brain damage," *Postgraduate Medical Journal*, vol. 77, no. 906, pp. 217–220, 2001.

[4] M. B. Zimmermann, "The adverse effects of mild-to-moderate iodine deficiency during pregnancy and childhood: a review," *Thyroid*, vol. 17, no. 9, pp. 829–835, 2007.

[5] G. Morreale De Escobar, M. J. Obregon, and F. E. Del Rey, "Is neuropsychological development related to maternal hypothyroidism or to maternal hypothyroxinemia?" *The Journal of Clinical Endocrinology & Metabolism*, vol. 85, no. 11, pp. 3975–3987, 2000.

[6] G. M. De Escobar, M. J. Obregón, and F. E. Del Rey, "Iodine deficiency and brain development in the first half of pregnancy," *Public Health Nutrition*, vol. 10, no. 12, pp. 1554–1570, 2007.

[7] V. J. Pop, J. L. Kuijpens, A. L. Van Baar et al., "Low maternal free thyroxine concentrations during early pregnancy are associated with impaired psychomotor development in infancy," *Clinical Endocrinology*, vol. 50, no. 2, pp. 147–155, 1999.

[8] D. Glinoer, "The regulation of thyroid function in pregnancy: pathways of endocrine adaptation from physiology to pathology," *Endocrine Reviews*, vol. 18, no. 3, pp. 404–433, 1997.

[9] S. J. Mandel, C. A. Spencer, and J. G. Hollowell, "Are detection and treatment of thyroid insufficiency in pregnancy feasible?" *Thyroid*, vol. 15, no. 1, pp. 44–53, 2005.

[10] D. Glinoer, P. De Nayer, F. Delange et al., "A randomized trial for the treatment of mild iodine deficiency during pregnancy: maternal and neonatal effects," *The Journal of Clinical Endocrinology & Metabolism*, vol. 80, no. 1, pp. 258–269, 1995.

[11] I. Velasco, M. Carreira, P. Santiago et al., "Effect of iodine prophylaxis during pregnancy on neurocognitive development of children during the first two years of life," *The Journal of Clinical Endocrinology & Metabolism*, vol. 94, no. 9, pp. 3234–3241, 2009.

[12] M. Qian, D. Wang, W. E. Watkins et al., "The effects of iodine on intelligence in children: a meta-analysis of studies conducted in China," *Asia Pacific Journal of Clinical Nutrition*, vol. 14, no. 1, pp. 32–42, 2005.

[13] E. N. Pearce, "What do we know about iodine supplementation in pregnancy?" *The Journal of Clinical Endocrinology & Metabolism*, vol. 94, no. 9, pp. 3188–3190, 2009.

[14] M. Abalovich, N. Amino, L. A. Barbour et al., "Management of thyroid dysfunction during pregnancy and post partum : an Endocrine Society clinical practice guideline," *The Journal of Clinical Endocrinology & Metabolism*, vol. 92, pp. S1–S47, 2007.

[15] H. W. Kang, J. H. No, J. H. Chung et al., "Prevalence, clinical and ultrasonographic characteristics of thyroid incidentalomas," *Thyroid*, vol. 14, no. 1, pp. 29–33, 2004.

[16] M. Andersson, B. De Benoist, F. Delange, and J. Zupan, "Prevention and control of iodine deficiency in pregnant and lactating women and in children less than 2-years-old: conclusions and recommendations of the Technical Consultation," *Public Health Nutrition*, vol. 10, no. 12, pp. 1606–1611, 2007.

[17] ICCIDD Newsletter, "Iodine requirements in pregnancy and infancy," *International Council For the Control of Iodine Deficiency Disorders*, vol. 23, pp. 1–2, 2007.

[18] G. Stilwell, P. J. Reynolds, V. Parameswaran, L. Blizzard, T. M. Greenaway, and J. R. Burgess, "The influence of gestational stage on urinary iodine excretion in pregnancy," *The Journal of*

Clinical Endocrinology & Metabolism, vol. 93, no. 5, pp. 1737–1742, 2008.

[19] P. Laurberg, S. Andersen, R. I. Bjarnadóttir et al., "Evaluating iodine deficiency in pregnant women and young infants—complex physiology with a risk of misinterpretation," *Public Health Nutrition*, vol. 10, no. 12, pp. 1547–1552, 2007.

[20] P. Caron, M. Hoff, S. Bazzi et al., "Urinary iodine excretion during normal pregnancy in healthy women living in the southwest of France: correlation with maternal thyroid parameters," *Thyroid*, vol. 7, no. 5, pp. 749–754, 1997.

[21] M. Alvarez-Pedrerol, M. Guxens, M. Mendez et al., "Iodine levels and thyroid hormones in healthy pregnant women and birth weight of their offspring," *European Journal of Endocrinology*, vol. 160, no. 3, pp. 423–429, 2009.

[22] J. Sánchez-Vega, F. E. del Rey, H. Fariñas-Seijas, and G. M. de Escobar, "Inadequate iodine nutrition of pregnant women from Extremadura (Spain)," *European Journal of Endocrinology*, vol. 159, no. 4, pp. 439–445, 2008.

[23] M. Moleti, V. P. L. Presti, M. C. Campolo et al., "Iodine prophylaxis using iodized salt and risk of maternal thyroid failure in conditions of mild iodine deficiency," *The Journal of Clinical Endocrinology & Metabolism*, vol. 93, no. 7, pp. 2616–2621, 2008.

[24] L. Brander, C. Als, H. Buess et al., "Urinary iodine concentration during pregnancy in an area of unstable dietary iodine intake in Switzerland," *Journal of Endocrinological Investigation*, vol. 26, no. 5, pp. 389–396, 2003.

[25] M. B. Zimmermann, I. Aeberli, T. Torresani, and H. Bürgi, "Increasing the iodine concentration in the Swiss iodized salt program markedly improved iodine status in pregnant women and children: a 5-y prospective national study," *The American Journal of Clinical Nutrition*, vol. 82, no. 2, pp. 388–392, 2005.

[26] Y. Fuse, T. Ohashi, S. Yamaguchi, M. Yamaguchi, Y. Shishiba, and M. Irie, "Iodine status of pregnant and post partum Japanese women: effect of iodine intake on maternal and neonatal thyroid function in an iodine sufficient area," *The Journal of Clinical Endocrinology & Metabolism*, vol. 96, no. 12, pp. 3846–3854, 2011.

[27] Y. Orito, H. Oku, S. Kubota et al., "Thyroid function in early pregnancy in Japanese healthy women: relation to urinary iodine excretion, emesis, and fetal and child development," *The Journal of Clinical Endocrinology & Metabolism*, vol. 94, no. 5, pp. 1683–1688, 2009.

[28] F. Delange, G. Benker, P. Caron et al., "Thyroid volume and urinary iodine in European schoolchildren: standardization of values for assessment of iodine deficiency," *European Journal of Endocrinology*, vol. 136, no. 2, pp. 180–187, 1997.

[29] J. E. Haddow, M. R. McClain, G. Lambert-Messerlian et al., "Variability in thyroid-stimulating hormone suppression by human chronic gonadotropin during early pregnancy," *The Journal of Clinical Endocrinology & Metabolism*, vol. 93, no. 9, pp. 3341–3347, 2008.

[30] H. Asakura, S. Watanabe, A. Sekiguchi, G. G. Power, and T. Araki, "Severity of hyperemesis gravidarum correlates with serum levels of reverse T3," *Archives of Gynecology and Obstetrics*, vol. 264, no. 2, pp. 57–62, 2000.

[31] M. C. Smith, A. P. Murdoch, L. A. Danielson, K. P. Conrad, and J. M. Davison, "Relaxin has a role in establishing a renal response in pregnancy," *Fertility and Sterility*, vol. 86, no. 1, pp. 253–255, 2006.

[32] D. Kapoor and T. H. Jones, "Smoking and hormones in health and endocrine disorders," *European Journal of Endocrinology*, vol. 152, no. 4, pp. 491–499, 2005.

[33] S. Hieronimus, P. Ferrari, J. Gal et al., "Relative impact of iodine supplementation and maternal smoking on cord blood thyroglobulin in pregnant women with normal thyroid function," *European Thyroid Journal*. In press.

[34] B. Shields, A. Hill, M. Bilous et al., "Cigarette smoking during pregnancy is associated with alterations in maternal and fetal thyroid function," *The Journal of Clinical Endocrinology & Metabolism*, vol. 94, no. 2, pp. 570–574, 2009.

[35] E. N. Pearce, E. Oken, M. W. Gillman et al., "Association of first-trimester thyroid function test values with thyroperoxidase antibody status, smoking, and multivitamin use," *Endocrine Practice*, vol. 14, no. 1, pp. 33–39, 2008.

[36] R. T. Zoeller, "Environmental chemicals impacting the thyroid: targets and consequences," *Thyroid*, vol. 17, no. 9, pp. 811–817, 2007.

[37] F. Brucker-Davis, P. Ferrari, M. Boda-Buccino et al., "Cord blood thyroid tests in boys born with and without cryptorchidism. Correlations with birth parameters and in utero xenobiotics exposure," *Thyroid*, vol. 21, no. 10, pp. 1133–1141, 2011.

10

Histopathological Changes of the Thyroid and Parathyroid Glands in HIV-Infected Patients

Rabia Cherqaoui,[1] **K. M. Mohamed Shakir,**[2] **Babak Shokrani,**[3] **Sujay Madduri,**[4] **Faria Farhat,**[5] **and Vinod Mody**[5]

[1] *Howard University Hospital, 2041 Georgia Avenue NW, Washington, DC 20060, USA*

[2] *Department of Endocrinology, National Naval Medical Center, 8901 Wisconsin Avenue, Bethesda, MD 20889, USA*

[3] *Department of Pathology, 2041 Georgia Avenue NW, Washington, DC 20060, USA*

[4] *Division of Endocrinology and Metabolism, 2041 Georgia Avenue NW, Washington, DC 20060, USA*

[5] *Division of Infectious Disease, Department of Internal Medicine, Howard University Hospital, 2041 Georgia Avenue NW, Washington, DC 20060, USA*

Correspondence should be addressed to Rabia Cherqaoui; cherqaoui_rabi@yahoo.com

Academic Editor: B. Stack

Objective. To study histopathology of the thyroid and parathyroid glands in HIV-infected African Americans in the United States. *Methods.* A retrospective review of 102 autopsy cases done by the Department of Pathology at Howard University Hospital from 1980 through 2007 was conducted. The histopathological findings of the thyroid and parathyroid glands were reviewed, both macroscopically and microscopically. A control group of autopsy patients with chronic non-HIV diseases was examined. *Results.* There were 71 males (70%) and 31 females (30%) with an average age of 38 years (range: 20–71 y). Thirteen patients with abnormal thyroid findings were identified. Interstitial fibrosis was the most common histological finding (4.9%), followed by thyroid hyperplasia (1.9%). Infectious disease affecting the thyroid gland was limited to 2.9% and consisted of mycobacterium tuberculosis, *Cryptococcus* neoformans, and cytomegalovirus. Kaposi sarcoma of the thyroid gland was present in only one case (0.9%). Parathyroid hyperplasia was the most common histological change noted in the parathyroid glands. Comparing the histological findings of cases and controls, we found a similar involvement of the thyroid, with a greater prevalence of parathyroid hyperplasia in HIV patients. *Conclusion.* Thyroid and parathyroid abnormalities are uncommon findings in the HIV-infected African American population.

1. Introduction

Human immunodeficiency virus (HIV) and Acquired Immune Deficiency Syndrome (AIDS) are associated with multiple endocrine abnormalities [1]. Several investigators have studied the metabolic derangements and reported the functional abnormalities with specific endocrine glands [2]. There is however scant literature regarding histopathology of the thyroid and parathyroid glands in patients with HIV and AIDS, particularly in African Americans (AA). Nevertheless, extensive literature is available on serum biochemical thyroid functions and calcium fluctuations in these patients. Euthyroid sick syndrome, hypothyroidism, hypocalcemia, impaired parathyroid hormone secretion, and vitamin D deficiency appear to be common among the adult HIV-infected patients [3–5].

We postulated that the thyroid and parathyroid glands would be involved in AIDS patients as evidenced by functional abnormalities and derangements seen in these patients. Our study is the first retrospective report to describe the histopathology of the thyroid and parathyroid glands in HIV-infected AA patients in an inner city hospital in the United States.

2. Materials and Methods

A retrospective review of histopathology findings of the thyroid and parathyroid glands at autopsy was conducted at a tertiary care teaching hospital during the year 1980 through 2007. One hundred and two HIV-infected patients who died after admission to Howard University Hospital were identified. The study was reviewed and approved by the Institutional Review Board.

At the time of autopsy, thyroid and parathyroid glands were examined macroscopically and microscopically. Two transverse sections of the thyroid gland were routinely performed. If pathological lesions were noted, multiple sections were performed. Histopathological diagnosis was confirmed by two certified pathologists. Sections were stained with hematoxylin and eosin. Other stains included periodic acid Schiff, Grocott's methenamine silver and Ziehl-Neelsen stain as necessary.

The starting time of the study coincided with the introduction of Highly Active Antiretroviral Treatment (HAART); hence, no many patients were on HAART. Additionally, one third of patients reviewed died before initiation of HAART. We could retrieve a CD4 count only in 20.5% of patients. Incomplete adherence to the prescribed regimen was common, as self-reported by patients as well as evidenced by the number of HIV associated opportunistic infections these patients harbored. We compared the histopathological findings to a control-group which included patients without HIV infection (31 females and 44 males) who died at the hospital from other causes. Chi-square test was used to calculate the significance of these observations.

3. Results

3.1. Patient Characteristics. One hundred and two autopsy cases were reviewed in this study. There were 71 males (70%) and 31 females (30%) with an average age of 38 (range: 20–71 years). The mean time from HIV diagnosis to death was 53 months (range: 1–144 months). Most of the patients had AIDS, as suggested by the number of opportunistic infections they had (% patients had AIDS defining illnesses). CD4 lymphocyte count was documented in 20.5% of patients with a median CD4 count of 50 cells/μL. Eighty patients (78.4%) did not receive Pneumocystis jiroveci prophylaxis. Thirty-four (33%) of patients were from the pre-HAART period (1980–1990). Fourteen patients were on HAART. Our series included 40 patients with intravenous drug abuse (39.2%), 23 (22.5%) with heterosexual risk, 23 (22.5%) with homosexual or bisexual risk, and 56 (55%) with undocumented sexual preference. It is to be noted that these high risk behavior patterns were not mutually exclusive.

A control group for thyroid histopathologic examination was obtained in 75 non-HIV-infected patients. Comparing the histological findings of cases and controls, we found similar involvement of the thyroid, with greater prevalence of parathyroid hyperplasia in HIV patients.

3.2. Pathologic Findings. The thyroid gland weighed between 3 to 40 g. Weights of parathyroid glands were not available. Thyroid gland findings are shown in Table 1. Thirteen patients (7 males and 6 females) had abnormal histopathology of the thyroid gland. The mean age was 41 years, with a range

TABLE 1: Summary of thyroid gland findings in HIV-infected patients and controls.

Thyroid*	HIV-infected patients N (%)	Non-HIV-infected patients N (%)	P value
Normal	89 (87.3)	65 (86.6)	ns
Abnormal (microscopic)	12 (11.8)	10 (13.3)	0.11
Abnormal (macroscopic)	2 (1.96)	7 (9.3)	0.05

*The numbers will not sum to 100% since the categories are not mutually exclusive.

TABLE 2: Summary of parathyroid glands findings in HIV-infected patients and controls.

Parathyroids**	HIV-infected patients N (%)	Non-HIV-infected patients N (%)	P value
Normal	69 (67.6)	72 (96)	ns
Abnormal (microscopic)	33 (32.3)	3 (4)	0.04
Abnormal (macroscopic)	2 (1.96)	2 (2.6)	0.96

**The numbers will not sum to 100% since the categories are not mutually exclusive.

of 30–62 years. Seven of these patients had a history of intravenous drug abuse. The mean time from HIV diagnosis to death was 65.8 months ranging from 6 to 132 months. Only 4 of 13 patients had a CD4 count available with a mean 64, range of 0–200. One patient in this group was receiving Pneumocystis jiroveci prophylaxis and 4 patients were on HAART. The mean body mass index (BMI) was 25 kg/m^2 with a range of 15–40 kg/m^2. The mean weight of the thyroid gland was 21.4 grams with a range of 3 to 32 grams.

The gross examination of the thyroid gland was unremarkable in 100 patients (98%). One patient had a macroscopically nodular thyroid gland while another patient had an atrophic thyroid gland. The latter patient had both macroscopic (atrophy) and microscopic abnormalities (fibrosis) (Table 1). In the control group, the macroscopic histopathologic analysis of the thyroid revealed 68 patients (90.6%) having a normal thyroid macroscopic examination (Table 1).

Histological diagnoses are summarized in Tables 3 and 4.

Interstitial fibrosis (Figure 1) was the most common histological finding identified in thyroid gland sections (4.9%), followed by thyroid hyperplasia (1.9%). Isolated mild interstitial fibrosis was found in 2 patients. Two patients had interstitial fibrosis associated with hyperplasia of the thyroid gland. One patient showed a moderate degree of fibrosis and atrophy of the thyroid gland. One case of colloid goiter and one case of thyroid adenoma were also identified at autopsy (Table 3).

Infections of the thyroid gland included cytomegalovirus (1 case), Mycobacterium tuberculosis (1 case), and *Cryptococcus* (1 case), (Figures 2 and 3).

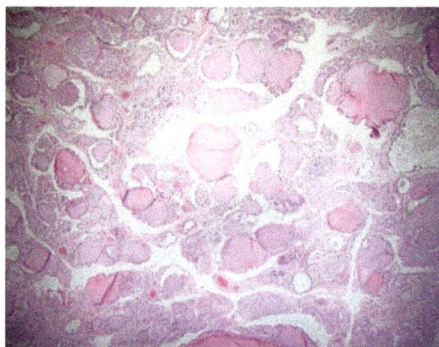

FIGURE 1: Microscopic section of the thyroid showing fibrosis of the interstitium (H&E, 400x).

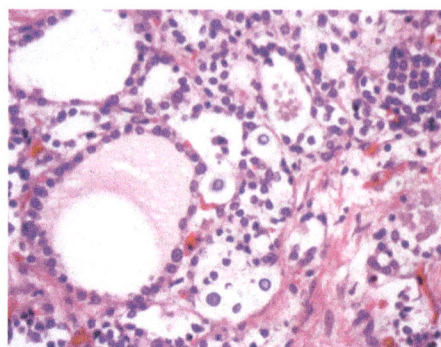

FIGURE 2: Microscopic section of the thyroid gland, (H&E) showing *Cryptococcus* with variation in size (400x).

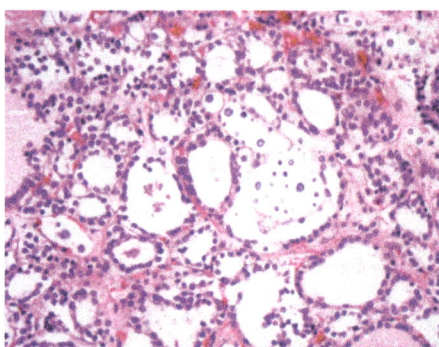

FIGURE 3: Microscopic section of the thyroid gland, (H&E) showing *Cryptococcus* (600x).

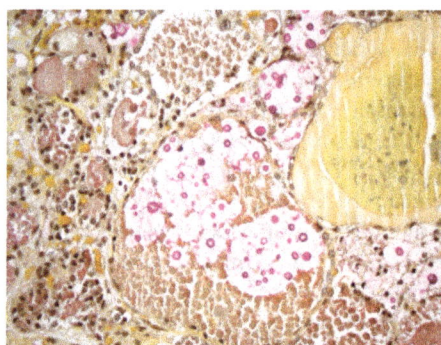

FIGURE 4: Microscopic section of the thyroid gland, mucin stain highlights yeast with thick capsule (400x).

TABLE 3: Histopathological findings in thyroid gland.

Histologic findings	Frequency HIV-infected patients (%)	Frequency Non-HIV-infected patients (%)
Nodular goiter	3 (2.7%)	6 (8%)
Cryptococcal infection	1 (0.9%)	1 (1.3%)
Mycobacterium Tuberculosis	1 (0.9%)	1 (1.3%)
Kaposi sarcoma	1 (0.9%)	0
CMV infection	1 (0.9%)	0
Interstitial fibrosis	5 (4.9%)	2 (2.6%)
Lymphocytic thyroiditis	0	2 (2.6%)
Papillary carcinoma	0	1 (1.3%)

TABLE 4: Histopathological findings in parathyroid glands.

Histologic findings	Frequency HIV-infected patients (%)	Frequency Non-HIV-infected patients (%)
Parathyroid hyperplasia	23 (22.5%)	2 (2.6%)
Nodular oncocytic hyperplasia	3 (2.9%)	0
CMV infection	3 (2.9%)	0
Fatty infiltration	2 (1.9%)	1 (1.3%)
Serous atrophy	2 (1.9%)	0

CMV: cytomegalovirus.

Furthermore, the most common systemic opportunistic infection in 13 of our patients with thyroid abnormalities was Mycobacterium avium complex infection (MAC) (38.4%) followed by Candida albicans (Figures 4 and 5). In the remaining HIV-infected patients without thyroid abnormalities, the most frequent opportunistic infection was Pneumocystis jiroveci (32.5%), followed equally by Candida and cytomegalovirus (19.1%).

Parathyroid glands involvement was noted in 32.1% of patients. Parathyroid hyperplasia was by far the most common histological finding accounting for 22.5% of cases followed by cytomegalovirus (CMV) infection of the parathyroid (2.9%) and nodular oncocytic hyperplasia (2.9%). Parathyroid hyperplasia was diagnosed if at least two of all four parathyroid glands were hyperplastic. Fatty infiltration (1.9%) and serous atrophy (1.9%) were also identified in the parathyroid glands (Table 4) (See Figures 6 and 7).

Most of these patients studied died of septic shock or respiratory failure (data not shown).

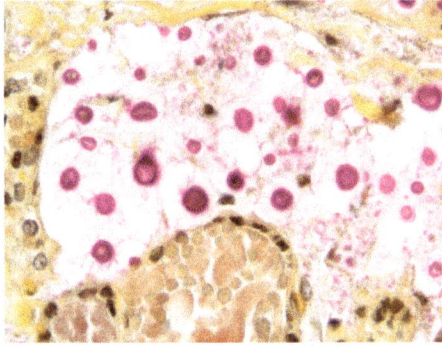

FIGURE 5: Microscopic section of the thyroid gland, mucin stain demonstrating thick capsule, and pleomorphic yeasts (1000x).

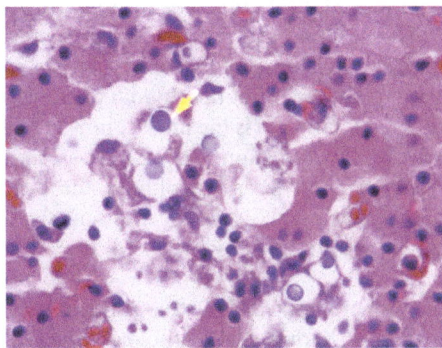

FIGURE 7: Microscopic section of the parathyroid gland, silver stain highlighting *Cryptococcus* with occasional narrow based budding (1000x).

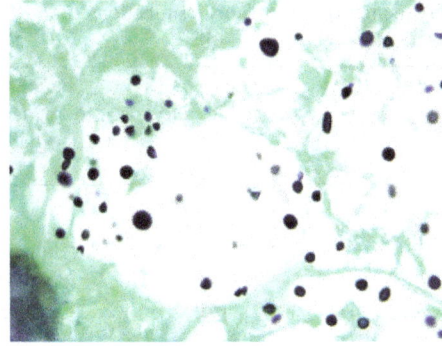

FIGURE 6: Microscopic section of the parathyroid gland showing *Cryptococcus* (yellow arrow). H&E (1000x).

Review of patient's data showed that abnormal pathological findings were found entirely in patients with ongoing illicit drug use.

The histological findings in control patients revealed cytological appearances consistent with benign thyroid nodular disease in 8% of control patients, interstitial fibrosis in 2.6%, lymphocytic thyroiditis in 2.6%, cryptococcal infection in 1.3%, papillary carcinoma in 1.3%, and mycobacterial tuberculosis in 1.3% of the control specimens (Table 3). The histological appearance of parathyroid glands from the control group did differ from the HIV group with 72 control patients (96%) showing normal histological appearance of the parathyroids as opposed 69 HIV-infected patients (67.6%) (Table 2).

4. Discussion

HIV infection and antiretroviral therapy can induce endocrine dysfunction. Patients with AIDS have increased prevalence of nonthyroidal illness, hypothyroidism, and abnormal serum parathyroid hormone (PTH) and serum calcium levels [4, 5]. These alterations in thyroid hormones and calcium homeostasis are rarely the result of a direct infection or infiltration of the thyroid and parathyroid glands. Although subclinical hypothyroidism has been recognized as more prevalent among HIV-infected individuals, it does not appear to have an autoimmune basis [6]. Graves's disease

subsequent to immune restoration due to HAART has been described and unlike the common infection-related immune reconstitution syndromes, it is usually diagnosed 12–36 months after HAART initiation [7]. Two studies from South America have described pathological changes in the thyroid gland in AIDS patients [8, 9]. However, no investigator has reported the histopathology of parathyroid glands in Human Immunodeficiency Virus (HIV) patients. This study represents the first detailed report of thyroid and parathyroid gland abnormalities in a HIV-infected African-American population in the United States.

Ethnicity-related differences in organ systems involvement in HIV patients have been described previously by Morgello et al. with cachexia, renal, cardiac and splenic involvement more frequent in blacks than in whites and/or Hispanic individuals [10]. Additionally, *Mycobacterium avium-intracellulare* (MAI) infection is also more commonly seen in blacks than in whites and/or Hispanic individuals [11]. However the exact explanation for these discrepancies is not clear.

Our findings are strikingly different from what have been published so far in terms of the frequency of thyroid involvement in HIV.

Basílio-De-Oliveira from Brazil reviewed autopsy cases of 100 AIDS patients [8]. The study included 72 white patients. Compared to our findings, thyroid involvement by infectious processes was significant. Mycobacterium tuberculosis infection of the thyroid gland was found in 23% of patients and cytomegalovirus (CMV) in 17%. Neoplastic involvement of the thyroid was also higher in frequency with Kaposi sarcoma (2%) and occult papillary carcinoma (4%) seen in patients. Histopathological lesions consisted mainly of interstitial fibrosis with follicular atrophy. Lima et al. studied forty-seven thyroids obtained at autopsy from 38 men and 9 women with AIDS in Brazil [9]. However, the ethnicity of the sample population was not documented. In contrast to our results, they identified greater frequency of infectious pathogens (14 cases, 29.7%) with five cases of mycobacterial infection (10.6%), four cases of histoplasmosis and cryptococcosis, and finally one case of paracoccidioidomycosis [11]. Their results were concordant with Basílio-De-Oliveira in regard to Mycobacterium infection being

TABLE 5: Frequency of opportunistic infections in HIV infected individuals.

Number of opportunistic infections	Patients with normal thyroid glands $n = 89$ (%)	Patients with abnormal thyroid glands $n = 13$ (%)
0	30 (33.7%)	1 (7.7%)
1	27 (30.3%)	6 (46.1%)
2	21 (23.5%)	4 (30.7%)
3	7 (7.8%)	2 (15.3%)
4	2 (2.2%)	0
5	1 (1.1%)	0
6*	1 (1.1%)	0

*MAC, cytomegalovirus, Cryptococcus, Candida, Pneumocystis jiroveci, and Herpes.

the most frequently detected agent. This may be due to the higher prevalence of mycobacteria in AIDS patients in Brazil [11, 12].

In postmortem examinations of these patients, thyroid pathology was common affecting 29 patients (61.3%), with nonspecific focal chronic inflammation affecting 14 cases (48.2%), colloid goiter in 5 cases (17.2%), and lipomatosis in 4 cases (13.7%). Lipomatosis was associated with atrophy (1 case), hyperplastic nodule (1 case), and histoplasmosis (1 case) [9].

In our study, the frequency of infectious etiology affecting the thyroid gland was limited to 2.9% (3 cases). There was only one case of cytomegalovirus (CMV), Cryptococcus, and tuberculosis. All our cases inclined to have occurred in the context of a widely 5 disseminated disease.

Several cases have been previously reported also as part of multiple organ involvement either antemortem or at autopsy [13–17]. In our series, some patients presented with multiple coexisting opportunistic infections. About 45% of patients in the HIV group with thyroid pathology had more than 2 opportunistic infections as opposed to 35% in the subgroup of HIV patients with normal thyroid histopathology (Table 5). Based on the limited number of patients, we cannot postulate a possible association between opportunistic infections and the occurrence of thyroid abnormalities.

While in previous case reports, Pneumocystis jiroveci has been a prominent cause of thyroiditis in HIV patients [18–21], particularly in patients on aerosolized pentamidine [22, 23], we did not identify this microorganism in any of our patients. This may be due to the fact that many patients presented to our hospital with symptoms suggestive of Pneumocystis jiroveci pneumonia and were treated promptly with trimethoprim-sulfamethoxazole leading to absence of histological evidence of this microorganism at autopsy.

This observation is consistent with other studies showing that after "curing" patients of their pneumocystis infections, biopsy specimens usually lack evidence of residual disease [24, 25].

Our most common finding was interstitial fibrosis seen in 5 of the 12 microscopic cases. Contempre et al. have linked thyroid fibrosis to transforming growth factor beta (TGF-beta) in which follicular cell necrosis occurs first followed

by thyroid fibrosis in the setting of selenium deficiency [26]. Similarly, interstitial fibrosis of the thyroid gland in our series could represent the histologic sequelae of previous inflammatory or infectious assaults coupled with an impaired tissue repair due to the underlying immunosuppression. In addition, Human Immunodeficiency Virus infection itself is associated with increased levels of transforming growth factor beta (TGF-beta) [27].

Of note, we identified two cases of thyroid hyperplasia which has been described as a normal response to alterations in the feedback mechanism of thyrotropin-releasing hormone and thyroid-stimulating hormone [28]. Additionally, it has been shown that HIV-1-infected inflammatory cells may release a mitogen protein (TAT) which enhances the production of growth factors including fibroblast growth factor (FGF-1 and FGF-2) and transforming growth factor-beta [29]. These fibroblast growth factors appear to be involved in the pathogenesis of thyroid hyperplasia [30].

Neoplastic involvement of the thyroid gland was present in one case. Kaposi sarcoma is the most common malignancy associated with HIV infection [31]. Kaposi sarcoma of the thyroid is uncommon, described only in the context of a widespread metastasis [32]. Its pathogenesis involves immunodeficiency, oncogenic DNA viruses, and the HIV-1 protein Tat [33].

Little is known about the relative contribution of illicit drugs use to the thyroid histopathology in HIV-infected populations. Our study suggests that ongoing drug use may impact thyroid tissue in HIV patients.

There is scant literature about the histopathology of the parathyroid glands in HIV patients. We identified parathyroid hyperplasia as the most common histological process (Table 4). The histologic appearance of parathyroid hyperplasia was hypercellularity with heterogenous cell proliferation but predominantly chief cells associated with reduced stromal fat and involving more than one gland.

This finding could be reflective of the secondary hyperparathyroidism resulting from the high prevalence of vitamin D deficiency in African American [34] in general and also specifically HIV-infected individuals [35, 36], although we do not have vitamin D levels in any of these patients. Both parathyroid and nodular oncocytic hyperplasia have been described as a feature of secondary hyperparathyroidism [37]. In the HIV population in particular, this process can also result from decreased serum calcium secondary to impairment in renal function, nutritional status, and chronic malabsorption.

Of note, a decrease of parathyroid hormone (PTH) level has also been previously reported in human immunodeficiency virus (HIV)-infected patients [38]. The mechanism might be related to antibodies against parathyroid cells. Using anti-Leu3a, a monoclonal antibody recognizing CD4, HIV-positive patients have been found to express CD4 molecule at the surface of parathyroid gland cells, indicating the possibility of either functional inhibition by anti-CD4 antibodies or direct infection by HIV [39].

In addition, current evidence indicates that HIV-infected persons have micronutrient deficiencies [40]. Therefore, the question of whether parathyroid hyperplasia could be related to possible micronutrient deficiency such as iodine deficiency remains to be established in HIV-infected subjects. Further research is needed to elucidate the role of micronutrient deficiencies on parathyroid pathology in HIV-infected subjects.

Our study findings must be interpreted in light of several limitations. First, our findings stem from a retrospective review of general autopsies in HIV-infected African American patients; hence, the small number of histologic sections might have influenced the microscopic findings recorded.

Larger studies focusing on thyroid and parathyroid are required to establish the prevalence of our findings.

Second, we were unable to analyze the thyroid function tests and the autoimmune status of our sample. One could argue that interstitial fibrosis is fairly non-specific and further prospective studies correlating histopathological findings with thyroid serologies for a better assessment of thyroid pathology in HIV African American population are needed.

5. Conclusion

We conclude that thyroid and parathyroid abnormalities are uncommon findings in the HIV-infected African American population. The most common characteristics of histopathology seen in the thyroid and parathyroid glands in these patients include interstitial fibrosis and parathyroid hyperplasia, respectively.

Abbreviations

HIV: Human Immunodeficiency Virus
AIDS: Acquired Immune Deficiency Syndrome
HAART: Highly Active Antiretroviral Treatment
BMI: Body mass index
CMV: Cytomegalovirus
MAI: *Mycobacterium avium-intracellulare*
PTH: Parathyroid hormone
MAC: Mycobacterium avium complex
TGF-beta: Transforming growth factor beta
FGF: Fibroblast growth factor
H&E: Hematoxylin and eosin stain.

References

[1] A. Danoff, "HIV and the thyroid—what every practicing endocrinologist needs to know," *Nature Clinical Practice Endocrinology and Metabolism*, vol. 2, no. 11, pp. 602–603, 2006.

[2] K. Samaras, "Metabolic consequences and therapeutic options in highly active antiretroviral therapy in human immunodeficiency virus-1 infection," *Journal of Antimicrobial Chemotherapy*, vol. 61, no. 2, pp. 238–245, 2008.

[3] D. E. Sellmeyer and C. Grunfeld, "Endocrine and metabolic disturbances in Human Immunodeficiency Virus infection and the Acquired Immune Deficiency Syndrome," *Endocrine Reviews*, vol. 17, no. 5, pp. 518–532, 1996.

[4] S. Beltran, F. Lescure, R. Desailloud et al., "Increased prevalence of hypothyroidism among human immunodeficiency virus-infected patients: a need for screening," *Clinical Infectious Diseases*, vol. 37, no. 4, pp. 579–583, 2003.

[5] E. W. Kuehn, H. J. Anders, J. R. Bogner, J. Obermaier, F. D. Goebel, and D. Schlöndorff, "Hypocalcaemia in HIV infection and AIDS," *Journal of Internal Medicine*, vol. 245, no. 1, pp. 69–73, 1999.

[6] S. Beltran, F.-X. Lescure, I. El Esper, J.-L. Schmit, and R. Desailloud, "Subclinical hypothyroidism in HIV-infected patients is not an autoimmune disease," *Hormone Research*, vol. 66, no. 1, pp. 21–26, 2006.

[7] C. J. Hoffmann and T. T. Brown, "Thyroid function abnormalities in HIV-infected patients," *Clinical Infectious Diseases*, vol. 45, no. 4, pp. 488–494, 2007.

[8] C. A. Basílio-De-Oliveira, "Infectious and neoplastic disorders of the thyroid in AIDS patients: an autopsy study," *The Brazilian Journal of Infectious Diseases*, vol. 4, no. 2, pp. 67–75, 2000.

[9] M. A. Lima, L. L. L. Freitas, C. Montandon, D. C. Filho, and M. L. Silva-Vergara, "The thyroid in acquired immunodeficiency syndrome," *Endocrine Pathology*, vol. 9, no. 3, pp. 217–223, 1998.

[10] S. Morgello, R. Mahboob, T. Yakoushina, S. Khan, and K. Hague, "Autopsy findings in a human immunodeficiency virus-infected population over 2 decades: influences of gender, ethnicity, risk factors, and time," *Archives of Pathology and Laboratory Medicine*, vol. 126, no. 2, pp. 182–190, 2002.

[11] M. de C Ramos, M. Jacques De Moraes, A. L. Calusni, G. N. Roscani, and E. Picolli Alves, "A retrospective bacteriological study of mycobacterial infections in patients with acquired immune deficiency syndrome (AIDS)," *The Brazilian Journal of Infectious Diseases*, vol. 4, no. 2, pp. 86–90, 2000.

[12] S. M. Nakatani, I. J. T. Messias-Reason, M. Burger, and C. A. Cunha, "Prevalence of Mycobacterium avium and Mycobacterium tuberculosis in blood cultures of Brazilian AIDS patients after introduction of highly active retroviral therapy," *Brazilian Journal of Infectious Diseases*, vol. 9, no. 6, pp. 459–463, 2005.

[13] A. H. Szporn, S. Tepper, and C. W. Watson, "Disseminated cryptococcosis presenting as thyroiditis. Fine needle aspiration and autopsy findings," *Acta Cytologica*, vol. 29, no. 3, pp. 449–453, 1985.

[14] L. Z. Goldani, A. P. Zavascki, and A. L. Maia, "Fungal thyroiditis: an overview," *Mycopathologia*, vol. 161, no. 3, pp. 129–139, 2006.

[15] A. M. Avram, C. A. Sturm, C. W. Michael, J. C. Sisson, and C. A. Jaffe, "Cryptococcal thyroiditis and hyperthyroidism," *Thyroid*, vol. 14, no. 6, pp. 471–474, 2004.

[16] T. S. Frank, V. A. LiVolsi, and A. M. Connor, "Cytomegalovirus infection of the thyroid in immunocompromised adults," *Yale Journal of Biology and Medicine*, vol. 60, no. 1, pp. 1–8, 1987.

[17] X. Zhang, D. El-Sahrigy, A. Elhosseiny, and M. R. Melamed, "Simultaneous cytomegalovirus infection and kaposi's sarcoma of the thyroid diagnosed by fine needle aspiration in an aids patient: a case report and first cytologic description of the two entities occurring together," *Acta Cytologica*, vol. 47, no. 4, pp. 645–648, 2003.

[18] R. Battan, P. Mariuz, M. C. Raviglione, M. T. Sabatini, M. P. Mullen, and L. Poretsky, "Pneumocystis carinii infection of the thyroid in a hypothyroid patient with AIDS: diagnosis by fine needle aspiration biopsy," *Journal of Clinical Endocrinology and Metabolism*, vol. 72, no. 3, pp. 724–726, 1991.

[19] M. McCarty, R. Coker, and E. Claydon, "Case report: Disseminated Pneumocystis carinii infection in a patient with

the acquired immune deficiency syndrome causing thyroid gland calcification and hypothyroidism," *Clinical Radiology*, vol. 45, no. 3, pp. 209–210, 1992.

[20] D. J. Drucker, D. Bailey, and L. Rotstein, "Thyroiditis as the presenting manifestation of disseminated extrapulmonary pneumocystis carinii infection," *Journal of Clinical Endocrinology and Metabolism*, vol. 71, no. 6, pp. 1663–1665, 1990.

[21] R. Guttler, P. A. Singer, S. G. Axline et al., "Pneumocystis carinii thyroiditis: report of three cases and review of the literature," *Archives of Internal Medicine*, vol. 153, no. 3, pp. 393–396, 1993.

[22] M. V. Ragni, A. Dekker, F. R. DeRubertis et al., "Pneumocystis carinii infection presenting as necrotizing thyroiditis and hypothyroidism," *American Journal of Clinical Pathology*, vol. 95, no. 4, pp. 489–493, 1991.

[23] A. E. Walts and H. E. Pitchon, "Pneumocystis carinii in FNA of the thyroid," *Diagnostic Cytopathology*, vol. 7, no. 6, pp. 615–617, 1991.

[24] C. H. Hsiao, S. H. Huang, S. F. Huang et al., "Autopsy findings on patients with AIDS in Taiwan," *Zhonghua Min Guo Wei Sheng Wu Ji Mian Yi Xue Za Zhi*, vol. 30, no. 3, pp. 145–159, 1997.

[25] C. M. Reichert, T. J. O'Leary, and D. L. Levens, "Autopsy pathology in the acquired immune deficiency syndrome," *American Journal of Pathology*, vol. 112, no. 3, pp. 357–382, 1983.

[26] B. Contempre, O. Le Moine, J. E. Dumont, J.-F. Denef, and M. C. Many, "Selenium deficiency and thyroid fibrosis. A key role for macrophages and transforming growth factor β (TGF-β)," *Molecular and Cellular Endocrinology*, vol. 124, no. 1-2, pp. 7–15, 1996.

[27] S. Amarnath, L. Dong, J. Li, Y. Wu, and W. Chen, "Endogenous TGF-β activation by reactive oxygen species is key to Foxp3 induction in TCR-stimulated and HIV-1-infected human CD4+CD25-T cells," *Retrovirology*, vol. 4, article 57, 2007.

[28] M. D. Perez-Montiel and S. Suster, "The spectrum of histologic changes in thyroid hyperplasia: a clinicopathologic study of 300 cases," *Human Pathology*, vol. 39, no. 7, pp. 1080–1087, 2008.

[29] S. R. Opalenik, J. T. Shin, J. N. Wehby, V. K. Mahesh, and J. A. Thompson, "The HIV-1 TAT protein induces the expression and extracellular appearance of acidic fibroblast growth factor," *The Journal of Biological Chemistry*, vol. 270, no. 29, pp. 17457–17467, 1995.

[30] S. D. Thompson, J. A. Franklyn, J. C. Watkinson, J. M. Verhaeg, M. C. Sheppard, and M. C. Eggo, "Fibroblast growth factors 1 and 2 and fibroblast growth factor receptor 1 are elevated in thyroid hyperplasia," *Journal of Clinical Endocrinology and Metabolism*, vol. 83, no. 4, pp. 1336–1341, 1998.

[31] Y. Aoki and G. Tosato, "Targeted inhibition of angiogenic factors in AIDS-related disorders," *Current Drug Targets*, vol. 3, no. 2, pp. 115–128, 2003.

[32] P. H. Krauth and J. F. Katz, "Kaposi's sarcoma involving the thyroid in a patient with AIDS," *Clinical Nuclear Medicine*, vol. 12, no. 11, pp. 848–849, 1987.

[33] G. Nunnari, J. A. Smith, and R. Daniel, "HIV-1 Tat and AIDS-associated cancer: targeting the cellular anti-cancer barrier?" *Journal of Experimental and Clinical Cancer Research*, vol. 27, no. 1, article 3, 2008.

[34] S. S. Harris, "Vitamin D and African Americans," *Journal of Nutrition*, vol. 136, no. 4, pp. 1126–1129, 2006.

[35] M. Rodríguez, B. Daniels, S. Gunawardene, and G. K. Robbins, "High frequency of vitamin D deficiency in ambulatory HIV-Positive patients," *AIDS Research and Human Retroviruses*, vol. 25, no. 1, pp. 9–14, 2009.

[36] C. J. P. van den Bout-van den Beukel, L. Fievez, M. Michels et al., "Vitamin D deficiency among HIV type 1-infected individuals in the Netherlands: effects of antiretroviral therapy," *AIDS Research and Human Retroviruses*, vol. 24, no. 11, pp. 1375–1382, 2008.

[37] R. V. Lloyd, B. R. Douglas, and W. F. Young Jr., *Endocrine Diseases, Atlas Nontumor Pathology First Series*, vol. 1, pp. 74–78, Armed Forces Institute of Pathology, Washington, DC, USA, 2002.

[38] P. Jaeger, S. Otto, R. F. Speck et al., "Altered parathyroid gland function in severely immunocompromised patients infected with human immunodeficiency virus," *Journal of Clinical Endocrinology and Metabolism*, vol. 79, no. 6, pp. 1701–1705, 1994.

[39] P. Hellman, A. Karlsson-Parra, L. Klareskog et al., "Expression and function of a CD4-like molecule in parathyroid tissue," *Surgery*, vol. 120, no. 6, pp. 985–992, 1996.

[40] P. K. Drain, R. Kupka, F. Mugusi, and W. W. Fawzi, "Micronutrients in HIV-positive persons receiving highly active antiretroviral therapy," *American Journal of Clinical Nutrition*, vol. 85, no. 2, pp. 333–345, 2007.

11

Thyroid Hormone Receptors in Two Model Species for Vertebrate Embryonic Development: Chicken and Zebrafish

Veerle M. Darras,[1] Stijn L. J. Van Herck,[1] Marjolein Heijlen,[1] and Bert De Groef[1, 2]

[1] *Division Animal Physiology and Neurobiology, Biology Department, Laboratory of Comparative Endocrinology, K.U.Leuven, 3000 Leuven, Belgium*
[2] *Department of Agricultural Sciences, Centre for Agribiosciences, La Trobe University, Bundoora, VIC 3086, Australia*

Correspondence should be addressed to Veerle M. Darras, veerle.darras@bio.kuleuven.be

Academic Editor: Michelina Plateroti

Chicken and zebrafish are two model species regularly used to study the role of thyroid hormones in vertebrate development. Similar to mammals, chickens have one thyroid hormone receptor α (TRα) and one TRβ gene, giving rise to three TR isoforms: TRα, TRβ2, and TRβ0, the latter with a very short amino-terminal domain. Zebrafish also have one TRβ gene, providing two TRβ1 variants. The zebrafish TRα gene has been duplicated, and at least three TRα isoforms are expressed: TRαA1-2 and TRαB are very similar, while TRαA1 has a longer carboxy-terminal ligand-binding domain. All these TR isoforms appear to be functional, ligand-binding receptors. As in other vertebrates, the different chicken and zebrafish TR isoforms have a divergent spatiotemporal expression pattern, suggesting that they also have distinct functions. Several isoforms are expressed from the very first stages of embryonic development and early chicken and zebrafish embryos respond to thyroid hormone treatment with changes in gene expression. Future studies in knockdown and mutant animals should allow us to link the different TR isoforms to specific processes in embryonic development.

1. Introduction

Thyroid hormones (THs) play an important role in development by controlling the growth and differentiation of almost every organ in the vertebrate body. They act mainly, although not exclusively, by binding to intracellular TH receptors (TRs), members of the nuclear receptor superfamily. TRs are ligand-inducible transcription factors that bind 3,5,3′-triiodothyronine (T_3) or with a lower affinity also 3,5,3′,5′-tetraiodothyronine or thyroxine (T_4). They function as homodimers or preferentially as heterodimers with other members of the same receptor family, notably the retinoid X receptors (RXRs). TRs recognize specific DNA sequences in the promoter region of TH-responsive genes and can bind to these TH response elements (TREs) even in the absence of ligand. Generally, unliganded TRs are bound to a set of corepressors leading to active repression of gene transcription. Ligand binding induces a conformational change, resulting in release of the corepressors and recruitment of coactivators and stimulation of gene transcription. The molecular mechanisms involved in TR-mediated gene transcription have recently been reviewed in more detail by other authors (e.g., [1–4]).

The first clear evidence for the need of THs in vertebrate development came from frogs, where THs control the transition from an aquatic larva to a terrestrial juvenile during metamorphosis. Since that time, THs have been shown to be involved not only in postnatal/posthatch development but also in earlier stages, both in mammals and in nonmammalian species. All vertebrate embryos have access to THs long before the embryonic thyroid gland starts hormone secretion, either by transplacental transfer in mammals [5] or by TH deposition in the yolk in other vertebrates [6, 7]. Whether or not these THs can influence early development largely depends on the presence and tissue-specific distribution of TRs in the species investigated. In this paper we try to summarize the information available for two nonmammalian model species for vertebrate embryonic development. The chicken is a long-established model for the study of early development. It has been a major model in embryology for more than a century and has recently become even more powerful thanks to the possibilities of gain- and loss-of-function technologies [8]. The zebrafish emerged more recently but became a mainstream model organism for the molecular aspects of development very rapidly, because it combines an external development and a relatively short generation time with several possibilities of genetic manipulation [9].

2. Different Isoforms of Nuclear TH Receptors

Vertebrates generally have two TR genes located on different chromosomes, encoding, respectively, thyroid hormone receptor alpha (TRα) and thyroid hormone receptor beta (TRβ). Due to ancestral gene duplication, some nonmammalian vertebrate species, including several fish, have two TRα-encoding genes [10]. Each TR consists of an amino-terminal regulatory domain, a central DNA-binding domain, and a carboxy-terminal hormone-binding domain. The latter not only binds THs, but is also involved in the interaction with corepressors and coactivators, and in the dimerisation of the receptors. The structure and function of TRs has been very well conserved throughout vertebrate evolution. They seem to originate from a single TR gene that has a common ancestry with a TR gene found in the cephalochordate *Amphioxus* and the sea squirt *Ciona*, and interestingly even in the trematode *Schistosoma*. This suggests that the origin of the TR gene goes back early in animal evolution [11, 12]. Each vertebrate TR gene typically gives rise to several variants through alternative splicing and the use of different transcription start sites. In rodents, this leads to three hormone-binding TRβ variants (TRβ1, TRβ2, and TRβ3) differing in their amino-terminal domain, one hormone-binding TRα variant (TRα1) and two TRα variants (TRα2 and TRα3) that have a different carboxy-terminus and are not capable of hormone binding. In addition, some truncated TRs have been identified (TR$\Delta\beta$3, TR$\Delta\alpha$1, and TR$\Delta\alpha$2) that have the capacity to bind THs but that cannot bind to TREs [1]. So far the number of TR isoforms identified in chicken and zebrafish is more restricted, but a more thorough investigation may considerably increase their number as happened in rodents over the last decades.

The presence of nuclear binding sites for T$_3$ was first shown in rat in the early seventies [13, 14]. Approximately ten years later, similar studies in chicken embryos showed that such binding sites were already present early in embryonic development, in liver, brain, and lung tissue [15–17]. In addition, these studies showed that shifts occurred in the K_a values for T$_3$ binding during development and that while nuclei purified from brain of 9-day-old embryos (E9) bound T$_3$ twice as good as T$_4$, this shifted to a 5-fold better binding of T$_3$ at E17 [16]. This led to the suggestion that maybe more than one type of binding site was present and that their relative abundance might change during development.

The first step to the identification of the molecular structure of TRs was made when it was shown in chicken and in rat that the cellular counterpart of the *v-erb-A* gene coded for a protein capable of binding T$_3$ with the same affinity as the previously identified nuclear binding sites [18, 19]. As a result, it became clear that the previously described chicken *c-erb-A* gene [20] was the gene for chicken TRα [18]. A few years later, a cDNA encoding a chicken TRβ was characterised. This cTRβ closely resembled the human and rat TRβ sequences identified at that time, but it had a much shorter amino-terminal domain [21, 22]. Shortly thereafter another TRβ with a longer amino-terminal domain was identified [23]. It closely resembled rat TRβ2 and was therefore named cTRβ2, while the previously identified shorter TRβ was named TRβ0 [23]. It was shown that TRβ2 was more efficient in transactivation of a reporter gene than TRβ0 [23, 24]. All three chicken TR isoforms have a functional hormone-binding domain and bind T$_3$ with higher affinity than T$_4$. No truncated or non-ligand-binding variants have been described so far. A comparison of the structure of the chicken and mouse TR variants is given in Figure 1.

Two TR genes were originally identified in zebrafish, TRα and TRβ, giving rise to the transcripts TRα1 and TRβ1 [26, 27]. Zebrafish TRα1 showed a high similarity with TRαs from other vertebrates, but it had 14 additional carboxy-terminal amino acids that were not found in any other known TR [26, 28]. Zebrafish TRβ1 had the typical structure of all other TRβs including the short amino-terminal domain [27, 29]. One year later, a second TRβ isoform was described that had a 9-amino acid insert in the hinge region between the DNA- and the ligand-binding domain [28], a feature found in several teleost TRβs but not in other vertebrate classes [30]. Comparison of the activity of the TRα and TRβ proteins suggested that TRβ1 transactivating activity was ligand-dependent and repressed in the absence of T$_3$, while TRα had constitutive transactivating activity in the absence of ligand [27, 31].

Only recently it was shown that due to ancestral gene duplication, zebrafish has two TRα genes and that they are both expressed [10, 32]. The originally identified TRα gene has therefore been renamed *thraa*, while the second one is called *thrab*. The *thraa* gene gives rise to at least two proteins: TRαA1 and TRαA1-2. TRαA1 corresponds to the original TRα1 with the carboxy-terminal extension while TRαA1-2 does not have this extension [32]. The so-called F domain extension does not alter the overall structure of TRαA1, but it reduces the transcriptional activity of the receptor by changing its affinity for the zebrafish coactivator NCoA2 [32]. The sequence of the ligand-binding domain of TRαB, the transcript encoded by the *thrab* gene, is very similar to the one of TRαA1-2, but based on the predicted sequence, it probably has a shorter amino-terminal domain and some splice variations that might have functional consequences [32]. All the zebrafish TRs mentioned above have a functional hormone-binding domain. However, there is some evidence for the presence of a TRβ2-like transcript that could encode a truncated TR with a complete DNA-binding domain but no ligand-binding domain [33]. A

cTRα 72% 97% 92% 90%
50 118 408

mTRα1
52 120 410

zTRαA1 45% 92% 86% 82%
56 124 427

zTRαA1-2 45% 92% 86% 82%
56 95% 124 97% 413

zTRαB 84% 94% 88% 89%
14 82 371

A/B C (DBD) D/E (LBD)

(a)

cTRβ0 95% 96% 95%
2 100% 68 100% 369

cTRβ2 95% 96% 77%
109 189 476

mTRβ1
94 174 461

mTRβ2 100% 100% 80%
108 188 475

zTRβ1-isoform 1 92% 89% 86%
100% 19 100% 99 386

zTRβ1-isoform 2 92% 89% 86%
19 99 377

A/B C (DBD) D/E (LBD)

(b)

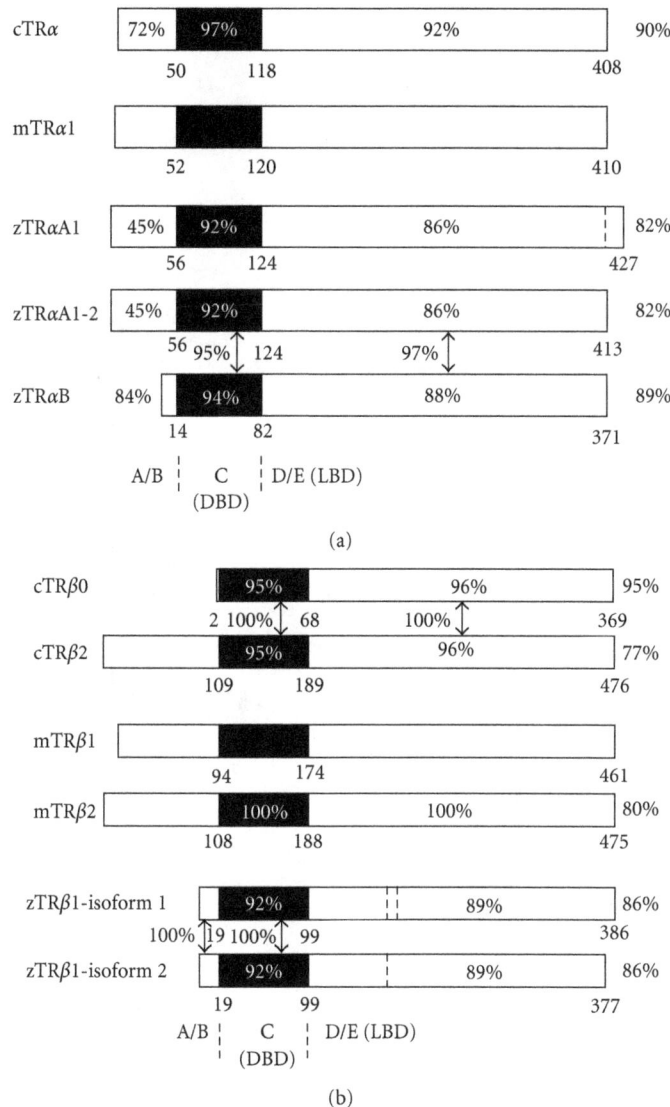

FIGURE 1: Comparison of mouse (m), chicken (c), and zebrafish (z) TR isoforms. (a) TRα variants and (b) TRβ variants. Truncated TR isoforms that do not bind T_3 are not included, nor are the TRβ3 variants that have only been found in rats. Numbering of amino acids is represented under each bar. Percentages within the bars are identities of that domain with the homologous domain of mTRα1 or mTRβ1, respectively. Percentages right of the bars give the overall similarity of the entire protein with the canonical mouse homolog. Percentages in between bars show the similarity between the respective domains. A/B: A and B domain; C (DBD): C domain or DNA-binding domain; D/E (LBD): D and E domain or ligand-binding domain. The dotted line in the D/E domain of zTRαA1 marks the first of the 14 additional carboxy-terminal amino acids not found in the other TRs. The dotted lines in the D/E domain of zTRβ1 isoform 1 delineate a 9-amino-acid insert that is missing in the equivalent location in zTRβ1 isoform 2 (also indicated with a dotted line). Comparisons were based on the following UniProtKB sequences: mTRα1 (P63058-2), mTRβ1 (P37242-1), mTRβ2 (P37242-2), cTRα1 (P04625), cTRβ0 (P68306), cTRβ2 (Q91003), zTRαA1 (Q98867-1), zTRα1-2 (Q98867-2), zTRαB (A0ST48), zTRβ1-isoform 1 (Q9PVE4-1), and zTRβ1-isoform 2 (Q9PVE4-2).

comparison of the structure of the zebrafish and mouse TR variants is given in Figure 1.

3. Expression and Distribution of TRs during Embryonic Development

The expression pattern of chicken and zebrafish TRs has so far been studied predominantly, if not exclusively, at the mRNA level using techniques like Northern blot analysis, *in situ* hybridisation (ISH), and quantitative reverse transcription polymerase chain reaction (qRT-PCR). While ISH is the only technique providing information on the cell-specific distribution pattern, qRT-PCR is by far the most sensitive one. This difference in detection limit has to be taken into account when comparing the results from different groups published over the years.

Chicken embryonic development takes three weeks from the beginning of incubation to hatching. Studies in early chick embryos have shown that TRα is expressed earlier

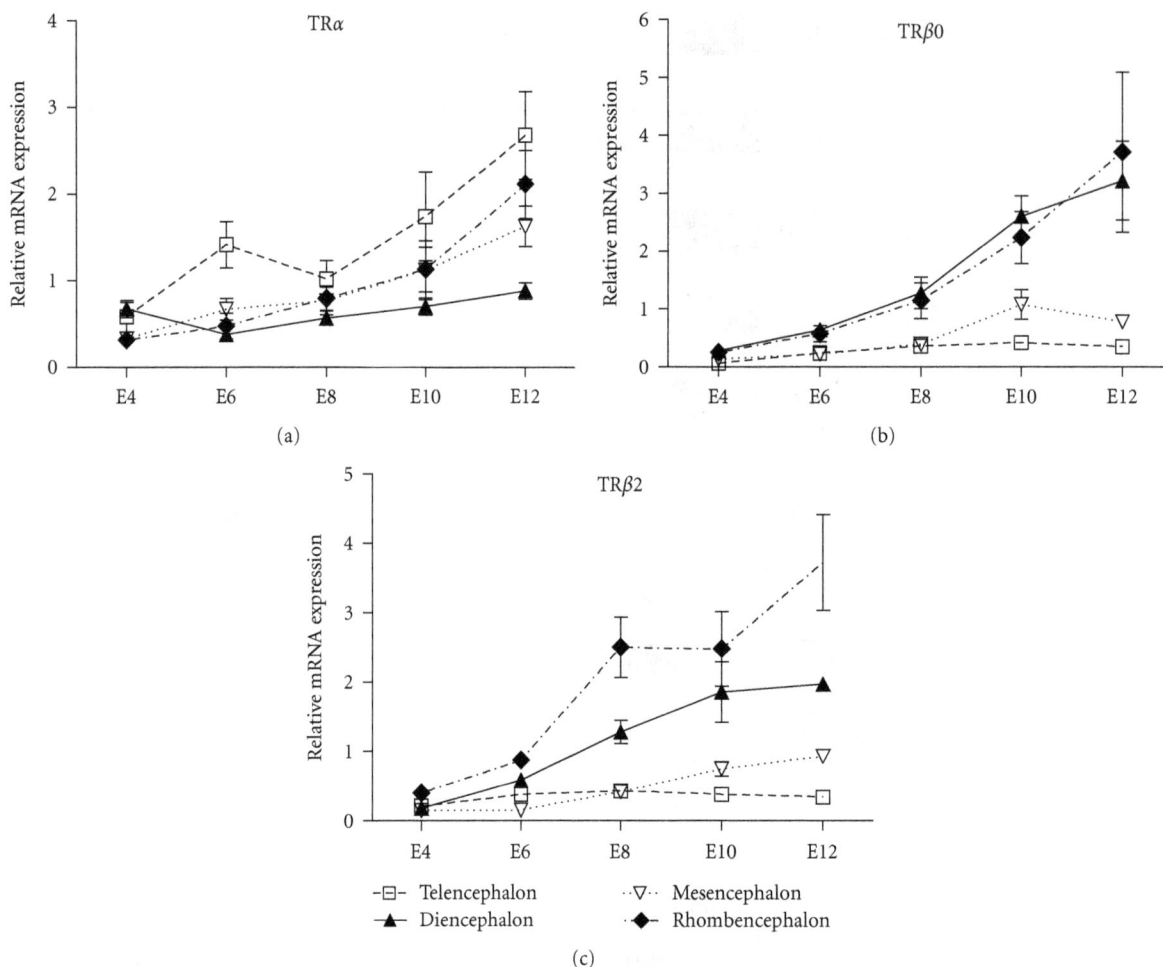

FIGURE 2: Ontogenetic pattern of TRα, TRβ0, and TRβ2 expression in different brain regions of 4- to 12-day-old chick embryos. Specific mRNA levels were measured by qRT-PCR and normalised against a combination of four housekeeping genes: β actin, GAPDH, β2 microglobulin, and cyclophilin A. Values represent the mean ± SEM for 6 independent samples per stage.

than TRβ. TRα mRNA was already detected on the first day of incubation and whole-mount ISH in embryos after 18 to 33 hours of incubation showed the highest expression in the neurectoderm [34]. At that time, TRβ expression was found to be extremely low [34]. This predominance of TRα at early stages was confirmed by Northern blot analysis showing the presence of TRα mRNA in brain, red blood cells and yolk sac at E4, while TRβ0 mRNA could only be detected from E7 onwards in yolk sac [21, 35]. Using an RNase protection assay, TRβ2 mRNA was first detected at E6, specifically in the retina [23]. Recently, qRT-PCR analysis by our own group demonstrated that all three known chicken TR variants are already expressed in brain at E4. Analysis of different brain regions from E4 up to E12 showed a clear and gradual increase of TRα mRNA levels in telencephalon, mesencephalon, and rhombencephalon (including cerebellum, pons, and myelencephalon), while the increase was marginal in diencephalon. In contrast, expression of both TRβ0 and TRβ2 clearly increased in diencephalon and rhombencephalon, whereas there was only a small increase in telencephalon and mesencephalon (Figure 2).

Several studies in older embryos have confirmed that TRα and TRβ are expressed in a spatiotemporal divergent pattern and that TRα is the most widely distributed isoform. Northern blot analysis in embryonic tissues from the second week of incubation onwards showed TRα expression in brain, eye, lung, kidney, heart, liver, intestine, muscle, spleen, red blood cells, and yolk sac [21]. The high expression in embryonic red blood cells confirmed earlier findings obtained by ISH [35]. The TRβ0 signal on Northern blot was restricted to brain, eye, lung, kidney, and yolk sac [21]. ISH on embryonic brain samples showed that both TRα and TRβ were predominantly expressed in cerebellum. However, while TRα was abundantly present in E15 and E19 cerebellum, TRβ0 expression was still faint at E19 and increased after hatching [36]. The same research group also found that during eye development, there was a shift from a relatively high TRβ2 expression to a predominance of TRβ0 towards the last days of embryonic development [21]. Our group again used qRT-PCR to analyse the expression of TRβ2 in tissues of late-stage embryos and early posthatch chicks. It was found, as in mammals, that TRβ2 expression was very restricted in peripheral tissues. At E18 this receptor was mainly expressed in brain, thyroid gland, pineal gland, pituitary gland, and retina, with a clear predominance in retina [37, 38]. More detailed analysis in diencephalon, pituitary, and thyroid gland showed a steady increase in expression from E14 up to E20. Then levels stabilised in diencephalon and pituitary, but they continued to increase in thyroid gland [38].

Zebrafish development from fertilisation to hatching only takes 3 days. The embryos are small and in most studies complete embryos have been pooled for RNA extraction and quantification of TR mRNA levels. Northern blot studies showed that TRαA1 mRNA was clearly present at the start of development but those levels rapidly dropped towards the early gastrula stage. This probably reflects the disappearance of maternal transcripts, since TRαA1 is only present in high amounts in ovary and testis of adult zebrafish [26, 32]. Zygotic expression of TRαA1 could be demonstrated after the mid-blastula transition about 3 hours postfertilisation (hpf) using RNase protection and qRT-PCR, but levels remained very low throughout embryonic and larval development [26, 32]. In contrast, after the disappearance of maternal TRαA1-2 and TRαB mRNA, zygotic expression of these TR isoforms was increased 5- and 28-fold, respectively, in larvae at 4 days post fertilisation (dpf) compared to embryos at 1 dpf [32]. Except for the recent study of Takayama and colleagues [32], the available RT-PCR expression data were all obtained using primers based exclusively on the *thraa* sequence and also do not allow to distinguish the different TRαA transcripts. Transcription levels for TRαA and TRβ have been compared during the first 12 cell cycles of the zebrafish zygote (0–4 hpf) using semiquantitative RT-PCR. The results showed that the level of maternal TRαA transcripts was higher than the level of TRβ1 transcripts, which were already degraded by the 2-cell stage. Zygotic expression of TRαA and TRβ1 transcripts could already be shown at the 8- to 16-cell stage, well before the mid-blastula transition and the increase in TRαA appeared to precede the increase in TRβ1 [27]. The same research group continued their studies at later stages, showing more or less stable expression of TRα at 1, 2, and 3 dpf, while TRβ, expression increased substantially between the early gastrula stage (5-6 hpf) and 2 dpf [39]. We measured TRαA expression by qRT-PCR at regular intervals during embryonic development, confirming relatively high mRNA levels at 8 hpf followed by low levels up till hatching [7]. For TRβ we found more or less stable mRNA levels throughout embryonic development, followed by a rapid increase around hatching [25] (Figure 3). Data of an ISH study for a wide range of nuclear receptors showed no or only baseline signal for TRα in zebrafish embryos, while TRβ was expressed from approximately 30 hpf onwards in the retina and from approximately 40 hpf onwards also in the mid- and hindbrain [10, 40].

4. TR-Mediated Actions of TH during Embryonic Development

Thyroid hormones play a major role in the development and maturation of most chicken organs, as is the case in all vertebrates. In addition THs are important in chicken

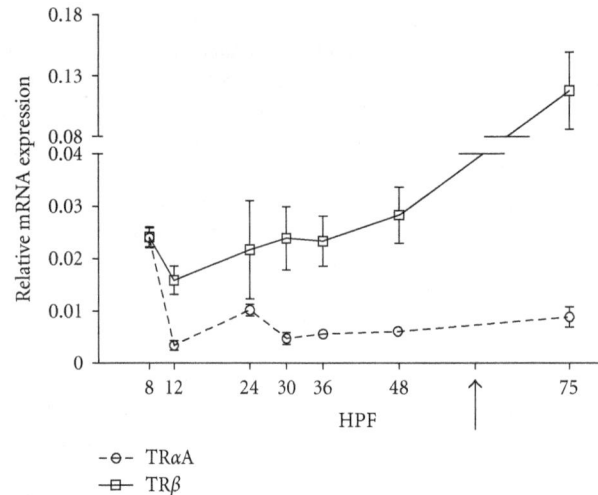

FIGURE 3: Expression of TRαA and TRβ in whole zebrafish embryos during the first three days post fertilisation. Specific mRNA levels were measured by qRT-PCR and normalised against the housekeeping gene Elongation factor 1α. Values represent the mean $\pm$ SEM for 3 independent samples (pools of 50–100 embryos) per stage. The arrow indicates the average time of hatching. HPF: hours post fertilisation. Data were taken from [7, 25].

for yolk sac retraction and hatching [41]. While it is clear that nuclear TR-mediated gene transcription is extremely important in the control of these developmental processes, little is known about the specific role of each of the different TR isoforms. In mammals, studies in transgenic mice have contributed substantially to our understanding of the role of each hormone-binding TR variant, leading to the conclusion that all of them seem to have both unique and redundant functions [42–44]. Given the high similarity of chicken TRα, TRβ0, and TRβ2 with mammalian TRα1, TRβ1, and TRβ2, this is probably also the case in chicken and a number of studies indeed point in that direction.

The relatively high expression of TRα in neurectoderm during the first two days of incubation suggests that this receptor plays an important role in the early development of the nervous system [34]. At this moment, it is still unclear whether the main function of TRs at that stage is repression of gene transcription in the unliganded state or whether the low amount of TH in the embryo is already controlling ligand-dependent stimulation of gene transcription. The latter is possible since T_3 was shown to be present in the embryo from the first day of incubation and administration of a high dose of T_3 disturbed the development of neural tube and brain [34]. We showed that E4 embryos efficiently take up THs from the yolk and injection of surplus hormone at that stage is capable of changing the expression of some TH-responsive genes, including TRs, in the embryonic brain, indicating that ligand-dependent control of gene transcription is possible at these early stages [45, and own unpublished results]. The upregulation of TR protein by T_3 found in hypothalamic neurons from E6 embryos kept in culture also points to the early effects of TH-dependent physiological actions of TRs [46].

The relatively high expression levels of TRβ2 at E6 and its progressive decrease later on suggest that this specific TR isoform is important for the early stages of retina development [23]. *In ovo* treatment of E7 to E12 embryos with T$_4$ accelerates the maturation of the cornea [47], but since all three TR isoforms are expressed in chicken eye by E9 [21, 23], this effect cannot be linked to a specific receptor subtype. Later in development, TRβ2 seems to be important in feedback regulation of the thyrotropic axis. We found that its expression level in diencephalon and in pituitary closely paralleled the increase in plasma T$_4$ from E14 towards a maximum at E20 and the decrease thereafter. Moreover, a 30 min *in vitro* exposure of E18 pituitaries to 10 or 100 nM T$_4$ or T$_3$ reduced TRβ2 expression by more than half [38]. This would agree with the role of TRβ2 described in the regulation of TSH and TRH production in mice [48, 49] and the negative effect of T$_3$ on the TRβ-mediated TRH transcription found in primary cultures of embryonic chick hypothalamic neurons transiently transfected with TRα or TRβ [50].

Describing the role of the different zebrafish TRs in embryonic development is hampered by the lack of information on their tissue-specific distribution in these early stages since the primers or probes used in many studies, including our own, do not allow to unequivocally identify the distinct transcripts. Moreover, while a multitude of genes have been knocked down using specific morpholino antisense oligomers to study their role in zebrafish embryonic development, the TR genes seem to have escaped notice. It has been suggested that at the beginning of development, in the absence of TH, TRαA1 functions mainly as a transcriptional repressor and that it may repress retinoic acid signalling in blastula- and gastrula-stage embryos [26]. Overexpression of TRαA1 in early development interfered with the role of retinoic acid in the establishment of the anteroposterior axis in the central nervous system and resulted in severe disruption of the rostral hindbrain [51]. However, although the zebrafish thyroid gland only starts hormone secretion around the time of hatching, zebrafish embryos take up THs from the egg yolk, and hormone-dependent stimulation of gene transcription may occur even in early embryos. We showed that when embryos were reared in medium containing 5 nM T$_3$, hormone levels in the embryos increased dramatically, concomitant with an acceleration of developmental rate and hatching. We also observed an increase in the expression of TRα in T$_3$-treated embryos at 48 hpf compared to controls, while TRβ expression was not altered [7]. Other investigators found that immersion in 5 nM T$_3$ first downregulated TRαA and TRβ1 levels, while continued treatment up to 72 hpf resulted in upregulation of expression of both genes [27]. The same group showed that T$_3$ treatment of zebrafish embryos starting at 48 hpf upregulated TRα and TRβ expression, whereas the drug amiodarone that can bind to TRs and antagonise their action strongly inhibited TRα and TRβ expression. This suggests that, as in early chicken embryos, TH can exert a positive autoregulatory feedback control on the transcription of its receptors [39]. This agrees with our studies where we knocked down the type 2 iodothyronine deiodinase, the enzyme converting T$_4$ to the receptor-active T$_3$. In these embryos, TRα expression was slightly lower at 24 hpf and 31 hpf compared to controls, and TRβ expression was clearly reduced [52].

5. Conclusions

As in other vertebrates, several TR isoforms have been identified in chicken and zebrafish. All of them appear to be fully functional receptors and so far no truncated TRs have been characterised. The different TR variants are expressed throughout embryonic development in spatiotemporal divergent patterns. As in mammals, there seems to be a predominance of TRα over TRβ expression at the early stages of embryonic development in both species. Before the embryonic thyroid gland becomes active, chicken and zebrafish embryos have access to THs from a maternal deposit in the yolk, and it has been shown that TH administration to early embryos can stimulate transcription of TH-dependent genes. However, as in mammals, it remains unclear whether the main action of TRs in the first stages of development is the repression of gene transcription in the unliganded form or the stimulation of gene transcription following ligand binding. We also need more data to be able to link the different TR isoforms to specific processes in embryonic development, particularly in zebrafish. In combination with data available from frogs and mammals, this will allow identifying isoform-specific actions that have been conserved throughout vertebrate evolution. Gene knockdown studies and the use of mutant embryos can certainly contribute to solve these questions in the near future. This will even further increase the attractiveness of these externally developing model species for functional genomics studies in relation to the role of THs and their receptors in human development and health.

References

[1] S. Y. Cheng, J. L. Leonard, and P. J. Davis, "Molecular aspects of thyroid hormone actions," *Endocrine Reviews*, vol. 31, no. 2, pp. 139–170, 2010.

[2] P. M. Yen, S. Ando, X. Feng, Y. Liu, P. Maruvada, and X. Xia, "Thyroid hormone action at the cellular, genomic and target gene levels," *Molecular and Cellular Endocrinology*, vol. 246, no. 1-2, pp. 121–127, 2006.

[3] N. Koibuchi, "Animal models to study thyroid hormone action in cerebellum," *Cerebellum*, vol. 8, no. 2, pp. 89–97, 2009.

[4] Y. B. Shi, "Dual functions of thyroid hormone receptors in vertebrate development: the roles of histone-modifying cofactor complexes," *Thyroid*, vol. 19, no. 9, pp. 987–999, 2009.

[5] G. M. De Escobar, M. J. Obregón, and F. E. Del Rey, "Role of thyroid hormone during early brain development," *European Journal of Endocrinology, Supplement*, vol. 151, no. 3, pp. U25–U37, 2004.

[6] M. Prati, R. Calvo, and G. M. De Escobar, "L-Thyroxine and 3,5,3′-triiodothyronine concentrations in the chicken egg and in the embryo before and after the onset of thyroid function," *Endocrinology*, vol. 130, no. 5, pp. 2651–2659, 1992.

[7] C. N. Walpita, S. Van der Geyten, E. Rurangwa, and V. M. Darras, "The effect of 3,5,3′-triiodothyronine supplementation on zebrafish (Danio rerio) embryonic development and

expression of iodothyronine deiodinases and thyroid hormone receptors," *General and Comparative Endocrinology*, vol. 152, no. 2-3, pp. 206–214, 2007.

[8] C. D. Stern, "The chick: a great model system becomes even greater," *Developmental Cell*, vol. 8, no. 1, pp. 9–17, 2005.

[9] P. Haffter and C. Nüsslein-Volhard, "Large scale genetics in a small vertebrate, the zebrafish," *International Journal of Developmental Biology*, vol. 40, no. 1, pp. 221–227, 1996.

[10] S. Bertrand, B. Thisse, R. Tavares et al., "Unexpected novel relational links uncovered by extensive developmental profiling of nuclear receptor expression," *PLoS Genetics*, vol. 3, no. 11, pp. 2085–2100, 2007.

[11] S. Bertrand, F. G. Brunet, H. Escriva, G. Parmentier, V. Laudet, and M. Robinson-Rechavi, "Evolutionary genomics of nuclear receptors: from twenty-five ancestral genes to derived endocrine systems," *Molecular Biology and Evolution*, vol. 21, no. 10, pp. 1923–1937, 2004.

[12] M. Schubert, F. Brunet, M. Paris, S. Bertrand, G. Benoit, and V. Laudet, "Nuclear hormone receptor signaling in amphioxus," *Development Genes and Evolution*, vol. 218, no. 11-12, pp. 651–665, 2008.

[13] J. H. Oppenheimer, D. Koerner, H. L. Schwartz, and M. I. Surks, "Specific nuclear triiodothyronine binding sites in rat liver and kidney," *Journal of Clinical Endocrinology and Metabolism*, vol. 35, no. 2, pp. 330–333, 1972.

[14] H. H. Samuels and J. S. Tsai, "Thyroid hormone action. Demonstration of similar receptors in isolated nuclei of rat liver and cultured GH_1 cells," *Journal of Clinical Investigation*, vol. 53, no. 2, pp. 656–659, 1974.

[15] D. Bellabarba and J. G. Lehoux, "Triiodothyronine nuclear receptor in chick embryo: nature and properties of hepatic receptor," *Endocrinology*, vol. 109, no. 4, pp. 1017–1025, 1981.

[16] D. Bellabarba, S. Bédard, S. Fortier, and J. G. Lehoux, "3,5,3'-triiodothyronine nuclear receptor in chick embryo. Properties and ontogeny of brain and lung receptors," *Endocrinology*, vol. 112, no. 1, pp. 353–359, 1983.

[17] M. A. Haidar and P. K. Sarkar, "Ontogeny, regional distribution and properties of thyroid-hormone receptors in the developing chick brain," *Biochemical Journal*, vol. 220, no. 2, pp. 547–552, 1984.

[18] J. Sap, A. Muñoz, and K. Damm, "The c-erb-A protein is a high-affinity receptor for thyroid hormone," *Nature*, vol. 324, no. 6098, pp. 635–640, 1986.

[19] C. Weinberger, C. C. Thompson, and E. S. Ong, "The c-erb-A gene encodes a thyroid hormone receptor," *Nature*, vol. 324, no. 6098, pp. 641–646, 1986.

[20] B. Vennstrom, "Isolation and characterization of chicken DNA homologous to the two putative oncogenes of avian erythroblastosis virus," *Cell*, vol. 28, no. 1, pp. 135–143, 1982.

[21] D. Forrest, M. Sjoberg, and B. Vennstrom, "Contrasting developmental and tissue-specific expression of α and β thyroid hormone receptor genes," *EMBO Journal*, vol. 9, no. 5, pp. 1519–1528, 1990.

[22] M. O. Showers, D. S. Darling, G. D. Kieffer, and W. W. Chin, "Isolation and characterization of a cDNA encoding a chicken β thyroid hormone receptor," *DNA and Cell Biology*, vol. 10, no. 3, pp. 211–221, 1991.

[23] M. Sjoberg, B. Vennstrom, and D. Forrest, "Thyroid hormone receptors in chick retinal development: differential expression of mRNAs for α and N-terminal variant β receptors," *Development*, vol. 114, no. 1, pp. 39–47, 1992.

[24] M. Sjöberg and B. Vennstrom, "Ligand-dependent and -independent transactivation by thyroid hormone receptor β2 is determined by the structure of the hormone response element," *Molecular and Cellular Biology*, vol. 15, no. 9, pp. 4718–4726, 1995.

[25] C.N. Walpita, *The use of zebrafish (Danio rerio) as a model organism to study the role of thyroid hormone in embryonic development of teleost fish*, Ph.D. thesis, K.U.Leuven, 2008.

[26] J. J. Essner, J. J. Breuer, R. D. Essner, S. C. Fahrenkrug, and P. B. Hackett, "The zebrafish thyroid hormone receptor α1 is expressed during early embryogenesis and can function in transcriptional repression," *Differentiation*, vol. 62, no. 3, pp. 107–117, 1997.

[27] Y. W. Liu, L. J. Lo, and W. K. Chan, "Temporal expression and T3 induction of thyroid hormone receptors α1 and β1 during early embryonic and larval development in zebrafish, Danio rerio," *Molecular and Cellular Endocrinology*, vol. 159, no. 1-2, pp. 187–195, 2000.

[28] O. Marchand, R. Safi, H. Escriva, E. Van Rompaey, P. Prunet, and V. Laudet, "Molecular cloning and characterization of thyroid hormone receptors in teleost fish," *Journal of Molecular Endocrinology*, vol. 26, no. 1, pp. 51–65, 2001.

[29] I. Jones, M. Srinivas, L. Ng, and D. Forrest, "The thyroid hormone receptor β gene: structure and functions in the brain and sensory systems," *Thyroid*, vol. 13, no. 11, pp. 1057–1068, 2003.

[30] E. R. Nelson and H. R. Habibi, "Molecular characterization and sex-related seasonal expression of thyroid receptor subtypes in goldfish," *Molecular and Cellular Endocrinology*, vol. 253, no. 1-2, pp. 83–95, 2006.

[31] D. M. Power, L. Llewellyn, M. Faustino et al., "Thyroid hormones in growth and development of fish," *Comparative Biochemistry and Physiology C*, vol. 130, no. 4, pp. 447–459, 2001.

[32] S. Takayama, U. Hostick, M. Haendel, J. Eisen, and B. Darimont, "An F-domain introduced by alternative splicing regulates activity of the zebrafish thyroid hormone receptor α," *General and Comparative Endocrinology*, vol. 155, no. 1, pp. 176–189, 2008.

[33] E. R. Nelson and H. R. Habibi, "Thyroid receptor subtypes: structure and function in fish," *General and Comparative Endocrinology*, vol. 161, no. 1, pp. 90–96, 2009.

[34] F. Flamant and J. Samarut, "Involvement of thyroid hormone and its α receptor in avian neurulation," *Developmental Biology*, vol. 197, no. 1, pp. 1–11, 1998.

[35] D. Hentzen, A. Renucci, D. le Guellec et al., "The chicken c-erbA proto-oncogene is preferentially expressed in erythrocytic cells during late stages of differentiation," *Molecular and Cellular Biology*, vol. 7, no. 7, pp. 2416–2424, 1987.

[36] D. Forrest, F. Hallböök, H. Persson, and B. Vennstrom, "Distinct functions for thyroid hormone receptors α and β in brain development indicated by differential expression of receptor genes," *EMBO Journal*, vol. 10, no. 2, pp. 269–275, 1991.

[37] S. V. H. Grommen, B. De Groef, E. R. Kühn, and V. M. Darras, "The use of real-time PCR to study the expression of thyroid hormone receptor β2 in the developing chicken," *Annals of the New York Academy of Sciences*, vol. 1040, pp. 328–331, 2005.

[38] S. V. H. Grommen, L. Arckens, T. Theuwissen, V. M. Darras, and B. De Groef, "Thyroid hormone receptor β2 is strongly up-regulated at all levels of the hypothalamo-pituitary-thyroidal axis during late embryogenesis in chicken," *Journal of Endocrinology*, vol. 196, no. 3, pp. 519–528, 2008.

[39] Y. W. Liu and W. K. Chan, "Thyroid hormones are important for embryonic to larval transitory phase in zebrafish," *Differentiation*, vol. 70, no. 1, pp. 36–45, 2002.

[40] B. Thisse et al., ZFIN database, http://zfin.org/cgi-bin/web-driver?MIval=aa-ZDB_home.apg.

[41] E. Decuypere, E. Dewil, and E. R. Kühn, "The hatching process and the role of hormones," in *Avian Incubation*, S. G. Tullett, Ed., pp. 239–256, Butterworth & Heineman, London, UK, 1990.

[42] P. J. O'Shea and G. R. Williams, "Insight into the physiological actions of thyroid hormone receptors from genetically modified mice," *Journal of Endocrinology*, vol. 175, no. 3, pp. 553–570, 2002.

[43] S. Y. Cheng, "Isoform-dependent actions of thyroid hormone nuclear receptors: lessons from knockin mutant mice," *Steroids*, vol. 70, no. 5–7, pp. 450–454, 2005.

[44] F. Flamant and L. Quignodon, "Use of a new model of transgenic mice to clarify the respective functions of thyroid hormone receptors in vivo," *Heart Failure Reviews*, vol. 15, no. 2, pp. 117–120, 2010.

[45] S. L. J. Van Herck, S. Geysens, P. Tylzanowski, and V. M. Darras, "Ontogeny of thyroid hormone transport and deiodination in the early chicken brain," submitted to *Endocrinology*.

[46] F. Lezoualc'h, A. Hassan, H. Abdel-Tawab, J. Puymirat, and B. A. Demeneix, "Precocious auto-induction of thyroid hormone receptors in embryonic chick hypothalamic neurons," *Neuroscience Letters*, vol. 180, no. 2, pp. 197–202, 1994.

[47] A. H. Conrad, Y. Zhang, A. R. Walker et al., "Thyroxine affects expression of KSPG-related genes, the carbonic anhydrase II gene, and KS sulfation in the embryonic chicken cornea," *Investigative Ophthalmology and Visual Science*, vol. 47, no. 1, pp. 120–132, 2006.

[48] E.D. Abel, R. S. Ahima, M. E. Boers, J. K. Elmquist, and F. E. Wondisford, "Critical role for thyroid hormone receptor β2 in the regulation of paraventricular thyrotropin-releasing hormone neurons," *Journal of Clinical Investigation*, vol. 107, no. 8, pp. 1017–1023, 2001.

[49] E. D. Abel, E. G. Moura, R. S. Ahima et al., "Dominant inhibition of thyroid hormone action selectively in the pituitary of thyroid hormone-receptor-β null mice abolishes the regulation of thyrotropin by thyroid hormone," *Molecular Endocrinology*, vol. 17, no. 9, pp. 1767–1776, 2003.

[50] F. Lezoualc'h, A. H. S. Hassan, P. Giraud, J. P. Loeffler, S. L. Lee, and B. A. Demeneix, "Assignment of the β-thyroid hormone receptor to 3,5,3'-triiodothyronine- dependent inhibition of transcription from the thyrotropin-releasing hormone promoter in chick hypothalamic neurons," *Molecular Endocrinology*, vol. 6, no. 11, pp. 1797–1804, 1992.

[51] J. J. Essner, R. G. Johnson, and P. B. Hackett, "Overexpression of thyroid hormone receptor α1 during zebrafish embryogenesis disrupts hindbrain patterning and implicates retinoic acid receptors in the control of hox gene expression," *Differentiation*, vol. 65, no. 1, pp. 1–11, 1999.

[52] C. N. Walpita, A. D. Crawford, E. D. R. Janssens, S. Van Der Geyten, and V. M. Darras, "Type 2 Iodothyronine deiodinase is essential for thyroid hormone-dependent embryonic development and pigmentation in zebrafish," *Endocrinology*, vol. 150, no. 1, pp. 530–539, 2009.

12

MicroRNA Role in Thyroid Cancer Development

Francesca Marini, Ettore Luzi, and Maria Luisa Brandi

Unit of Metabolic Bone Diseases, Department of Internal Medicine, University of Florence, Viale Pieraccini 6, 50139 Florence, Italy

Correspondence should be addressed to Maria Luisa Brandi, m.brandi@dmi.unifi.it

Academic Editor: Daniel Christophe

MicroRNAs (miRNAs) are endogenous noncoding RNAs that negatively regulate gene expression by binding the 3′ noncoding region of the messenger RNA targets inducing their cleavage or blocking the protein translation. They play important roles in multiple biological and metabolic processes, including developmental timing, signal transduction, and cell maintenance and differentiation. Their deregulation can predispose to diseases and cancer. miRNA expression has been demonstrated to be deregulated in many types of human tumors, including thyroid cancers, and could be responsible for tumor initiation and progression. In this paper we reviewed the available data on miRNA deregulation in different thyroid tumors and describe the putative role of miRNA in thyroid cancer development.

1. Introduction

MicroRNAs (miRNAs) are endogenous single-stranded non-coding RNAs of about 22 nucleotides which suppress gene expression by selectively binding to the complementary 3′ untranslated region (3′-UTR) of messenger RNAs (mRNAs) through base-pairing. They play important roles in multiple biological and metabolic processes, such as cell differentiation, proliferation, and survival. Presently, miRNAs are considered one of the most important regulators of gene expression at posttranscriptional level, and it has been estimated that over one third of all human genes could be targeted by miRNAs [1]. Moreover, miRNAs are strongly conserved even among different species, strengthening the hypothesis of their important roles in many essential biological processes.

Recent studies have also supported a role of miRNAs in the initiation and progression of human malignancies. The analysis of global miRNA expression in cancer patients showed different patterns of miRNA overexpression or downregulation in cancer versus normal tissues [2] in several human tumors, such as colorectal neoplasia [3], B cell chronic lymphocytic leukaemia [4, 5], B cell lymphoma [6], lung cancer [7], breast cancer [8], and glioblastoma [9, 10]. The involvement of miRNAs in human cancer is probably due to the fact that >50% of miRNA genes are located at chromosomal fragile sites or common break point sites or within regions of deletion or amplification that are generally altered in human tumors [11]. The deregulation of miRNA expression is suspected to be an important regulator of tumor development and progression in several human tissues. The overexpression of specific miRNAs could lead to the repression of tumor suppressor gene expression, and conversely the downregulation of specific miRNAs could result in an increase of oncogene expression; both these situations induce subsequent malignant effects on cell proliferation, differentiation, and apoptosis that lead to tumor growth and progress.

Experimental evidence demonstrated that the majority of miRNAs present lower expression levels in tumors compared to normal tissues, independent of the cell type. Global miRNA expression is higher in normal tissues compared to their tumoral counterparts or to cancer cell lines. In addition, poorly differentiated tumors present a lower global level of miRNA expression compared to more differentiated tumors [12]. All these data are consistent with the hypothesis that a higher global miRNA expression is associated with cellular differentiation. The reduction of global miRNA expression may reduce cell differentiation that is the hallmark of all human cancers.

2. miRNA Transcription, Maturation, and Mechanisms of Action

miRNAs are transcribed as long, poly-adenylated, and capped primary transcripts (pri-miRNAs) that are cleaved, at nuclear level, to ~60–70 nucleotide hairpin-shaped intermediates (pre-miRNAs) by the nuclear RNase III Drosha [13]. Following nuclear processing by Drosha, pre-miRNAs are exported to the cytoplasm by the nuclear transport receptor exportin-5 [14]. At cytoplasmic level pre-miRNAs are processed into ~22 nucleotide miRNA duplexes by the cytoplasmic RNase III Dicer [15]. These double-stranded products are unwound by a still unidentified helicase and incorporated as single-stranded RNAs (guide strand) into a ribonucleoprotein complex, known as the RNA-induced silencing complex (RISC) [16]. Which of the two RNA strands is incorporated in the RISC is determined by the stability of the base pairs at the 5′ end of the duplex; the other strand is degraded. The incorporate guide strand leads the RISC to the complementary sequence in the 3′-UTR of target mRNA, negatively regulating gene expression at the posttranscriptional level by targeting the 3′-UTR region of the mRNAs. Nucleotides 2–8 (referred to as "seed") of the mature miRNAs are evolutionary conserved and result in being crucial in determining target specificity. miRNAs can downregulate gene expression by two distinct posttranscriptional mechanisms: mRNA cleavage or translational repression. The choice of mechanism is determined only by the identity of the mRNA target and the degree of miRNA-mRNA complementarity: miRNA will specify induce the cleavage of mRNA if the target has sufficient complementarity to the miRNA itself, or it will repress translation if the mRNA does not have sufficient complementarity [17, 18] (Figure 1). In the first case miRNA may act as small interfering RNAs (siRNAs) and it cleaves mRNA targets between the nucleotides pairing to positions 10 and 11 of the miRNA [19, 20]; after the cleavage of the target the miRNA remains intact and can guide the recognition and destruction of other mRNAs [17]. Conversely, the reduced complementarity between miRNA and its target mRNA generally creates mismatches and bulges in the central region of the miRNA-mRNA duplex (at positions 10–12 of the mature miRNA sequence) that prevent the siRNA-like cleavage of target mRNA. miRNA-mediated translational repression can be regulated both at initiation level or at postinitiation level of the translation process. In the initiation block the RISC complex inhibits translation by interfering with eIEF4F-cap recognition and 40S small ribosomal subunit recruit or by preventing the assembly of the 60S subunit to form the 80S ribosomal complex. In the postinitial block RISC may inhibit ribosome elongation, inducing ribosome drop-off or facilitating proteolysis of the nascent polypeptides [21].

Recently, it has been hypothesized a role of miRNAs in the upregulation of protein translation. A recent study [22] showed that miR-369-3 linked the AU-rich elements (AREs) of the TNFα mRNA to upregulate translation, through direct base pairing between miR-369-3 "seed" region and complementary ARE regions, under cell cycle arrest conditions. The authors hypothesized that miRNAs may switch between translation repression or activation based on cell cycle status: in proliferating cells they repress translation while under cell cycle arrest they promote translation.

Another study [23] indicated a possible role of miRNAs in positive activation of translation. The authors found that miR-10a interacted with the 5′ untranslated region (5′-UTR) of the mRNAs encoding ribosomal proteins to enhance their translation. Moreover, miR-10a resulted in being capable of both translation repression through 3′-UTR binding or of translation promotion via 5′-UTR binding of different mRNA targets. These data suggest that the same miRNA may exert different effects depending on the site of interaction with its targets.

3. Identification of miRNA Targets

Identification of miRNA targets and of their specific interaction sites is fundamental in the comprehension of miRNA roles in the regulation of biological processes as well as in the development of human malignancies.

Some algorithms, such as miRanda (http://www.microrna.org/microrna/home.do), TargetScan (http://www.targetscan.org/), or PicTar (http://pictar.mdc-berlin.de/), have been developed for the computational prediction of miRNA targets. All these bioinformatic predictions are primarily based, and limited, on conserved interactions involving the miRNA "seed" region and the 3′-UTRs of target mRNAs. A limitation of these prediction programs is that they are not able to reveal novel aspects of miRNA target recognition. False-positive predictions can be eliminated by experimental validation studies but false-negative predictions remain often unsolved.

Experimental approaches to miRNA target identification have mainly focused on analyses of both transcriptome and proteome expression arrays in cells in which a single miRNA has been overexpressed or inhibited. Effects on endogenous target protein levels serve as a good indicator to validate the miRNA-target interaction. However, this approach suffers from a limitation: in fact when a miRNA is introduced, by transfection, in high concentrations into a cell, this may effect the observed effect on target mRNA and generate false-positive results, since the level of translation repression is strongly dependent not only on miRNA and mRNA target complementarity but also on both the amount of target mRNA and the amount of available miRNA in the cell [24].

A direct evidence that a miRNA binds a specific target mRNA can be obtained by formaldehyde cross-linking of the miRNA to its targets [22] or by 4-thiouridine-modified miRNAs [23], both these techniques allow the subsequent mapping of the exact site of binding using primer extension.

4. miRNA Deregulation in Thyroid Tumors

Thyroid tumors represent a good model for studying multi-step cancer development in epithelial cells as they comprise a range of lesions with different degrees of malignancy: from benign differentiated and noninvasive adenomas to malignant undifferentiated anaplastic invasive carcinomas.

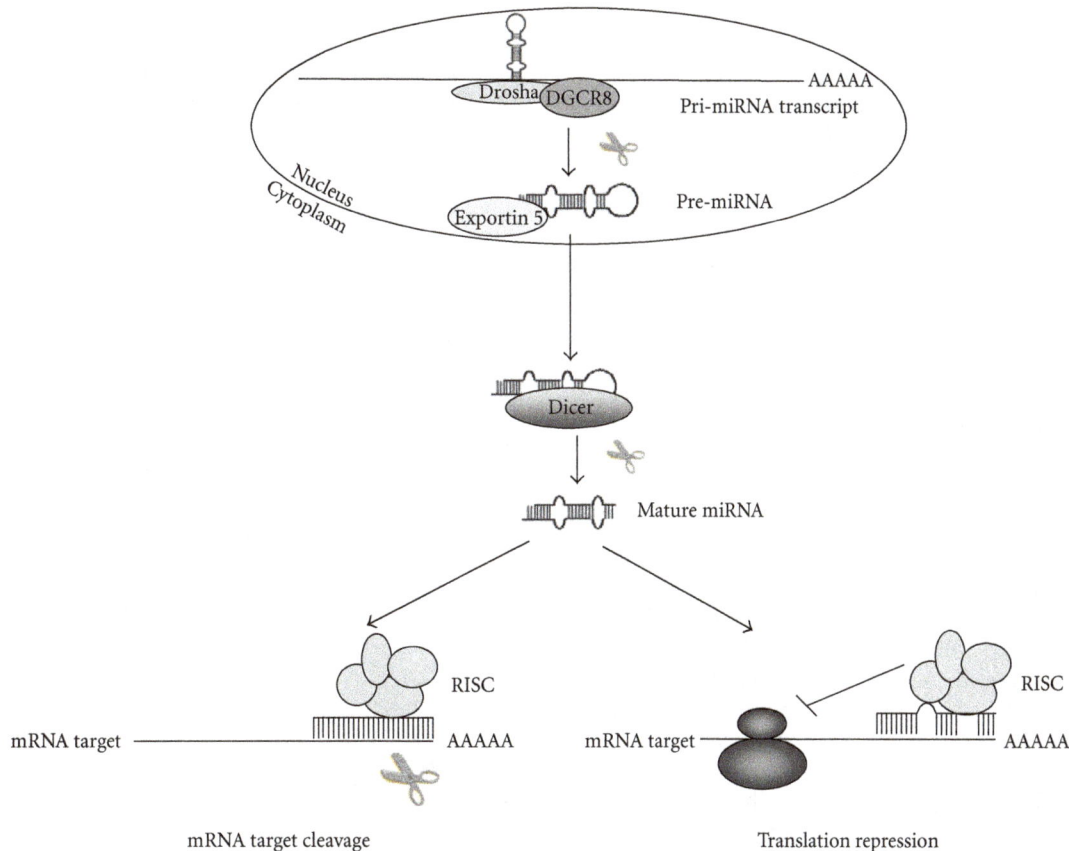

FIGURE 1: Model for miRNA biogenesis and functional mechanisms. miRNA genes are transcribed by RNA polymerase II (pol II) into primary transcripts (pri-miRNAs) that are cleaved by the Drosha-DGCR8 complex to 60–70 nt pre-miRNAs. Pre-miRNAs are then transported to the cytoplasm by exportin-5 and there processed by the endonuclease Dicer to generate a double-stranded mature miRNA of about 21–23 nt. After a strand selection/separation process, the mature miRNA is incorporated into the RISC complex while the other strand is degraded. RISC complex will recognize and mediate cleavage or repression of specific mRNAs.

The two most common thyroid tumors are papillary thyroid carcinoma (PTC) and follicular thyroid carcinoma (FTC), accounting, respectively, for about 80% and 15% of all cases, both well differentiated and originating from thyroid follicular cells. PTCs are often multifocal, characterized by classical papillary architecture, and they usually metastasize to the regional lymph nodes. FTCs are often unifocal, encapsulated, and they usually metastasize via the vascular system to lungs and bones. Both these tumors may progress to poorly differentiated carcinoma or to completely nondifferentiated anaplastic carcinoma. Anaplastic thyroid carcinomas (ATCs) are very rare thyroid cancers (2–5% of all cases), extremely undifferentiated and highly aggressive. Medullary thyroid carcinoma (MTC) is a rare thyroid tumor, accounting for less than 5% of all thyroid cancers, that originates from the thyroid intrafollicular C cells.

Several independent studies have analyzed miRNA expression in numerous and different types of thyroid tumors, evidencing a miRNA deregulation in cancer tissues compared to their normal counterparts [25–38]; in thyroid tumors 32% of all known human miRNAs resulted in being upregulated and 38% to be downregulated with more than a 2-fold change as compared to normal tissues [39]. Moreover,

the miRNA expression profile presents a significant variability between different kinds of thyroid cancers, even if they originate from the same type of thyroid cells [25, 39]. C-cell-derived MTC has a miRNA expression profile significantly different from those of thyroid tumors originating from follicular cells; but also papillary carcinomas, conventional follicular adenomas and carcinomas, and oncocytic follicular adenomas and carcinomas, all originating from follicular cells, show different and specific miRNA expression profiles. At the moment the exact biological roles of miRNAs in thyroid carcinogenesis remain to be fully elucidated but it seems reasonable that the distinctive pattern of miRNA expression in thyroid tumors compared to normal thyroid tissue may be useful in diagnosis and/or therapy of thyroid neoplasia and that different miRNA expression patterns in different types of thyroid tumors could be useful tools for their classification.

However, the majority of miRNA profiling studies do not provide an estimate of miRNA abundance in normal thyroid tissues and in thyroid tumors. Today, it is recognized that only the most abundantly expressed miRNAs are able to occupy a substantial fraction of their mRNA targets, affecting their translation. The magnitude of translation repression is strongly dependent on the number of miRNA-RISC complexes with respect to the amount of target mRNA molecules. It is hypothesizable that, among all the misregulated miRNAs, only those which are abundantly overexpressed or strongly downregulated are involved in thyroid tumorigenesis. The most abundantly expressed miRNAs in human healthy thyroid gland are listed in Table 1; data are derived from http://www.mirz.unibas.ch/cloningprofiles/ using the "visualization of miRNA expression profiles" tool.

5. The Role of MicroRNAs in Papillary Thyroid Carcinoma

Some studies analyzed the miRNA expression profile in PTCs [26–32] (Table 2).

Comparing global miRNA expression in human PTCs versus unaffected thyroid tissue He et al. [26] individuated a set of five miRNAs (miR-146, miR-221, miR-222, miR-21, and miR-181a) that were significantly overexpressed in PTCs compared to the adjacent normal tissue. Particularly, three of them, miR-146, miR-221, and miR-222, showed 11- to 19-fold higher level in tumor tissues. The probe sequence of miR-146 used in the miRNA array chip was designed for miR-146a isoform, located on human chromosome 5. Recently a second isoform, named miR-146b, has been described on human chromosome 10. These two miRNAs differ only for two nucleotides in the sequence of their mature forms. Using primers for premature forms of miR-146a and miR-146b, no expression of miR-146a was detected in thyroid tissues by RT-PCR analysis, while a significant overexpression of miR-146b was found in PTC tumor samples as confirmed also by Northern blot for mature miR-146b. Deregulation of miR-146b, miR-221, and miR-222 in the thyroid may be a crucial component of PTC initiation and development. The putative target of these miRNAs was suspected to be KIT, a tyrosine kinase receptor that plays an important role in cell growth and differentiation, acting as an oncogene in many cancers [41, 42]. Nevertheless, neoplastic transformation has been shown to be associated with either overexpression or downregulation of c-KIT in different tissues [43–45]. In PTC tissues in which miR-146b, miR-221, and miR-222 were strongly overexpressed there was a downregulation of KIT transcript and KIT protein. In 50% of cases the reduced expression of KIT was associated with germline single-nucleotide changes in both the two recognition sites of KIT for miR-221 and miR-222 (3′-UTR region of KIT) and for miR-146b (exon 18 of KIT). In conclusion, the upregulation of these five specific miRNAs, and particularly of miR-146b, miR-221, and miR-222, and the subsequent downregulation of KIT seem to be involved in PTC pathogenesis, and sequence changes in miRNA target genes can contribute to their regulation.

c-KIT is frequently expressed in benign thyroid adenomas and goiters, while its expression results in being lowered in about 60% of FTCs and completely absent in PTCs and ATCs. Moreover, the absence of c-KIT expression has been demonstrated also in metastases from primary thyroid tumors, indicating that the modulation of this tyrosine

TABLE 1: Most abundantly expressed miRNAs in human healthy thyroid gland. The table reports the most abundantly expressed miRNAs in human normal thyroid gland; data are derived from http://www.mirz.unibas.ch/cloningprofiles/. The tool screened a total of 768 human miRNAs. Only miRNAs with an abundance value over 3.0 have been reported in the table.

miRNA	Abundance value in thyroid gland
let-7b	56.0
let-7a	52.0
miR-143	47.0
miR-126	39.0
let-7i	32.5
let-7c	29.5
miR-125b	29.0
miR-16	27.0
miR-200c	24.5
miR-26a	23.6666666
let-7f	21.5
miR-23b	16.0
miR-24	14.0
miR-99a	13.0
miR-29a	12.0
miR-30d	12.0
miR-451	12.0
miR-23a	11.0
miR-15a	9.0
miR-27b	9.0
miR-30c	9.0
miR-21	8.0
miR-27a	8.0
miR-30a	8.0
miR-100	8.0
miR-191	8.0
let-7e	7.0
let-7g	6.0
miR-99b	6.0
miR-125a-5p	6.0
miR-145	6.0
miR-195	5.0
let-7d	4.0
miR-25	4.0
miR-206	4.0
miR-10b	3.0
miR-22	3.0
miR-138	3.0
miR-152	3.0
miR-423-3p	3.0

kinase receptor is not dependent on the thyroid microenvironment but is associated to the transformed malignant cell phenotype [46]. To date, the biological significance of loss of c-KIT in thyroid tumors is not elucidated. Surprisingly, the depletion of c-KIT expression in thyroid tumors in contrast with the gain of function of other tyrosine kinase

TABLE 2: Studies of deregulation of miRNA expression profile in thyroid tumors. The table reports a list of published studies on the deregulation of miRNA expression profile in different kinds of thyroid tumors. Type of analyzed thyroid samples, used analysis methods and individuated upregulated or downregulated miRNAs in thyroid tumors are depicted in the table.

Thyroid tumor type	Analyzed samples	Methods	Tumor upregulated miRNAs	Tumor downregulated miRNAs	Reference
PTC	20 fresh PTC tissues versus 20 normal adjacent normal thyroid tissues	Global miRNA microarray, quantitative RT-PCR and Northern blots	miR-146b, miR-221, and miR-222	—	He et al. [26]
PTC	30 fresh PTC tissues versus 10 normal thyroid tissues	Global miRNA microarray, quantitative RT-PCR, and Northern blots	miR-181b, miR-221, and miR-222	—	Pallante et al. [27]
PTC	20 formalin-fixed paraffin-embedded PTC tissues versus 20 formalin-fixed paraffin-embedded multinodular goiter	Global miRNA microarray and quantitative RT-PCR	miR-21, miR-31, miR-34a, miR-172, miR-181a, miR-181b, miR-213, miR-221, miR-222, miR-223, and miR-224	miR-19b-1,2, miR-30a-5p, miR-30c, miR-130b, miR-145sh, miR-218, miR-292-as, miR-300, and miR-345	Tetzlaff et al. [28]
PTC versus non-PTC	84 formalin-fixed paraffin-embedded tissues and 40 ex vivo aspirate specimens of PTC and non-PTC tumors (follicular adenoma, follicular carcinoma hyperplastic nodules)	Quantitative RT-PCR	miR-146b, miR-221, and miR-222	—	Chen et al. [29]
PTC	28 BRAF mutated PTC tissues versus 26 BRAF wild-type PTC tissues	Quantitative RT-PCR	No difference between mutated and nonmutated PTC	No difference between mutated and nonmutated PTC	Sheu et al. [31]
PTC	100 PTC tissues versus 16 paired normal thyroid control	Quantitative RT-PCR	miR-146b, miR-221, and miR-222	—	Chou et al. [32]
PTC	2 PTC cell lines bearing a RET mutation versus normal thyroid cell lines	Global miRNA microarray	miR-34a, miR-96, miR-99a, miR-100, miR-125b, miR-128b, miR-130b, miR-139, miR-141, miR-142-3p, miR-146, miR-148, miR-185, miR-200a, miR-200b, miR-211, miR-213, miR-216, and let-7d	miR-15a, miR-34c, miR-107, miR-127, miR-135b, miR-145, miR-149, miR-154, miR-181a, miR-218, miR-299, miR-302b, miR-302c, miR-323, and miR-370	Cahill et al. [40]

TABLE 2: Continued.

Thyroid tumor type	Analyzed samples	Methods	Tumor upregulated miRNAs	Tumor downregulated miRNAs	Reference
FTC	22 FTC samples versus 20 FA and 4 normal control thyroid tissues	Global miRNA microarray and quantitative RT-PCR	miR-192, miR-197, miR-328, and miR-346	—	Weber et al. [33]
FTC PTC, other thyroid tumor variants	A 60-fresh-thyroid tumor and normal samples (23 PTCs, 9 FTCs, 8 FAs, 4 ATCs, 4 poorly differentiated carcinomas, 2 MTCs, 5 hyperplastic nodules, and 5 normal thyroid tissues) and 62 fine-needle aspiration samples	Quantitative RT-PCR	PTC: miR-31, miR-122a, miR-146b, miR-155, miR-187, miR-205, miR-221, miR-222, and miR-224 Conventional FA: miR-190, miR-205, miR-210, miR-224, miR-328, miR-339, and miR-342 Oncocytic FA: miR-31, miR-183, miR-203, miR-221, miR-224, and miR-339 Conventional FTC: miR-146b, miR-155, miR-187, miR-221, miR-222, and miR-224 Oncocytic FTC: miR-183, miR-187, miR-197, miR-221, miR-222, and miR-339 Poorly differentiated carcinomas: miR-129, miR-146b, miR-183, miR-187, miR-221, miR-222, and miR-339 ATC: miR-137, miR-155, miR-187, miR-205, miR-214, miR-221, miR-222, and miR-224 MTC: miR-9, miR-10a, miR-124a, miR-127, miR-129, miR-137, miR-154, miR-224, miR-323, and miR-370	—	Nikiforova et al. [25]
ATC	ATC tissues versus normal thyroid tissues	Global miRNA microarray, quantitative RT-PCR, Northern blots, and in situ hybridization	—	miR-26a, miR-30a-5p, miR-30d, and miR-125b	Visone et al. [34]
ATC	10 ATC and 5 FTC cell lines, 3 ATC and 8 PTC tissues versus normal thyroid samples	Quantitative RT-PCR	miR-21, miR-146b, miR-221, and miR-222	miR-26a, miR-138, miR-219, and miR-345	Mitomo et al. [38]
ATC	ATC cell lines and ATC cancer lesions versus normal thyroid tissues	Global miRNA microarray, quantitative RT-PCR, and Northern blots	miR-17-3p, miR-17-5p, miR-18a, miR-19a, miR-19b, miR-20a, and miR-92-1	—	Takakura et al. [37]
ATC	ATC tissues versus PTC and FTC tissues	Global miRNA microarray and quantitative RT-PCR	—	miR-30 and miR-200	Braun et al. [35]

receptors such as c-RET and c-MET or of oncogenes such as *c-RAS*, suggesting that different tyrosine kinase receptor signaling pathways may exert opposite biological effects in a given cell type, alternatively controlling mitogenesis or cell differentiation. It is hypothesizable that, in thyroid tissue, the c-KIT signaling pathway may control some aspects of the thyrocyte differentiation rather than cell proliferation.

Pallante et al. [27] analyzed the global miRNA expression profile in 30 human PTCs versus 10 normal thyroid tissues using a microarray chip containing 368 human precursor and mature miRNA oligonucleotide probes, accounting for 245 human and mouse miRNA genes and including all the three miR-181 human isoforms (miR-181a, miR-181b, and miR-181c). The analysis revealed an altered miRNA expression profile that distinguished PTCs from normal thyroid tissues: five miRNAs (miR-221, miR-222, miR-213, miR-220, and miR-181b) were overexpressed in the neoplastic tissues. However, a recent work by Chiang et al. [47] strongly suggested that miR-220 is not a miRNA, and miR-213 is not recognized as a miRNA in the miRNA database (http://www.mirbase.org/). The study of Pallante et al. found that miR-221, miR-222, and miR-181b resulted in being abundantly expressed in PTCs, while their expression was only weakly detectable in the healthy thyroid tissues, with the overexpression of miR-221 reaching up to 70-fold increase. overexpression of miR-181b has been also confirmed by quantitative RT-PCR analysis using a couple of primers specifically designed for precursor of the miR-181b isoform to exclude a false-positive result for miR-181b, due to possible cross-hybridization of probes for the miR-181a and miR-181c isoforms in the microarray chip. The authors also demonstrated that miR-221 and miR-222 downregulated the level of c-KIT in PTCs confirming data previously published [41]. In addition, a human thyroid carcinoma cell line transfected with a vector over-expressing miR-221 showed a significant increase of cell growth, and, conversely, the inhibition of miR-221 function by antisense oligonucleotide transfection in the same cell line resulted in a significant reduction of cell growth [27]. The results of these functional studies, together with the previously reported expression data, suggest a critical role of miR-221 in thyroid carcinoma cell growth and, thus, probably in the process of papillary thyroid carcinogenesis.

A study of Tetzlaff et al. [28] analyzed global miRNA expression profile by microarray chip (including known miRNAs from human, mouse, rat, and predicted/candidate human miRNAs) in a series of PTC formalin-fixed paraffin-embedded (FFPE) samples versus benign proliferative multinodular goiters (MNGs). The analysis revealed a set of 13 upregulated miRNAs and a set of 26 downregulated miRNAs. Misregulation has been validated by real-time RT-PCR, in an independent series of tumoral tissues, only for miR-21, miR-31, miR-221, and miR-222, with miR-221 and miR-222 showing a strong upregulation in PTCs compared to independent set of MNGs. Data from this study confirmed miR-221 and miR-222 to be altered in PTCs, as previously described in fresh tissue analyses [26, 27] and, mostly, supported the possibility to use FFPE tumor tissues to analyze miRNA expression when fresh tissues are not

available or to perform retrospective studies. The author demonstrated the possibility to extract sufficient miRNA from FFPE tissues using a miRNA labeling method for total RNA extracts (All Total Nucleid Acid Isolation SyStem, Ambion) that bypassed the need for miRNA enrichment and reduced the amount of starting samples, followed by an ammonium acetate/ethanol precipitation.

A recent study by Chen et al. [29] analyzed the expression of a selected set of miRNAs by quantitative RT-PCR in PTCs, non-PTC lesions (follicular adenoma, follicular carcinoma hyperplastic nodules), and normal thyroid tissue. They evidenced an overexpression of miR-146b, miR-221, and miR-222 in PTCs compared to both non-PTC group and healthy controls, but with miR-221 and miR-222 presenting a substantial overlap between different tumor groups. The authors concluded that the expression analysis of miR-221 and miR-222 cannot be resolving in distinguishing PTCs from other tumoral lesions. Conversely, miR-146b resulted in being consistently and specifically overexpressed in classical PTCs, suggesting this miRNA as a possible diagnostic tool to identify PTCs from other thyroid tumors. Putative targets of miR-146b are the nuclear factor-κB (*NF-κB*), the interleukin-1 receptor-associated kinase 1 (*IRAK1*), and the tumor necrosis factor receptor-associated factor 6 (*TRAF6*), whose role in thyroid carcinogenesis has not yet been elucidated.

Mutations of the *BRAF* gene are implicated in the pathogenesis of PTC through the constitutive activation of the MAPK pathway; classical PTCs are often *BRAF* mutation positive while follicular PTCs are almost always *BRAF* mutation negative [48]. Chen et al. [29] found also that miR146b overexpression is common both in classical and follicular variants of PTCs, independently by the *BRAF* mutation status, suggesting this overexpression as a late event in the PTC progression and probably important for the definition of a complete carcinoma phenotype. This result has been confirmed also by Sheu et al. [31] who analyzed, in a series of 221 PTCs, if the *BRAF V600E* mutational status was correlated to the miRNA expression profile. They found no difference in the expression of five miRNAs (miR-146b, miR-181b, miR-21, miR-221, and miR-222) between *BRAF* mutated PTCs and wild-type PTCs. In addition, this study confirmed the overexpression of miR-146b, miR-221, and miR-222 as a useful tool to diagnostic PTCs.

More recently, Chou et al. [32] measured the expression of miR-146b, miR-221, and miR-222 in 100 cases of PTCs finding that their expression levels were associated with extra-thyroidal invasion. In particular miR-146b resulted in being highly expressed in tumors with high risk features and with the *BRAF V600E* mutation.

Results from all these studies agreed with the fact that miR-221 and miR-222 are both overexpressed in PTCs compared to normal thyroid tissue. Functional analysis on miR-221 function in human PTC-derived cell lines indicated a direct role of this miRNA in PTC carcinogenesis. A vector-induced miR-221 overexpression in these cell lines resulted in a higher number of cell colonies compared to negative control transfected cells; conversely, the block of miR-221 function by antisense oligonucleotide caused a significant reduction in cell proliferation [27]. A subsequent study investigated which pathways or molecular targets were regulated by miR-221 and miR-222 [49]. Some bioinformatic programs suggested the *CDKN1B* (*p27^{kip1}*) gene, an important regulator of cell cycle that inhibits the initiation of the S phase, as the putative target of miR-221 and miR-222. This study demonstrated that miR-221 and miR-222 negatively regulate the p27^{kip1} protein levels in Hela cells and thyroid carcinoma cells by binding to two specific target sites in the 3′-UTR of the *p27^{kip1}* gene. Transfection of TPC-1, thyroid papillary carcinoma cell line, with vectors for the overexpression of miR-221 and miR-222 resulted in decreased p27^{kip1} protein levels. Conversely, inhibition of miR-221 and miR-222 expression by specific 2′-O-Me-221 and 2′-O-Me-222 antisense oligonucleotides increased the p27^{kip1} protein levels. In both transfection experiments no significant variation of p27^{kip1} mRNA expression was observed. Results from this study strongly suggested that the overexpression of miR-221 and miR-222 in tumor thyroid cells could be responsible for the posttranscriptional negative regulation of p27^{kip1} protein expression, inducing cells to enter the S phase of cell cycle and, thus, increasing cell growth.

The *RET* oncogene mutations occur in about 43% of PTCs [50], constitutively activating the MAPK signal and promoting carcinogenesis. These mutations are responsible for the deregulation of thyroid cell proliferation and differentiation and for cell tumoral transformation. Cahill et al. [40] investigated miRNA expression in two human PTC cell lines bearing a *RET* mutation, compared to normal thyroid cell lines, finding that 21 miRNAs were significantly overexpressed (miR-34a, miR-96, miR-99a, miR-100, miR-125b, miR-128b, miR-130b, miR-139, miR-141, miR-142-3p, miR-146, miR-148, miR-185, miR-200a, miR-200b, miR-211, miR-213, miR-216 and let-7d) and 14 miRNAs were downregulated (miR-15a, miR-34c, miR-107, miR-127, miR-135b, miR-145, miR-149, miR-154, miR-181a, miR-218, miR-299, miR-302b, miR-302c, miR-323, and miR-370) in tumor cell lines when compared to normal thyroid. These differentially expressed miRNAs potentially regulate genes involved in thyroid functions, and their deregulation could be implicated in thyroid carcinoma progression.

A functional study of Ricarte-Filho et al. [36] investigated the involvement of the let-7f miRNA, recently associated to RAS protein level reduction in lung tumor, in PTC development. The authors found that, in thyroid *RET*-mutated cell lines, the enhanced expression of *RET* oncogene reduced the expression of let-7f. The stable transfection of *RET*-mutated TPC-1 cell line with vector for the overexpression of let-7f inhibited the MAPK activation and reduced cell proliferation. In particular, let-7f increases the expression of thyroid cell differentiation markers such as the TITF1 transcription factor, a key factor in normal thyroid development, and, thus, let-7f is fundamental for the correct regulation of thyroid cell growth and differentiation and the reduced expression of let-7f in *RET*-mutated thyroid cells is responsible for cell dedifferentiation during PTC malignant progression. Interestingly, let-7f, together with the miRNA let-7 family, is one of the most expressed miRNAs in healthy thyroid gland (Table 1), further suggesting its crucial role in

normal thyroid development and functionality. All these data suggested let-7f acting as a tumor suppressor and indicated this miRNA as a potential therapeutic agent in patients with PTCs bearing a *RET* mutation.

6. The Role of MicroRNAs in Follicular Thyroid Carcinoma

Only two studies have analyzed the miRNA expression alteration in FTCs [25, 33] (Table 2).

In 2006 Weber et al. [33] investigated if miRNAs are differentially expressed between human follicular thyroid carcinomas (FTCs) and follicular adenomas (FAs) testing two high-density miRNA expression arrays on 23 FTCs versus 20 FA samples and 4 normal thyroid controls. Four miRNAs (miR-192, miR-197, miR-328, and miR-346) resulted in being overexpressed in FTCs compared to FAs. None of these miRNAs have previously been associated with other thyroid neoplasia and appear to be specific for FTC phenotype. Two of them, miR-197 and miR-346, have been validated also by quantitative real-time RT-PCR that confirmed their significant overexpression in carcinomas compared to adenomas and healthy tissue. These two miRNAs may participate in the transformation of follicular tumors from benign to malignant status, and they and their target genes may provide novel molecular markers to differentiate malignant (FTCs) from benign (FAs) follicular thyroid neoplasia. The effects of these two deregulated miRNAs have been functionally investigated using two human thyroid cancer cell lines, FTC133 and K5, a human papillary thyroid cancer cell line, NPA87, and a human embryonic kidney cell line, HEK293T as control. The induction of miR-197 and miR-346 overexpression induced cell proliferation *in vitro*, whereas their inhibition led to cell growth arrest in both FTC133 and K5 cell lines, but not in NPA87 cell line, confirming that the deregulation of miR-197 and miR-346 is a marker of FTC phenotype but not of PTC phenotype. *In silico* analyses indicated putative targets of miR-197 and miR-346 that have been validated also by *in vitro* functional analyses. *EFEMP2* (fibulin 4), a protein involved in stabilization and organization of extracellular matrix structures that exerts tumor suppressor functions [51, 52], is inhibited by miR-346 overexpression. Activin A receptor type 1 (*ACVR1*), a potent inhibitor of cell growth in several human cell types including thyroid epithelium [53], and tetraspanin 3 (*TSPAN3*), whose exact biological role in tumors is still unknown, are both downexpressed as a consequence of miR-197 overexpression. Moreover, the authors performed functional studies also on miR-221 and miR-222 demonstrating that they do not have a role in FTC tumorigenesis.

More recently, Nikiforov et al. [25] compared miRNA expression profiles of principal types of thyroid cancers, finding a distinctive expression pattern associated to follicular thyroid tumors: miR-155, miR-187, miR-221, miR-222, and miR-224 resulted in being highly overexpressed in conventional FTCs, while miR-183, miR-187, miR-197, miR-221, miR-222, and miR-339 were overexpressed in the FTC oncocytic variants.

7. The Role of MicroRNAs in Anaplastic Thyroid Carcinoma

Few studies have analyzed the miRNA expression profiles in ATCs [34, 35, 37, 38] (Table 2).

Visone et al. [34] analyzed the miRNA expression of ATCs using a miRNA microarray chip, finding a significant down-expression of miR-26a, miR-30a-5p, miR-30d, and miR-125b in ATCs compared to normal thyroid samples. These data have been further validated by quantitative RT-PCR, Northern blot analyses, and *in situ* hybridization. Induced overexpression of miR-26a and miR-125b in two human ATC-derived cell lines resulted in cell growth inhibition, suggesting a role of these two miRNAs in negative cell cycle regulation and that their downregulation could be involved in thyroid tumorigenesis. No effect on cell proliferation was observed after induction of miR-30d and miR-30a-5p overexpression in the same ATC-derived cell lines. miR-26a influences cell cycle progression by negatively regulating the expression of *EZH2* oncogene, an epigenetic gene silencer involved in neoplastic development. Recently, Sander et al. [54] suggested miR-26a acting as a potential tumor suppressor in MYC-induced tumors, since overexpression of miR-26a in murine lymphoma cell lines reduced cell proliferation by increasing the percentage of cells in G1 phase. miR-125b resulted in being deregulated in several human tumors, suggesting a role of miR-125b in human carcinogenesis [55–57]. An upregulation of miR-125b expression reduced the proliferation of the CD133-positive glioma cells and arrested the cell cycle at the G1/S transition level [58], through the downregulation of CDK6 and CDC25A, respectively, a cyclin-dependent kinase positively regulating the transition from the G0/G1 phase to the S phase of the cell cycle and a positive regulator of G1/S transition by dephosphorylation and activation of cyclin-CDK complexes. Both CDK6 and CDC25A have been previously reported to modulate the G1/S transition in human embryonic stem cells [59]. Recently, Liang et al. [60] demonstrated that miR-125b suppresses hepatocarcinoma cell proliferation both *in vitro* and *in vivo* and that this miRNA increases the expression of p21Cip1/Waf1, arresting cell cycle at the G1 phase.

Another study [38] examined the expression of miRNAs in ATC-derived cell lines versus PTC-derived cell lines as well as ATC tissue samples versus PTC tissue samples, finding that miR-21, miR-146b, miR-221, and miR-222 were overexpressed, while miR-26a, miR-138, miR-219, and miR-345 were downregulated in ATC cell lines and tissues. Moreover, since miR-138 resulted in being the unique miRNA that showed a different expression profile between ATCs and other follicular cell-derived thyroid tumors, the authors investigated its putative role in ATC tumorigenesis, demonstrating that miR-138 could directly target the human telomerase reverse transcriptase (*hTERT*) gene at posttranscriptional level. hTERT is a catalytic subunit of telomerase that results in being overexpressed in primary ATCs compared to PTCs and associated with cell dedifferentiation and increased metastatic potential [61]. The upregulation of hTERT, subsequent to miR-138 downregulation, could be responsible for malignant progression of well-differentiated PTCs toward undifferentiated ATCs. Since miR-138 downregulation seemed to be strongly associated with the ATC phenotype, this miRNA could be useful as a diagnostic tool for ATC recognition and it may contribute to the development of novel treatment strategy for ATCs.

Takakura et al. [37] reported a group of seven miRNAs (miR-17-3p, miR-17-5p, miR-18a, miR-19a, miR-19b, miR-20a, and miR-92-1), compressively named as miR-17-92 cluster, to be overexpressed in ATC cell lines and ATC cancer lesions compared to adjacent thyroid normal tissues. To investigate functional role of these deregulated miRNAs in ATC tumorigenesis, human ATC cell lines have been induced to silence these miRNAs expression by transfection with specific miRNA antisenses. Inhibition of miR-17-3p expression totally suppressed cell growth and induced apoptosis by the strong activation of caspases 3 and 9. Suppression of miR17-5p or miR-19a caused a strong reduction of cell proliferation, not associated with apoptosis or caspase activation. Moreover, inhibition of miR17-5p, but not of miR-19a, was also responsible for cell senescence. miR-17-5p and miR-19a target, respectively, retinoblastoma 1 (*RB1*) and phosphatase and tensin homolog (*PTEN*) genes as confirmed by the fact that the expression of RB1 and PTEN proteins was increased in cells transfected with miR-17-5p and miR-19a inhibitors. Mutations of *PTEN* gene are associated with Cowden syndrome characterized by breast and thyroid tumors. *PTEN* acts as a tumor suppressor, negatively regulating cell growth by the repression of the cyclin-dependent kinase inhibitor p27^{kip1} expression. A reduced expression of PTEN protein is associated with thyroid cancer development [62, 63], and PTEN inactivation is associated with undifferentiated malignant ATCs, rather than other thyroid tumor types [64]. Therefore, the overexpression of miR-19a (and of its isoform miR-19b) might be responsible for *PTEN* posttranscriptional downregulation and subsequent increased cell growth in ATCs. In addition, downregulation of tumor suppressor activity of *RB1* by overexpression of miR-17-5p could further contribute to increased tumor cell proliferation. Selective inhibitors of miR-17-3p, miR-17-5p, and miR-19a demonstrated to significantly reduce cell growth in ATC-derived cell lines, and inhibitor of miR-17-3p also induced cell death. Therefore, these inhibitors could represent valid therapeutic approaches for the treatment of ATCs.

Very recently, Braun et al. [35] identified two miRNAs, miR-30 and miR-200, which were significantly downexpressed in ATCs compared to PTCs and FTCs. overexpression of these two miRNAs in mesenchymal ATC-derived cell lines reduced their invasive and metastatic potential, negatively regulating the expression of the mesenchymal-epithelial transition (MET) proteins. Conversely, inhibition of endogenous miR-200 expression was sufficient to induce the inverse process, the epithelial-mesenchymal transition (EMT) responsible for tumor cell invasiveness and metastatic potential. miR-200 targets the ZEB1 and ZEB2, both repressors of the E-cadherin (CDH1) gene expression. Park et al. [65] demonstrated, in 60 human cell lines conserved at the Nation Cancer Institute, a significant association between miR-200 expression and E-cadherin-vimentin ratio. Induced overexpression of miR-200 caused the upregulation of

E-cadherin in tumor cell lines and reduced their motility and invasiveness. Conversely, the inhibition of miR-200 reduced E-cadherin expression, increased expression of vimentin, and induced EMT. All these data suggested miR-200 as a key factor of the epithelial phenotype in cancer cells that could be used as therapeutic agent to reduce the rates of invasive and metastatic thyroid carcinomas.

8. The Role of MicroRNAs in Medullary Thyroid Carcinoma

Only one study [25] has analyzed the miRNA expression in MTCs compared to other thyroid tumors and normal thyroid tissue, finding a set of 10 specific miRNAs (miR-9, miR-10a, miR-124a, miR-127, miR-129, miR-137, miR-154, miR-224, miR-323, and miR-370) upregulated in this tumor type. No functional studies have been yet performed.

9. Conclusion and Future Perspectives

miRNAs are powerful key regulators of gene expression in many fundamental cellular processes such as proliferation, differentiation, and apoptosis. Deregulation of miRNA expression was observed in the initiation, development, and malignant progression of numerous human tumors [2–10]. miRNA expression profiles resulted in being different not only between tumors and healthy tissues but also between different histopathological lesions of the same tissue, between tumors at different stages of malignancy, and between primary tumors and metastases. Therefore, miRNA expression profiles may become useful novel biomarkers for tumor diagnostic and histological characterization. Recent findings suggested that miRNA expression profiles could enable classifying poorly characterized human tumors that can not be accurately classified only by the classical mRNA expression patterns [66]. Moreover, since differences in miRNA expression are, in some cases, associated with the prognosis, analysis of miRNA expression profiles could help also in the therapeutic management of patients.

Very recent data supported the possibility to use circulating miRNAs (plasma, serum, urine, or other body fluids) as a novel class of biomarkers to diagnose tumors, as expression patterns of circulating miRNAs are different between normal tissues and cancers and peculiar miRNA expression profiles are specifically associated with certain types of tumors [67]. In addition, circulating miRNAs present the advantage to be stable molecules with a great resistance to RNase activity that can be easily dosed by noninvasive techniques.

Moreover, since miRNAs regulate cancer cell proliferation, differentiation, apoptosis, and invasiveness, miRNAs and their biological targets could be potential targets of therapeutic genetic strategies in human tumors to interfere with cancer initiation and progression. miRNAs are possible targets for a RNA-based therapy both by positively modulating the expression of specific miRNAs *in vivo* using expression vectors [68] and/or by inhibiting miRNA expression by transfecting specific 2′-O-methyl-modified antisense RNA (antagomirs) [69].

Acknowledgments

This work was supported by unrestricted grants from Fondazione Ente Cassa di Risparmio di Firenze and Fondazione F.I.R.M.O. Raffaella Becagli to M. L. Brandi.

References

[1] B. P. Lewis, C. B. Burge, and D. P. Bartel, "Conserved seed pairing, often flanked by adenosines, indicates that thousands of human genes are microRNA targets," *Cell*, vol. 120, no. 1, pp. 15–20, 2005.

[2] G. A. Calin and C. M. Croce, "MicroRNA-cancer connection: the beginning of a new tale," *Cancer Research*, vol. 66, no. 15, pp. 7390–7394, 2006.

[3] M. Z. Michael, S. M. O'Connor, N. G. Van Holst Pellekaan, G. P. Young, and R. J. James, "Reduced accumulation of specific MicroRNAs in colorectal neoplasia," *Molecular Cancer Research*, vol. 1, no. 12, pp. 882–891, 2003.

[4] G. A. Calin, C. G. Liu, C. Sevignani et al., "MicroRNA profiling reveals distinct signatures in B cell chronic lymphocytic leukemias," *Proceedings of the National Academy of Sciences of the United States of America*, vol. 101, no. 32, pp. 11755–11760, 2004.

[5] G. A. Calin, M. Ferracin, A. Cimmino et al., "A microRNA signature associated with prognosis and progression in chronic lymphocytic leukemia," *The New England Journal of Medicine*, vol. 353, no. 17, pp. 1793–1801, 2005.

[6] P. S. Eis, W. Tam, L. Sun et al., "Accumulation of miR-155 and BIC RNA in human B cell lymphomas," *Proceedings of the National Academy of Sciences of the United States of America*, vol. 102, no. 10, pp. 3627–3632, 2005.

[7] J. Takamizawa, H. Konishi, K. Yanagisawa et al., "Reduced expression of the let-7 microRNAs in human lung cancers in association with shortened postoperative survival," *Cancer Research*, vol. 64, no. 11, pp. 3753–3756, 2004.

[8] M. V. Iorio, M. Ferracin, C. G. Liu et al., "MicroRNA gene expression deregulation in human breast cancer," *Cancer Research*, vol. 65, no. 16, pp. 7065–7070, 2005.

[9] S. A. Ciafrè, S. Galardi, A. Mangiola et al., "Extensive modulation of a set of microRNAs in primary glioblastoma," *Biochemical and Biophysical Research Communications*, vol. 334, no. 4, pp. 1351–1358, 2005.

[10] J. A. Chan, A. M. Krichevsky, and K. S. Kosik, "MicroRNA-21 is an antiapoptotic factor in human glioblastoma cells," *Cancer Research*, vol. 65, no. 14, pp. 6029–6033, 2005.

[11] G. A. Calin, C. Sevignani, C. D. Dumitru et al., "Human microRNA genes are frequently located at fragile sites and genomic regions involved in cancers," *Proceedings of the National Academy of Sciences of the United States of America*, vol. 101, no. 9, pp. 2999–3004, 2004.

[12] J. Lu, G. Getz, E. A. Miska et al., "MicroRNA expression profiles classify human cancers," *Nature*, vol. 435, no. 7043, pp. 834–838, 2005.

[13] Y. Lee, C. Ahn, J. Han et al., "The nuclear RNase III Drosha initiates microRNA processing," *Nature*, vol. 425, no. 6956, pp. 415–419, 2003.

[14] R. Yi, Y. Qin, I. G. Macara, and B. R. Cullen, "Exportin-5 mediates the nuclear export of pre-microRNAs and short hairpin RNAs," *Genes and Development*, vol. 17, no. 24, pp. 3011–3016, 2003.

[15] G. Hutvagner, J. McLachlan, A. E. Pasquinelli, E. Balint, T. Tuschl, and P. D. Zamore, "A cellular function for the RNA-interference enzyme dicer in the maturation of the let-7 small temporal RNA," *Science*, vol. 293, no. 5531, pp. 834–838, 2001.

[16] G. Tang, "siRNA and miRNA: an insight into RISCs," *Trends in Biochemical Sciences*, vol. 30, no. 2, pp. 106–114, 2005.

[17] G. Hutvagner and P. D. Zamore, "A microRNA in a multiple-turnover RNAi enzyme complex," *Science*, vol. 297, no. 5589, pp. 2056–2060, 2002.

[18] Y. Zeng and B. R. Cullen, "Sequence requirements for micro RNA processing and function in human cells," *RNA*, vol. 9, no. 1, pp. 112–123, 2003.

[19] C. Llave, Z. Xie, K. D. Kasschau, and J. C. Carrington, "Cleavage of Scarecrow-like mRNA targets directed by a class of Arabidopsis miRNA," *Science*, vol. 297, no. 5589, pp. 2053–2056, 2002.

[20] S. Yekta, I. H. Shih, and D. P. Bartel, "MicroRNA-directed cleavage of HOXB8 mRNA," *Science*, vol. 304, no. 5670, pp. 594–596, 2004.

[21] M. R. Fabian, N. Sonenberg, and W. Filipowicz, "Regulation of mRNA translation and stability by microRNAs," *Annual Review of Biochemistry*, vol. 79, pp. 351–379, 2010.

[22] S. Vasudevan, Y. Tong, and J. A. Steitz, "Switching from repression to activation: microRNAs can up-regulate translation," *Science*, vol. 318, no. 5858, pp. 1931–1934, 2007.

[23] U. A. Ørom, F. C. Nielsen, and A. H. Lund, "MicroRNA-10a binds the 5′UTR of ribosomal protein mRNAs and enhances their translation," *Molecular Cell*, vol. 30, no. 4, pp. 460–471, 2008.

[24] J. G. Doench and P. A. Sharp, "Specificity of microRNA target selection in translational repression," *Genes and Development*, vol. 18, no. 5, pp. 504–511, 2004.

[25] M. N. Nikiforova, G. C. Tseng, D. Steward, D. Diorio, and Y. E. Nikiforov, "MicroRNA expression profiling of thyroid tumors: biological significance and diagnostic utility," *Journal of Clinical Endocrinology and Metabolism*, vol. 93, no. 5, pp. 1600–1608, 2008.

[26] H. He, K. Jazdzewski, W. Li et al., "The role of microRNA genes in papillary thyroid carcinoma," *Proceedings of the National Academy of Sciences of the United States of America*, vol. 102, no. 52, pp. 19075–19080, 2005.

[27] P. Pallante, R. Visone, M. Ferracin et al., "MicroRNA deregulation in human thyroid papillary carcinomas," *Endocrine-Related Cancer*, vol. 13, no. 2, pp. 497–508, 2006.

[28] M. T. Tetzlaff, A. Liu, X. Xu et al., "Differential expression of miRNAs in papillary thyroid carcinoma compared to multinodular goiter using formalin fixed paraffin embedded tissues," *Endocrine Pathology*, vol. 18, no. 3, pp. 163–173, 2007.

[29] Y. T. Chen, N. Kitabayashi, X. K. Zhou, T. J. Fahey III, and T. Scognamiglio, "MicroRNA analysis as a potential diagnostic tool for papillary thyroid carcinoma," *Modern Pathology*, vol. 21, no. 9, pp. 1139–1146, 2008.

[30] C. Wilson, "Cancer: microRNA expression provides clues about the aggressiveness of papillary thyroid carcinoma," *Nature Reviews Endocrinology*, vol. 6, no. 8, p. 416, 2010.

[31] S. Y. Sheu, F. Grabellus, S. Schwertheim, K. Handke, K. Worm, and K. W. Schmid, "Lack of correlation between BRAF V600E mutational status and the expression profile of a distinct set of miRNAs in papillary thyroid carcinoma," *Hormone and Metabolic Research*, vol. 41, no. 6, pp. 482–487, 2009.

[32] C. K. Chou, R. F. Chen, F. F. Chou et al., "MiR-146b is highly expressed in adult papillary thyroid carcinomas with high

risk features including extrathyroidal invasion and the BRAF mutation," *Thyroid*, vol. 20, no. 5, pp. 489–494, 2010.

[33] F. Weber, R. E. Teresi, C. E. Broelsch, A. Frilling, and C. Eng, "A limited set of human MicroRNA is deregulated in follicular thyroid carcinoma," *Journal of Clinical Endocrinology and Metabolism*, vol. 91, no. 9, pp. 3584–3591, 2006.

[34] R. Visone, P. Pallante, A. Vecchione et al., "Specific microRNAs are downregulated in human thyroid anaplastic carcinomas," *Oncogene*, vol. 26, no. 54, pp. 7590–7595, 2007.

[35] J. Braun, C. Hoang-Vu, H. Dralle, and S. Hüttelmaier, "Downregulation of microRNAs directs the EMT and invasive potential of anaplastic thyroid carcinomas," *Oncogene*, vol. 29, no. 29, pp. 4237–4244, 2010.

[36] J. C. M. Ricarte-Filho, C. S. Fuziwara, A. S. Yamashita, E. Rezende, M. J. Da-Silva, and E. T. Kimura, "Effects of let-7 microRNA on cell growth and differentiation of papillary thyroid cancer," *Translational Oncology*, vol. 2, no. 4, pp. 236–241, 2009.

[37] S. Takakura, N. Mitsutake, M. Nakashima et al., "Oncogenic role of miR-17-92 cluster in anaplastic thyroid cancer cells," *Cancer Science*, vol. 99, no. 6, pp. 1147–1154, 2008.

[38] S. Mitomo, C. Maesawa, S. Ogasawara et al., "Downregulation of miR-138 is associated with overexpression of human telomerase reverse transcriptase protein in human anaplastic thyroid carcinoma cell lines," *Cancer Science*, vol. 99, no. 2, pp. 280–286, 2008.

[39] M. N. Nikiforova, S. I. Chiosea, and Y. E. Nikiforov, "MicroRNA expression profiles in thyroid tumors," *Endocrine Pathology*, vol. 20, no. 2, pp. 85–91, 2009.

[40] S. Cahill, P. Smyth, S. P. Finn et al., "Effect of ret/PTC 1 rearrangement on transcription and post-transcriptional regulation in a papillary thyroid carcinoma model," *Molecular Cancer*, vol. 5, article 70, 2006.

[41] L. K. Ashman, "The biology of stem cell factor and its receptor C-kit," *International Journal of Biochemistry and Cell Biology*, vol. 31, no. 10, pp. 1037–1051, 1999.

[42] Y. Kitamura and S. Hirota, "Kit as a human oncogenic tyrosine kinase," *Cellular and Molecular Life Sciences*, vol. 61, no. 23, pp. 2924–2931, 2004.

[43] P. G. Natali, M. R. Nicotra, M. F. Di Renzo et al., "Expression of the c-Met/HGF receptor in human melanocytic neoplasms: demonstration of the relationship to malignant melanoma tumour progression," *British Journal of Cancer*, vol. 68, no. 4, pp. 746–750, 1993.

[44] P. G. Natali, M. R. Nicotra, A. B. Winkler, R. Cavaliere, A. Bigotti, and A. Ullrich, "Progression of human cutaneous melanoma is associated with loss of expression of c-kit proto-oncogene receptor," *International Journal of Cancer*, vol. 52, no. 2, pp. 197–201, 1992.

[45] R. Matsuda, T. Takahashi, S. Nakamura et al., "Expression of the c-kit protein in human solid tumors and in corresponding fetal and adult normal tissues," *American Journal of Pathology*, vol. 142, no. 1, pp. 339–346, 1993.

[46] P. G. Natali, M. T. Berlingieri, M. R. Nicotra et al., "Transformation of thyroid epithelium is associated with loss of c-kit receptor," *Cancer Research*, vol. 55, no. 8, pp. 1787–1791, 1995.

[47] H. R. Chiang, L. W. Schoenfeld, J. G. Ruby et al., "Mammalian microRNAs: experimental evaluation of novel and previously annotated genes," *Genes and Development*, vol. 24, no. 10, pp. 992–1009, 2010.

[48] A. J. Adeniran, Z. Zhu, M. Gandhi et al., "Correlation between genetic alterations and microscopic features, clinical manifestations, and prognostic characteristics of thyroid papillary

carcinomas," *American Journal of Surgical Pathology*, vol. 30, no. 2, pp. 216–222, 2006.

[49] R. Visone, L. Russo, P. Pallante et al., "MicroRNAs (miR)-221 and miR-222, both overexpressed in human thyroid papillary carcinomas, regulate p27 protein levels and cell cycle," *Endocrine-Related Cancer*, vol. 14, no. 3, pp. 791–798, 2007.

[50] A. Fusco and M. Santoro, "20 years of RET/PTC in thyroid cancer: clinico-pathological correlations," *Arquivos Brasileiros de Endocrinologia e Metabologia*, vol. 51, no. 5, pp. 731–735, 2007.

[51] W. S. Argraves, L. M. Greene, M. A. Cooley, and W. M. Gallagher, "Fibulins: physiological and disease perspectives," *EMBO Reports*, vol. 4, no. 12, pp. 1127–1131, 2003.

[52] W. M. Gallagher, L. M. Greene, M. P. Ryan et al., "Human fibulin-4: analysis of its biosynthetic processing and mRNA expression in normal and tumour tissues," *FEBS Letters*, vol. 489, no. 1, pp. 59–66, 2001.

[53] K. M. Schulte, C. Jonas, R. Krebs, and H. D. Röher, "Activin A and activin receptors in thyroid cancer," *Thyroid*, vol. 11, no. 1, pp. 3–14, 2001.

[54] S. Sander, L. Bullinger, K. Klapproth et al., "MYC stimulates EZH2 expression by repression of its negative regulator miR-26a," *Blood*, vol. 112, no. 10, pp. 4202–4212, 2008.

[55] M. V. Iorio, M. Ferracin, C. G. Liu et al., "MicroRNA gene expression deregulation in human breast cancer," *Cancer Research*, vol. 65, no. 16, pp. 7065–7070, 2005.

[56] B. J. Henson, S. Bhattacharjee, D. M. O'Dee, E. Feingold, and S. M. Gollin, "Decreased expression of miR-125b and miR-100 in oral cancer cells contributes to malignancy," *Genes Chromosomes and Cancer*, vol. 48, no. 7, pp. 569–582, 2009.

[57] T. Ichimi, H. Enokida, Y. Okuno et al., "Identification of novel microRNA targets based on microRNA signatures in bladder cancer," *International Journal of Cancer*, vol. 125, no. 2, pp. 345–352, 2009.

[58] L. Shi, J. Zhang, T. Pan et al., "MiR-125b is critical for the suppression of human U251 glioma stem cell proliferation," *Brain Research*, vol. 1312, pp. 120–126, 2010.

[59] X. Zhang, I. Neganova, S. Przyborski et al., "A role for NANOG in G1 to S transition in human embryonic stem cells through direct binding of CDK6 and CDC25A," *Journal of Cell Biology*, vol. 184, no. 1, pp. 67–82, 2009.

[60] L. Liang, C.-M. Wong, Q. Ying et al., "MicroRNA-125b suppressed human liver cancer cell proliferation and metastasis by directly targeting oncogene LIN28B2," *Hepatology*, vol. 52, no. 5, pp. 1731–1740, 2010.

[61] Y. Ito, H. Yoshida, C. Tomoda et al., "Telomerase activity in thyroid neoplasms evaluated by the expression of human telomerase reverse transcriptase (hTERT)," *Anticancer Research*, vol. 25, no. 1 B, pp. 509–514, 2005.

[62] O. Gimm, A. Perren, L. P. Weng et al., "Differential nuclear and cytoplasmic expression of PTEN in normal thyroid tissue, and benign and malignant epithelial thyroid tumors," *American Journal of Pathology*, vol. 156, no. 5, pp. 1693–1700, 2000.

[63] P. Bruni, A. Boccia, G. Baldassarre et al., "PTEN expression is reduced in a subset of sporadic thyroid carcinomas: evidence that PTEN-growth suppressing activity in thyroid cancer cells is mediated by p27(kip1)," *Oncogene*, vol. 19, no. 28, pp. 3146–3155, 2000.

[64] T. Frisk, T. Foukakis, T. Dwight et al., "Silencing of the PTEN tumor-suppressor gene in anaplastic thyroid cancer," *Genes Chromosomes and Cancer*, vol. 35, no. 1, pp. 74–80, 2002.

[65] S. M. Park, A. B. Gaur, E. Lengyel, and M. E. Peter, "The miR-200 family determines the epithelial phenotype of cancer cells by targeting the E-cadherin repressors ZEB1 and ZEB2," *Genes and Development*, vol. 22, no. 7, pp. 894–907, 2008.

[66] J. Lu, G. Getz, E. A. Miska et al., "MicroRNA expression profiles classify human cancers," *Nature*, vol. 435, no. 7043, pp. 834–838, 2005.

[67] K. Zen and C. Y. Zhang, "Circulating microRNAs: a novel class of biomarkers to diagnose and monitor human cancers," *Medicinal Research Reviews*. In press.

[68] R. A. Dickins, M. T. Hemann, J. T. Zilfou et al., "Probing tumor phenotypes using stable and regulated synthetic microRNA precursors," *Nature Genetics*, vol. 37, no. 11, pp. 1289–1295, 2005.

[69] J. Krützfeldt, N. Rajewsky, R. Braich et al., "Silencing of microRNAs in vivo with 'antagomirs'," *Nature*, vol. 438, no. 7068, pp. 685–689, 2005.

13

EGF and TGF-β1 Effects on Thyroid Function

Gabriella Mincione,[1,2] Maria Carmela Di Marcantonio,[1]

Chiara Tarantelli,[1] Sonia D'Inzeo,[3] Arianna Nicolussi,[3]

Francesco Nardi,[3] Caterina Francesca Donini,[3] and Anna Coppa[3]

[1] *Department of Oncology and Experimental Medicine, University "G. d'Annunzio" Chieti-Pescara, 66013 Chieti, Italy*
[2] *Center of Excellence on Aging, Ce.S.I., "G. d'Annunzio" University Foundation, 66013 Chieti, Italy*
[3] *Department of Experimental Medicine and Department of Radiological Sciences Oncology and Anatomical Pathology,*
 Sapienza University of Rome, Viale Regina Elena, 324, 00161 Rome, Italy

Correspondence should be addressed to Anna Coppa, anna.coppa@uniroma1.it

Academic Editor: Guillermo Juvenal

Normal epithelial thyroid cells in culture are inhibited by TGF-β1. Instead, transformed thyroid cell lines are frequently resistant to its growth inhibitory effect. Loss of TGF-β responsiveness could be due to a reduced expression of TGF-β receptors, as shown in transformed rat thyroid cell lines and in human thyroid tumors, or to alterations of other genes controlling TGF-β signal transduction pathway. However, in thyroid neoplasia, a complex pattern of alterations occurring during transformation and progression has been identified. Functionally, TGF-β1 acts as a tumor suppressor in the early stage of transformation or as a tumor promoter in advanced cancer. This peculiar pleiotropic behaviour of TGF-β may result from cross-talk with signalling pathways mediated by other growth factors, among which EGF-like ligands play an important role. This paper reports evidences on TGF-β1 and EGF systems in thyroid tumors and on the cross-talk between these growth factors in thyroid cancer.

1. Introduction

Thyroid gland homeostasis is maintained through a fine regulation of thyrocyte growth and differentiation. This regulation occurs through complex interactions between thyroid-stimulating hormone (TSH) and other growth factors and cytokines [1]. Evidence supports the role of transforming growth factor-beta 1 (TGF-β1) and epidermal growth factor- (EGF-) like ligands in the regulation of thyroid proliferation and differentiation, given the numerous information focused on mechanism of signal transduction and cross-talk. It is emerging the concept that the basis behind the pleiotropic nature of TGF-β in the context of cell-type and tumorigenesis derived probably from differences in the mechanism of such cross-talk.

The TGF-β superfamily, which includes TGF-β$_s$, activins, and bone morphogenetic proteins (BMPs), is a multi-functional dimeric proteins family that regulates growth, differentiation and extracellular matrix production in many different cell types [2]. In epithelial cells, TGF-β acts as a tumor suppressor by inhibiting cell growth or by regulating cellular differentiation or apoptosis.

EGF is the prototype of a large family of peptides that consists of about a dozen members and has an essential role in embryonic development as well as in inducing cell growth. Mutations in the kinase domain of EGFR/ErbB1 (epidermal growth factor receptor) and ErbB2 are responsible of ligand-independent activation of cytoplasmic signal transducers that regulate motility, adhesion, protection from apoptosis, and transformation [3].

TGF-β and EGF are physiological regulators of thyroid cell differentiation and proliferation. TGF-β is normally expressed and secreted by thyrocytes, acting as a potent inhibitor of thyroid cell growth [4]. EGF, instead, acts as a strong mitogen for follicular thyroid cells [5]. Any alterations of these two factors or their signalling pathways may play an important role in the stepwise transition towards malignancy, including the ability to become, at least partially, resistant to growth inhibition, to proliferate without dependence on growth factors, to replicate without limit, to invade, and to metastasize. TGF-β1 appears to have a dual effect in tumorigenesis. It can act as a tumor suppressor in the pretumor stage, and as a tumor promoter in late stage of tumorigenesis. It is likely that during tumorigenesis, as a result of genetic and/or epigenetic changes, the balance between those opposing functions of TGF-β1 changes resulting in a switch to tumor promotion; however, the precise mechanism for this switch remains to be clarified [6]. In this paper we focused our attention on the role of EGF and TGF-β in the control of proliferation and differentiation of thyroid cells.

2. Thyroid Cell Regulation by Growth Factors

Physiological regulation of thyroid cell growth and function involves a complex network of factors that act through endocrine, paracrine, or autocrine mechanisms. The proliferation and differentiation of thyroid epithelial cells are under the control of a positive systemic signal, TSH, and a negative locally produced signal, TGF-β. The main function of the thyroid is the formation, storage, and secretion of thyroid hormones tightly controlled by TSH, but requiring insulin/insulin-like growth factor I (IGF-I) [7]. The steps leading to the thyroid hormone formation include thyroglobulin (TG) synthesis and transport to the lumen of thyroid follicles, the iodide uptake by the sodium iodide symporter (NIS), iodination of TG, and coupling of TG iodotyrosine residues by the thyroperoxidase (TPO). In rat thyroid cells, the expression of the TG, TPO, NIS, and TSH receptor (TSHR) is under the control of thyroid-restricted transcription factors, such as thyroid transcription factor-1 (TTF-1) [8], that plays the most important role in the expression of all the genes, Pax-8, and TTF-2 [9, 10].

TSH, through the activation of its receptor, has been shown to stimulate more than one signal transduction pathway, the main of which being the adenylcyclase/cAMP (cyclic adenosine monophosphate) pathway. cAMP seems to account for the mitogenic effects of TSH in human thyroid cells, mediated by the activation of cAMP-dependent protein kinases [11]. TSH-induced cAMP also appears to play a central role in iodide uptake and metabolism in the dog follicular cells [12], in *TG* and *TPO* gene expression in rat follicular cells [13]. Although TSH is the major regulator of thyroid growth and functions, it has been shown that a number of growth factors affect the proliferation and function of thyroid epithelial cells. In fact, TSH effects can be potentiated by several growth factors such as insulin and IGF-I in rat thyroid cells in culture [14]. Insulin or IGF-I synergizes with TSH to induce thyroid cell growth and to maintain specialized cell functions [11]. There is evidence that *TSHR* and *TG* gene expression are regulated by insulin/IGF-I as well as TSH in a rat thyroid cell line (FRTL-5) [15, 16]. Moreover, an important regulator of thyroid growth that stimulates proliferation *in vitro* includes EGF.

3. Epidermal Growth Factor-Related Ligands and Their Receptors

EGF is the prototype of a large family of peptides structurally related by possessing an EGF-like domain that consists of 6 cysteine residues capable of forming three disulfide-bonded intramolecular loops. These ligands are expressed in the extracellular domain of transmembrane proteins and are generated by regulated proteolysis to yield growth factors that contain 49–85 amino acids. The components of the EGF-like growth factors family are functionally related on the basis of binding to the members of the tyrosine kinase ErbB family (EGFR/ErbB1, ErbB2, ErbB3, and ErbB4) and are divided into three groups: the first includes EGF, transforming growth factor-alpha (TGF-α) and amphiregulin, which all bind specifically to EGFR/ErbB1. A second group includes betacellulin, heparin-binding EGF (HB-EGF), and epiregulin binding to both EGFR/ErbB1 and ErbB4, while the third group comprises the neuregulin family, differentiated by their binding to ErbB3 and ErbB4 (NRG1 and NRG2) or only to ErbB4 (NRG3 and NRG4) [17]. All four human receptors share four extracellular domains with high structural homology, a single transmembrane spanning helix, and a cytoplasmic portion that contains a conserved but not equally functional tyrosine kinase domain. Only the EGFR/ErbB1 and ErbB4 are fully functional in terms of ligand binding and kinase activity. ErbB2 fails to bind any of the known ErbB ligands but contributes its potent kinase activity to all possible heterodimers. ErbB3 has an impaired kinase activity and relies on the kinase activity of its heterodimerization partners for activation. Heterodimers of ErbB2 and ErbB3 are the most potent ErbB pair in mitogenic signalling [17–19].

After ligand binding, ErbB receptors achieve activation by forming homo- or heterodimeric receptor complexes. The dimerization of ErbB receptors represents the most important mechanism that drives transformation. Dimeric receptors become catalytically active and are able to phosphorylate the cytoplasmic receptor domain that serves as docking site for a variety of signalling molecules whose recruitment leads to the activation of intracellular pathways controlling diverse genetic programs. The two major signalling pathways activated by ErbB receptors are the mitogen-activated protein kinases (MAPKs) pathway which stimulates proliferation, and Phosphatidylinositol 3-kinases/AKT (PI3K-AKT) pathway which promotes cell survival (Figure 1). The specific combination of ErbB receptors in the dimer defines the downstream signalling network as well as the intensity and the duration of the stimulation. Indeed, heterodimers that involve ErbB3 stimulates the activation of PI3K pathway [20].

Amplification, overexpression and gene mutation of EGFR/ErbB1 and ErbB2 have been found in various human cancers [17, 21]. EGFR/ErbB1 is overexpressed in bladder, breast, head and neck, kidney, nonsmall cell lung, and prostate cancers [22]. Three truncated forms of the EGFR/ErbB1 have been described [23] among which the EGFRvIII (variant III) lacks the majority of the ectodomain and does not bind EGF. This variant is the most common in glioblastoma multiforme and also occurs in lung, breast,

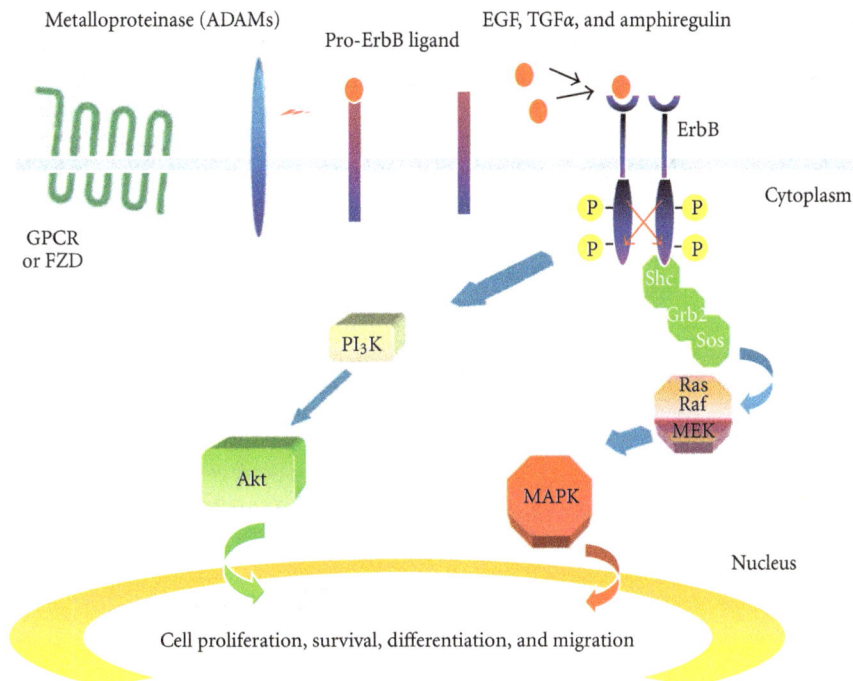

FIGURE 1: Mechanisms of action of ErbB receptor. In tumor cells, ErbB receptor tyrosine kinases are activated by autocrine or paracrine production of EGF family ligands. Autocrine ligand production results from the activation of G-protein coupled receptors (GPCRs) or frizzled (FZD) receptor which causes the metalloproteinases-mediated cleavage and release of pro-EGF-related ligands (ectodomain shedding). Binding of ligands to the extracellular domain of ErbB receptors leads to receptor dimerization, autophosphorylation, and activation of several downstream signalling pathways. In particular, tyrosine-phosphorylated ErbB receptors bind the adaptor proteins Shc and Grb2 leading to Sos recruitment and Ras/MAPK pathway activation. The PI3K/Akt pathway is stimulated through recruitment of the p85 adaptor subunit of PI3K to the receptor.

ovarian, and prostate cancer [24]. ErbB2 protein is overexpressed in breast cancer due to gene amplification in 15%–30% of invasive ductal breast cancers and overexpression correlates with poor prognosis and disease progression [25]. A number of studies have shown mutations in the kinase domain of EGFR/ErbB1 and ErbB2 [3, 21]. Intragenic somatic mutations in the *ErbB2* gene were reported in 5% of nonsmall cell lung cancer, 5% of gastric carcinomas, 3% of colorectal carcinomas, and 5% of breast carcinomas [26–28]. Accumulating evidence has suggested that also ErbB3 plays a critical role in cancer. Overexpression of ErbB3 often accompanies EGFR/ErbB1 or ErbB2 overexpression and has been frequently detected in a variety of cancers, including those of the breast [29], colon [30], stomach [31], ovary [32], and pancreas [33]. In ErbB2-driven cancers, ErbB3 functions as an intimate signalling partner that promotes the transforming potency of ErbB2, usually by activating the PI3K/AKT pathway [34]. ErbB4 receptor is made in at least four different full-length isoforms as a consequence of alternative mRNA splicing [35]. It has both oncogenic and tumor suppressive functions. Supporting a role in promoting growth, overexpression of ErbB4 enhances growth of human breast cancer cells [36] and transforms mouse mammary epithelial cells to form tumors *in vitro* and *in vivo* [37]. Supporting a suppressive role for mammary tumor growth activation of ErbB4 in breast cancer cells has been associated with cell-cycle arrest, differentiation, and apoptosis *in vitro* [38].

4. Epidermal Growth Factor-Related Ligands and Their Receptors in Thyroid

EGF is synthesized by thyroid gland and is able to induce thyroid cell proliferation in several species together with the loss of thyroid specific functions [5]. Moreover, EGF enhances the migration and invasiveness of papillary thyroid cancer [5, 39–41]. Accordingly, *in vitro* growth was inhibited when either neutralizing anti-TGF-α or anti-EGFR/ErbB1 antibodies were applied to thyroid carcinoma cell lines [42]. A correlation between the staining intensity of EGF and recurrence has been found statistically significant in a set of human papillary thyroid tumors, indicating EGF as a predictor of papillary thyroid carcinoma aggressiveness [43]. Follicular epithelial thyroid cells expressed weakly TGF-α protein, whereas 66% of hyperplastic thyroid nodules, 100% of thyroid adenocarcinomas, and all cases of papillary, follicular, and medullary carcinomas displayed intense staining for TGF-α. A parallel pattern of staining was observed for the EGFR/ErbB1 in these tissues, suggesting the potential for an *in vivo* autocrine loop [44]. Papillary carcinomas and their lymph node metastases coexpressed EGFR/ErbB1 and EbB2 mRNA transcripts at a higher level than in normal thyroid tissues [45]. Moreover, in the same histotype of cancer, it has also been demonstrated the coexpression of TGF-α and EGFR/ErbB1 mRNA transcripts at higher levels than in non-neoplastic thyroid tissues [46].

Rat thyroid epithelial cells transformed with K-ras oncogene were found to express high levels of ErbB4 receptor and Neuregulin-1 (HRG/NDF/NRG1) ligand compared to rat thyroid epithelial control cells. Treatment of K-ras transformed thyroid cells with neutralizing antibody against NRG1 reduced by 50% cell proliferation, demonstrating the presence of an active NRG1 protein secreted in the supernatant by the cells. These data indicate that in K-ras rat thyroid epithelial cells, the growth factor NRG1 signals through the heterodimer ErbB2/ErbB4 receptors in an autocrine fashion [47]. Nevertheless, in human papillary carcinomas the protein overexpression and nuclear localization of the NRG1 precursor isoform compared to normal thyroid tissues was not associated with the expression of ErbB receptors, while the expression of neuregulin-$\beta3$ (Hrg$\beta3$) was significantly correlated to ErbB3 protein expression, indicating this receptor as the cognate one [48].

EGFR/ErbB1 was higher expressed in anaplastic and papillary thyroid cancers than in normal thyroid tissues. In particular, Bergstrom et al. [49] have shown that EGFR/ErbB1 was expressed in all six anaplastic thyroid carcinomas examined and it was constitutive phosphorylated in 3 of the 6 cell lines tested. Song [50] has demonstrated that EGFR/ErbB1 was expressed in 90% of papillary carcinomas analyzed. Moreover, the role of EGFR/ErbB1 in stimulating the growth of thyroid tumors has been highlighted by the capability of Gefitinib, a small molecule inhibitor of EGFR/ErbB1, to reduce the growth of papillary, follicular, and anaplastic thyroid cancer cells [51, 52]. By immunohistochemical analyses, cytoplasmic immunopositivity of EGFR/ErbB1 was observed in papillary carcinomas, while no nuclear positivity for EGF and EGFR/ErbB1 was demonstrated. A study by Akslen et al. significantly associated cytoplasmatic EGFR/ErbB1 with the increased risk of recurrent tumor. Nuclear positivity for EGF and EGFR/ErbB1 was demonstrated to be a feature of both follicular adenomas and follicular carcinomas [53, 54].

The role of the ErbB2 proto-oncogene in thyroid carcinoma has been controversially discussed. It has been reported that high levels of ErbB2 mRNA expression correlated with lymph node metastasis in papillary carcinoma [45]. Studies by Utrilla et al. [55] and Haugen et al. [56] showed that there are marked differences in the pattern of ErbB2 immunoreactivity depending on the tumor type. The investigators demonstrated positivity for papillary carcinomas and negativity for follicular adenomas and follicular carcinomas, but they showed controversial results about medullary carcinomas. Moreover, ErbB2 was not detected in papillary carcinomas by immunohistochemistry [57]. Some studies investigated ErbB2 correlation with prognosis. Sugg et al. [58] found ErbB2 staining correlation with degree of differentiation, while Gumurdulu et al. [59] demonstrated that further investigations on ErbB2 role in thyroid tumors are required for determination of prognosis. Other studies have associated cytoplasmatic reactivity with patient's sex in tumor [60] or with development of metastasis [61].

Few studies analyzed all ErbB family members and their implication in thyroid tumors. Wiseman et al. [62] showed that EGFR/ErbB1, ErbB2, ErbB3, and ErbB4 were expressed in 76%, 2%, 57%, and 73% of differentiated thyroid carcinomas analyzed (90 cases of papillary and 6 cases of follicular carcinomas examined), respectively. Moreover, EGFR/ErbB1 and ErbB3 showed significantly increased expression, while ErbB4 showed significantly decreased expression in these tumors compared with benign thyroid lesions. ErbB3 expression correlated with the presence of lymph node metastases, tumor type, and higher N stage; the expression of ErbB4 correlated with lower T stage. Kato et al. [63] demonstrated that the transcription level of *ErbB2* and *ErbB3* genes was increased in papillary carcinomas compared to normal tissues, suggesting that the expression of an ErbB2-ErbB3 heterodimer may correlate with the aggressiveness of a thyroid tumor. Interestingly, coexisting protein overexpression of EGFR/ErbB1, ErbB2, ErbB3, and ErbB4 was demonstrated in 64% of papillary thyroid carcinomas providing numerous possibilities for functional receptor interactions [64].

5. TGF-β Effects on Thyroid Cell Physiology

TGF-β is synthesized as an inactive precursor that can be activated by different proteases produced by thyrocytes. Its expression is upregulated during TSH-induced thyroid hyperplasia in rats, suggesting that an increased local expression of TGF-$\beta1$, during thyroid hyperplasia, may contribute to the temporal stabilization of goiter size [65]. TGF-β signalling is propagated via cell surface serine/threonine kinases, TGF-β type I receptor (TβRI) and TGF-β type II receptor (TβRII). Both receptors are expressed on thyrocytes at equimolar amount [66] and, upon ligand binding by type II receptor, TβRI is recruited to an heteromeric complex and phosphorylated by TβRII, thus activating its serine/threonine kinase in order to phosphorylate the transcription factors R-Smad$_s$ (Smad2 and Smad3). The phosphorylated Smad2 or Smad3 associate with the common partner Co-Smad, Smad4, forming complexes that accumulate in the nucleus, where they regulate target genes expression either by interacting with other transcription factors and coactivators or corepressors or by directly binding to defined sequences in the promoter [67]. In contrast to R-Smad$_s$ and Co-Smad, the Inhibitory Smad$_s$ (I-Smad$_s$), including Smad6 and Smad7, bind to TβRI and compete with R-Smad$_s$ for activation by TβRI resulting in the inhibition of TGF-β signalling [68, 69]. A Smad ubiquitin regulatory factor 1 (Smurf1), being a HECT-type E3 (Homologous to the E6-AP C Terminus) ubiquitin ligase, interacts with inhibitory Smad7 and induces cytoplasmic localization of Smad7. Smurf1, then, associates with TβRI and enhances the turnover of this receptor [70] (Figure 2).

TGF-β is the important negative regulator of thyrocyte: it antagonizes the mitogenic effects of the main growth factors in cultured cells of human [65, 71], dog [72], pig [73], and rat origin [4, 74]. TGF-β delays progression during the mid–late G1 phase by directly controlling cyclin D1-3 levels and preventing the relocalization of p27/kip1 inhibitor from cyclin E/cdk2 to cyclin D3/cdk4 complexes [72, 74]. TGF-β has been shown to downregulate the expression of thyroid-specific genes in the majority of species. The iodide

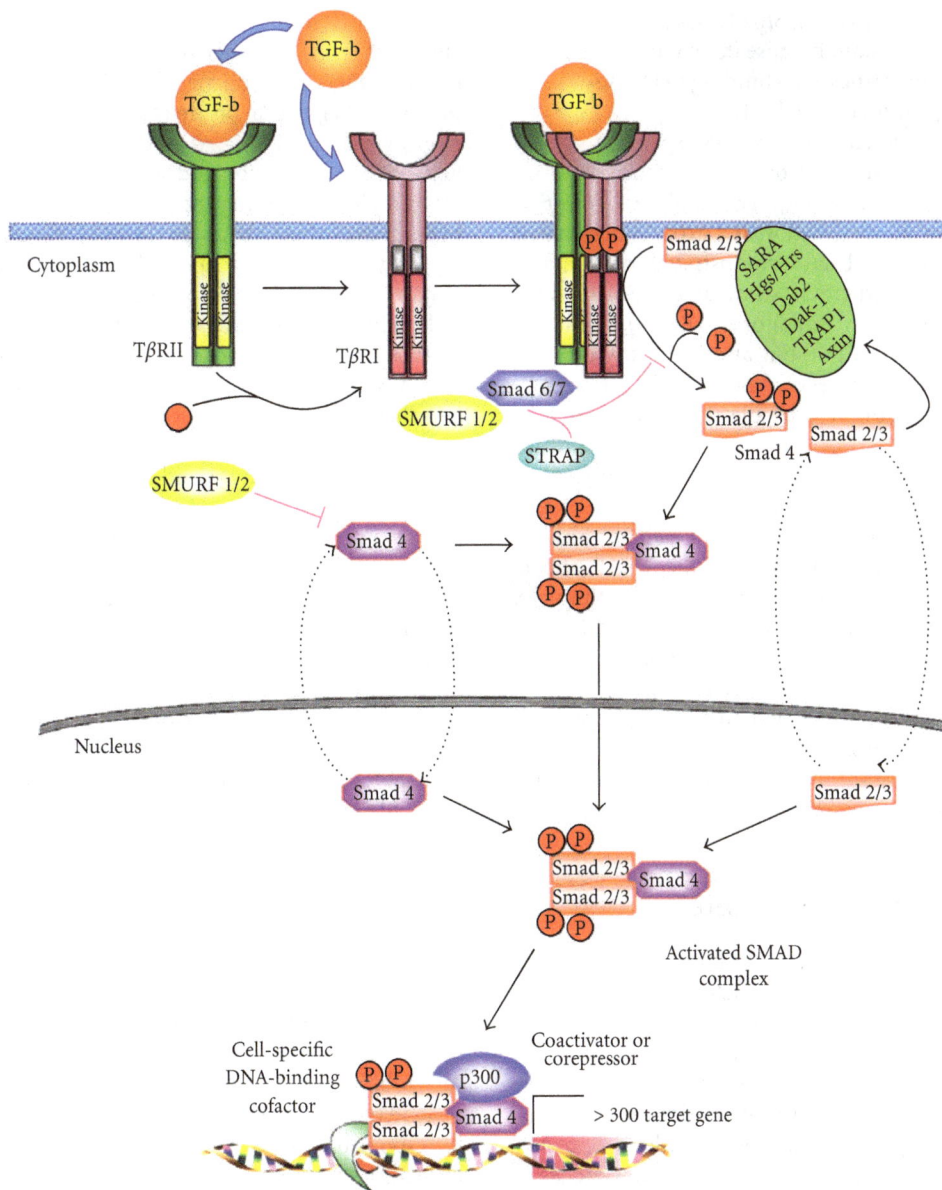

FIGURE 2: Intracellular signal transduction of TGF-β signalling. TGF-β ligand binds to TβRI and TβRII to constitute active heterodimers that possess serin-threonin kinase activity. Activated TβRI phosphorylates Smad2 and Smad3, which in turn form a complex with Smad4. Smad2 or Smad3/Smad4 complex translocates into the nucleus where interacts with other DNA-binding transcription factors, coactivators and corepressors, regulating the transcription of target genes.

trapping is inhibited in rat thyroid cells by blocking the protein kinase A (PKA) pathway, but not the PKA-induced DNA synthesis [75]. Moreover, we have demonstrated that the overexpression of ErbB2 in FRTL-5 cells, responsible of the resistance to the inhibitory action of TGF-β on cell proliferation, does not affect the inhibition of iodide uptake caused by TGF-β [66]. This effect was likely due in part to the inhibition of the expression of NIS mRNA and its protein [76, 77] and in part to the inhibition of the expression and activity of the Na+/I- ATPase, an enzyme that plays a key role in iodide uptake [78]. Similar responses have also been observed in porcine cell cultures, where TGF-β inhibits iodide uptake and metabolism, cAMP formation,

and T4 release [41]. In human thyroid primary cultures, TGF-β inhibits most effects of cAMP on gene expression [79]. The rat thyroid cell lines represent a good model to study the TGF-β action in regulating the TG expression respect to porcine thyroid follicular cells where, TGF-β has no effect [80]. In the FRTL-5 rat thyroid epithelial cell line, the addition of TGF-β inhibits Pax8 mRNA causing a decreased formation of Pax8/DNA complexes, both with or without the addition of TSH that is responsible of the TGFβ1-induced suppression of *TG* gene expression [81]. In the same cells, it has been demonstrated that the inhibition of TG biosynthesis and TSHR expression by TGF-β1 could be counterbalanced by blocking the nuclear translocation of

Smad2 and Smad4 [82]. Instead, Smad3 has a key role in the reduction of NIS expression, because its physical interaction with Pax8 in turn diminishes Pax8 binding to DNA sequence involved in the regulation of NIS [83].

In porcine thyroid cells cultured in suspension, TGF-β counteracts TSH positive effect on folliculogenesis causing an inversion of cell polarity [84]. The ability of TGF-β to modulate cytoskeleton organization and extracellular matrix protein distribution has been demonstrated not only in porcine thyroid cells, where it stimulates the expression of plasminogen activator inhibitor-1 (PAI-1), clusterin, trombospondin-1 [80, 85, 86], but also in rat thyroid cells [87]. Finally, in the same cellular model TGF-β1 inhibits the major histocompatibility complex (MHC) class I by regulating two elements at the transcription start site of the flanking region and increases the downstream regulatory element (DRE) binding of an ubiquitously expressed Y-box protein, termed TSEP-1 (TSHR suppressor element-binding Protein-1), an important suppressor of the TSHR and of MHC class I and class II expression [88]. TGF-β1 stimulates monocyte chemoattractant Protein-1 (MCP-1) and colony-stimulating factor (CSF) [89], as well as endothelin and its receptors in human thyroid follicular cells [90].

Therefore, it can be concluded that TGF-β exerts an important effect on thyroid cells in all the species tested, inhibiting the proliferation and function and modulating extracellular matrix (ECM) formation.

6. Role of TGF-β in Thyroid Cancer

The inhibition of cellular proliferation is one of the primary action of the TGF-β signalling. This factor is involved in the regulation of other numerous cellular functions as embryogenesis, differentiation, apoptosis, angiogenesis, immunosuppression, and wound-healing process [91]. Given the multifunctional role of TGF-β, any aberration of its normal signalling cascade may have wide-ranging pathologic consequences. Yet, paradoxically, TGF-β also modulates processes such as cell invasion and microenvironment modification that cancer cells may exploit to their advantage. Consequently, the output of a TGF-β response is highly contextual throughout development, across different tissues, and also in cancer [92].

Thyroid cancer incidence has significantly increased during the past decades [93], and it has become one of the ten leading cancer types in females being more frequent than ovarian, urinary, bladder, or pancreas cancer [94]. Although the majority of thyroid cancers have an excellent prognosis, there are a small percentage of cases that show an extensive local invasion and distant metastases, which frequently do not respond to standard treatments and have a worsened prognosis. The genetic basis for the initiation and development of the common type of thyroid cancer, papillary thyroid carcinoma (PTC), is well characterized. It has been demonstrated that the activation of oncogenes like RAS, BRAF, RET/PTC, and PI3K/AKT plays an important role in thyroid tumorigenesis [95]. However, it is also interesting to underscore the differences among the tumors arising from

the different mutations. Studies *in vitro* and *in vivo* have clearly shown that other oncoproteins, like EGF and TGF-β, exert their own oncogenic drive, conferring a distinct biological behaviour on thyroid tumors. The homoeostasis of growth in differentiated epithelia reflects a critical balance between the promotion and suppression of cell division. The thyroid gland is among the most common sites of epithelial hyperplasia, affecting up to 15% of the adult population, typically presenting as "sporadic" or multinodular nontoxic Goiter (MNTG), the hyperplastic gland usually contains well-defined nodules of varying size, surrounded by a normal epithelium. A wide range of studies has revealed evidence for an involvement of several autocrine growth stimulators and their receptors in the progression of MNTG. Prominent among these is TGF-β, and a lack of response to TGF-β inhibitory action in thyroid cells may be responsible for some cases of MNTG in human cells [71]. In rats, thyroid hyperplasia induced by iodide deficiency and goitrogen is accompanied by an increase in TGF-β1 expression and the arrest of goiter growth after 4 weeks. This surprising result is thought to reflect a critical role of TGF-β1 in stabilizing goiter mass [65, 96]. This would suggest that the increase in TGF-β1 levels observed during goiter induction might be a mechanism to counteract the goitrogenic effect of endogenous TSH [65, 97]. Instead, in a group of patients with either papillary adenomas ($n = 14$) or carcinomas ($n = 14$), not significant changes in blood levels of TGF-β1 have been observed compared to normal controls [98].

Increased expression of TGF-β, NFkB (nuclear factor of κB), and CDC42, compared to the normal thyroid tissue, has been demonstrated in a group of human papillary thyroid carcinomas, analyzed by oligonucleotide microarray of microscopically dissected intratumoral samples from central and invasive regions. These data together with reduced levels of mRNAs encoding proteins involved in cell-cell adhesion and communication and an overexpression of vimentin strongly support the hypothesis that the TGF-β, responsible of epithelial mesenchymal transition (EMT) induction, increases the tumor invasiveness in papillary thyroid carcinomas [95].

Perturbations of TGF-β signalling are central to tumorigenesis and tumor progression. TβRII is commonly inactivated through mutation and loss of heterozygosity (LOH) in several types of carcinoma [99]. Lazzereschi et al. [100], have obtained similar results in a series of human thyroid tumors, from benign lesions (adenomas) to neoplastic lesions of increasing aggressiveness (papillary and follicular carcinomas) up to the extremely aggressive anaplastic tumors. Northern blot analyses demonstrated a statistically significant reduction (about 2-3-fold less) of TβRII expression in papillary thyroid carcinomas in comparison with the respective healthy tissues. Immunostaining of the formalin-fixed sections with specific anti-TβRII antibodies substantiates these data, clearly demonstrating that the greatest reduction in TβRII immunoreactivity was found in the highly malignant, undifferentiated anaplastic thyroid tumors. A comparative study performed in different types of epithelial thyroid carcinomas of patients from different regions of the world demonstrated a strong decrease of TβRII expression in follicular cancer of patients from China, Japan, and USA (50%, 55%, and 90% respectively). In papillary thyroid carcinoma TβRII was decreased in 75%, 77% and 96% of patients from Japan, China, and USA, respectively. Finally, in undifferentiated cancer, the reduction of TβRII expression was observable in 83% of patients from USA and in 100% of patients from China [101].

Inactivating mutations in Smad2 and 4 are frequently found in some cancers [102]. In a group of 20 follicular thyroid neoplasms, classified as 11 adenomas and 9 minimally invasive follicular carcinomas, according to current pathological criteria, Smad2 expression investigated by immunohistochemistry has been lost, while TβRII expression was lost in 78%. These data indicate that the downregulation of TβRII remains the major consistent abnormality in thyroid carcinomas that may be used to differentiate minimally invasive carcinomas from adenomas, while the downregulation of Smad2 could be another mechanism by which carcinomas become independent from TGFβ–mediated growth inhibition [103].

The tumor suppressor role of TβRII has been demonstrated in vitro in a model of K-ras transformed rat thyroid cells, where the overexpression of TβRII induces not only a partial reversion of malignant phenotype restoring the sensitivity to TGF-β, but also a significant reduction in spontaneous and lung artificial metastases when transplanted in athymic nude mice [104]. In this model, the overexpression of TβRII is essential to reduce the invasive potential and to modulate the adhesive and migratory cell behaviours by controlling the integrin functions rather than integrin receptor expression [105]. The inhibitory action of TGF-β1 on cellular migration, invasion, and adhesion is present in a set of human PTC and follicular thyroid carcinoma (FTC) cell lines, while inhibition of TGFβ-induced cell growth is maintained only in FTC cell lines [106]. Other authors demonstrated that in human papillary thyroid carcinoma cell line TPC-1, these effects are probably due to the lower level of Smads 2, 3, and 4 associated to an increase in Smad7 expression [107]. Otherwise, the altered expression of TGF-β pathway proteins not always is responsible of resistance to the TGF-β action. A human anaplastic carcinoma cell line, despite the activity of receptors signalling, Smad2 phosphorylation and nuclear translocation of Smad2/4 complexes, is strongly resistant to the TGF-β action, suggesting that other signalling mechanisms might be related to the escape from TGF-β sensitivity [108].

Sensitivity to TGF-β is impaired in thyroid tumors and escape from TGF-β action is actively selected during thyroid tumor development. Destruction of the TGF-β signalling at the level of Smad genes is common in human carcinomas, the deficiencies of Smad4 have been hypothesized to underlie TGF-β resistance of tumor cells and to strongly accelerate the malignant progression of neoplastic lesions initiated by other oncogenic stimuli [92]. Lazzereschi et al. [109] showed, for the first time, the mutational and the expression status of Smad4 in a consistent number of thyroid tumors of different histotypes, demonstrating the high frequency of Smad4 abnormalities (27%) in thyroid tumors, comparable only with Smad4 mutation frequency in tumors arising from the gastrointestinal tract, both sporadic and inherited. The high frequency of alterations in Smad4 sequence led the authors to propose that these changes may constitute a nearly and frequent event in thyroid tumors natural history. Smad4 inactivation in tumors is generally a late event linked to progression to overt carcinoma. In human papillary thyroid cell lines, TPC-1 and BCPAP, it has been recently demonstrated a strong reduction in the level of SMAD4 protein, which is responsible for an alteration of TGF-β signalling and for some of the TGF-β-mediated biological effects. The overexpression of Smad4, restoring TGF-β signal transduction, determines a significant increase of antiproliferative response to TGF-β, reduces the invasive behaviour of these cells as well as is responsible of a significant increase of E-cadherin expression, indicating that the level of SMAD4 is a critical regulator of these processes. To remark the important role of SMAD4 in thyroid carcinogenesis contributes also the finding obtained by immunohistochemistry that 7 out of 23 (30%) PTC tumor samples, including 1 case of follicular variant of PTC$_s$, present a weak and focal intensity of SMAD4 staining compared to normal tissue from the opposite lobe [110].

The stability of TβRI represents an important regulatory mechanism for TGF-β signalling both in cell culture studies and in vivo models. TGF-β receptors are ubiquitinated and degraded through the action of several cooperating protein complexes containing E3 ligases as well as other important regulators of protein degradation. The I-Smad$_s$ regulate many of these complexes, orchestrating both ubiquitination and de-ubiquitination [111]. The levels of Smurf1 and Smad7 are overexpressed in the anaplastic thyroid carcinoma cell line [112], and an increase of SMAD7 expression has been found in a group of papillary and follicular carcinomas with respect to benign pathologies, indicating SMAD7 as another SMAD involved in thyroid tumorigenesis [113].

It is known that TGF-β's role in human cancer appears both complex and context depended. Depending on the tumor type and the stage of tumor progression, it can exercite strong tumor suppressive or tumor-promoting functions. More recently, it has been demonstrated that also in thyroid cells, as well as in the skin tumors, or in metastatic colon cancer [114], TGF-β can acts as tumor-promoting factor. The expression of BRAFV660E, in normal rat thyrocytes and in fifty cases of human PTC determines a reduction of NIS expression and an increase of TGF-β secretion, suggesting an hyperactivation of TGF-β signalling, responsible of the pro-tumorigenic activity [115].

The aberrant microRNA (miR) expression, involved in the cell growth suppressive function, has been demonstrated in a large number of follicular thyroid neoplasias [116]. More recently, a new important function of TGF-β, involving the regulation of expression of miR levels (miR-200 and miR-30), has been discovered in human anaplastic thyroid carcinoma (ATC). ATCs represent a more aggressive type of thyroid cancer arising from mesenchymal de-/transdifferentiation of epithelial thyroid cells that rapidly invade the adjacent tissue. The main function of miR-200 and miR-30 is to negatively regulate the EMT process in follicular cells. The low levels of miR-200 and miR-30 in ATCs respect to that observed in thyroid normal tissues, in PTCs or in FTCs, strongly suggest that the invasive potential of ATC is due to enhancement of EMT process. In addition, it has been demonstrated that the reduction of miR-200 and miR-30 in these carcinomas is caused by a strong activation of TGF-β signalling due to an upregulation of TβRI and Smad2. Therefore, the authors not only propose a novel molecular panel to identify ATCs, but also they suggest the inhibition of TGF-β signalling represent a new likely approach for the treatment of these carcinomas [117].

7. Growth Factors Cross-Talk in Thyroid: Role of TGF-β and EGF Systems in the Regulation of Thyroid Growth

Complex and apparently redundant interactions between hormones and growth factors regulate thyroid cell proliferation and differentiation. However, information about the cross-talk between different growth factors that regulate thyroid cell growth is limited. Ariga et al. [118] studied the signalling pathway through which the synergistic actions between IGF-I and TSH are mediated in FRTL-5 cells. Also, TGF-β1 and IGF-I appear to interact and have opposite effects on the growth of rat thyroid cells [75]. In particular, TGF-β1 attenuates IGF-I-stimulated MAPK phosphorylation through inhibition of IRS-1 (insulin receptor substrate-1) tyrosine phosphorylation, IRS-1/Grb2/Sos complex formation and CrkII tyrosine phosphorylation thus leading to the suppression of FRTL-5 cell growth [119]. ErbB ligands and ErbB receptors provide a complex and multilayered network of signalling that is deregulated in many human tumors. However, several are the causes and mechanisms of uncontrolled signalling by ErbB receptors suggesting that differences exist within the ErbB family in the mechanism of regulation but also in the cross-talk with other growth factors.

TGF-β is involved in two opposing activities: it is able to function as a growth inhibitor at early stages of carcinogenesis and as a growth promoter at later stages of neoplasia when tumor cells that have developed the capability to bypass the tumor inhibitor function of TGF-β, paradoxically, may use it for tumor progression by means of multiple mechanisms. Overexpression of TGF-β ligands has been reported in most cancers [120] and correlates with markers of a more metastatic phenotype and/or a poor patient outcome. This dual role of TGF-β is believed to result from molecular cross-talk with a complex network of signalling pathways involving either direct effects on tumor cells or paracrine effects on other cells [121]. Several reports provided evidence that TGF-β can collaborate with EGF/ErbB receptors system. Indeed, it has been shown that Smads proteins may cross-talk with mitogenic growth-factor signalling through receptor tyrosine kinase-induced MEK/MAPK protein kinases both in a synergistic (MEK1-induced Smad2 phosphorylation) [122] or an antagonistic interplay (MAPK-induced Smad1 phosphorylation) [123, 124]. In tumors, ErbB receptors and their

ligands promote growth and confer apoptosis resistance, thus overcoming TGF-β1 growth inhibition and apoptotic effect. Indeed, in rat hepatocytes an autocrine loop of TGF-β in cells that have undergone EMT, induces an upregulation of EGFR/ErbB1 ligands by promoting their shedding through the activation of ADAM17 (a disintegrin and metalloprotease 17) and thus allowing some cells to escape from TGFβ-induced pro-apoptotic effect [125, 126]. A further mechanistic insight on the conversion of the function of TGF-β from tumor suppressor to tumor promoter has been provided by the evidence that the EGF signalling pathway may enhance TGF-β responses. EGF increases the stability of TβRII thus preventing full loss of TβRII expression in late stage of cancers, and thereby permits some of the direct oncogenic behaviour of TGF-β during tumor progression [127]. Uttamsingh et al. [128] showed that in conjunction with EGF, TGF-β1 helps to augment migration, invasion and anchorage-independent growth of intestinal epithelial cells, in agreement with reports indicating that activation of TGF-β signalling promotes pulmonary metastasis of mammary tumors in neu transgenic mice [129]. Moreover, the elevated and prolonged activation of ERK/MAPK and its requirement for EGF and TGFβ1-induced EMT and migration/invasion of intestinal cells is in agreement with that between ErbB2 and TGF-β1 in mammary epithelial cells [130]. In fibroblasts, TGF-β induces the upregulation of ErbBs ligands and activation of cognate receptors via the canonical Smad pathway, thus allowing the induction of fibroblast cell morphologic transformation and anchorage-independent growth [131].

Contrasting to this *plethora* of data on cross-talk between EGF and TGF-β1 signals, there are very few results in the literature relating the interconnection between EGF and TGF-β signalling pathways in thyroid cancer cells.

Rat thyroid epithelial cells overexpressing the ErbB2 proto-oncogene are not transformed *in vitro* but no longer depend on TSH for cell growth and become resistant to the growth inhibitory effects of TGF-β1, thus suggesting that ErbB2 proto-oncogene, when overexpressed, is able to interfere and cross-talk with growth factors that control in a positive and negative manner the thyroid cell proliferation [132]. Using collagen gel-cultured porcine follicles, Nilsson et al. [133] demonstrated that the morphoregulatory effects of EGF are highly influenced by TGF-β1. In particular, TGF-β1 inhibits EGF-induced thyrocytes proliferation, but it synergizes with EGF in the stimulation of cell migration. This latter effect could be due to the known role of TGF-β1 to regulate the cell-matrix interactions, by stimulating the synthesis of extracellular matrix components, inhibiting proteases and inducing changes of integrin synthesis. However, contrasting to these results, TGF-β1 inhibited both EGF-induced mitogenesis and motogenesis in rabbit corneal epithelial cells [134] indicating that the modulation by TGF-β1 of EGF responses differs among epithelial cell types.

Moreover, in a follicular thyroid cancer cell line lacking endogenous TSHR, EGF, and TGF-β have been shown to enhance VEGF (vascular endothelial growth factor) secretion. Since the loss of the TSHR is characteristic of anaplastic thyroid cancer, which usually exhibits significantly increased VEGF expression and a high degree of angiogenesis compared with differentiated thyroid cancer, the finding of VEGF stimulation by EGF and TGF-β, highlights the important role of these growth factors in thyroid tumor progression and aggressiveness [135]. Preliminary data from our laboratory demonstrate that cotreatment with EGF and TGF-β1 results in opposite effects in human thyroid cancer cell lines. Indeed, TGF-β1 inhibits EGF-mediated migration in invasion/wound healing assay, while a synergistic effect between TGF-β1 and EGF is observed in anchorage-independent growth assay. These findings demonstrate that cell invasion and anchorage-independent growth capability involve different factors and molecular mechanisms (Mincione G. et al., unpublished results).

8. Conclusions

The findings described in this paper support the hypothesis that a network formed by the EGF/ErbBs system and TGF-β pathway is involved in the pathogenesis and progression of thyroid tumors. Further understanding of the complexity of cross-talk between these pathways in thyroid disease related to gain of function of ErbB, inactivation of growth suppression function, or activation of tumor promoter activity of TGF-β1 will offer a broader spectrum of points of intervention and will lead to continued advances in thyroid cancer treatment.

References

[1] G. Vassart and J. E. Dumont, "The thyrotropin receptor and the regulation of thyrocyte function and growth," *Endocrine Reviews*, vol. 13, no. 3, pp. 596–611, 1992.

[2] D. M. Kingsley, "The TGF-beta superfamily: new members, new receptors, and new genetic tests of function in different organisms," *Genes and Development*, vol. 8, no. 2, pp. 133–146, 1994.

[3] S. E. Wang, A. Narasanna, M. Perez-Torres et al., "HER2 kinase domain mutation results in constitutive phosphorylation and activation of HER2 and EGFR and resistance to EGFR tyrosine kinase inhibitors," *Cancer Cell*, vol. 10, no. 1, pp. 25–38, 2006.

[4] G. Colletta, A. M. Cirafici, and A. Di Carlo, "Dual effect of transforming growth factor beta on rat thyroid cells: inhibition of thyrotropin-induced proliferation and reduction of thyroid-specific differentiation markers," *Cancer Research*, vol. 49, no. 13, pp. 3457–3462, 1989.

[5] L. M. Asmis, H. Gerber, J. Kaempf, and H. Studer, "Epidermal growth factor stimulates cell proliferation and inhibits iodide uptake of FRTL-5 cells in vitro," *Journal of Endocrinology*, vol. 145, no. 3, pp. 513–520, 1995.

[6] J. Massaguè, S. W. Blain, and R. S. Lo, "TGFbeta signaling in growth control, cancer, and heritable disorders," *Cell*, vol. 103, no. 2, pp. 295–309, 2000.

[7] J. E. Dumont, C. Maenhaut, and F. Lamy, "Control of thyroid cell proliferation and goitrogenesis," *Trends in Endocrinology and Metabolism*, vol. 3, no. 1, pp. 12–17, 1992.

[8] A. M. Musti, V. M. Ursini, E. V. Avvedimento, V. Zimarino, and R. D. Lauro, "A cell type specific factor recognizes the rat thyroglobulin promoter," *Nucleic Acids Research*, vol. 15, no. 20, pp. 8149–8166, 1987.

[9] M. Zannini, V. Avantaggiato, E. Biffali et al., "TTF-2, a new forkhead protein, shows a temporal expression in the developing thyroid which is consistent with a role in controlling the onset of differentiation," *EMBO Journal*, vol. 16, no. 11, pp. 3185–3197, 1997.

[10] M. Zannini, H. Francis-Lang, D. Plachov, and R. Di Lauro, "Pax-8, a paired domain-containing protein, binds to a sequence overlapping the recognition site of a homeodomain and activates transcription from two thyroid-specific promoters," *Molecular and Cellular Biology*, vol. 12, no. 9, pp. 4230–4241, 1992.

[11] P. P. Roger, M. Taton, J. Van Sande, and J. E. Dumont, "Mitogenic effects of thyrotropin and adenosine 3′,5′-monophosphate in differentiated normal human thyroid cells in vitro," *Journal of Clinical Endocrinology and Metabolism*, vol. 66, no. 6, pp. 1158–1165, 1988.

[12] S. Filetti and B. Rapoport, "Autoregulation by iodine of thyroid protein synthesis: influence of iodine on amino acid transport in cultured thyroid cells," *Endocrinology*, vol. 114, no. 4, pp. 1379–1385, 1984.

[13] B. Van Heuverswyn, A. Leriche, J. Van Sande, J. E. Dumont, and G. Vassart, "Transcriptional control of thyroglobulin gene expression by cyclic AMP," *FEBS Letters*, vol. 188, no. 2, pp. 192–196, 1985.

[14] D. Tramontano, G. W. Cushing, A. C. Moses, and S. H. Ingbar, "Insulin-like growth factor-I stimulates the growth of rat thyroid cells in culture and synergizes the stimulation of DNA synthesis induced by TSH and Graves'-IgG," *Endocrinology*, vol. 119, no. 2, pp. 940–942, 1986.

[15] P. Santisteban, L. D. Kohn, and R. Di Lauro, "Thyroglobulin gene expression is regulated by insulin and insulin-like growth factor I, as well as thyrotropin, in FRTL-5 thyroid cells," *Journal of Biological Chemistry*, vol. 262, no. 9, pp. 4048–4052, 1987.

[16] M. Saji, T. Akamizu, M. Sanchez et al., "Regulation of thyrotropin receptor gene expression in rat FRTL-5 thyroid cells," *Endocrinology*, vol. 130, no. 1, pp. 520–533, 1992.

[17] Y. Yarden and M. X. Sliwkowski, "Untangling the ErbB signalling network," *Nature Reviews Molecular Cell Biology*, vol. 2, no. 2, pp. 127–137, 2001.

[18] R. Pinkas-Kramarski, L. Soussan, H. Waterman et al., "Diversification of Neu differentiation factor and epidermal growth factor signaling by combinatorial receptor interactions," *EMBO Journal*, vol. 15, no. 10, pp. 2452–2467, 1996.

[19] D. Graus-Porta, R. R. Beerli, J. M. Daly, and N. E. Hynes, "ErbB-2, the preferred heterodimerization partner of all ErbB receptors, is a mediator of lateral signaling," *EMBO Journal*, vol. 16, no. 7, pp. 1647–1655, 1997.

[20] M. Alimandi, A. Romano, M. C. Curia et al., "Cooperative signaling of ErbB3 and ErbB2 in neoplastic transformation and human mammary carcinomas," *Oncogene*, vol. 10, no. 9, pp. 1813–1821, 1995.

[21] S. V. Sharma, D. W. Bell, J. Settleman, and D. A. Haber, "Epidermal growth factor receptor mutations in lung cancer," *Nature Reviews Cancer*, vol. 7, no. 3, pp. 169–181, 2007.

[22] D. S. Salomon, R. Brandt, F. Ciardiello, and N. Normanno, "Epidermal growth factor-related peptides and their receptors in human malignancies," *Critical Reviews in Oncology/Hematology*, vol. 19, no. 3, pp. 183–232, 1995.

[23] R. Zandi, A. B. Larsen, P. Andersen, M.-T. Stockhausen, and H. S. Poulsen, "Mechanisms for oncogenic activation of the epidermal growth factor receptor," *Cellular Signalling*, vol. 19, no. 10, pp. 2013–2023, 2007.

[24] D. K. Moscatello, M. Holgado-Madruga, A. K. Godwin et al., "Frequent expression of a mutant epidermal growth factor receptor in multiple human tumors," *Cancer Research*, vol. 55, no. 23, pp. 5536–5539, 1995.

[25] D. J. Slamon, G. M. Clark, S. G. Wong, W. J. Levin, A. Ullrich, and W. L. McGuire, "Human breast cancer: correlation of relapse and survival with amplification of the HER-2/neu oncogene," *Science*, vol. 235, no. 4785, pp. 177–182, 1987.

[26] J. W. Lee, Y. H. Soung, S. H. Seo et al., "Somatic mutations of ERBB2 kinase domain in gastric, colorectal, and breast carcinomas," *Clinical Cancer Research*, vol. 12, no. 1, pp. 57–61, 2006.

[27] P. Stephens, C. Hunter, G. Bignell et al., "Lung cancer: intragenic ERBB2 kinase mutations in tumours," *Nature*, vol. 431, no. 7008, pp. 525–526, 2004.

[28] H. Shigematsu, T. Takahashi, M. Nomura et al., "Somatic mutations of the HER2 kinase domain in lung adenocarcinomas," *Cancer Research*, vol. 65, no. 5, pp. 1642–1646, 2005.

[29] R. Naidu, M. Yadav, S. Nair, and M. K. Kutty, "Expression of c-erbB3 protein in primary breast carcinomas," *British Journal of Cancer*, vol. 78, no. 10, pp. 1385–1390, 1998.

[30] C. A. Maurer, H. Friess, B. Kretschmann et al., "Increased expression of erbB3 in colorectal cancer is associated with concomitant increase in the level of erbB2," *Human Pathology*, vol. 29, no. 8, pp. 771–777, 1998.

[31] M. Kobayashi, A. Iwamatsu, A. Shinohara-Kanda, S. Ihara, and Y. Fukui, "Activation of ErbB3-PI3-kinase pathway is correlated with malignant phenotypes of adenocarcinomas," *Oncogene*, vol. 22, no. 9, pp. 1294–1301, 2003.

[32] T. Rajkumar, G. W. H. Stamp, C. M. Hughes, and W. J. Gullick, "c-erbB3 protein expression in ovarian cancer," *Journal of Clinical Pathology*, vol. 49, no. 4, pp. M199–M202, 1996.

[33] H. Friess, L. Wang, Z. Zhu et al., "Growth factor receptors are differentially expressed in cancers of the papilla of vater and pancreas," *Annals of Surgery*, vol. 230, no. 6, pp. 767–775, 1999.

[34] T. Holbro, R. R. Beerli, F. Maurer, M. Koziczak, C. F. Barbas III, and N. E. Hynes, "The ErbB2/ErbB3 heterodimer functions as an oncogenic unit: ErbB2 requires ErbB3 to drive breast tumor cell proliferation," *Proceedings of the National Academy of Sciences of the United States of America*, vol. 100, no. 15, pp. 8933–8938, 2003.

[35] T. T. Junttila, M. Sundvall, J. A. Määttä, and K. Elenius, "ErbB4 and its isoforms: selective regulation of growth factor responses by naturally occurring receptor variants," *Trends in Cardiovascular Medicine*, vol. 10, no. 7, pp. 304–310, 2000.

[36] J. A. Määttä, M. Sundvall, T. T. Junttila et al., "Proteolytic cleavage and phosphorylation of a tumor-associated ErbB4 isoform promote ligand-independent survival and cancer cell growth," *Molecular Biology of the Cell*, vol. 17, no. 1, pp. 67–79, 2006.

[37] C. C. Lynch, T. Vargo-Gogola, M. D. Martin, B. Fingleton, H. C. Crawford, and L. M. Matrisian, "Matrix metalloproteinase 7 mediates mammary epithelial cell tumorigenesis through the ErbB4 receptor," *Cancer Research*, vol. 67, no. 14, pp. 6760–6767, 2007.

[38] R. S. Muraoka-Cook, L. S. Caskey, M. A. Sandahl et al., "Heregulin-dependent delay in mitotic progression requires HER4 and BRCA1," *Molecular and Cellular Biology*, vol. 26, no. 17, pp. 6412–6424, 2006.

[39] T. Hoelting, A. E. Siperstein, O. H. Clark, and Q.-Y. Duh, "Epidermal growth factor enhances proliferation, migration, and invasion of follicular and papillary thyroid cancer in vitro and in vivo," *Journal of Clinical Endocrinology and Metabolism*, vol. 79, no. 2, pp. 401–408, 1994.

[40] B. F. van der Laan, J. L. Freeman, and S. L. Asa, "Expression of growth factors and growth factor receptors in normal and tumorous human thyroid tissues," *Thyroid*, vol. 5, no. 1, pp. 67–73, 1995.

[41] G. Bechtner, D. Schopohl, M. Rafferzeder, R. Gärtner, and U. Welsch, "Stimulation of thyroid cell proliferation by epidermal growth factor is different from cell growth induced by thyrotropin or insulin-like growth factor I," *European Journal of Endocrinology*, vol. 134, no. 5, pp. 639–648, 1996.

[42] B. Gabler, T. Aicher, P. Heiss, and R. Senekowitsch-Schmidtke, "Growth inhibition of human papillary thyroid carcinoma cells and multicellular spheroids by anti-EGF-receptor antibody," *Anticancer Research*, vol. 17, no. 4, pp. 3157–3159, 1997.

[43] Y. Mizukami, A. Nonomura, T. Hashimoto et al., "Immunohistochemical demonstration of epidermal growth factor and c-myc oncogene product in normal, benign and malignant thyroid tissues," *Histopathology*, vol. 18, no. 1, pp. 11–18, 1991.

[44] V. Gorgoulis, D. Aninos, C. Priftis et al., "Expression of epidermal growth factor, transforming growth factor-alpha and epidermal growth factor receptor in thyroid tumors," *In Vivo*, vol. 6, no. 3, pp. 291–296, 1992.

[45] R. Aasland, J. R. Lillehaug, R. Male, O. Josendal, J. E. Varhaug, and K. Kleppe, "Expression of oncogenes in thyroid tumours: coexpression of c-erbB2/neu and c-erbB," *British Journal of Cancer*, vol. 57, no. 4, pp. 358–363, 1988.

[46] D. R. Haugen, L. A. Akslen, J. E. Verhaug, and J. R. Lillehaug, "Demonstration of a TGF-alpha-EGF-receptor autocrine loop and c-myc protein over-expression in papillary thyroid carcinomas," *International Journal of Cancer*, vol. 55, no. 1, pp. 37–43, 1993.

[47] G. Mincione, A. Piccirelli, D. Lazzereschi, D. S. Salomon, and G. Colletta, "Heregulin-dependent autocrine loop regulates growth of K-ras but not erbB-2 transformed rat thyroid epithelial cells," *Journal of Cellular Physiology*, vol. 176, no. 2, pp. 383–391, 1998.

[48] O. Fluge, L. A. Akslen, D. R. F. Haugen, J. E. Varhaug, and J. R. Lillehaug, "Expression of heregulins and associations with the ErbB family of tyrosine kinase receptors in papillary thyroid carcinomas," *International Journal of Cancer*, vol. 87, no. 6, pp. 763–770, 2000.

[49] J. D. Bergstrom, B. Westermark, and N.-E. Heldin, "Epidermal growth factor receptor signaling activates met in human anaplastic thyroid carcinoma cells," *Experimental Cell Research*, vol. 259, no. 1, pp. 293–299, 2000.

[50] B. Song, "Immunohistochemical demonstration of epidermal growth factor receptor and ceruloplasmin in thyroid diseases," *Acta Pathologica Japonica*, vol. 41, no. 5, pp. 336–343, 1991.

[51] B. A. Schiff, A. B. McMurphy, S. A. Jasser et al., "Epidermal growth factor receptor (EGFR) is overexpressed in anaplastic thyroid cancer, and the EGFR inhibitor gefitinib inhibits the growth of anaplastic thyroid cancer," *Clinical Cancer Research*, vol. 10, no. 24, pp. 8594–8602, 2004.

[52] S. Hoffmann, S. Gläser, A. Wunderlich et al., "Targeting the EGF/VEGF-R system by tyrosine-kinase inhibitors-a novel antiproliferative/antiangiogenic strategy in thyroid cancer," *Langenbeck's Archives of Surgery*, vol. 391, no. 6, pp. 589–596, 2006.

[53] L. A. Akslen, A. O. Myking, H. Salvesen, and J. E. Varhaug, "Prognostic impact of EGF-receptor in papillary thyroid

carcinoma," *British Journal of Cancer*, vol. 68, no. 4, pp. 808–812, 1993.

[54] U. Marti, C. Ruchti, J. Kämpf et al., "Nuclear localization of epidermal growth factor and epidermal growth factor receptors in human thyroid tissues," *Thyroid*, vol. 11, no. 2, pp. 137–145, 2001.

[55] J. C. Utrilla, I. Martin-Lacave, M. V. San Martin, J. M. Fernandex-Santos, and H. Galera-Davidson, "Expression of c-erbB-2 oncoprotein in human thyroid tumours," *Histopathology*, vol. 34, no. 1, pp. 60–65, 1999.

[56] D. R. F. Haugen, L. A. Akslen, J. E. Varhaug, and J. R. Lillehaug, "Expression of c-erbB-2 protein in papillary thyroid carcinomas," *British Journal of Cancer*, vol. 65, no. 6, pp. 832–837, 1992.

[57] T. Murakawa, H. Tsuda, T. Tanimoto, T. Tanabe, S. Kitahara, and O. Matsubara, "Expression of KIT, EGFR, HER-2 and tyrosine phosphorylation in undifferentiated thyroid carcinoma: implication for a new therapeutic approach," *Pathology International*, vol. 55, no. 12, pp. 757–765, 2005.

[58] S. L. Sugg, S. Ezzat, L. Zheng, I. B. Rosen, J. L. Freeman, and S. L. Asa, "Cytoplasmic staining of erbB-2 but not mRNA levels correlates with differentiation in human thyroid neoplasia," *Clinical Endocrinology*, vol. 49, no. 5, pp. 629–637, 1998.

[59] D. Gumurdulu, A. Uguz, S. Erdogan, I. Tuncer, and O. Demircan, "Expression of c-erbB-2 oncoprotein in different types of thyroid tumors: an immunohistochemical study," *Endocrine Research*, vol. 29, no. 4, pp. 465–472, 2003.

[60] L. A. Akslen and J. E. Varhaug, "Oncoproteins and tumor progression in papillary thyroid carcinoma: presence of epidermal growth factor receptor, c-erbB-2 protein, estrogen receptor related protein, p21-ras protein, and proliferation indicators in relation to tumor recurrences and patient survival," *Cancer*, vol. 76, no. 9, pp. 1643–1654, 1995.

[61] R. Kremser, P. Obrist, G. Spizzo et al., "Her2/neu overexpression in differentiated thyroid carcinomas predicts metastatic disease," *Virchows Archiv*, vol. 442, no. 4, pp. 322–328, 2003.

[62] S. M. Wiseman, O. L. Griffith, A. Melck et al., "Evaluation of type 1 growth factor receptor family expression in benign and malignant thyroid lesions," *The American Journal of Surgery*, vol. 195, no. 5, pp. 667–673, 2008.

[63] S. Kato, T. Kobayashi, K. Yamada et al., "Expression of erbB receptors mRNA in thyroid tissues," *Biochimica et Biophysica Acta*, vol. 1673, no. 3, pp. 194–200, 2004.

[64] D. R. F. Haugen, L. A. Akslen, J. E. Varhaug, and J. R. Lillehaug, "Expression of c-erbB-3 and c-erbB-4 proteins in papillary thyroid carcinomas," *Cancer Research*, vol. 56, no. 6, pp. 1184–1188, 1996.

[65] A. Logan, C. Smith, G. P. Becks, A. M. Gonzalez, I. D. Phillips, and D. J. Hill, "Enhanced expression of transforming growth factor-β1 during thyroid hyperplasia in rats," *Journal of Endocrinology*, vol. 141, no. 1, pp. 45–57, 1994.

[66] A. Coppa, G. Mincione, S. Mammarella, A. Ranieri, and G. Colletta, "Epithelial rat thyroid cell clones, escaping from transforming growth factor beta negative growth control, are still inhibited by this factor in the ability to trap iodide," *Cell Growth and Differentiation*, vol. 6, no. 3, pp. 281–290, 1995.

[67] L. Attisano and J. L. Wrana, "Smads as transcriptional co-modulators," *Current Opinion in Cell Biology*, vol. 12, no. 2, pp. 235–243, 2000.

[68] T. Imamura, M. Takase, A. Nishihara et al., "Smad6 inhibits signalling by the TGF-beta superfamily," *Nature*, vol. 389, no. 6651, pp. 622–626, 1997.

[69] A. Nakao, M. Afrakhte, A. Morén et al., "Identification of Smad7, a TGFbeta-inducible antagonist of TGFbeta signalling," *Nature*, vol. 389, no. 6651, pp. 631–635, 1997.

[70] C. Suzuki, G. Murakami, M. Fukuchi et al., "Smurf1 regulates the inhibitory activity of Smad7 by targeting Smad7 to the plasma membrane," *Journal of Biological Chemistry*, vol. 277, no. 42, pp. 39919–39925, 2002.

[71] B. Grubeck-Loebenstein, G. Buchan, R. Sadeghi et al., "Transforming growth factor beta regulates thyroid growth. Role in the pathogenesis of nontoxic goiter," *Journal of Clinical Investigation*, vol. 83, no. 3, pp. 764–770, 1989.

[72] F. Depoortere, I. Pirson, J. Bartek, J. E. Dumont, and P. P. Roger, "Transforming growth factor beta(1) selectively inhibits the cyclic AMP-dependent proliferation of primary thyroid epithelial cells by preventing the association of cyclin D3-cdk4 with nuclear p27(kip1)," *Molecular Biology of the Cell*, vol. 11, no. 3, pp. 1061–1076, 2000.

[73] A. Franzén, E. Piek, B. Westermark, P. ten Dijke, and N.-E. Heldin, "Expression of transforming growth factor-beta1, activin A, and their receptors in thyroid follicle cells: negative regulation of thyrocyte growth and function," *Endocrinology*, vol. 140, no. 9, pp. 4300–4310, 1999.

[74] C. Carneiro, C. V. Alvarez, J. Zalvide, A. Vidal, and F. Domínguez, "TGF-beta1 actions on FRTL-5 cells provide a model for the physiological regulation of thyroid growth," *Oncogene*, vol. 16, no. 11, pp. 1455–1465, 1998.

[75] X.-P. Pang, M. Park, and J. M. Hershman, "Transforming growth factor-beta blocks protein kinase-A-mediated iodide transport and protein kinase-C-mediated DNA synthesis in FRTL-5 rat thyroid cells," *Endocrinology*, vol. 131, no. 1, pp. 45–50, 1992.

[76] A. Kawaguchi, M. Ikeda, T. Endo, T. Kogai, A. Miyazaki, and T. Onaya, "Transforming growth factor-beta1 suppresses thyrotropin-induced Na^+/I^- symporter messenger RNA and protein levels in FRTL-5 rat thyroid cells," *Thyroid*, vol. 7, no. 5, pp. 789–794, 1997.

[77] A. E. Pekary and J. M. Hershman, "Tumor necrosis factor, ceramide, transforming growth factor-beta1, and aging reduce Na^+/I^- symporter messenger ribonucleic acid levels in FRTL-5 cells," *Endocrinology*, vol. 139, no. 2, pp. 703–712, 1998.

[78] A. E. Pekary, S. R. Levin, D. G. Johnson, L. Berg, and J. M. Hershman, "Tumor necrosis factor-alpha (TNF-alpha) and transforming growth factor-beta 1 (TGF-beta 1) inhibit the expression and activity of Na + /K(+)-ATPase in FRTL-5 rat thyroid cells," *Journal of Interferon and Cytokine Research*, vol. 17, no. 4, pp. 185–195, 1997.

[79] M. Taton, F. Lamy, P. P. Roger, and J. E. Dumont, "General inhibition by transforming growth factor beta 1 of thyrotropin and cAMP responses in human thyroid cells in primary culture," *Molecular and Cellular Endocrinology*, vol. 95, no. 1-2, pp. 13–21, 1993.

[80] D. Claisse, I. Martiny, B. Chaqour et al., "Influence of transforming growth factor beta1 (TGF-beta1) on the behaviour of porcine thyroid epithelial cells in primary culture through thrombospondin-1 synthesis," *Molecular and Cellular Endocrinology*, vol. 112, part 9, pp. 1405–1416, 1999.

[81] H.-C. Kang, M. Ohmori, N. Harii, T. Endo, and T. Onaya, "Pax-8 is essential for regulation of the thyroglobulin gene by transforming growth factor-beta1," *Endocrinology*, vol. 142, no. 1, pp. 267–275, 2001.

[82] A. Nicolussi, S. D'Inzeo, M. Santulli, G. Colletta, and A. Coppa, "TGF-beta control of rat thyroid follicular cells differentiation," *Molecular and Cellular Endocrinology*, vol. 207, no. 1-2, pp. 1–11, 2003.

[83] E. Costamagna, B. García, and P. Santisteban, "The functional interaction between the paired domain transcription factor Pax8 and Smad3 is involved in transforming growth factor-beta repression of the sodium/iodide symporter gene," *Journal of Biological Chemistry*, vol. 279, no. 5, pp. 3439–3446, 2004.

[84] N. Delorme, C. Remond, H. Sartelet et al., "TGFbeta1 effects on functional activity of porcine thyroid cells cultured in suspension," *Journal of Endocrinology*, vol. 173, no. 2, pp. 345–355, 2002.

[85] G. Kotlarz, Y. Wegrowski, L. Martiny, P. J. Declerck, and G. Bellon, "Enhanced expression of plasminogen activator inhibitor-1 by dedifferentiated thyrocytes," *Biochemical and Biophysical Research Communications*, vol. 295, no. 3, pp. 737–743, 2002.

[86] Y. Wegrowski, C. Perreau, L. Martiny, B. Haye, F. X. Maquart, and G. Bellon, "Transforming growth factor beta-1 up-regulates clusterin synthesis in thyroid epithelial cells," *Experimental Cell Research*, vol. 247, no. 2, pp. 475–483, 1999.

[87] C. Garbi, G. Colletta, A. M. Cirafici, P. C. Marchisio, and L. Nitsch, "Transforming growth factor-beta induces cytoskeleton and extracellular matrix modifications in FRTL-5 thyroid epithelial cells," *European Journal of Cell Biology*, vol. 53, no. 2, pp. 281–289, 1990.

[88] G. Napolitano, V. Montani, C. Giuliani et al., "Transforming growth factor-beta1 down-regulation of major histocompatibility complex class I in thyrocytes: coordinate regulation of two separate elements by thyroid-specific as well as ubiquitous transcription factors," *Molecular Endocrinology*, vol. 14, no. 4, pp. 486–505, 2000.

[89] M. Matsumura, N. Banba, S. Motohashi, and Y. Hattori, "Interleukin-6 and transforming growth factor-beta regulate the expression of monocyte chemoattractant protein-1 and colony-stimulating factors in human thyroid follicular cells," *Life Sciences*, vol. 65, no. 12, pp. PL129–PL135, 1999.

[90] Y.-C. L. Tseng, S. Lahiri, S. Jackson, K. D. Burman, and L. Wartofsky, "Endothelin binding to receptors and endothelin production by human thyroid follicular cells: effects of transforming growth factor-beta and thyrotropin," *Journal of Clinical Endocrinology and Metabolism*, vol. 76, no. 1, pp. 156–161, 1993.

[91] M. J. Truty and R. Urrutia, "Basics of TGF-beta and pancreatic cancer," *Pancreatology*, vol. 7, no. 5-6, pp. 423–435, 2007.

[92] J. Massagué, "TGFβ in cancer," *Cell*, vol. 134, no. 2, pp. 215–230, 2008.

[93] L. Davies and H. G. Welch, "Increasing incidence of thyroid cancer in the United States, 1973–2002," *Journal of the American Medical Association*, vol. 295, no. 18, pp. 2164–2167, 2006.

[94] A. Jemal, R. Siegel, E. Ward, T. Murray, J. Xu, and M. J. Thun, "Cancer statistics, 2007," *CA: A Cancer Journal for Clinicians*, vol. 57, no. 1, pp. 43–66, 2007.

[95] V. Vasko, A. V. Espinosa, W. Scouten et al., "Gene expression and functional evidence of epithelial-to-mesenchymal transition in papillary thyroid carcinoma invasion," *Proceedings of the National Academy of Sciences of the United States of America*, vol. 104, no. 8, pp. 2803–2808, 2007.

[96] S. P. Bidey, D. J. Hill, and M. C. Eggo, "Growth factors and goitrogenesis," *Journal of Endocrinology*, vol. 160, no. 3, pp. 321–332, 1999.

[97] M. A. Pisarev, L. Thomasz, and G. J. Juvenal, "Role of transforming growth factor beta in the regulation of thyroid function and growth," *Thyroid*, vol. 19, no. 8, pp. 881–892, 2009.

[98] D. Vesely, J. Astl, P. Lastuvka, P. Matucha, I. Sterzl, and J. Betka, "Serum levels of IGF-I, HGF, TGFbeta1, bFGF and VEGF in thyroid gland tumors," *Physiological Research*, vol. 53, no. 1, pp. 83–89, 2004.

[99] L. Levy and C. S. Hill, "Alterations in components of the TGF-beta superfamily signaling pathways in human cancer," *Cytokine and Growth Factor Reviews*, vol. 17, no. 1-2, pp. 41–58, 2006.

[100] D. Lazzereschi, A. Ranieri, G. Mincione, S. Taccogna, F. Nardi, and G. Colletta, "Human malignant thyroid tumors displayed reduced levels of transforming growth factor beta receptor type II messenger RNA and protein," *Cancer Research*, vol. 57, no. 10, pp. 2071–2076, 1997.

[101] Y. Imamura, L. Jin, J. P. Grande et al., "Analysis of TGF-β and TGF-β-RII in thyroid neoplasms from the United States, Japan, and China," *Endocrine Pathology*, vol. 9, no. 3, pp. 209–216, 1998.

[102] J. Seoane, "Escaping from the TGFbeta anti-proliferative control," *Carcinogenesis*, vol. 27, no. 11, pp. 2148–2156, 2006.

[103] J. West, T. Munoz-Antonia, J. G. Johnson, D. Klotch, and C. A. Muro-Cacho, "Transforming growth factor-beta type II receptor and Smad proteins in follicular thyroid tumors," *Laryngoscope*, vol. 110, no. 8, pp. 1323–1327, 2000.

[104] A. Turco, A. Coppa, S. Aloe et al., "Overexpression of transforming growth factor beta-type II receptor reduces tumorigenicity and metastatic potential of K-ras-transformed thyroid cells," *International Journal of Cancer*, vol. 80, no. 1, pp. 85–91, 1999.

[105] A. Nicolussi, S. D'Inzeo, A. Gismondi, and A. Coppa, "Reduction of invasive potential in K-ras-transformed thyroid cells by restoring of TGF-β pathway," *Clinical and Experimental Metastasis*, vol. 23, no. 5-6, pp. 237–248, 2006.

[106] T. Hölting, A. Zielke, A. E. Siperstein, O. H. Clark, and Q.-Y. Duh, "Transforming growth factor-beta 1 is a negative regulator for differentiated thyroid cancer: studies of growth, migration, invasion, and adhesion of cultured follicular and papillary thyroid cancer cell lines," *Journal of Clinical Endocrinology and Metabolism*, vol. 79, no. 3, pp. 806–813, 1994.

[107] S. E. Matsuo, S. G. Leoni, A. Colquhoun, and E. T. Kimura, "Transforming growth factor-beta1 and activin A generate antiproliferative signaling in thyroid cancer cells," *Journal of Endocrinology*, vol. 190, no. 1, pp. 141–150, 2006.

[108] N. E. Heldin, D. Bergström, A. Hermansson et al., "Lack of responsiveness to TGF-beta1 in a thyroid carcinoma cell line with functional type I and type II TGF-beta receptors and Smad proteins, suggests a novel mechanism for TGF-beta insensitivity in carcinoma cells," *Molecular and Cellular Endocrinology*, vol. 153, no. 1-2, pp. 79–90, 1999.

[109] D. Lazzereschi, F. Nardi, A. Turco et al., "A complex pattern of mutations and abnormal splicing of Smad4 is present in thyroid tumours," *Oncogene*, vol. 24, no. 34, pp. 5344–5354, 2005.

[110] S. D'Inzeo, A. Nicolussi, A. Ricci et al., "Role of reduced expression of SMAD4 in papillary thyroid carcinoma,"

Journal of Molecular Endocrinology, vol. 45, no. 4, pp. 229–244, 2010.

[111] A. Moustakas and C. H. Heldin, "The regulation of TGFbeta signal transduction," *Development*, vol. 136, no. 22, pp. 3699–3714, 2009.

[112] J. M. Cerutti, K. N. Ebina, S. E. Matsuo, L. Martins, R. M. B. Maciel, and E. T. Kimura, "Expression of Smad4 and Smad7 in human thyroid follicular carcinoma cell lines," *Journal of Endocrinological Investigation*, vol. 26, no. 6, pp. 516–521, 2003.

[113] S. E. Matsuo, A. P. Z. Fiore, S. M. Siguematu et al., "Expression of SMAD proteins, TGF-beta/activin signaling mediators, in human thyroid tissues," *Arquivos Brasileiros de Endocrinologia & Metabologia*, vol. 54, no. 4, pp. 406–412, 2010.

[114] D. Padua and J. Massagué, "Roles of TGFbeta in metastasis.," *Cell Research*, vol. 19, no. 1, pp. 89–102, 2009.

[115] G. Riesco-Eizaguirre, I. Rodríguez, A. De La Vieja et al., "The BRAFV600E oncogene induces transforming growth factor beta secretion leading to sodium iodide symporter repression and increased malignancy in thyroid cancer," *Cancer Research*, vol. 69, no. 21, pp. 8317–8325, 2009.

[116] R. Visone, P. Pallante, A. Vecchione et al., "Specific microRNAs are downregulated in human thyroid anaplastic carcinomas," *Oncogene*, vol. 26, no. 54, pp. 7590–7595, 2007.

[117] J. Braun, C. Hoang-Vu, H. Dralle, and S. Hüttelmaier, "Downregulation of microRNAs directs the EMT and invasive potential of anaplastic thyroid carcinomas," *Oncogene*, vol. 29, no. 29, pp. 4237–4244, 2010.

[118] M. Ariga, T. Nedachi, M. Akahori et al., "Signalling pathways of insulin-like growth factor-I that are augmented by cAMP in FRTL-5 cells," *Biochemical Journal*, vol. 348, part 2, pp. 409–416, 2000.

[119] G. Mincione, D. L. Esposito, M. C. Di Marcantonio, A. Piccirelli, A. Cama, and G. Colletta, "TGF-β1 modulation of IGF-I signaling pathway in rat thyroid epithelial cells," *Experimental Cell Research*, vol. 287, no. 2, pp. 411–423, 2003.

[120] A. B. Roberts and L. M. Wakefield, "The two faces of transforming growth factor β in carcinogenesis," *Proceedings of the National Academy of Sciences of the United States of America*, vol. 100, no. 15, pp. 8621–8623, 2003.

[121] G. Torre-Amione, R. D. Beauchamp, H. Koeppen et al., "A highly immunogenic tumor transfected with a murine transforming growth factor type beta 1 cDNA escapes immune surveillance," *Proceedings of the National Academy of Sciences of the United States of America*, vol. 87, no. 4, pp. 1486–1490, 1990.

[122] M. P. De Caestecker, W. T. Parks, C. J. Frank et al., "Smad2 transduces common signals from receptor serinethreonine and tyrosine kinases," *Genes and Development*, vol. 12, no. 11, pp. 1587–1592, 1998.

[123] M. Kretzschmar, J. Doody, and J. Massagué, "Opposing BMP and EGF signalling pathways converge on the TGF-β family mediator Smad1," *Nature*, vol. 389, no. 6651, pp. 618–622, 1997.

[124] M. Kretzschmar, J. Doody, I. Timokhina, and J. Massagué, "A mechanism of repression of TGFfβ/Smad signaling by oncogenic Ras," *Genes and Development*, vol. 13, no. 7, pp. 804–816, 1999.

[125] M. M. Murillo, G. del Castillo, A. Sánchez, M. Fernández, and I. Fabregat, "Involvement of EGF receptor and c-Src in the survival signals induced by TGF-β1 in hepatocytes," *Oncogene*, vol. 24, no. 28, pp. 4580–4587, 2005.

[126] G. del Castillo, M. M. Murillo, A. Alvarez-Barrientos et al., "Autocrine production of TGF-β confers resistance to apoptosis after an epithelial-mesenchymal transition process in hepatocytes: role of EGF receptor ligands," *Experimental Cell Research*, vol. 312, no. 15, pp. 2860–2871, 2006.

[127] K. Song, T. L. Krebs, and D. Danielpour, "Novel permissive role of epidermal growth factor in transforming growth factor β (TGF-β) signaling and growth suppression. Mediation by stabilization of TGF-β receptor type II," *Journal of Biological Chemistry*, vol. 281, no. 12, pp. 7765–7774, 2006.

[128] S. Uttamsingh, X. Bao, and K. T. Nguyen, "Synergistic effect between EGF and TGF-β1 in inducing oncogenic properties of intestinal epithelial cells," *Oncogene*, vol. 27, no. 18, pp. 2626–2634, 2008.

[129] P. M. Siegel, W. Shu, R. D. Cardiff, W. J. Muller, and J. Massagué, "Transforming growth factor β signaling impairs Neu-induced mammary tumorigenesis while promoting pulmonary metastasis," *Proceedings of the National Academy of Sciences of the United States of America*, vol. 100, no. 14, pp. 8430–8435, 2003.

[130] S. E. Seton-Rogers and J. S. Brugge, "ErbB2 and TGF-beta: a cooperative role in mammary tumor progression?" *Cell Cycle*, vol. 3, no. 5, pp. 597–600, 2004.

[131] M. Andrianifahanana, M. C. Wilkes, C. E. Repellin et al., "ERBB receptor activation is required for profibrotic responses to transforming growth factor β," *Cancer Research*, vol. 70, no. 19, pp. 7421–7430, 2010.

[132] G. Mincione, M. Cirafici, D. Lazzereschi, S. Pepe, F. Ciardiello, and G. Colletta, "Loss of thyrotropin regulation and transforming growth factor beta-induced growth arrest in erbB-2 overexpressing rat thyroid cells," *Cancer Research*, vol. 53, no. 22, pp. 5548–5553, 1993.

[133] M. Nilsson, T. Dahlman, B. Westermark, and K. Westermark, "Transforming growth factor-β promotes epidermal growth factor-induced thyroid cell migration and follicle neoformation in collagen gel separable from cell proliferation," *Experimental Cell Research*, vol. 220, no. 2, pp. 257–265, 1995.

[134] H. Mishima, M. Nakamura, J. Murakami, T. Nishida, and T. Otori, "Transforming growth factor-beta modulates effects of epidermal growth factor on corneal epithelial cells," *Current Eye Research*, vol. 11, no. 7, pp. 691–696, 1992.

[135] S. Hoffmann, L. C. Hofbauer, V. Scharrenbach et al., "Thyrotropin (TSH)-induced production of vascular endothelial growth factor in thyroid cancer cells in vitro: evaluation of TSH signal transduction and of angiogenesis-stimulating growth factors," *Journal of Clinical Endocrinology & Metabolism*, vol. 89, no. 12, pp. 6139–6145, 2004.

14

Controversies in the Management and Followup of Differentiated Thyroid Cancer: Beyond the Guidelines

Hala Ahmadieh and Sami T. Azar

Division of Endocrinology, Department of Internal Medicine, American University of Beirut Medical Center,

3 Dag Hammarskjold Plaza, New York, NY 10017, USA

Correspondence should be addressed to Sami T. Azar, sazar@aub.edu.lb

Academic Editor: Maria Grazia Chiofalo

Thyroid cancer is among the most common endocrine malignancies. Genetic and environmental factors play an important role in the pathogenesis of differentiated thyroid cancer. Both have good prognosis but with frequent recurrences. Cancer staging is an essential prognostic part of cancer management. There are multiple controversies in the management and followup of differentiated thyroid cancer. Debate still exists with regard to the optimal surgical approach but trends toward a more conservative approach, such as lobectomy, are being more favored, especially in papillary thyroid cancer, of tumor sizes less than 4 cm, in the absence of other high-risk suggestive features. Survival of patients with well-differentiated thyroid cancer was adversely affected by lymph node metastases. Prophylactic central LN dissection did improve accuracy in staging and decrease postop TG level, but it had no effect on small-sized tumors. Conservative approach was more applied with regard to the need and dose of radioiodine given postoperatively. There have been several advancements in the management of radioiodine resistant advanced differentiated thyroid cancers. Appropriate followup is required based on risk stratification of patients postoperatively. Many studies are still ongoing in order to reach the optimal management and followup of differentiated thyroid cancer.

1. Incidence and Prevalence of Thyroid Cancer

Thyroid cancer is one of the most common endocrine malignancies currently present. The estimated new thyroid cancer cases in the United States in 2012 are 56,460 and there are around 1780 deaths from thyroid cancer [1]. Incidence of thyroid cancer has been increasing. This could be related to the earlier detection of thyroid cancer with the current use of imaging and the use of FNA of all suspicious thyroid nodules. It is important to note that the overall 10-year mortality for DTC is low at about 7% but the recurrence rate occurrence is higher, causing considerable anxiety among patients and treating physicians. The current paper focuses on the controversies in the initial management and subsequent followup of well-differentiated thyroid cancer.

2. Pathogenesis of Differentiated Thyroid Cancer

Papillary and follicular thyroid carcinomas are the two histological subtypes of differentiated thyroid cancer. Both are indolent and have good prognosis overall. The biological behavior of these two carcinomas differ significantly, where papillary thyroid carcinoma is known to frequently metastasize to regional lymph nodes, whereas follicular thyroid carcinoma more frequently metastasizes to distant organs such as the lung, bone, and brain. Pathogenesis of differentiated thyroid carcinoma is multifactorial with both genetic and environmental factors playing an important role. For unknown reasons, it was found to be 2–4 times more common in women. Previous exposure to ionizing radiation including external irradiation of the neck would increase the incidence of thyroid cancer especially the papillary type. It was noted that there is a five- and two-fold increase of thyroid cancer incidence in obese men and women, respectively. In areas with adequate iodine intake differentiated thyroid carcinoma accounts for more than 80% of cases of thyroid cancer with the papillary type being the most common. In iodine deficient area there is a relative increase in the incidence of follicular and anaplastic thyroid cancer [2].

In recent years, the molecular basis of thyroid carcinogenesis has been investigated. In papillary thyroid carcinoma, BRAF mutations account for 45% of the cases with a higher prevalence in the "tall cell" differentiated forms. RET/PTC rearrangement was also found to account for 25–30% of papillary thyroid carcinoma cases. Point mutations of Ras gene and PAX 8/PPAR$_y$ rearrangement account for the majority of follicular thyroid carcinomas. Distant metastasis at the time of diagnosis was the most important prognostic factor for both papillary and follicular thyroid carcinomas. Extrathyroidal extension and lymph node metastasis were important prognostic factors for papillary thyroid carcinoma while the grade of invasiveness and carcinoma differentiation were important to evaluate the biological behavior of follicular thyroid cancer [3].

3. Staging of Differentiated Thyroid Cancer

Cancer staging is an essential prognostic and integral part of cancer management. 17 different staging systems were described for patients with thyroid carcinoma [5]. The most currently used is the 6th edition TNM (tumor, node, and metastasis) staging, proposed by The American Joint Committee on Cancer (AJCC) and the International Union against Cancer Committee (UICC). Patients whose age is less than 45 years can be either Stage I or II with the only difference between the two stages is the absence or presence of metastasis. However, in older patients, nodal metastasis would classify those patients as stage III patients while distant metastasis would classify them as stage IV [6, 7]. It is important to note that the AJCC TNM classification to define thyroid cancer was recently criticized because it was considered that it may be too optimistic to classify younger patients this way. Effect of age and disease extent on mortality was examined in the AJCC staging system using survival data obtained from SEER Program from 1973 to 2005, with the aim of determining whether risk stratification did portray outcomes of DTC for young patients specifically. In multivariate analysis, 50% increased mortality was found for every decade from age 40 to 90, with this effect being more pronounced in women. When TNM staging applied for those above, the age of 45 years was applied to those less than 45 years and it was noted that there was an increased mortality for those now reclassified as stage III or IV based on LN involvement and tumor spread outside the thyroid but without distant metastases. However, the limitations of this study was that it did not analyze recurrence which is, of course, something more frequent than mortality in DTC [8]. Other important staging systems include the AGES (Age, Grade, Extent, Size) [9], the MACIS (Metastasis,

Age, Completeness of resection, Invasion, Size) [10], both proposed by the Mayo Clinic, and both stratify patients into four risk groups, and the AMES (Age, Metastasis, Extension, Size) [11] proposed by the Lahey clinic, in addition to many other important staging systems as well. It was shown that after 20 years of diagnosis of differentiated thyroid cancer, the two most important prognostic factors were male gender and having the follicular type of thyroid cancer [12].

4. Controversies in the Management of Differentiated Thyroid Cancer

Initial management of differentiated thyroid cancer consists of thyroidectomy and, in certain cases, radioactive iodine therapy to ablate remnant remaining tissue and perhaps metastatic cancer. These are generally followed by long-term therapy with thyroxine with the aim of reducing circulating levels of thyrotropin (thyroid stimulating hormone, TSH) below normal. Revised American thyroid association guidelines were published in 2009 that looked at optimal management and follow up of differentiated thyroid cancer [13]. However, there are still controversies involving the optimal extent of initial surgery, the indications for prophylactic central lymph node dissection, the need for radioiodine therapy and the dose required, the degree of TSH suppression and its importance, and the aid of molecular markers to determine the risk of malignancy especially for indeterminate FNA samples.

4.1. Proper Extent of Initial Surgery. Extent of disease does affect outcome in patients with papillary thyroid carcinoma. Conflicting data exists in the literature regarding the optimal surgical approach for patients with differentiated thyroid cancer due to the fact that there are still no prospective, randomized studies addressing the issue specifically. ATA revised guidelines in 2009 stated that "for patients with thyroid cancer >1 cm, the initial surgical procedure should be a near-total or total thyroidectomy unless there are contraindications to this surgery. Thyroid lobectomy alone may be sufficient treatment for small (<1 cm), low-risk, unifocal, intrathyroidal papillary carcinomas in the absence of prior head and neck irradiation or radiologically or clinically involved cervical nodal metastases" [13]. Similarly, the 2007 British Guidelines for the management of thyroid cancer mentioned that "patients with a papillary thyroid cancer (PTC) more than 1 cm in diameter or with high-risk follicular thyroid cancer (FTC) should undergo near-total or total thyroidectomy". However, it was mentioned that "patients with low-risk PTC and even FTC ≤1 cm in diameter may be treated with thyroid lobectomy alone" [14]. A study looked at whether total thyroidectomy, as compared to lobectomy, would result in decreased recurrence and improved long-term survival in 52,173 patients who underwent surgery for papillary thyroid carcinoma. 82.9% of those patients underwent total thyroidectomy while 17.1% underwent lobectomy. A 10-year recurrence rate was 4.6% in tumors <1 cm, 7.1% in 1.0–1.9 cm, 8.6% in 2.0–2.9 cm, 11.6% in 3.0–3.9 cm, 17.2% in 4.0–7.9 cm, and 24.8% in tumors >8.0 cm. For those patients whose tumor size was less than 1 cm extent of surgery had no impact on recurrence or survival, while for those patients with tumor size more than 1 cm lobectomy resulted in higher risk of recurrence and death ($P = 0.04$) [15]. Another retrospective review of 289 patients, selected for either thyroid lobectomy ($n = 72$) or total thyroidectomy ($n = 217$), without radioactive iodine remnant ablation, and followed by a single experienced endocrinologist with modern disease detection tools, in a tertiary referral center, was developed at the Memorial Sloan-Kettering Cancer Center (MSKCC). After a 5-year followup, disease recurrence was detected in 2.3% (5/217) of patients treated with total thyroidectomy, without radioactive iodine remnant ablation, and in 4.2% (3/72) of patients treated with thyroid lobectomy alone. Size of the primary tumor, presence of cervical lymph node metastases and American Thyroid Association risk category were all statistically significant predictors of recurrence. Changes in serum thyroglobulin were not helpful in identifying persistent/recurrent structural disease presence. In addition it was found that 88% (7/8) of patients who had recurrent disease were rendered clinically disease-free with additional therapies [16]. A recent study, utilizing the Surveillance, Epidemiology, and End Results program database of the National Cancer Institute, questioned the validity of the most recent ATA guidelines regarding the extent of surgery for papillary thyroid cancer. This study included 22,724 patients with papillary thyroid cancer, of which 5964 patients underwent lobectomy with a median followup of 9 years. Multivariate analysis showed no survival difference between patients who underwent total thyroidectomy versus lobectomy for all tumor sizes (<1 cm, 1–1.9 cm, 2–2.9 cm, 3–3.9 cm, and >4 cm. It was also shown that increased age, increased tumor size, extrathyroidal extent, and positive nodal status displayed significantly worse disease specific survival and overall survival ($P < 0.001$ [17]). The debate regarding the extent of surgery in patients with papillary thyroid carcinoma persists and a well-designed prospective randomized study is needed in order to clarify whether less strict approach should be applied in such cases even for those patients whose tumor size is more than 1 cm.

4.2. Prophylactic versus Therapeutic Central LN Dissection. Presence of LN metastasis has a negative outcome in general and can be identified preoperatively or during operation. Prophylactic neck dissection is defined as the removal of seemingly normal lymph nodes apparent as per ultrasound and during surgery. Prophylactic central LN dissection would improve accuracy in staging, decreases postoperative TG level, can be performed safely as total thyroidectomy alone in experienced hands leading sometimes to avoidance of further operations in central neck, and may lead to lower recurrence and improved mortality. The other rationale to perform prophylactic central LN dissection is the questionable ability of the preoperative ultrasound or intraoperative assessment to adequately evaluate the central neck compartment [18–20]. However, it may lead to a higher rate of hypoprathyroidism that was reported in one study to occur in up to 14% of patients after prophylactic central LN dissection as opposed

to 1-2% after total thyroidectomy, and the higher possibility of recurrent laryngeal injury, with the absence of level 1 data of lower recurrence and improved survival [18]. Hence, a current widely debated subject in PTC patients is whether prophylactic central neck dissection (PCND) should be done in patients who are found to have clinically negative nodes by ultrasound, on physical exam, and during intraoperative assessment.

Some studies have shown no difference in survival in those patients who underwent lymphadenectomy versus those who did not [21]. On the other hand, a large multi-institutional study looked of how the presence of lymph node disease would adversely affect the outcome in 19,918 patients with papillary and follicular thyroid carcinomas using Surveillance, Epidemiology, and End Results (SEER) database, which is a large scale sample of 14 percent of the U.S. population. Using a multivariate analysis it was shown that those patients whose age is more than 45 years, who had the presence of distant metastasis, tumors of large size size >4 cm, and lymph node metastasis did significantly have predicted poor outcome. Overall survival at 14 years was 82 per cent for patients with node negative as opposed to 79 per cent for node positive patients ($P < 0.05$); hence, survival of those patients with well-differentiated thyroid cancer was adversely affected by lymph node metastases where they were at greater risk of recurrence and death [22]. Moreover, a retrospective study was done over a period of 12 month, which included patients before year 2002, when the initial management included total thyroidectomy and radioiodine therapy for papillary thyroid cancer, and patients managed after the year 2002, where management was modified to include prophylactic central LN dissection in addition to total thyroidectomy. Those patients with regional LN metastasis had higher stimulated thyroglobulin levels at one year followup if no prophylactic central LN dissection was done. In addition, more complete lymphadenectomy was associated with a lowering of thyroglobulin levels overall [23].

Recently in a study including 115 patients an aggressive approach to papillary thyroid cancer was adapted, with prophylactic bilateral level dissection of LNs (level VI) and in some cases, ipsilateral symmetrical levels II, III, and IV dissections, in patients with small papillary thyroid cancer, who had negative preoperative neck ultrasound. Mean size of PTC was 12.5 mm and extension of tumor beyond thyroid capsule was found in 29% of patients, with central LNs found to be involved in 45% of patients, and lateral LNs involved in 47% of patients. 58% of patients underwent radioiodine therapy afterwards, in those PTC tumors larger than 18 mm with lymph node metastases, or having aggressive histology and younger age (<18 years). Prophylactic lymph node dissection modified the indication for radioiodine ablation in 30% of patients. At 1-year followup all patients had negative neck ultrasound examinations, and 97% had an undetectable stimulated serum thyroglobulin [24].

These opposing findings in retrospective studies continue the current and do not provide a uniform approach in the management of PTC; however, a current prospective multicenter clinical trial has been submitted to the National

Institute of Health trying to look at the benefits and risks of an ipsilateral prophylactic central LN dissection. ATA guidelines consider prophylactic central LN dissection in patients with T3 and T4 tumors but not in those who has smaller tumors [13]. The Japanese association of endocrinology recommends prophylactic central LN dissection based on clinic-pathological features rather than treating all patients uniformly in the same way [25].

4.3. Radioactive Iodine Ablation. In addition to the current controversy regarding the extent of surgery and the need for prophylactic central LN dissection, the need for postoperative radioactive iodine (RAI) ablation is also a current widely debated subject. RAI therapy is used as an adjunct to surgery, to eradicate occult persistent or metastatic disease, with the aim of reducing the risk of recurrence and improving mortality. Differentiated thyroid cancer, especially papillary thyroid cancer, has an excellent prognosis overall, that is why the need for postoperative RAI therapy has been questioned. As per ATA guidelines, RAI is recommended in patients with gross extrathyroidal extension, known distant metastases, and for tumors more than 4 cm. For patients whose tumors are 1 to 4 cm, a selective approach is recommended. RAI is not recommended for tumors less than 1 cm even if multifocal but micro-PTC and no high-risk features present [13]. Some even advocate no RAI ablation for well-differentiated PTC for tumors between 1 and 4 cm who have less than 3–5 metastatic cervical lymph nodes that are less than 5 mm in diameter [26]. On the other hand, British guidelines mentioned that "majority of patients with a tumor more than 1 cm in diameter, who have undergone a near-total/total thyroidectomy, should have 131I ablation" [14]. A recent retrospective study revisited the issue of RAI ablation and analyzed 289 patients, of which 74% were low risk and 26% were intermediate risk according to the ATA risk stratification study, from the Memorial Sloan-Kettering Cancer Center. 75% of patients were treated with total thyroidectomy and 25% treated with lobectomy. Selective central neck lymph node dissection was done in 5% of those patients. It was shown that only 2% of those treated with total thyroidectomy and 4% with lobectomy who did not have RAI therapy recurred. Even when tumors >1 cm were only analyzed, the recurrence rate following total thyroidectomy without RAI remained low at 4% [16].

With regards to the dose of RAI needed, larger doses of RAI therapy (100–200 mCi) are considered appropriate, if residual microscopic disease is suspected, or aggressive tumor histology detected. As for distant metastatic, disease a "fixed-dose" regimen is the most widely used, with 150 mCi for cervical and higher doses in the range of 200–250 mCi for pulmonary metastases or skeletal metastases [27]. As for the optimal dose of RAI therapy needed in those patients at low risk, a recent randomized phase 3 trial compared two thyrotropin stimulation methods (thyroid hormone withdrawal and the use of recombinant human thyrotropin) and two different radiodine doses (I131) (1.1 GBq and 3.7 GBq), in a 2-by-2 design, in 752 patients with low-risk differentiated thyroid cancer, where patients were included

if they had pT1 (tumor diameter ≤ 1 cm) and N1 or Nx, pT1 (with tumor diameter >1 to 2 cm) and any N stage, or pT2N0 with absent distant metastasis. Thyroid ablation was equivalent between different I131 doses and between different thyrotropin stimulation methods [28]. Another recent study showed the same outcome as the previous study where patients aged 16 to 80 with T1 to T3 tumor size, with possible spread to LN, but no metastasis, underwent low-versus high-dose RAI, in combination with either TSH alfa or TH withdrawal prior, and it was shown that the success rates were comparable in all groups of patients ranging between 85 and 89% [29].

4.4. Molecular Markers to Aid in Malignancy Diagnosis in Indeterminate FNA Samples. The expansion of knowledge regarding genetic mutations in thyroid cancers has led to the use of molecular markers as an indicator of prognosis and for the malignancy diagnosis especially in indeterminate FNA samples (BRAF, RAS, RET/PTC, and PAX8/PPARγ) [2]. Recent large prospective studies have emphasized the ability of genetic markers (BRAF, RAS, RET/PTC, and PAX8/PPARγ) and protein markers (galectin-3) to significantly improve and affect the preoperative diagnostic accuracy especially for patients who have indeterminate thyroid nodules [30–34]. Moreover, the use of such molecular markers was further recommended by the 2009 revised ATA guidelines where the sensitivity of malignant diagnosis in FNA thyroid nodules was found to be increased from 44% to 80%, when comparing cytology alone to cytology combined with molecular testing for the markers in most of those studies. One of those studies showed that the sensitivity of malignant diagnosis in FNA increased from 60%, with cytology alone, to 90% with cytology and molecular testing for BRAF, RAS, RET, TRK, and PPARγ mutations [33]. It can be concluded that the best current preoperative tool for thyroid cancer is the cytological examination of molecular markers of FNA biopsies from indeterminate thyroid nodules.

5. Controversies in the Followup of Differentiated Thyroid Cancer

5.1. Role of TSH Suppressive Therapy. Thyroid hormone suppression is now a recognized treatment for patients with differentiated thyroid cancer. In 2002, the first meta-analysis was published regarding TSH suppressive therapy but included 10 studies with small series of patients. This meta-analysis concluded that treatment with high thyroxine doses was effective in decreasing recurrence but it had little importance with regards to the overall survival [35]. Then in 2006, a study stratified the effect of this therapeutic approach and found that this approach had no effect on survival in stage I low-risk patients, but patients staged II, III, and IV did have worse survival when TSH level was maintained more than 3 mU/L [36]. The revised ATA guidelines state that "in patients with persistent disease, the serum TSH should be maintained below 0.1 mU/L indefinitely in the absence of specific contraindications." They also added that "in patients who are clinically and biochemically free of disease but who presented with high-risk disease, consideration should be given to maintaining TSH suppressive therapy to achieve serum TSH levels of 0.1–0.5 mU/L for 5–10 years" but "in patients free of disease, especially those at low risk for recurrence, the serum TSH may be kept within the low normal range (0.3–2 mU/L). They further mentioned that "in patients who have not undergone remnant ablation who are clinically free of disease and have undetectable suppressed serum Tg and normal neck US, the serum TSH may be allowed to rise to the low normal range (0.3–2 mU/L)" [13]. Moreover, British guidelines recommended that in those patients being treated with 131I, levothyroxine therapy should be added three days later, with the aim of suppressing serum thyroid-stimulating hormone (TSH) to <0.1 mIU/L. In patients confirmed to be low risk, a serum TSH <0.5 mIU/L was considered acceptable [14]. It is important to mention that the only randomized prospective study conducted to date, recently published, assessed the efficacy of thyroid hormone suppressive therapy, where they randomized 400 patients undergoing surgery for DTC into a group treated with thyroxine to achieve TSH suppression, while other group of patients treated to maintain TSH within the normal range. The authors found that after a mean followup of 7 years, there was no significant difference between the two groups in regard to disease-free time, relapse, and time of relapse, distant metastases, overall mortality, or specific mortality [37]. In addition it was noted that TSH suppressive therapy was not without risk. A recent review noted increased incidence of kidney, pancreas, ovarian, and breast cancers [38]. Large epidemiological studies, including 29,000 patients, in Norway, monitored for 9 years after having suppressed TSH levels to less than 0.5 Mu/L, noted increased cancer incidence (hazard ratio 1.34) [39]. It was postulated that integrin activation by THs was responsible for promoting angiogenesis by thyroid hormones through the activation of mitogen-activated protein kinase (or MAPK pathway) [40].

Therefore the beneficial role of TSH suppressive therapy is questioned, given the recent randomized study that failed to show any benefit for TSH suppressive therapy, in addition to its possible overall increased risk to other cancer developments.

5.2. Diagnostic Imaging for the Followup of DTC.

The 3-to-12-month monitoring of patients with extrathyroidal invasion or local-regional nodal metastases using ultrasound of neck and serum thyroglobulin should be performed on all patients with differentiated thyroid cancer as per ATA guidelines [13]. It is worth noting that sometimes elevated thyroglobulin or thyroglobulin antibody is found along with negative radioactive iodine scan and in such cases ultrasound is definitely recommended and this could be indicative of nonradioiodine avid residual or recurrent disease. It was found that half of the patients with negative radioiodine scan have recurrent disease based on the use of ultrasound, which can accurately identify lesions in the neck even as small as 3 mm [41]. Other imaging techniques

that can be used in followup of certain patients include CT scan of the neck with IV contrast, CT scan of the chest, and magnetic resonance imaging (MRI) although the sensitivity of these imaging techniques are inferior to ultrasound, and they are frequently used if ultrasound is not available, or if deep posterior disease suspected. Fluorodeoxyglucose positron-emission tomography (FDG-PET or PET)/CT imaging is useful for the detection of radioiodine negative and thyroglobulin positive thyroid cancer which tends to have higher glucose metabolism and this points to tumor dedifferentiation [42, 43]. TSH stimulates 18FDG uptake by differentiated thyroid carcinoma making it more sensitive. However, a large multicenter study showed that rh TSH stimulated PET-CT changed treatment plan in only 6% of cases [44].

5.3. Long-Term Followup and Stratification of DTC Patients.

As shown in Table 1 Patients can be risk stratified at 6 months followup based on their unstimulated and stimulated thyroglobulin level, thyroglobulin antibodies, neck exam, neck ultrasound, diagnostic radioiodine scans, use of other cross-sectional imaging like CT scans, MRI, or PET into having excellent, acceptable, and incomplete response [4].

Patients who are considered to have excellent response based on undetectable thyroglobulin including stimulated thyroglobulin, normal neck ultrasound, negative radioiodine scan, and negative scans (CT, MRI, or PET) can be followed with yearly physical exam and yearly suppressed thyroglobulin with no need for stimulated thyroglobulin. Patients who had acceptable response, meaning detectable suppressed thyroglobulin < 1 ng/mL, stimulated thyroglobulin < 10 ng/mL, nonspecific changes in neck ultrasound including few subcentimetric LNs, and negative radioiodine scans, can be followed with yearly physical exam, suppressed and stimulated thyroglobulin yearly for at least another 3 years. Patients who have incomplete response, due to increased suppressed TG > 1 ng/mL, increased stimulated thyroglobulin > 10 ng/mL with cervical LNs > 1 cm, positive radioiodine scan, and positive other imaging modalities including CT, MRI, or PET, should be referred for additional therapies [4]. This was clearly shown in Table 2. On the other hand, based on expert opinion, British guidelines mentioned that serum thyroglobulin should be checked in all postoperative patients with differentiated thyroid cancer six weeks after surgery and stimulated thyroglobulin indicated 6 months after 131I ablation. They also added that postablation whole-body scan, done after stopping levothyroxine for four weeks, should be considered 3–10 days after 131I ablation. However, in low-risk patients, the measurement of stimulated thyroglobulin without a diagnostic 131I WBS may be adequate. In such cases, it was recommended that ultrasonography of the neck 6–12 months after thyroidectomy is indicated. As for the long-term recurrence, proposed by the British guidelines, annual clinical examination, annual measurement of serum Tg and TSH, diagnostic imaging and FNA as indicated are required [14].

TABLE 1: Variables determined during follow-up that predict response to therapy (Tg → thyroglobulin) (adapted from [4]).

	Excellent response	Acceptable response	Incomplete response
Suppressed Tg	Undetectable	Detectable but <1 ng/mL	>1 ng/mL
Stimulated Tg	Undetectable	<10 ng/mL	>10 ng/mL
Trend in suppressed Tg	Remains undetectable	Declining	Stable or rising
Anti-Tg antibodies	Absent	Absent or declining	Persistent or rising
Neck examination	Normal	Normal	Palpable disease
Neck ultrasonography	No evidence of disease	Nonspecific changes in thyroid bed, Stable millimeter sized cervical LN even if abnormal by US criteria	Evidence of structurally significant recurrent/persistent disease in the thyroid bed (>1 cm), cervical lymph nodes (>1 cm), or distant metastases, particularly if structurally progressive or FDG avid
Diagnostic RAI WBS	No evidence for RAI avid disease	No evidence for RAI avid disease, very faint uptake in thyroid bed only	Persistent/recurrent RAI avid disease present
Cross-sectional imaging (MRI, CT)	No evidence of disease	Non-specific changes	Structural disease present
FDG PET scanning	No evidence of disease	Non-specific changes consistent with normal variants or inflammatory changes	FDG avid disease present

TABLE 2: Follow-up strategy based on risk groups (adapted from [4]).

	Initial estimate of risk of recurrence first 2 years of followup incomplete response		
Suppressed Tg	Low risk Q 6 months	Intermediate risk Q 6 months	High risk Q 6 months
Stimulated Tg	Not required	<10 ng/mL	>10 ng/mL
Neck ultrasound	Q year × 2	Q year × 2	Q year × 2
Diagnostic RAI WBS	Not required	1-2 years	1-2 years
Cross-sectional imaging (MRI, CT)	Not required	Not required	If Tg elevated or high clinical suspicion
	Secondary risk stratification response to therapy assessment		
Ongoing followup	Yearly physical examination, yearly suppressed Tg	Yearly physical examination, yearly suppressed Tg, stimulated Tg to document undetectable Tg on suppression, continued observation/assessment of indeterminate structural abnormalities for at least another 2-3 years	Consider additional cross-sectional imaging, possibly FDG PET scan and the need for additional therapy

5.4. Management of Advanced or Metastatic Thyroid Cancer.
Surgery in advanced thyroid carcinomas is the best modality used for recurrent neck metastases, since most recurrences are seen in the thyroid bed or regional lymph nodes. This is usually followed by further radioactive iodine, especially if the recurrence is radioiodine avid, along with thyroid hormone suppression. If the gross tumors are not radioactive iodine avid then further postoperative radioactive iodine will be of limited benefit. Surgery is also considered for isolated metastases in bone and brain. External beam radiotherapy (EBRT) may be an effective adjuvant therapy in patients with locally invasive papillary carcinoma who are 45 years of age and older [45, 46]. British guidelines noted that external beam radiotherapy can occasionally be used in patients with pT4 tumours (TNM staging) who have residual disease in the neck not amenable to surgery, especially in tumours not taking up 131I. In addition it was found to have a possible role as a palliative measure in patients with advanced local or distant disease [14]. Patients who are found to have brain metastasis can be treated with surgery which was found in one study to improve median survival from four to 22 months in patients who had 1 or more brain metastases. Radioiodine therapy and/or external beam radiotherapy should be considered after surgical resection

with the concomitant use of steroids. External beam radiation therapy (EBRT) or gamma knife radiosurgery and IV bisphosphonates has also been used for patients with painful bony metastasis [47, 48]. Clinical trials should be considered the first-line therapy for patients who are considered to have nonavid radioactive iodine response. Systemic chemotherapy has been tried in widespread progressive disease that is radioiodine resistant but has not been shown to be effective to date [49]. Several tyrosine kinase inhibitors have been tried until now with a partial response ranging between 13% and 50% [50–52].

References

[1] American Cancer Society, *Cancer Facts & Figures 2012*, American Cancer Society, Atlanta, Ga, USA, 2012.

[2] F. Giusti, A. Falchetti, F. Franceschelli, F. Marini, A. Tanini, and M. L. Brandi, "Thyroid cancer: current molecular perspectives," *Journal of Oncology*, vol. 2010, Article ID 351679, 17 pages, 2010.

[3] F. Pacini, M. G. Castagna, L. Brilli, and G. Pentheroudakis, "Differentiated thyroid cancer: ESMO clinical recommendations for diagnosis, treatment and follow-up," *Annals of Oncology*, vol. 20, no. 4, pp. 143–146, 2009.

[4] R. Tuttle, R. Leboeuf, and A. R. Shaha, "Medical management of thyroid cancer: a risk adapted approach," *Journal of Surgical Oncology*, vol. 97, no. 8, pp. 712–716, 2008.

[5] B. H. H. Lang, C. Y. Lo, W. F. Chan, K. Y. Lam, and K. Y. Wan, "Staging systems for papillary thyroid carcinoma: a review and comparison," *Annals of Surgery*, vol. 245, no. 3, pp. 366–378, 2007.

[6] A. R. Shaha, "TNM classification of thyroid carcinoma," *World Journal of Surgery*, vol. 31, no. 5, pp. 879–887, 2007.

[7] F. L. Greene, D. L. Page, I. D. Fleming et al., Eds., *AJCC Cancer Staging Handbook: TNM Classification of Malignant Tumors*, Springer, New York, NY, USA, 6th edition, 2002.

[8] H. Tran Cao, L. Johnston, D. Chang, and M. Bouvet, "The AJCC TNM staging underestimates risk in young patients with more aggressive differentiated thyroid cancer," *Clinical Thyroidology*, vol. 24, no. 6, 2012.

[9] I. D. Hay, C. S. Grant, W. F. Taylor, and W. M. McConahey, "Ipsilateral lobectomy versus bilateral lobar resection in papillary thyroid carcinoma: a retrospective analysis of surgical outcome using a novel prognostic scoring system," *Surgery*, vol. 102, no. 6, pp. 1088–1095, 1987.

[10] I. D. Hay, E. J. Bergstralh, J. R. Goellner et al., "Predicting outcome in papillary thyroid carcinoma: development of a reliable prognostic scoring system in a cohort of 1779 patients surgically treated at one institution during 1940 through 1989," *Surgery*, vol. 114, no. 6, pp. 1050–1058, 1993.

[11] B. Cady, R. Rossi, I. Hay, K. H. Cohn, and N. W. Thompson, "An expanded view of risk-group definition in differentiated thyroid carcinoma," *Surgery*, vol. 104, no. 6, pp. 947–953, 1988.

[12] L. E. Johnston, H. S. Tran Cao, D. C. Chang, and M. Bouvet, "Sociodemographic predictors of survival in differentiated thyroid cancer: results from the SEER database," *ISRN Endocrinology*, vol. 2012, Article ID 384707, 8 pages, 2012.

[13] D. S. Cooper, G. M. Doherty, B. R. Haugen et al., "Revised American thyroid association management guidelines for patients with thyroid nodules and differentiated thyroid cancer," *Thyroid*, vol. 19, no. 11, pp. 1167–1214, 2009.

[14] P. Perros, S. Clarke, J. Franklyn et al., "Guidelines for the management of thyroid cancer," British Thyroid Association, 2007.

[15] K. Y. Bilimoria, D. J. Bentrem, C. Y. Ko et al., "Extent of surgery affects survival for papillary thyroid cancer," *Annals of Surgery*, vol. 246, no. 3, pp. 375–381, 2007.

[16] F. Vaisman, A. Shaha, S. Fish, and R. Tuttle, "Initial therapy with either thyroid lobectomy or total thyroidectomy without radioactive iodine remnant ablation is associated with very low rates of structural disease recurrence in properly selected patients with differentiated thyroid cancer," *Clinical Endocrinology*, vol. 75, no. 1, pp. 112–119, 2011.

[17] A. H. Mendelsohn, D. A. Elashoff, E. Abemayor, and M. A. St John, "Surgery for papillary thyroid carcinoma: is lobectomy enough?" *Archives of Otolaryngology—Head and Neck Surgery*, vol. 136, no. 11, pp. 1055–1061, 2010.

[18] E. L. Mazzaferri, G. M. Doherty, and D. L. Steward, "The pros and cons of prophylactic central compartment lymph node dissection for papillary thyroid carcinoma," *Thyroid*, vol. 19, no. 7, pp. 683–689, 2009.

[19] J. M. Stulak, C. S. Grant, D. R. Farley et al., "Value of preoperative ultrasonography in the surgical management of initial and reoperative papillary thyroid cancer," *Archives of Surgery*, vol. 141, no. 5, pp. 489–496, 2006.

[20] W. T. Shen, L. Ogawa, D. Ruan, I. Suh, Q. Y. Duh, and O. H. Clark, "Central neck lymph node dissection for papillary thyroid cancer: the reliability of surgeon judgment in predicting which patients will benefit," *Surgery*, vol. 148, no. 2, pp. 398–403, 2010.

[21] J. L. Roh, J. Y. Park, and C. I. Park, "Total thyroidectomy plus neck dissection in differentiated papillary thyroid carcinoma patients: pattern of nodal metastasis, morbidity, recurrence, and postoperative levels of serum parathyroid hormone," *Annals of Surgery*, vol. 245, no. 4, pp. 604–610, 2007.

[22] Y. D. Podnos, D. Smith, L. D. Wagman, and J. D. I. Ellenhorn, "The implication of lymph node metastasis on survival in patients with well-differentiated thyroid cancer," *American Surgeon*, vol. 71, no. 9, pp. 731–734, 2005.

[23] M. Sywak, L. Cornford, P. Roach, P. Stalberg, S. Sidhu, and L. Delbridge, "Routine ipsilateral level VI lymphadenectomy reduces postoperative thyroglobulin levels in papillary thyroid cancer," *Surgery*, vol. 140, no. 6, pp. 1000–1007, 2006.

[24] S. Bonnet, D. Hartl, S. Leboulleux et al., "Prophylactic lymph node dissection for papillary thyroid cancer less than 2 cm: implications for radioiodine treatment," *The Journal of Clinical Endocrinology and Metabolism*, vol. 94, no. 4, pp. 1162–1167, 2009.

[25] H. Takami, Y. Ito, T. Okamoto, and A. Yoshida, "Therapeutic strategy for differentiated thyroid carcinoma in japan based on a newly established guideline managed by Japanese society of thyroid surgeons and Japanese association of endocrine surgeons," *World Journal of Surgery*, vol. 35, no. 1, pp. 111–121, 2011.

[26] H. Tala and R. Tuttle, "Contemporary post surgical management of differentiated thyroid carcinoma," *Clinical Oncology*, vol. 22, no. 6, pp. 419–429, 2010.

[27] C. Durante, N. Haddy, E. Baudin et al., "Long-term outcome of 444 patients with distant metastases from papillary and

follicular thyroid carcinoma: benefits and limits of radioiodine therapy," *The Journal of Clinical Endocrinology and Metabolism*, vol. 91, no. 8, pp. 2892–2899, 2006.

[28] M. Schlumberger, B. Catargi, I. Borget et al., "Strategies of radioiodine ablation in patients with low-risk thyroid cancer," *The New England Journal of Medicine*, vol. 366, no. 18, pp. 1663–1673, 2012.

[29] U. Mallick, C. Harmer, B. Yap et al., "Ablation with low-dose radioiodine and thyrotropin alfa in thyroid cancer," *The New England Journal of Medicine*, vol. 366, no. 18, pp. 1674–1685, 2012.

[30] W. Moses, J. Weng, I. Sansano et al., "Molecular testing for somatic mutations improves the accuracy of thyroid fine-needle aspiration biopsy," *World Journal of Surgery*, vol. 34, no. 11, pp. 2589–2594, 2010.

[31] T. J. Musholt, C. Fottner, M. M. Weber et al., "Detection of papillary thyroid carcinoma by analysis of BRAF and RET/PTC1 mutations in fine-needle aspiration biopsies of thyroid nodules," *World Journal of Surgery*, vol. 34, no. 11, pp. 2595–2603, 2010.

[32] Y. E. Nikiforov, D. L. Steward, T. M. Robinson-Smith et al., "Molecular testing for mutations in improving the fine-needle aspiration diagnosis of thyroid nodules," *The Journal of Clinical Endocrinology and Metabolism*, vol. 94, no. 6, pp. 2092–2098, 2009.

[33] S. Cantara, M. Capezzone, S. Marchisotta et al., "Impact of proto-oncogene mutation detection in cytological specimens from thyroid nodules improves the diagnostic accuracy of cytology," *The Journal of Clinical Endocrinology and Metabolism*, vol. 95, no. 3, pp. 1365–1369, 2010.

[34] C. Franco, V. Martínez, J. P. Allamand et al., "Molecular markers in thyroid fine-needle aspiration biopsy: a prospective study," *Applied Immunohistochemistry and Molecular Morphology*, vol. 17, no. 3, pp. 211–215, 2009.

[35] N. J. McGriff, G. Csako, L. Gourgiotis, L. C. Guthrie, F. Pucino, and N. J. Sarlis, "Effects of thyroid hormone suppression therapy on adverse clinical outcomes in thyroid cancer," *Annals of Medicine*, vol. 34, no. 7-8, pp. 554–564, 2002.

[36] J. Jonklaas, N. J. Sarlis, D. Litofsky et al., "Outcomes of patients with differentiated thyroid carcinoma following initial therapy," *Thyroid*, vol. 16, no. 12, pp. 1229–1242, 2006.

[37] I. Sugitani and Y. Fujimoto, "Does postoperative thyrotropin suppression therapy truly decrease recurrence in papillary thyroid carcinoma? A randomized controlled trial," *The Journal of Clinical Endocrinology and Metabolism*, vol. 95, no. 10, pp. 4576–4583, 2010.

[38] C. Zafón, "TSH-suppressive treatment in differentiated thyroid cancer. A dogma under review," *Endocrinología y Nutrición*, vol. 59, no. 2, pp. 125–130, 2012.

[39] A. I. Hellevik, B. O. Åsvold, T. Bjøro, P. R. Romundstad, T. I. L. Nilsen, and L. J. Vatten, "Thyroid function and cancer risk: a prospective population study," *Cancer Epidemiology Biomarkers and Prevention*, vol. 18, no. 2, pp. 570–574, 2009.

[40] J. J. Bergh, H. Y. Lin, L. Lansing et al., "Integrin $\alpha_V\beta_3$ contains a cell surface receptor site for thyroid hormone that is linked to activation of mitogen-activated protein kinase and induction of angiogenesis," *Endocrinology*, vol. 146, no. 7, pp. 2864–2871, 2005.

[41] A. Antonelli, P. Miccoli, M. Ferdeghini et al., "Role of neck ultrasonography in the follow-up of patients operated on for thyroid cancer," *Thyroid*, vol. 5, no. 1, pp. 25–28, 1995.

[42] U. Feine, R. Lietzenmayer, J. P. Hanke, J. Held, H. Wöhrle, and W. Müller-Schauenburg, "Fluorine-18-FDG and iodine-131-iodide uptake in thyroid cancer," *Journal of Nuclear Medicine*, vol. 37, no. 9, pp. 1468–1472, 1996.

[43] W. Wang, H. Macapinlac, S. M. Larson et al., "[^{18}F]-2-fluoro-2-deoxy-D-glucose positron emission tomography localizes residual thyroid cancer in patients with negative diagnostic 131I whole body scans and elevated serum thyroglobulin levels," *The Journal of Clinical Endocrinology and Metabolism*, vol. 84, no. 7, pp. 2291–2302, 1999.

[44] S. Leboulleux, P. R. Schroeder, N. L. Busaidy et al., "Assessment of the incremental value of recombinant thyrotropin stimulation before 2-[18F]-fluoro-2-deoxy-D-glucose positron emission tomography/computed tomography imaging to localize residual differentiated thyroid cancer," *The Journal of Clinical Endocrinology and Metabolism*, vol. 94, no. 4, pp. 1310–1316, 2009.

[45] R. W. Tsang, J. D. Brierley, W. J. Simpson, T. Panzarella, M. K. Gospodarowicz, and S. B. Sutcliffe, "The effects of surgery, radioiodine, and external radiation therapy on the clinical outcome of patients with differentiated thyroid carcinoma," *Cancer*, vol. 82, no. 2, pp. 375–388, 1998.

[46] J. Farahati, C. Reiners, M. Stuschke et al., "Differentiated thyroid cancer. Impact of adjuvant external radiotherapy in patients with perithyroidal tumor infiltration (stage pT4)," *Cancer*, vol. 77, no. 1, pp. 172–180, 1996.

[47] C. F. A. Eustatia-Rutten, J. A. Romijn, M. J. Guijt et al., "Outcome of palliative embolization of bone metastases in differentiated thyroid carcinoma," *The Journal of Clinical Endocrinology and Metabolism*, vol. 88, no. 7, pp. 3184–3189, 2003.

[48] Y. Orita, I. Sugitani, K. Toda, J. Manabe, and Y. Fujimoto, "Zoledronic acid in the treatment of bone metastases from differentiated thyroid carcinoma," *Thyroid*, vol. 21, no. 1, pp. 31–35, 2011.

[49] F. Santini, V. Bottici, R. Elisei et al., "Cytotoxic effects of carboplatinum and epirubicin in the setting of an elevated serum thyrotropin for advanced poorly differentiated thyroid cancer," *The Journal of Clinical Endocrinology and Metabolism*, vol. 87, no. 9, pp. 4160–4165, 2002.

[50] A. Ravaud, C. de la Fouchardière, F. Courbon et al., "Sunitinib in patients with refractory advanced thyroid cancer: the THYSU phase II trial," *Journal of Clinical Oncology*, vol. 26, article 6058, 2008.

[51] K. C. Bible, R. C. Smallridge, W. J. Maples et al., "Endocrine Malignancies Disease Oriented Group, Mayo Phase 2 Consortium; Mayo Clinic, Rochester, MN; Mayo Clinic, Jacksonville, FL; National Cancer Institute, Bethesda, MD. Phase II trial of pazopanib in progressive, metastatic, iodine-insensitive differentiated thyroid cancers," *Journal of Clinical Oncology*, vol. 27, article 3521, 2009.

[52] N. Busaidy and M. Cabanillas, "Differentiated thyroid cancer: management of patients with radioiodine nonresponsive disease," *Journal of Thyroid Research*, vol. 2012, Article ID 618985, 12 pages, 2012.

15

Preoperative Thyrotropin Serum Concentrations Gradually Increase from Benign Thyroid Nodules to Papillary Thyroid Microcarcinomas Then to Papillary Thyroid Cancers of Larger Size

Carles Zafon,[1] Gabriel Obiols,[1] Juan Antonio Baena,[2] Josep Castellví,[3] Belen Dalama,[1] and Jordi Mesa[1]

[1] Department of Endocrinology, Hospital General Universitari Vall d'Hebron, Pg. Vall d'Hebron 119-129, 08035 Barcelona, Spain
[2] Department of Surgery, Unit of Endocrinological Surgery, Hospital General Universitari Vall d'Hebron, 08035 Barcelona, Spain
[3] Department of Pathology, Hospital General Universitari Vall d'Hebron, 08035 Barcelona, Spain

Correspondence should be addressed to Carles Zafon, 26276czl@comb.cat

Academic Editor: Nikola Bešič

We evaluated the preoperative serum thyrotropin (TSH) levels in 386 patients operated on for nodular thyroid disease (NTD). TSH levels for cases with final benign disease and differentiated thyroid carcinoma (DTC) were compared. No evidence of cancer was detected in 310 patients (80.3%), whereas malignancy was present in 76 cases (19.7%). Mean TSH concentration was 1.36 ± 1.62 mU/L in benign patients and 2.08 ± 2.1 in cases with malignant lesions ($P = 0.0013$). The group of malignancy was subdivided in papillary thyroid carcinoma (PTMC) versus thyroid cancer of larger size (TCLS). Mean TSH was 1.71 ± 1.52 in PTMC and 2.42 ± 2.5 in TCLS. Significant differences were found when all groups (benign, PTMC and TCLS) were compared ($P < 0.001$). However, pairwise comparisons between them showed that differences were only significant between benign and TCLS groups ($P < 0.01$). In conclusion, TSH levels were higher in patients with a final diagnosis of DTC. Moreover, it appears that there exists an increment in tumor size as a function of increment in the TSH level.

1. Introduction

Treatment of differentiated thyroid carcinomas (DTCs) includes total thyroidectomy, followed by removing affected (and nonaffected) lymph nodes in the central compartment of the neck, radioiodine for ablation of thyroid remnants or metastases, and suppressive treatment with L-thyroxine [1]. A supraphysiologic dose of thyroid hormone to suppress the secretion of endogenous thyroid-stimulating hormone (TSH) is associated with a longer relapse-free survival, overall survival, and carcinoma-related death [2]. The rationale for this approach is that TSH is the main regulator of thyrocyte differentiation and growth, and this capacity is retained in cancer cells of DTCs [3].

Furthermore, in recent years it has been shown that serum TSH concentration is an independent predictor of thyroid malignancy [4]. Several clinical studies have reported that higher levels of TSH are associated with an increased incidence of thyroid cancer in patients with nodular thyroid disease (NTD). It is currently not clear whether TSH is involved in the development of thyroid cancer, in the progression of thyroid cancer, or both [5]. Two reports have demonstrated that higher preoperative serum TSH levels are associated with more advanced cancer stages at the time of diagnosis [6, 7]. Moreover, Gerschpacher et al. [8] found that the TSH level is not elevated in subjects with papillary thyroid carcinoma (PTC) measuring ≤1 cm in size, a subset of tumors referred to as papillary thyroid microcarcinomas (PTMCs). Together, these findings support the notion that TSH may contribute to tumor progression.

The present study was conducted to determine the preoperative serum TSH levels in a group of patients who underwent surgery for NTD. TSH concentrations were correlated with the final histological diagnosis, defined

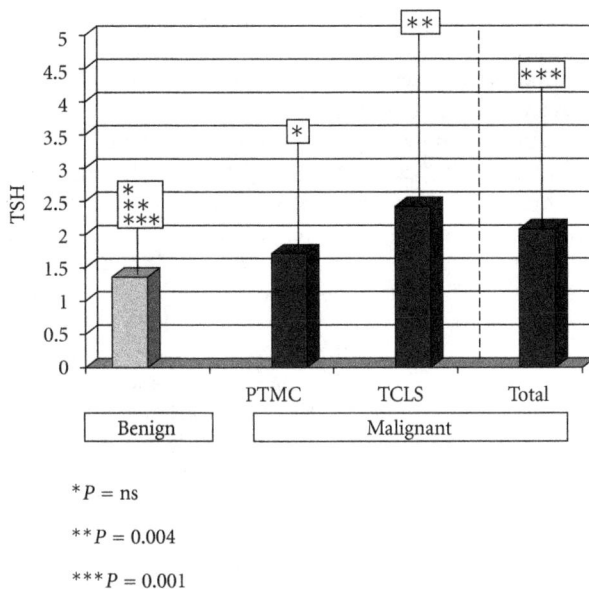

*P = ns

**P = 0.004

***P = 0.001

FIGURE 1: TSH concentrations in the different study groups. PTMC: papillary thyroid microcarcinoma and TCLS: thyroid carcinoma of larger size).

as the presence or absence of malignancy. Moreover, the group of malignancies was subdivided between patients with PTMCs and patients with thyroid cancers of larger size (TCLS).

2. Material and Methods

From January 2006 to December 2009, 438 patients underwent thyroid surgery for NTD. Patients (i) with known thyroid cancer, (ii) without an available serum TSH concentration within 1 year before surgery, (iii) with a final histological diagnosis other than DTC (e.g., medullary thyroid cancer or anaplastic thyroid cancer), and (iv) hyperthyroidism due to the Graves disease were not included. Three hundred eighty-six patients were eligible for the study.

All patients had a solitary thyroid nodule or a multinodular goiter detected by clinical examination, ultrasound scan (US), or both. Preoperatively, thyroid USs confirmed NTD in all cases. A fineneedle aspiration biopsy (FNAB) was performed for thyroid nodules > 1 cm, or nodules < 1 cm with suspicious US features. Thyroidectomy was prescribed for patients with malignant, suspicious, or repetitive indeterminate nodules according to FNAB results. Moreover, surgery was indicated for benign disease when local symptoms were present or for esthetic reasons.

All patients had a serum TSH level within 1 year before surgery measured by an automated immunochemiluminescent assay (Immulite 2500; Siemens, Los Angeles, Calif, USA). The normal range was 0.4–4.0 mU/L.

Statistical analysis was performed to determinate whether or not there were differences in age and TSH levels between patients diagnosed with benign lesions, compared with those diagnosed with thyroid cancer. Furthermore, the group of

patients with malignancies was subdivided into PTMCs and TCLS. Age was evaluated as a continuous variable. The TSH concentration was evaluated as a continuous variable and categorically within the following 3 ranges: <0.4 mU/L (subclinical hyperthyroidism); 0.4–4.0 mU/L (euthyroidism); >4.0 mU/L (subclinical hypothyroidism). The Student's t-test was used for numerical variables. The Fisher's exact test was used for categorical variables. The nonparametric Kruskall-Wallis test was used to determinate whether there were significant differences between patients with benign, PTMCs, and TCLS. Afterwards, Bonferroni's adjustment for multiple comparisons was applied to the pairwise comparisons of groups. Values were reported as the mean ± SEM. A P value < 0.05 was considered statistically significant.

3. Results

There were 386 patients who met the inclusion criteria. The final pathology data showed no evidence of malignancy in 310 patients (80.3%), whereas malignant lesions were present in 76 cases (19.7%).

The benign group included 250 females (80.6%) and 60 males (19.4%). The mean age at the time of diagnosis was 54.4 ± 14.2 years. There were 247 (79.7%) patients with multinodular goiter and 63 (20.3%) patients with thyroid nodule. Histological features of chronic thyroiditis were present in 75 (24.2%) patients.

DTC was diagnosed in 60 females (78.9%) and 16 males (21.1%). The mean age at the time of diagnosis was 49.3 ± 14.4 years. There was a significant difference in age between both groups (P = 0.005). There were 45 (59.2%) patients with multinodular goiter and 31 (28.2%) patients with thyroid nodule. Histological features of chronic thyroiditis were present in 18 (23.7%) patients. In the cohort of patients with malignancies, PTMCs were demonstrated in 36 patients (47.3%) and TCLS in the remaining 40 patients (PTC, n = 37; follicular thyroid carcinoma, n = 3; mean tumor size 25.21 ± 11.8 mm). The mean age in the patients with PTMCs was 52.1 ± 14.7 years, and 46.8 ± 13.8 years in the patients with TCLS.

Figure 1 shows the TSH concentrations in the different study groups. The preoperative mean TSH level in the 310 patients with no evidence of malignancy was 1.36 ± 1.62 mU/L, whereas the mean TSH concentration in the group of 76 patients with malignancies was 2.08 + 2.1 mU/L (P = 0.0013). Thus, the TSH levels were higher in patients with a final diagnosis of DTC. Among the set of patients with malignant nodules, mean TSH was 1.71 ± 1.52 mU/L in patients with PTMCs and 2.42 ± 2.5 mU/L in patients with TCLS. Statistical significance was found when the three groups (benign, PTMCs, and TCLS) were compared (P < 0.001). However, pairwise comparisons between them showed that differences in TSH were only significant between benign and TCLS groups (P < 0.01).

Seventy-four (23.9%) patients with benign nodules were classified as subclinical hyperthyroidism (TSH < 0.4 mU/L). This diagnosis was only detected in 10 patients (13.1%) with malignancies (P = 0.027). In contrast, 8 patients

TABLE 1: Distribution of patients according to TSH categories: <0.4 mU/L (subclinical hyperthyroidism); 0.4–4.0 mU/L (euthyroidism); >4.0 mU/L (subclinical hypothyroidism). PTMC: papillary thyroid microcarcinoma and TCLS: thyroid carcinoma of larger size.

TSH levels (mU/L)	Benign	PTMC	TCLS	Total malignant	All cases
<0.4	74	6	4	10	84
0.4–4.0	225	28	30	58	283
>4.0	11	2	6	8	19

(10.6%) with thyroid cancer were diagnosed with subclinical hypothyroidism (TSH > 4 mU/L), whereas this profile existed in 11 patients (3.5%) with benign lesions ($P = 0.01$). In summary, in patients with subclinical hyperthyroidism, normal TSH concentration and subclinical hypothyroidism malignancy rate were 12%, 20.5%, and 42%, respectively, (Table 1).

When we excluded all patients with TSH out of the normal range, the association between the TSH level and the final histology remained significant. The mean TSH level in the 225 patients with no evidence of malignancy and a normal TSH was 1.47 ± 0.8 mU/L, whereas the mean TSH level in the 58 patients with malignancies was 1.8 ± 0.8 mU/L ($P = 0.009$). Among this last group, mean TSH level was 1.75 ± 0.8 mU/L in patients with PTMCs and 1.84 ± 0.9 mU/L in patients with TCLS. Again, these differences were not significant. However, the TSH levels were significantly different between the group with benign lesions and a normal TSH level and patients with TCLS and a normal TSH level ($P = 0.026$). Finally, there were not significant differences among groups related to the presence of chronic thyroiditis.

4. Discussion

Several epidemiologic studies have confirmed that during the last decade, the incidence of DTC, and especially PTC, has increased worldwide [9, 10]. Furthermore, this highest incidence has been observed in tumors <1 cm in size, that is, PTMCs [11]. PTMCs exhibit significant differences in the mode of presentation from papillary tumors of larger size. Although PTMCs exhibit a more benign behavior [12], some authors suggest that there exists a subgroup of PTMCs that can be aggressive, requiring therapeutic management similar to larger tumors.

Boelaert et al. [4] reported, for the first time, that the TSH serum concentration could be an independent predictor of thyroid malignancy. The authors found that the risk of diagnosis of DTC rises in parallel with TSH serum levels. Moreover, they derived a formula for risk of malignancy based on the TSH level. Thereafter, these findings were subsequently confirmed by others. Haymart et al. [7] found that the preoperative mean TSH level is significantly higher in patients with a final diagnosis of thyroid cancer. The same group has shown that this relationship is independent from age [13]. Jonklaas et al. [14] reported that this

association remained in a strictly euthyroid population (after subclinical hypo- and hyperthyroidism cases were excluded) who underwent thyroid surgery for NTD. In this regard, Polyzos et al. [15] confirmed that TSH levels are predictive of malignancy only within a normal range because they did not find this association in patients with subclinical hypothyroidism. Jin et al. [16] have found that in patients with NTD, a serum TSH level < 0.9 has a probability of malignancy of approximately 10%, whereas in those patients with a serum TSH > 5.5, the rate of cancer is 65%. Recently, in a large series, Fiore et al. [17] reported that patients with nodular goiter treated with L-thyroxine had a significantly lower prevalence of PTC diagnosed by cytology. Moreover, the same authors reported that TSH levels were higher in patients with PTC than in benign NTD [6].

Two reports have demonstrated that a higher preoperative serum TSH was not only associated with the risk of DTC, but also associated with a more advanced stage of cancer at the time of diagnosis [6, 7]. In contrast, the association between TSH levels and PTMCs has not been extensively analyzed. In the series by Haymart et al. [7], the authors performed an analysis of the subset of tumors < 1 cm in size. Although the number of cases was very low, an increased risk of cancer persisted with a higher TSH in patients with PTMCs until the TSH was ≥ 5.00 mU/L. Recently, Gerschpacher et al. [8] compared the preoperative serum TSH concentrations between a cohort of 33 patients with PTMCs and a control group of 54 patients in which the thyroid gland was removed for medullary thyroid carcinoma or C-cell hyperplasia. The authors found no significant differences and concluded that the TSH level is not elevated in patients with PTMCs.

To our knowledge, the present paper is the first study that has not only compared TSH concentrations in patients with benign and malignant lesions, but also in PTMCs and TCLS. We have confirmed that the TSH level is significantly different between benign nodules and DTCs. These differences have persisted when comparing benign lesions and carcinomas > 1 cm in size, and when comparing all three groups. It appears that there exists an increment in tumor size as a function of increment in the TSH level. Thus, benign lesions have the lowest TSH levels, PTMCs have intermediate concentrations, and DTCs of larger size are associated with the highest levels of TSH. However, though the escalatory increment of TSH between the three groups of patients is evident, statistical analysis shows that differences are not significant, probably due to the small number of cases with cancer. According to these results, we suggest that TSH participates in the carcinogenesis of PTC, it is possibly that it acts as a growth factor and could be one of the parameters that determines the size of DTCs. In this regard, recently, Franco et al. [18] have found that TSH signaling pathway may predispose thyroid cells to BRAF-induced transformation, in mice with a thyroid-specific knockin of oncogenic Braf (LSL-$Braf^{V600E}$/TPO-Cre).

It is interesting to note that in our cohort, all patients underwent thyroid surgery. Thus, diagnoses of DTCs or benign thyroid disease were based on surgical pathologic results in all of the cases analyzed. In contrast, the diagnosis was established with FNAB results in other series without confirmatory histological results. For example, in the study by Boelaert et al. [4], only 37% of patients had definitive pathologic results. The final histological results were available in 21.6% of the patients in the series of Polyzos et al. [15]. Thus, in those series, it is possible that all of the microcarcinomas were not detected.

Unfortunately, information about thyroid antibodies was not analysed because there were no data in approximately one quarter of patients. However, histological preparations were examined, in order to verify the presence or not of autoimmune chronic thyroiditis. In this regard, we did not observe any differences between groups.

Finally, it is well known the predominantly benign nature of thyroid autonomous nodules. Moreover, in patients with autonomous nodules, TSH concentrations were decreased or suppressed. In our study, the association between TSH level and final histology remained significant after patients with subclinical hypo- and hyperthyroidism were excluded.

In summary, we have shown that TSH levels were higher in patients with a final diagnosis of DTC. Moreover, it appears that there exists an increment in tumor size as a function of increment in the TSH level. Although the role of the TSH level in the development and/or progression of thyroid cancer remains controversial, our results support the hypothesis that the TSH level might be involved in the progression, that is, the size, of an existing DTC.

References

[1] D. S. Cooper, G. M. Doherty, B. R. Haugen et al., "Revised American thyroid association management guidelines for patients with thyroid nodules and differentiated thyroid cancer," *Thyroid*, vol. 19, no. 11, pp. 1167–1214, 2009.

[2] B. Biondi and D. S. Cooper, "Benefits of thyrotropin suppression versus the risks of adverse effects in differentiated thyroid cancer," *Thyroid*, vol. 20, no. 2, pp. 135–146, 2010.

[3] C. García-Jiménez and P. Santisteban, "TSH Signalling and Cancer," *Arquivos Brasileiros de Endocrinologia e Metabologia*, vol. 51, no. 5, pp. 654–671, 2007.

[4] K. Boelaert, J. Horacek, R. L. Holder, J. C. Watkinson, M. C. Sheppard, and J. A. Franklyn, "Serum thyrotropin concentration as a novel predictor of malignancy in thyroid nodules investigated by fine-needle aspiration," *Journal of Clinical Endocrinology and Metabolism*, vol. 91, no. 11, pp. 4295–4301, 2006.

[5] K. Boelaert, "The association between serum TSH concentration and thyroid cancer," *Endocrine-Related Cancer*, vol. 16, no. 4, pp. 1065–1072, 2009.

[6] E. Fiore, T. Rago, M. A. Provenzale et al., "Lower levels of TSH are associated with a lower risk of papillary thyroid cancer in patients with thyroid nodular disease: thyroid autonomy may play a protective role," *Endocrine-Related Cancer*, vol. 16, no. 4, pp. 1251–1260, 2009.

[7] M. R. Haymart, D. J. Repplinger, G. E. Leverson et al., "Higher serum thyroid stimulating hormone level in thyroid nodule patients is associated with greater risks of differentiated thyroid cancer and advanced tumor stage," *Journal of Clinical Endocrinology and Metabolism*, vol. 93, no. 3, pp. 809–814, 2008.

[8] M. Gerschpacher, C. Göbl, C. Anderwald, A. Gessl, and M. Krebs, "Thyrotropin serum concentrations in patients with papillary thyroid microcancers," *Thyroid*, vol. 20, no. 4, pp. 389–392, 2010.

[9] L. Davies and H. G. Welch, "Increasing incidence of thyroid cancer in the United States, 1973-2002," *Journal of the American Medical Association*, vol. 295, no. 18, pp. 2164–2167, 2006.

[10] L. Leenhardt, P. Grosclaude, and L. Chérié-Challine, "Increased incidence of thyroid carcinoma in france: a true epidemic or thyroid nodule management effects? Report from the french thyroid cancer committee," *Thyroid*, vol. 14, no. 12, pp. 1056–1060, 2004.

[11] R. Lloyd, R. de Lellis, P. Heitz et al., *World Health Organization Classification of Tumors: Pathology and Genetics of Tumors of the Endocrine Organs*, IARC Press, Lyon, France, 2004.

[12] S. Noguchi, H. Yamashita, S. Uchino, and S. Watanabe, "Papillary microcarcinoma," *World Journal of Surgery*, vol. 32, no. 5, pp. 747–753, 2008.

[13] M. R. Haymart, S. L. Glinberg, J. Liu, R. S. Sippel, J. C. Jaume, and H. Chen, "Higher serum TSH in thyroid cancer patients occurs independent of age and correlates with extrathyroidal extension," *Clinical Endocrinology*, vol. 71, no. 3, pp. 434–439, 2009.

[14] J. Jonklaas, H. Nsouli-Maktabi, and S. J. Soldin, "Endogenous thyrotropin and triiodothyronine concentrations in individuals with thyroid cancer," *Thyroid*, vol. 18, no. 9, pp. 943–952, 2008.

[15] S. A. Polyzos, M. Kita, Z. Efstathiadou et al., "Serum thyrotropin concentration as a biochemical predictor of thyroid malignancy in patients presenting with thyroid nodules," *Journal of Cancer Research and Clinical Oncology*, vol. 134, no. 9, pp. 953–960, 2008.

[16] J. Jin, R. Machekano, and C. R. McHenry, "The utility of preoperative serum thyroid-stimulating hormone level for predicting malignant nodular thyroid disease," *American Journal of Surgery*, vol. 199, no. 3, pp. 294–298, 2010.

[17] E. Fiore, T. Rago, M. A. Provenzale et al., "L-thyroxine-treated patients with nodular goiter have lower serum TSH and lower frequency of papillary thyroid cancer: results of a cross-sectional study on 27 914 patients," *Endocrine-Related Cancer*, vol. 17, no. 1, pp. 231–239, 2010.

[18] A. T. Franco, R. Malaguarnera, S. Refetoff et al., "Thyrotrophin receptor signaling dependence of Braf-induced thyroid tumor initiation in mice," *Proceedings of the National Academy of Sciences of the United States of America*, vol. 108, no. 4, pp. 1615–1620, 2011.

16

Symptoms and Signs Associated with Postpartum Thyroiditis

Maureen Groer[1] and Cecilia Jevitt[2]

[1] University of South Florida College of Nursing, 12910 Bruce B. Downs Boulevard, Tampa, FL 33612, USA
[2] Yale University School of Nursing, P.O. Box 27399, West Haven, CT 06515-7399, USA

Correspondence should be addressed to Maureen Groer; mgroer@health.usf.edu

Academic Editor: Brendan C. Stack Jr.

Background. Postpartum thyroiditis (PPT) is a common triphasic autoimmune disease in women with thyroid peroxidase (TPO) autoantibodies. This study evaluated women's thyroid disease symptoms, physical findings, stress levels, and thyroid stimulating hormone (TSH) levels across six postpartum months in three groups, TPO negative, TPO positive, and PPT positive women. *Methods.* Women were recruited in midpregnancy ($n = 631$) and TPO status was determined which then was used to form the three postpartum groups. The three groups were compared on TSH levels, thyroid symptoms, weight, blood pressure, heart rate, a thyroid exam, and stress scores. *Results.* Fifty-six percent of the TPO positive women developed PPT. Hypothyroid group (F (2, 742) = 5.8, P = .003) and hyperthyroid group (F (2, 747) = 6.6, P = .001) subscale scores differed by group. Several symptoms and stress scores were highest in the PPT group. *Conclusions.* The normal postpartum is associated with many symptoms that mimic thyroid disease symptoms, but severity is greater in women with either TPO or PPT positivity. While the most severe symptoms were generally seen in PPT positive women, even TPO positive women seem to have higher risk for these signs and symptoms.

1. Introduction

The postpartum is considered a vulnerable time for the development or recurrence of some autoimmune diseases (ADs), particularly those caused by excessive T helper 1 (Th1) lymphocyte mediated processes (eg. rheumatoid arthritis (RA)), multiple sclerosis (MS), and postpartum thyroiditis (PPT). These ADs often ameliorate during pregnancy but then exacerbate or occur for the first time in the postpartum period [1]. This is thought to be due to the return of Th1 mediated immunity, which is suppressed in pregnancy [2]. The most common postpartum autoimmune disease (AD) is postpartum thyroiditis (PPT), a thyroid dysfunction that occurs within the first year after delivery or miscarriage [3]. PPT occurs during the early postpartum in approximately half of women who have autoantibodies to the enzyme, thyroid peroxidase, during the first trimester of pregnancy [4]. Thyroid peroxidase is a microsomal enzyme that is required in the synthesis of thyroid hormone, but many women who have this autoantibody remain euthyroid. PPT usually has a triphasic course, from euthyroidism, to a short hyperthyroid phase (22%) followed by a longer period of

hypothyroidism (48%) and a recovery to euthyroidism [5]. Variants of this course occur. Recently it has been shown that up to fifty percent of women with PPT remain hypothyroid at one year [6]. There is significant risk for women with PPT (up to 50%) to develop permanent thyroid disease over time [3, 6]. The pathophysiology involves Th1 cells, autoantibodies, and autoreactive T helper 2 (Th2) cells that promote antithyroid autoantibody production. Cytotoxic T cells and NK cells also participate in a direct destruction of the gland [7]. TPO autoantibodies are able to bind to thyrocytes and activate complement, which sets in motion antibody dependent cytotoxic mechanisms which involve further destruction of the thyrocytes.

Symptoms that women with PPT experience are thought to be related to the phase of disease. PPT symptoms during the hyperthyroid phase are usually short-lived and in the hypothyroid phase are particularly likely to be under-diagnosed, as many women consider their experiences as "normal" postpartum symptoms. Routine TPO antibody screening is not done in pregnancy and many TPO positive women have no or subclinical symptoms of thyroid dysfunction, so risk for PPT cannot be predicted for the individual untested woman unless she has had a previous episode of the disease.

We examined differences across the course of the postpartum in TPO positive women compared to a TPO negative comparison group. A list of common symptoms of hypo- and hyperthyroidism was constructed, and women reported on the occurrence and severity of each symptom at 7 consecutive postpartum assessments. The current report compares symptoms, TSH levels, other hormones, and physical findings in three groups, TPO negative, TPO positive, and PPT positive women across six postpartum months.

2. Method

Institutional Review Board (IRB) approval was achieved and informed consent gathered at the initiation of the study. Pregnant women ($n = 631$) were recruited at prenatal clinics. Study participants were women first measured for the TPO autoantibody after the first trimester and before 25 weeks of gestation and identified as either TPO positive or negative at that time. Exclusion criteria included the following: age less than 18 or older than 45 years; known autoimmune disease; previous thyroid disease; HIV positivity; use of medications that affect immunity; chronic diseases, such as diabetes; serious mental illness, such as bipolar disorder, schizophrenia, untreated depression, or unresolved perinatal bereavement; body mass index (BMI) <20; history of hyperemesis; current multiple gestation; current pregnancy product of *in vitro* fertilization (IVF); fetal abnormalities; and being unable to participate in a six-month postpartum followup. All TPO positive ($n = 63$) women who were identified in pregnancy were invited into the postpartum phase of the study, while a sample of TPO negative women ($n = 568$) were selected by a random number generator to participate as the comparison group in the postpartum phase ($n = 72$). TPO status was determined by ELISA (ORGENTEC, Mainz, Germany) according to kit directions using standards and controls and done in duplicate. The coefficient of variation was always less than 5%. TPO antibody titer greater than 20 IUs was used as the cutoff value for positivity. TSH levels were also measured in all TPO positive women at the initial pregnancy blood draw. Women were not informed of their TPO status until the end of the study, or unless they experienced PPT and needed referral.

3. Materials and Procedure

Women recruited into this study received a home visit by a research nurse one week after giving birth and then monthly for postpartum months 1 through 6. At each postpartum home visit, participants received a targeted physical examination (thyroid gland palpation, blood pressure, heart rate, and weight). Detailed data were gathered on breastfeeding and smoking, alcohol consumption, and exercise. They also completed a thyroid disease symptom list. This list consisted of 19 items and participants rated occurrence of symptoms as not present (0), mild (1), moderate (2), severe (3), or very severe (4) (Table 1). The list was developed by the investigators based

TABLE 1: Demographic characteristics by group.

	TPO negative	TPO positive	PPT positive
Income	9% < $4999	.6% < $4999	1.1% < $4999
	31% > $69,999	38% > $69,999	38% > $69,999
BMI	29.7	32.1	28.3
Breastfeeding	52%	70%	56%
Smoking	8%	1.6%	0%
Parity	1.03	1.00	1.00

on a review of literature on symptoms of thyroid disease, a review of older clinical screening instruments which were deemed too difficult to use in the home setting [8], and consultation with an endocrinologist.

The Perceived Stress Scale (PSS) [9] was used to assess levels of self-reported stress and was completed at each postpartum visit. The 14-item version of the scale evaluates perceptions of stress using a Likert scale ranging from 0 (never) to 4 (very often). The internal consistency reliability has been reported to be .84 to .86 in young adults. Congruent and criterion validity for the scale has been demonstrated to be excellent, although predictive validity declines over time [9].

A venipuncture was performed and 15 mLs of blood were drawn into heparinized vacutainers. The blood was transported to the laboratory within 2 hours. Blood samples were centrifuged at 1200 g for 25 minutes at 4°C and plasma aliquoted into Eppendorf tubes and frozen at −80°C until later analysis in batches. TSH (ALPCO, Salem, N.H.) was always measured at each visit for the TPO positive women, regardless of symptoms, and assayed according to kit directions. TPO negative women with severity scores on the thyroid screening list indicating occurrence of hyper- or hypothyroid symptoms also had TSH levels measured. PPT was assessed as possible when a TSH level of less than 0.3 or more than 3.0 mIU/L occurred. This is the level chosen for screening of thyroid disease in adults [10] and during pregnancy [11]. Women meeting these criteria were referred to their health care providers for further diagnosis and treatment. They continued in the study after referral. The research nurse who made the postpartum home visits and the research participants were blinded to TPO status.

Statistical analysis was performed using SPSS v. 22. Data were analyzed descriptively and examined for normality and transformed if necessary. One way analysis of variance was computed on symptom subscale scores and PSS scores by group. Spearman correlations were used for correlations between TSH levels and signs and symptoms. A P value of <.05 was considered significant for these tests. Kruskal-Wallis analyses were performed on individual symptoms by group with a pairwise comparison test for post-hoc analyses. Bonferroni corrections were made for multiple comparisons with a $P < .003$ considered significant for these tests. Reliabilities (α) were calculated for the symptoms on the thyroid checklist hyperthyroid symptoms and hypothyroid symptoms subscales.

4. Results

TPO positivity was found in 63 of the 631 (10%) participants at the pregnancy measurement point. All but two of the TSH titers on these TPO positive women were in the euthyroid range when measured in the plasma samples collected in pregnancy (mean $1.46 \pm .21$; range 0.16–4.6 mIU/mL). Of the 63 TPO positive women, 46 agreed to be in the postpartum followup. The reasons for not participating in the postpartum follow-up study included moving to a different location, lack of interest in the study, and being lost to followup. The demographics of the TPO positive women who did not participate were not different than those who did participate. Of these 46 TPO positive participants, 26 (56.2%) developed PPT during the first six months of the postpartum. There were 4 TPO negative women who developed symptoms and signs of thyroid disease, including out of range TSH levels. These women were not included in the analysis as they could have developed another thyroid disease such as Graves' disease. The research was described to participants as a study of immunity and hormones. However, if a woman became PPT positive, she was informed of this result and referrals were made to her health care provider, so from that point on she did know her status.

TSH levels were either below 0.3 mIU/mL or above 3.0 mIU/mL for a woman to be classified as having potential PPT. Thirteen had elevated TSH (hypothyroid) and thirteen had low TSH (hyperthyroid) at time of identification of possible PPT (Figure 1). While we attempted to assure followup with health care providers and potential further diagnostic testing for these women, we found that there is a common lack of knowledge about PPT by primary care providers, and few responded to our inquiries about follow-up diagnosis and treatment. In addition, some women had low incomes and no health care available for followup. For purposes of the study we classified TPO positive women as having likely developed PPT when a change (often dramatic) from normal TSH levels to levels outside the normal range occurred at one of the monthly visits and remained abnormal thereafter. No PPT positive woman, even those few who underwent medical referral and treatment, became euthyroid after being classified as PPT positive during the six-month course of the study. Only two PPT positive women were prescribed levothyronine and they continued in the study until the sixth month. Removing these women from the analysis had no effect on the results.

There were no differences in ethnicity by TPO status or PPT positivity status. Table 1 depicts sociodemographic variables by group. None of the differences were statistically significant.

The thyroid symptom list had both common hyperthyroid and hypothyroid symptoms which were grouped and analyzed as symptom severity subscales. Table 2 shows symptoms categorized as being most associated with hypothyroidism or hyperthyroidism. The hyperthyroidism scale was comprised of 9 items (maximum severity score = 36) and the hypothyroidism scale had 10 items (maximum severity score = 40). The Cronbach's α for the hyperthyroid symptom subscale was .70 and for the hypothyroid subscale was .77.

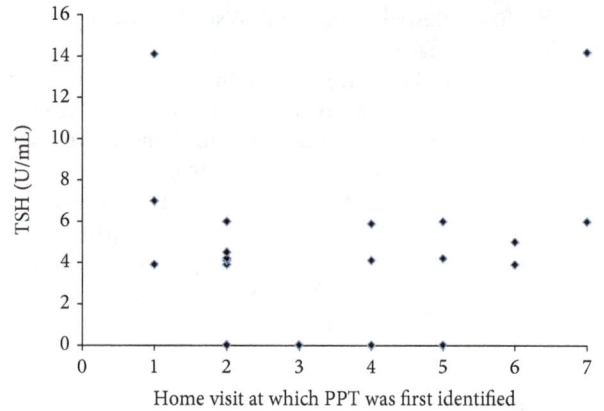

FIGURE 1: TSH levels in plasma at the time at which TPO positive women were first identified as PPT positive. Home visit 1 was at 1-week postpartum and the following time intervals were from month 1 through 6.

TABLE 2: Thyroid symptom screening.

Lack of energy	0	1	2	3	4
Irritability	0	1	2	3	4
Nervousness	0	1	2	3	4
Sweating	0	1	2	3	4
Dry skin	0	1	2	3	4
Shaking hands	0	1	2	3	4
Depression	0	1	2	3	4
Heat intolerance	0	1	2	3	4
Dry hair	0	1	2	3	4
Puffy face	0	1	2	3	4
Hair falling out	0	1	2	3	4
Weight loss	0	1	2	3	4
Constipation	0	1	2	3	4
Aches and pains	0	1	2	3	4
Tingling or numbness	0	1	2	3	4
Cold intolerance	0	1	2	3	4
Poor memory	0	1	2	3	4
Lack of concentration	0	1	2	3	4
Palpitations	0	1	2	3	4

bold items comprise the hypothyroid subscale; non bold items comprise the hyperthyroid subscale.
0: no presence of symptom; 1: mild; 2: moderate; 3: severe; 4: very severe.

At time of first identification of PPT status, the mean score on the hypothyroid subscale was 8.5 ± 7.3 (SD) and on the hyperthyroid subscale was 5.4 ± 5.0 (SD). Comparisons of scores in the period before a woman became PPT positive showed a score of 6.75 ± 5.5 for the hypothyroid subscale and 6.87 ± 5.78 for the hyperthyroid scale, and these were not statistically significantly different from the values at identification of PPT positivity. However, the mean TSH of $1.52 \pm .8$ (SD) preceding the identification of PPT was significantly different ($t = -3.0$, $P = .005$) than the TSH at identification of presence of PPT (3.95 ± 3.96 (SD)).

Figures 2(a) and 2(b) depict the means of the hypothyroid and hyperthyroid subscale scores across the postpartum for

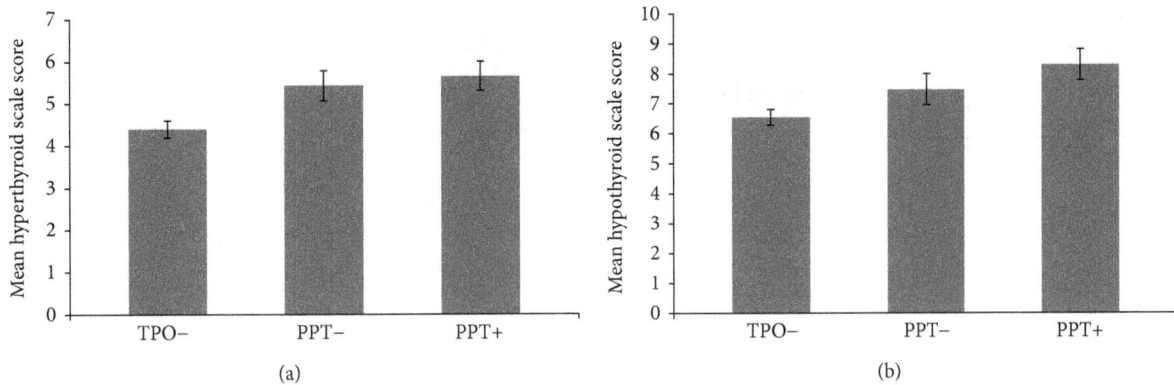

FIGURE 2: (a) Hypothyroid subscale scores by group. Error bars are standard errors of the mean. (b) Hyperthyroid subscale scores by group. Error bars are standard errors of the mean.

each group. A one-way between groups analysis of variance was conducted to explore the effect of group (TPO negative, TPO positive without PPT, and PPT positive) on the mean hypothyroid and hyperthyroid subscale scores. There was a statistically significant difference at the $P = .003$ level in hypothyroid subscale scores [$F(2, 742) = 5.8, P = .003$]. Post-hoc comparisons using the Tukey HSD test indicated that the mean score for the hypothyroid subscale was significantly higher for the PPT positive group (8.29) compared to the TP0 negative group (6.53), but not significantly different than the TPO positive, PPT negative group (7.47). With regard to the hyperthyroid subscale, there was a statistically significant difference in scores at the $P = .001$ level [$F(2, 747) = 6.6, P = .001$]. Post-hoc analysis found that there were significant differences in the hyperthyroid subscale scores comparing TPO negative women (4.39) with both TPO positive PPT negative (5.43) and PPT positive (5.65) groups.

All groups reported experiencing symptoms and there were no dramatic differences by group in the frequency of reporting any symptom experience (Table 3). Table 4 depicts the frequency of women who reported that a symptom was either "severe" or "very severe." Correcting for multiple comparisons by using a Bonferroni correction ($P < .003$), six symptom severities were significantly different by group (lack of energy, shaking hands, heat intolerance, cold intolerance, poor memory, and lack of concentration). All significant symptom severities were higher in both TPO positive and PPT positive groups compared to TPO negative women.

Twelve TPO positive women had palpable thyroid glands and 5 PPT positive women and two TPO positive, PPT negative, women had visible goiters. The five goiters in PPT positive women were associated with extremely low TSH levels in three women and high levels in two women.

Mean PSS scores were significantly different by group [$F(2, 755) = 11.1, P < .001$]. Post-hoc analysis showed that PPT positive women had higher mean scores across the postpartum (22.5) compared to TPO negative women (19.3) ($P < .001$). However, the difference between PPT positive and TPO positive, PPT negative women (20.8) was not significant ($P = .15$).

TABLE 3: Percent of women reporting any symptoms on thyroid symptom checklist by TPO and PPT status.

Symptom	TPO negative	TPO positive	TPO positive PPT positive
Lack of energy	68.4%	74.6%	78%
Irritability	49.6%	54.4%	61.9%
Nervousness	32.7%	37.9%	37.1%
Weight loss	44.5%	24.3%	48.7%
Sweating	31.5%	32%	38.6%
Shaking hands	11.6%	15.5%	10.7%
Palpitations	11.2%	11.7%	10.2%
Heat intolerance	31.9%	36.9%	41.6%
Dry hair	34.1%	34.9%	35.5%
Puffy face	13.2%	17.6%	14.2%
Dry skin	50.6%	55.3%	51.3%
Hair falling out	38.4%	54.4%	34%
Constipation	37.9%	37.9%	35.5%
Aches and pains	48.6%	44%	52.3%
Tingling or numbness	17.9%	13.6%	21.8%
Cold intolerance	32.8%	26.2%	21.2%
Poor memory	49.8%	48.5%	57.4%
Lack of concentration	44.4%	49.5%	57.9%
Depression	21.5%	29.1%	33.5%

In the sample as a whole, TSH levels were correlated with heart rate ($r = .124, P < .05$), systolic blood pressure ($r = .164, P < .01$), diastolic blood pressure ($r = .22, P < .001$), and BMI ($r = .15, P < .02$). The scores on hyper- versus hypothyroid subscales were not significantly correlated with TSH levels.

5. Discussion

Many postpartum women feel exhausted, depressed, and not able to concentrate. Even physical symptoms such as

TABLE 4: Comparisons of frequencies of "severe or vey severe" symptom reports on thyroid symptom checklist by group.

Symptom	TPO negative (a)	TPO positive PPT negative (b)	PPT positive (c)
Lack of energy	13.2%	18%	18% (**a, c)
Irritability	9.5%	5.9%	11.4%
Nervousness	5%	5.2%	8.6%
Weight loss	3.9%	5.9%	8.0%
Sweating	4.4%	5.9%	9.2%
Shaking hands	1.8%	1.5%	6.1% (**b, c)
Palpitations	0.08%	0%	1.2%
Heat Intolerance	5.5%	8.2%	8.6% (**a, c)
Dry hair	5.1%	10.4%	12.3%
Puffy face	0.08%	0.08%	0.06%
Dry skin	11.9%	9.7%	12.8%
Hair falling out	13.5%	14.1%	14.7%
Constipation	7.1%	12.7%	13.5%
Aches and pains	10.4%	11.1%	11.7%
Tingling or numbness	3%	4.4%	2.5%
Cold intolerance	3.3%	2.2%	6.7% (**b, c)
Poor memory	6.4%	10.4%	13.5% (**a, c)
Lack of concentration	6.0%	4.4%	12.8% (**b, c)
Depression	3.3%	8.3%	6.1%

**indicate $P < 0.003$.

hair falling out were reported as occurring by a third of postpartum women who were TPO negative in the study. Certainly postpartum women are often dealing with many demands and stressors [12–14]. Differentiating the "normal" postpartum experience from the experience of women with thyroid disease cannot rely on symptom reports. However, severity of symptoms was clearly different for both groups of TPO positive women. The TPO positive women who did not develop thyroiditis were different in hypo- and hyperthyroid subscale scores compared to TPO negative women. They also had significant differences in particular symptom severities. The presence of measurable thyroid autoantibodies, whether or not PPT develops, indicates an autoimmune perturbation in the gland even in euthyroid women. We and others have reported that the presence of TPO autoantibodies alone may be associated with postpartum depression [15, 16]. Thyroid inflammation could have subtle effects on neurological function.

When PPT does develop, it is unlike other autoimmune diseases in that it is reversible, although many women who develop PPT go on to later chronic hypothyroidism. It is also an unusual disease in that as yet unknown postpartum physiological changes unmask the disease in susceptible women. The observation that perceived stress was significantly higher in the PPT group is noteworthy. The distress associated with the disease is likely additive with the usual stressors associated with the postpartum.

This study should raise the awareness of providers to the need to screen for TPO autoantibodies, since these women appear to be experiencing more postpartum distress and are at risk for development of PPT. Screening for TPO autoantibodies is currently not a clinical recommendation for all pregnant women and therefore many cases of PPT are missed. In our study, of the 26 who were identified with PPT, only two would have returned to their health care provider based on their perceptions of the severity of their symptoms. Even with referrals being made for all the PPT positive women in the study, only two were actually treated. Treatment could have included thyroid hormone replacement, antidepressants, and supportive care, but the usual approach was to watch and wait. The return to euthyroidism after PPT does not necessarily herald a healthy thyroid gland, as the risk for permanent thyroid disease as well as recurrence of PPT in subsequent pregnancies is very significant [17]. In addition, the quality of life for women with PPT as well as those who are TPO positive is likely to be impaired by severity of some of the symptoms we measured as well as by general perceived stress. Clearly there is a need for health care providers to be more aware of this condition, as it may appear after the usual 6-week postpartum visit and then may be present in the primary care setting.

6. Limitations

There are several important limitations to this study. The number of participants with PPT was small. The thyroid symptom list may have inadequately captured the symptoms of PPT, and the symptom and stress data were self-report. The designation of PPT status was based on a change from normal range TSH levels to out of range levels, without a full thyroid panel and clinical diagnosis. Women who became PPT positive were so informed and thus this may have influenced their responses in subsequent home visits.

Additional studies are needed to determine the most appropriate symptom screenings useful in diagnosing PPT. However, these data should prompt clinicians to investigate thyroid function when women report severe exhaustion, sleep disturbances, weight gain, and hair loss in the postpartum period. Attributing these symptoms to normal postpartum occurrences can cause unnecessary suffering for some new mothers.

Authors' Contribution

Dr. Groer was the P.I. on the R01 grant that funded this research. She analyzed all data and prepared the paper draft. Dr. Jevitt was the Co-I on the R01 grant that funded this research. She provided critical review and suggestions to the paper.

Acknowledgment

The authors acknowledge the NIH funding, R01NR05000.

References

[1] I. J. Elenkov, J. Hoffman, and R. L. Wilder, "Does differential neuroendocrine control of cytokine production govern the expression of autoimmune diseases in pregnancy and the postpartum period?" *Molecular Medicine Today*, vol. 3, no. 9, pp. 379–383, 1997.

[2] S. Saito, A. Nakashima, T. Shima, and M. Ito, "Th1/Th2/Th17 and regulatory T-cell paradigm in pregnancy," *The American Journal of Reproductive Immunology*, vol. 63, no. 6, pp. 601–610, 2010.

[3] S. Gaberšček and K. Zaletel, "Thyroid physiology and autoimmunity in pregnancy and after delivery," *Expert Review of Clinical Immunology*, vol. 7, no. 5, pp. 697–707, 2011.

[4] J. H. Lazarus, A. B. Parkes, and L. D. Premawardhana, "Postpartum thyroiditis," *Autoimmunity*, vol. 35, no. 3, pp. 169–173, 2002.

[5] M. H. Samuels, "Subacute, silent, and postpartum thyroiditis," *Medical Clinics of North America*, vol. 96, no. 2, pp. 223–233, 2012.

[6] A. Stagnaro-Green, A. Schwartz, R. Gismondi, A. Tinelli, T. Mangieri, and R. Negro, "High rate of persistent hypothyroidism in a large-scale prospective study of postpartum thyroiditis in Southern Italy," *The Journal of Clinical Endocrinology and Metabolism*, vol. 96, no. 3, pp. 652–657, 2011.

[7] A. F. Muller, H. A. Drexhage, and A. Berghout, "Postpartum thyroiditis and autoimmune thyroiditis in women of childbearing age: recent insights and consequences for antenatal and postnatal care," *Endocrine Reviews*, vol. 22, no. 5, pp. 605–630, 2001.

[8] S. Kalra, S. K. Khandelwal, and A. Goyal, "Clinical scoring scales in thyroidology: a compendium," *Indian Journal of Endocrinology and Metabolism*, vol. 15, supplement 2, pp. S89–S94, 2011.

[9] S. Cohen, T. Kamarck, and R. Mermelstein, "A global measure of perceived stress," *Journal of Health and Social Behavior*, vol. 24, no. 4, pp. 385–396, 1983.

[10] H. J. Baskin, R. H. Cobin, D. S. Duick et al., "American Association of Clinical Endocrinologists medical guidelines for clinical practice for the evaluation and treatment of hyperthyroidism and hypothyroidism," *Endocrine Practice*, vol. 8, no. 6, pp. 457–469, 2002.

[11] A. Stagnaro-Green, M. Abalovich, E. Alexander et al., "Guidelines of the American Thyroid Association for the diagnosis and management of thyroid disease during pregnancy and postpartum," *Thyroid*, vol. 21, no. 10, pp. 1081–1125, 2011.

[12] M. Groer, M. Davis, K. Casey, B. Short, K. Smith, and S. Groer, "Neuroendocrine & immune relationships in postpartum fatigue," *MCN The American Journal of Maternal/Child Nursing*, vol. 30, no. 2, pp. 133–138, 2005.

[13] M. W. Groer, M. W. Davis, and J. Hemphill, "Postpartum stress: current concepts and the possible protective role of breastfeeding," *Journal of Obstetric, Gynecologic, and Neonatal Nursing : JOGNN / NAACOG*, vol. 31, no. 4, pp. 411–417, 2002.

[14] C. M. Jevitt, M. W. Groer, N. F. Crist, L. Gonzalez, and V. D. Wagner, "Postpartum stressors: a content analysis," *Issues in Mental Health Nursing*, vol. 33, no. 5, pp. 309–318, 2012.

[15] M. W. Groer and J. H. Vaughan, "Positive thyroid peroxidase antibody titer is associated with dysphoric moods during pregnancy and postpartum," *Journal of Obstetric, Gynecologic, & Neonatal Nursing*, vol. 42, no. 1, pp. E26–E32, 2013.

[16] J. H. Lazarus, R. Hall, S. Othman et al., "The clinical spectrum of postpartum thyroid disease," *QJM*, vol. 89, no. 6, pp. 429–435, 1996.

[17] J. H. Lazarus, "Thyroid dysfunction: reproduction and postpartum thyroiditis," *Seminars in Reproductive Medicine*, vol. 20, no. 4, pp. 381–388, 2002.

17

Management of Differentiated Thyroid Cancer in Pregnancy

Syed Ali Imran[1] and Murali Rajaraman[2]

[1] Division of Endocrinology and Metabolism, Dalhousie University, Halifax, NS, Canada B3H 2Y9
[2] Department of Radiation Oncology, Dalhousie University, Halifax, NS, Canada B3H 2Y9

Correspondence should be addressed to Syed Ali Imran, ali.imran@dal.ca

Academic Editor: Bijay Vaidya

In young women, differentiated thyroid cancer is the second most common malignancy diagnosed around the time of pregnancy. Management of thyroid cancer during pregnancy poses distinct challenges due to concerns regarding maternal and fetal well-being. In most cases surgery can be safely delayed until after delivery and with adequate management and outcome of pregnancy in women with thyroid cancer is excellent. Ideally these patients should be managed by a multidisciplinary team, and management plan should be determined by a consensus between the patient and the healthcare team.

1. Introduction

With the rising incidence of differentiated thyroid cancer (DTC), particularly in younger women, DTC is the second most common cancer diagnosed around the time of pregnancy with a prevalence of 14 per 100,000 [1]. Normal physiological changes occurring during pregnancy and concerns regarding fetal well-being pose distinct challenges to all aspects of DTC management. This paper reviews various facets of DTC management during pregnancy based on the published evidence and extensive clinical experience of the authors.

2. Is Pregnancy a Risk Factor for Thyroid Cancer?

Since DTC has a threefold higher incidence in women of reproductive age [2], an association between estrogen, human chorionic gonadotropin (HCG), and DTC has long been speculated. Several studies have suggested an association between the risk of DTC and high parity [3, 4], and there is also evidence that use of fertility agent, clomiphene, in parous women is associated with a higher risk of DTC [5]. The data regarding an association between estrogen and DTC, however, are inconsistent, with some studies reporting a pro-proliferative effect of estrogen on thyroid cancer cell lines [6], while others showing a stimulatory effect of estrogen on normal and adenomatous thyroid only, but not on thyroid cancer [7]. The clinical data are also conflicting; one study reported a higher risk of DTC in women exposed to estrogen-containing oral contraceptive and postmenopausal hormone replacement therapy [8], while another study reported no association between the use of exogenous estrogens and DTC [9]. Similar discordance exists in data regarding the outcome of DTC diagnosed during pregnancy; for instance, one study suggests that DTC diagnosed during pregnancy is associated with poorer prognosis and is more likely to have positive ERα expression as compared to tumours diagnosed in nongravidic period [10], while another retrospective study comparing the outcome of DTC diagnosed in pregnant women with age-matched controls showed no significant difference in cancer recurrence or cancer-related death [11]. The data regarding the effect of HCG on DTC are also nonconfirmatory. Although rising HCG during pregnancy has a stimulatory effect on thyroid hormone production, there is no evidence to date linking HCG with DTC. In a large cohort of women treated with fertility drugs, the use of HCG was not associated with a higher risk of DTC [5]. In summary, therefore, epidemiologic data suggest an association between high parity and risk of DTC; but there is lingering unclarity regarding the outcome of DTC that is diagnosed during pregnancy.

3. Management of Thyroid Cancer during Pregnancy

The management of DTC during pregnancy generally falls into two clinical scenarios. One includes those women who are diagnosed de novo with DTC during pregnancy, while the other includes women with previous history of DTC who have either become pregnant or are planning pregnancy. Both groups present distinct therapeutic challenges requiring specific clinical approach based on disease stage, patient preference, and stage of pregnancy.

3.1. Thyroid Surgery during Pregnancy. For most women with newly diagnosed DTC or those with resectable macro-scopic recurrence, a decision about whether or not to perform surgery during pregnancy has to be made. This question is perhaps the biggest source of vexation for patients and physicians alike. So far there has been no prospective study comparing the outcome of DTC in women undergoing surgery during pregnancy versus those where surgery was delayed until after delivery. A retrospective, cross-sectional study comparing 201 pregnant women undergoing thyroid and parathyroid surgery with age-matched nonpregnant controls reported that pregnant women had significantly longer hospital stay, higher hospital costs, and higher rates of general and endocrine complications [12]. Another large survey of almost thirteen thousand pregnant women reported a significantly higher risk of spontaneous abortion in women who underwent surgery during gestation compared with those who did not have surgery [13]. However, the risk of surgery during pregnancy must be balanced against patients' anxiety and perceived concern of tumour growth in case surgery is delayed for several months. This question was addressed through a retrospective study [11] that compared outcomes of DTC in 61 pregnant women with 528 age-matched nonpregnant controls. Of pregnant women with DTC, one underwent surgery in the first trimester, twelve in the second, and one in the third trimester, while most of the patients underwent surgery after delivery. After a median followup of 22.4 years, no significant differences in recurrence were observed between women who underwent surgery during or after pregnancy.

Currently there is no consensus about the optimum timing of surgery for DTC in pregnancy [14], and individualized decisions are generally based on patients' wishes and other risk factors, though most would agree that, in the absence of aggressive disease, it is reasonable to delay surgery until after delivery [15]. On the other hand, if surgery is to be considered, for example, in case of large tumour, compressive symptoms, aggressive pathological or clinical features, rapid enlargement of tumor, or patients' concern, it should be performed in the second trimester before 24-week gestation [14] primarily due to an increased risk of spontaneous abortion when surgery is performed in the first trimester [13].

In our interdisciplinary clinic setting (attended by an endocrinologist, surgeon, and a radiation oncologist), we stratify individual patient-risk based on several factors such as cytological features (in case of newly identified DTC), pathological aggressiveness and previous tumor behavior (in case of recurrence), rapidity of growth, compressive symptoms, and ultrasound features while also taking into account patient's wishes and concerns and the obstetrician's opinion before reaching a consensus. In the absence of any high-risk features, we would normally prefer to delay surgery until after delivery but we closely monitor patients throughout pregnancy by performing neck ultrasound scans during each trimester.

3.2. Radioiodine Therapy and Pregnancy. Radioiodine (^{131}I) administration during pregnancy is contraindicated due to the sequelae of exposing the embryo or fetus to high doses of radiation which include fetal hypothyroidism, attention deficit disorders, memory impairment, mental retardation, malformations, growth changes, induction of malignancies including leukemia, and lethal changes [16]. Women scheduled to have radioiodine therapy should exclude pregnancy with appropriate testing beforehand [14].

^{131}I should not be given to nursing women [14] due to the significant accumulation of ^{131}I in the lactating breast and its excretion in breast milk [16]. As most thyroid cancers are slow growing, delaying ^{131}I therapy to allow breastfeeding for a short duration may be considered through discussions between the patient and the treating physician. Postpartum ^{131}I therapy should be deferred for at least 6–8 weeks after lactating women have stopped breastfeeding [14]. There is a paucity of reliable data on the kinetics of ^{131}I excretion in breast milk. Therefore, after ^{131}I therapy, it is recommended that breastfeeding should only be resumed with the birth of another child [17, 18]. In order to avoid stagnation of ^{131}I in the lactating breast and minimize the risk of breast radiation exposure, suppression of lactation through dopaminergic agents has been utilized but this should only be used very cautiously [14] after discussion with the patient. Although one large study suggested a possible increase in miscarriage rate if conception occurred within 6 months of ^{131}I therapy [19], subsequent studies failed to confirm adverse outcomes for pregnancies or offspring related to previous ^{131}I therapy [20]. A conservative recommendation is that women receiving radioiodine therapy should avoid pregnancy for 6–12 months [14] to prevent any increase in risk of infertility, miscarriage, or fetal malformation [21].

3.3. Thyroid Hormone Replacement during Pregnancy. Most women undergoing subtotal or total thyroidectomy for DTC require thyroid hormone replacement. Adequate thyroid hormone levels are crucial for maternal and fetal well-being, and several studies have reported that even mild hypothyroidism during pregnancy is associated with both adverse maternal and fetal outcomes. For instance, one study showed that children of women with undiagnosed hypothyroidism during pregnancy had lower IQ score than their age-matched controls [22]. In another study of women without overt thyroid dysfunction, the risk of miscarriage, fetal or neonatal death increased by 60% with every doubling in TSH concentration [23]. However, the data regarding low TSH in pregnancy is relatively reassuring, and, in a large survey of 25,765 women of which 433 had subclinical hyperthyroidism, low TSH was not associated with adverse outcomes [24].

The two major challenges in assessing and replacing thyroid hormones during pregnancy are emulating various physiological changes occurring in the thyroid gland during pregnancy and limitations of the commonly utilized laboratory tests for testing thyroid function. The thyroid gland undergoes remarkable changes during pregnancy. A rising HCG in early pregnancy, due to its similarity to thyroid-stimulating hormone (TSH), promotes the release of thyroid hormones which consequently leads to a transient drop in serum TSH values. At the same time, an increasing estrogen level causes two- to threefold rise in thyroid-binding globulin which alters the measured levels of total thyroxine (T4) and triiodothyronine (T3) and to some extent free thyroid hormones as well [25], thus limiting the usefulness of thyroid hormone measurement. This is further complicated by the fact that there can be a wide interassay variability in measured thyroid hormones during pregnancy [26]. Several other factors such as gestational age and singleton versus multiple-birth pregnancy can also alter thyroid hormone levels, in particular serum TSH values [27, 28]. A large survey of over thirteen thousand pregnant women reported a much tighter reference range for TSH especially in early pregnancy (2.5th and 95th percentiles of 0.1 mIU/L and 2.5 mIU/L, resp.), as compared with general population [27]. Based on these physiological variations, it is ideal to use gestational age-specific reference ranges expressed as multiples of the median, instead of reference values based on general population; however, most commercial assays do not quote pregnancy-specific reference values. Recently more elaborate techniques such as liquid chromatography-tandem mass spectrometry and equilibrium dialysis have been utilized to assess serum T4 in pregnancy [29, 30], but, apart from being much more expensive and time consuming, the correlation between free T4 measured through these techniques and serum TSH in pregnancy remains poor [29]. Furthermore, the requirement for thyroid hormone replacement increases by as much as 20–40% during pregnancy starting as early as the first few weeks of gestation [31, 32]. Due to its long half-life, T4 administration can take as much as 4–6 weeks before reaching a steady state in plasma.

With these multiple factors, pursuing a narrow therapeutic TSH target during pregnancy can be quite challenging. One study looked at the effect of empirically increasing the dose of thyroxin replacement immediately upon confirmation of pregnancy and concluded that giving an extra two tablets of thyroxin each week significantly reduces the risk of maternal hypothyroidism during the first trimester and mimics the normal physiology [33]. One caveat with this study was that patients who were athyreotic, those requiring a prepregnancy thyroxin dose of at least 100 μg/d,

and those with prepregnancy serum TSH concentrations below 1.5 mIU/liter had the highest risk for developing TSH suppression and required subsequent dose modifications after the initial intervention.

In our centre, whenever possible, we typically begin the management of these patients with proper prepregnancy counseling by informing our patients about the rationale for more frequent TSH testing and the need for dose adjustment. In addition, we make patients aware of the possibility of reduced thyroxin absorption with commonly used prepregnancy supplements such as iron and calcium and advise to take them separately from their thyroxin. Those who are already taking suppressive TSH therapy and are planning to get pregnant are typically advised to reduce the dose of thyroxin aiming for a TSH in the range of 0.5–2.5 mIU/L. Upon confirmation of pregnancy, the dose is increased by an additional two tablets each week if TSH is ≥1.5 mIU/L and by one tablet if TSH is <1.5 mIU/L. Serum TSH levels are checked every 4–6 weeks and the dose adjusted to achieve and maintain TSH in the range of 0.5–2.5 mIU/L during pregnancy.

3.4. Followup of Thyroid Cancer during Pregnancy. Most pregnant women with low-risk DTC require little more than routine TSH monitoring and periodic clinical examination during pregnancy. Radioactive iodine scan or stimulated thyroglobulin (Tg) estimation through either thyroid hormone withdrawal or recombinant TSH (Thyrogen) is not justifiable in pregnancy. Several studies have reported that although serum Tg levels can vary significantly during each trimester, the overall values remain well within the normal nonpregnant range [34–36].

In our centre, we devise our followup strategy for such patients based on their risk factors. Pregnant women with low-risk DTC who were regarded free of disease prior to pregnancy, aside from their thyroxin dose adjustment, are followed on a three monthly (once in each trimester) basis with an unstimulated Tg, and a thorough neck examination is conducted at each visit. Those women who have high-risk DTC or had documented recurrence of DTC prior to pregnancy are followed more rigorously on a three monthly basis with unstimulated Tg and neck ultrasonography. Normal reference ranges for serum Tg are irrelevant for followup of such patients, and decision regarding cancer progress is based on their prepregnancy Tg levels as well as ultrasonography findings.

4. The Role of Multidisciplinary Team in Management of Thyroid Cancer

Outside specialist centers, DTC patients have traditionally been managed by a variety of specialties which leads to an inconsistent and fragmented care, borne out by several studies from various centers [37–39]. Patient surveys have also confirmed poor and inconsistent coordination of thyroid cancer care among different caregivers [40]. Over the past decade, several centers of excellence have developed models of multidisciplinary teams comprising surgeons, radiologists, pathologists, endocrinologists, and allied specialists to deliver coordinated care within hospitals which ensures that each individual patient gets appropriate treatment decision made by a team of experts [41]. In our centre, all DTC patients (including pregnant females) are assessed and followed by a team of specialists including a surgeon, an endocrinologist, a radiation oncologist, a dietitian, specialist nurses and, in case of pregnant women, the team works closely with an obstetrician and gynecologist. In our opinion, pregnant women with DTC should ideally be referred to a specialist centre but, in the absence of such facility, management decisions should be made through close cooperation of all caregivers and the patient.

References

[1] L. H. Smith, B. Danielsen, M. E. Allen, and R. Cress, "Cancer associated with obstetric delivery: results of linkage with the California cancer registry," *American Journal of Obstetrics and Gynecology*, vol. 189, no. 4, pp. 1128–1135, 2003.

[2] A. Jemal, R. Siegel, E. Ward, T. Murray, J. Xu, and M. J. Thun, "Cancer statistics, 2007," *CA: A Cancer Journal for Clinicians*, vol. 57, no. 1, pp. 43–66, 2007.

[3] O. Kravdal, E. Glattre, and T. Haldorsen, "Positive correlation between parity and incidence of thyroid cancer: new evidence based on complete Norwegian birth cohorts," *International Journal of Cancer*, vol. 49, no. 6, pp. 831–836, 1991.

[4] S. Preston-Martin, L. Bernstein, and M. C. Pike, "Thyroid cancer among young women related to prior thyroid disease and pregnancy history," *British Journal of Cancer*, vol. 55, no. 2, pp. 191–195, 1987.

[5] C. G. Hannibal, A. Jensen, H. Sharif, and S. K. Kjaer, "Risk of thyroid cancer after exposure to fertility drugs: results from a large Danish cohort study," *Human Reproduction*, vol. 23, no. 2, pp. 451–456, 2008.

[6] M. L. Lee, G. G. Chen, A. C. Vlantis, G. M. K. Tse, B. C. H. Leung, and C. A. Van Hasselt, "Induction of thyroid papillary carcinoma cell proliferation by estrogen is associated with an altered expression of Bcl-xL," *Cancer Journal*, vol. 11, no. 2, pp. 113–121, 2005.

[7] L. Del Senno, E. Degli Uberti, S. Hanau, R. Piva, R. Rossi, and G. Trasforini, "In vitro effects of estrogen on tgb and c-myc gene expression in normal and neoplastic human thyroids," *Molecular and Cellular Endocrinology*, vol. 63, no. 1-2, pp. 67–74, 1989.

[8] A. M. McTiernan, N. S. Weiss, and J. R. Daling, "Incidence of thyroid cancer in women in relation to reproductive and hormonal factors," *American Journal of Epidemiology*, vol. 120, no. 3, pp. 423–435, 1984.

[9] W. J. Mack, S. Preston-Martin, L. Bernstein, D. Qian, and M. Xiang, "Reproductive and hormonal risk factors for thyroid cancer in Los Angeles County females," *Cancer Epidemiology Biomarkers and Prevention*, vol. 8, no. 11, pp. 991–997, 1999.

[10] G. Vannucchi, M. Perrino, S. Rossi et al., "Clinical and molecular features of differentiated thyroid cancer diagnosed during pregnancy," *European Journal of Endocrinology*, vol. 162, no. 1, pp. 145–151, 2010.

[11] M. Moosa and E. L. Mazzaferri, "Outcome of differentiated thyroid cancer diagnosed in pregnant women," *Journal of Clinical Endocrinology and Metabolism*, vol. 82, no. 9, pp. 2862–2866, 1997.

[12] S. Kuy, S. A. Roman, R. Desai, and J. A. Sosa, "Outcomes following thyroid and parathyroid surgery in pregnant women," *Archives of Surgery*, vol. 144, no. 5, pp. 399–406, 2009.

[13] J. B. Brodsky, E. N. Cohen, and B. W. Brown, "Surgery during pregnancy and fetal outcome," *American Journal of Obstetrics and Gynecology*, vol. 138, no. 8, pp. 1165–1167, 1980.

[14] D. S. Cooper, G. M. Doherty, B. R. Haugen et al., "Revised American thyroid association management guidelines for patients with thyroid nodules and differentiated thyroid cancer," *Thyroid*, vol. 19, no. 11, pp. 1167–1214, 2009.

[15] R. P. Owen, K. J. Chou, C. E. Silver et al., "Thyroid and parathyroid surgery in pregnancy," *European Archives of Oto-Rhino-Laryngology*, vol. 267, pp. 1825–1835, 2010.

[16] C. A. Gorman, "Radioiodine and pregnancy," *Thyroid*, vol. 9, no. 7, pp. 721–726, 1999.

[17] E. B. Silberstein, A. Alavi, H. R. Balon et al., "Society of Nuclear Medicine Procedure Guideline for Therapy of Thyroid Disease with Iodine-131 (Sodium Iodide) Version 2.0," http://interactive.snm.org/index.cfm?PageID=805.

[18] "Release of patients administered radioactive material," US nuclear regulatory commission, Regulatory Guide 8.39, April 1997, http://www.nucmed.com.

[19] M. Schlumberger, F. De Vathaire, C. Ceccarelli et al., "Exposure to radioactive iodine-131 for scintigraphy or therapy does not preclude pregnancy in thyroid cancer patients," *Journal of Nuclear Medicine*, vol. 37, no. 4–6, pp. 606–612, 1996.

[20] J. P. Garsi, M. Schlumberger, C. Rubino et al., "Therapeutic administration of I for differentiated thyroid cancer: radiation dose to ovaries and outcome of pregnancies," *Journal of Nuclear Medicine*, vol. 49, no. 5, pp. 845–852, 2008.

[21] E. H. Holt, "Care of the pregnant thyroid cancer patient," *Current Opinion in Oncology*, vol. 22, no. 1, pp. 1–5, 2010.

[22] J. E. Haddow, G. E. Palomaki, W. C. Allan et al., "Maternal thyroid deficiency during pregnancy and subsequent neuropsychological development of the child," *New England Journal of Medicine*, vol. 341, no. 8, pp. 549–555, 1999.

[23] N. Benhadi, W. M. Wiersinga, J. B. Reitsma, T. G. M. Vrijkotte, and G. J. Bonsel, "Higher maternal TSH levels in pregnancy are associated with increased risk for miscarriage, fetal or neonatal death," *European Journal of Endocrinology*, vol. 160, no. 6, pp. 985–991, 2009.

[24] B. M. Casey, J. S. Dashe, C. E. Wells, D. D. McIntire, K. J. Leveno, and F. G. Cunningham, "Subclinical hyperthyroidism and pregnancy outcomes," *Obstetrics and Gynecology*, vol. 107, no. 2, pp. 337–341, 2006.

[25] R. H. Lee, C. A. Spencer, J. H. Mestman et al., "Free T4 immunoassays are flawed during pregnancy," *American Journal of Obstetrics and Gynecology*, vol. 200, no. 3, pp. 260.e1–260.e6, 2009.

[26] E. Berta, L. Samson, A. Lenkey et al., "Evaluation of the thyroid function of healthy pregnant women by five different hormone assays," *Pharmazie*, vol. 65, no. 6, pp. 436–439, 2010.

[27] J. S. Dashe, B. M. Casey, C. E. Wells et al., "Thyroid-stimulating hormone in singleton and twin pregnancy: importance of gestational age-specific reference ranges," *Obstetrics and Gynecology*, vol. 106, no. 4, pp. 753–757, 2005.

[28] J. E. Haddow, G. J. Knight, G. E. Palomaki, M. R. McClain, and A. J. Pulkkinen, "The reference range and within-person variability of thyroid stimulating hormone during the first and second trimesters of pregnancy," *Journal of Medical Screening*, vol. 11, no. 4, pp. 170–174, 2004.

[29] J. Jonklaas, N. Kahric-Janicic, O. P. Soldin, and S. J. Soldin, "Correlations of free thyroid hormones measured by

tandem mass spectrometry and immunoassay with thyroid-stimulating hormone across 4 patient populations," *Clinical Chemistry*, vol. 55, no. 7, pp. 1380–1388, 2009.

[30] B. Yue, A. L. Rockwood, T. Sandrock, S. L. La'ulu, M. M. Kushnir, and A. W. Meikle, "Free thyroid hormones in serum by direct equilibrium dialysis and online solid-phase extraction-liquid chromatography/tandem mass spectrometry," *Clinical Chemistry*, vol. 54, no. 4, pp. 642–651, 2008.

[31] E. K. Alexander, E. Marqusee, J. Lawrence, P. Jarolim, G. A. Fischer, and P. R. Larsen, "Timing and magnitude of increases in levothyroxine requirements during pregnancy in women with hypothyroidism," *New England Journal of Medicine*, vol. 351, no. 3, pp. 241–310, 2004.

[32] S. J. Mandel, P. R. Larsen, E. W. Seely, and G. A. Brent, "Increased need for thyroxine during pregnancy in women with primary hypothyroidism," *New England Journal of Medicine*, vol. 323, no. 2, pp. 91–96, 1990.

[33] L. Yassa, E. Marqusee, R. Fawcett, and E. K. Alexander, "Thyroid hormone early adjustment in pregnancy (The THERAPY) trial," *Journal of Clinical Endocrinology and Metabolism*, vol. 95, no. 7, pp. 3234–3241, 2010.

[34] O. P. Soldin, R. E. Tractenberg, J. G. Hollowell, J. Jonklaas, N. Janicic, and S. J. Soldin, "Trimester-specific changes in maternal thyroid hormone, thyrotropin, and thyroglobulin concentrations during gestation: trends and associations across trimesters in iodine sufficiency," *Thyroid*, vol. 14, no. 12, pp. 1084–1090, 2004.

[35] Y. Hara, T. Tanikawa, and Y. Sakatsume, "Decreased serum thyroglobulin levels in the late stage of pregnancy," *Acta Endocrinologica*, vol. 113, no. 3, pp. 418–423, 1986.

[36] K. Kamikubo, T. Komaki, S. Nakamura, S. Sakata, K. Yasuda, and K. Miura, "Theoretical consideration of the effects of dilution on estimates of free thyroid hormones in serum," *Clinical Chemistry*, vol. 30, no. 5, pp. 634–636, 1984.

[37] S. A. Hundahl, I. D. Fleming, A. M. Fremgen, and H. R. Menck, "A National Cancer Data Base report on 53,856 cases of thyroid carcinoma treated in the U.S., 1985–1995," *Cancer*, vol. 83, no. 12, pp. 2638–2648, 1998.

[38] M. P. J. Vanderpump, L. Alexander, J. H. B. Scarpello, and R. N. Clayton, "An audit of the management of thyroid cancer in a district general hospital," *Clinical Endocrinology*, vol. 48, no. 4, pp. 419–424, 1998.

[39] S. Hölzer, C. Reiners, K. Mann et al., "Patterns of care for patients with primary differentiated carcinoma of the thyroid gland treated in Germany during 1996," *Cancer*, vol. 89, no. 1, pp. 192–201, 2000.

[40] http://www.thyroid-cancer-alliance.org.

[41] "Improving Outcomes in Head and Neck Cancer," The Manual, National Institute of Clinical Excellence, November 2004, http://www.nice.org.uk.

18

Differentiated Thyroid Cancer: Management of Patients with Radioiodine Nonresponsive Disease

Naifa Lamki Busaidy and Maria E. Cabanillas

Department of Endocrine Neoplasia and Hormonal Disorders, University of Texas MD Anderson Cancer Center, 1515 Holcombe Boulevard, Unit 1461, Houston, TX 77030, USA

Correspondence should be addressed to Naifa Lamki Busaidy, nbusaidy@mdanderson.org

Academic Editor: Mingzhao M. Xing

Differentiated thyroid carcinoma (papillary and follicular) has a favorable prognosis with an 85% 10-year survival. The patients that recur often require surgery and further radioactive iodine to render them disease-free. Five percent of thyroid cancer patients, however, will eventually succumb to their disease. Metastatic thyroid cancer is treated with radioactive iodine if the metastases are radioiodine avid. Cytotoxic chemotherapies for advanced or metastatic noniodine avid thyroid cancers show no prolonged responses and in general have fallen out of favor. Novel targeted therapies have recently been discovered that have given rise to clinical trials for thyroid cancer. Newer aberrations in molecular pathways and oncogenic mutations in thyroid cancer together with the role of angiogenesis in tumor growth have been central to these discoveries. This paper will focus on the management and treatment of metastatic differentiated thyroid cancers that do not take up radioactive iodine.

1. Introduction

Thyroid carcinoma is the most common endocrine malignancy with a prevalence of 335,000 and incidence of 37,200 in the United States in 2009 [1]. Differentiated thyroid carcinoma, namely papillary and follicular thyroid carcinoma, makes up about 94% of these cases. Despite the generally good prognosis of thyroid carcinoma, about 5% of patients will develop metastatic disease which fails to respond to radioactive iodine, exhibiting a more aggressive behavior. These patients will die of their disease [1–4].

85% of patients with differentiated thyroid carcinomas are cured with surgery, radioactive iodine, and TSH suppression. Of those that recur, the vast majority will recur in the neck, and best treatment options are surgical with potential further radioactive iodine. A small percentage of patients will develop or present with metastases and are more difficult to treat. When metastases have radioiodine avidity, prognosis is better, and further radioactive iodine may be used. However, when multiple doses of radioactive iodine have been tried or the patient has nonradioactive iodine avid disease, other options need to be considered. This paper will aim to discuss the treatment options of those patients with nonradioiodine avid, recurrent, or metastatic differentiated thyroid cancer.

2. Diagnosis of Recurrent/Metastatic Disease Extent

Screening ultrasound of the neck and tumor marker (thyroglobulin) should be performed on all patients with differentiated thyroid cancer, per accepted guidelines [5]. The finding of an elevated thyroglobulin or thyroglobulin antibody in the face of a negative radioactive iodine scan is indicative of non-radioiodine avid residual or recurrent disease. Both ultrasound of the neck and thin spiral CT of the chest should be performed for detection of disease. If symptoms occur or the thyroglobulin is out of proportion to the amount of disease seen, other imaging can be ordered as dictated by the clinical scenario. Other imaging modalities include MRI of the brain, spine, bone scan, and ^{18}FDG-PET/CT scans. Table 1 summarizes the imaging modalities used in thyroid cancer surveillance.

TABLE 1: Imaging modalities for RAI-refractory recurrent disease.

Imaging study	Utility	Pros	Cons
Ultrasound neck	Detection of neck disease	Sensitive; ability to biopsy	Operator dependent; difficult to detect invasive disease and disease in the posterior neck
CT	Detection of local and metastatic disease	Sensitive; less operator dependent	Radiation exposure; risk of renal injury with contrast; delays in radioiodine administration
MRI	Detection of local and metastatic disease	Sensitive for CNS disease; no radiation exposure	Difficult to tolerate in some patients; risk of nephrogenic systemic fibrosis (NSF) in patients with renal failure; contraindicated in patients with certain metal devices or implants
FDG-PET scan	Detection of metastatic disease and providing prognostic information	Sensitive when used with CT	Detects FDG-avid disease only

2.1. Role of Ultrasound. Ultrasonography (U/S) of the neck (thyroid bed and cervical neck compartments), as opposed to RAI scans, is recommended in the followup of these patients. This shift in practice is due to the fact that many recurrent tumors lose the ability to capture iodine, leading to false negatives. As many as half of the patients with findings of recurrence on U/S may have no uptake on radioiodine scanning or may have an undetectable serum thyroglobulin [6].

Recurrence of papillary thyroid carcinoma is most commonly in the neck (thyroid bed and lymph nodes), and hence, ultrasound is the mainstay of routine followup of these patients. U/S can be used to accurately diagnose and identify lesions in the neck as small as 3 mm. Routine use of U/S in the 3- to 12-month monitoring of patients with extrathyroidal invasion or local-regional nodal metastases [7, 8] is now recommended as part of consensus guidelines [5]. Although U/S can aid in distinguishing benign lesions from malignant lesions, FNA (U/S guided) is most helpful to definitively prove recurrent cancer. Thyroglobulin can be measured in the washout of the needle taken from neck lymph nodes [9–11]. This is especially helpful in cases where the FNA specimen is nondiagnostic.

2.2. CT and MRI. Other imaging techniques that can be used in individual cases of thyroid cancer followup include CT scan of the neck with IV contrast, CT scan of the chest, and magnetic resonance imaging (MRI). MRI and CT scan of the neck play important roles in the detection of recurrent disease although the sensitivity of these is not as well established as ultrasound for the detection of true thyroid cancer recurrences in the neck. CT and MRI of the neck are not recommended for routine use in the detection of recurrent disease but have the advantage of being much less operator dependent. If good ultrasonography is not readily available or deep posterior neck disease is suspected, CT and MRI of the neck can be used for the detection of disease.

The most common place for papillary thyroid carcinoma to metastasize outside the neck is the chest. CT scan of

the chest may show macro- and micronodular pulmonary metastases that do not routinely take up iodine. This cross-sectional imaging of the chest is used for long-term followup when lung metastases are known or suspected based on elevations in thyroglobulin.

CT and MRI scans of other less commonly found sites of distant metastases include imaging of the brain, spine, abdomen, and pelvis as the clinical scenario dictates based on symptoms, clinical suspicion, or prior to initiation of various therapies.

2.3. [18]FDG PET-CT. Fluorodeoxyglucose positron-emission tomography (FDG-PET or PET)/CT imaging is an increasingly more useful tool in the detection of radioiodine-negative, thyroglobulin-positive thyroid cancer [12–15]. Thyroid carcinomas with little to no iodine activity tend to have higher glucose metabolism and positive FDG-PET scans [12, 16, 17]. This tends to be representative of tumor dedifferentiation. Patients with larger volumes of FDG-avid disease or higher SUVs are less likely to respond to radioiodine and have a higher mortality over a 3-year followup compared with the patients with no FDG uptake [18, 19]. Tumors that take up radioactive iodine are less likely to yield positive FDG PET scans [20].

PET/CT scans can be used for detection of occult recurrences or metastases [16, 21, 22] or to provide information about the biology of the metastatic disease and prognostic information. The latter is not standard practice, but several studies have now shown that FDG-PET correlates with the overall survival [14, 15, 21]. This information may be helpful to decide which patients warrant systemic treatment for their metastatic disease if they are refractory/resistant to radioactive iodine or have reached the maximum benefit from this treatment.

[18]FDG-PET has been approved for reimbursement for the detection of occult thyroid cancer in patients who have a thyroglobulin greater than 10 ng/mL and have negative radioiodine imaging. [18]FDG-PET CTs are also used in those

TABLE 2: Therapeutic modalities for RAI-refractory recurrent disease.

	Indication	Pros	Cons
Surgery	Surgically resectable local recurrences; metastasectomy	Potential for cure	Potential significant morbidity
External beam radiation	Adjuvant: neck Therapeutic and palliative: metastatic sites	Decrease in recurrence, progression, and pain	May preclude future neck surgery; dysphagia and xerostomia; secondary malignancies
PEIT	Locally recurrent disease in patients at high risk for morbidity and mortality from surgical resection	Potential for avoidance of surgery	Local pain; injury to local structures; unknown effect on survival and recurrence
Systemic chemotherapy (including TKIs)	Unresectable, RAI-refractory, metastatic disease	May slow progression of disease; may alleviate disease symptoms	Significant adverse events; unknown effect on survival

PEIT: percutaneous ethanol injection therapy; TKI: tyrosine kinase inhibitors.

patients whose cancers are very poorly differentiated and make no thyroglobulin.

The overall sensitivity, specificity, and accuracy of ^{18}F-FDG PET/CT in one series of 59 patients with radioiodine-negative, thyroglobulin-positive, recurrent disease were 68.4%, 82.4%, and 73.8%, respectively [23]. Other studies have shown a sensitivity of 70–95% and a specificity of 77–100% [12, 13]. FDG-PET is not sensitive enough to detect subcentimeter metastases, as it is common in metastatic papillary thyroid carcinoma and should be used in conjunction with CT chest imaging.

TSH stimulates ^{18}FDG uptake by differentiated thyroid carcinoma [24], suggesting that PET scans may be more sensitive after TSH stimulation with rhTSH or withdrawal of thyroid hormone [24–26]. While rhTSH-stimulated PET-CT identified more total FDG-avid lesions compared to non-stimulated FDG-PET CT in a large multicenter study, it changed treatment planning only 6% of the time [27].

False positives, such as infections or granulomatous diseases/sarcoid or postoperative changes due to inflammation, amongst others, have been reported in thyroid cancer about 11–25% of the time suggesting that the malignant nature of the disease should be confirmed prior to further therapy [27–30].

3. Treatment of Advanced or Metastatic Thyroid Cancer

Most patients with differentiated thyroid cancers are rendered free of disease after surgery, radioactive iodine, and thyroid hormone suppression. Approximately 15–20% of patients will recur locoregionally or have distant metastases. Although it is the most effective medical treatment for differentiated thyroid carcinoma, only about 50–80% of primary tumors and their metastases take up radioactive iodine [7, 31–34], rendering this therapy ineffective in most cases. Thus, other treatment modalities such as surgery, external beam radiation, percutaneous ethanol injection therapy (PEIT), and systemic chemotherapy are indicated. Table 2 summarizes the indications for each of these therapies.

3.1. Surgery. Surgery in advanced thyroid carcinomas is most commonly used for recurrent neck metastases and metastasectomies in selected sites. Recurrences in the neck are most commonly seen in the thyroid bed or regional lymph nodes. Although most occur within the first five years after diagnosis, late recurrences do occur. In one study with 40-year followup, 35% of patients recurred. Two-thirds of them were within the first decade after initial therapy, and two thirds were locoregional [35].

Surgery is considered first-line therapy in patients with gross nodal or recurrent neck disease. This can be followed by further radioactive iodine (if the recurrent tumors took up radioiodine prior to surgery) and thyroid hormone suppression. One-third to one half of patients may be free of disease in short-term followup [36]. If the gross tumors do not take up radioactive iodine from previous posttreatment scans or preoperative radioiodine scans are negative, further postoperative radioactive iodine will be of limited benefit and may increase the side effects of further iodine. Adverse events from further radioactive iodine include xerostomia, nasolacrimal duct obstruction, and secondary malignancies [37–42].

Surgery alone with complete ipsilateral compartmental dissections of involved areas or modified neck dissections as opposed to "berry picking" or selective lymph node resection procedures or ethanol ablation may be of benefit [43, 44]. It is not evident that recurrent locoregional disease in the setting of distant metastatic disease should be resected, unless there is airway or an other vital structural compromise. If the tumors invade the upper aerodigestive tract, a combined treatment modality of surgery and ^{131}I (if tumors take up radioactive iodine) and/or adjuvant external beam radiotherapy is advised [45–48]. Due to potential morbidity from surgical resection of recurrent disease, these patients should be referred to centers with expertise in this area.

Surgery is also considered for isolated metastases, metastases in bone (especially if long bones, spine, or weight bearing), and brain (see Section 3.3 below).

3.2. External Beam Radiotherapy. External beam radiotherapy (EBRT) has a very specific role in the treatment of papillary thyroid carcinoma. Although it is somewhat controversial, retrospective studies have shown that it may be an effective adjuvant therapy to prevent local-regional recurrence in patients 45 years of age and older with locally invasive papillary carcinoma after surgery [49, 50]. Ten-year local relapse-free rates (93% versus 78%) and disease-specific survival rates (100% versus 95%) were higher in a subgroup of patients with papillary histology and presumed microscopic disease treated with EBRT [49]. Doses in the range of 40–50 Gy may aid in local-regional control in patients with papillary thyroid carcinoma who are over 45 years of age and have incomplete resection near the aerodigestive tract and/or those with gross extrathyroidal invasion with presumed microscopic residual disease. EBRT is generally avoided in patients under 45 years of age both because of their good prognosis and the potential late side effects of therapy including secondary malignancies. External beam radiation may also preclude further surgery in the future if the tumor recurs.

Acute complications of external beam radiotherapy include esophagitis and tracheitis. Long-term complications include neck fibrosis, xerostomia, dental decay, osteoradionecrosis, and the risk of tracheal stenosis [34]. Newer techniques to deliver radiation with fewer adverse events are being used in the treatment of cancer, including intensity-modulated radiation therapy (IMRT). Limited data in thyroid cancer with short-term followup suggests similar outcomes and may reduce chronic morbidity relative to conventional EBRT [51]. Many centers currently use IMRT as the radiation treatment of choice for thyroid carcinomas requiring EBRT [52].

3.3. Metastatic Sites Requiring Special Attention.

Although most patients with metastatic disease will need systemic therapy, metastatic disease to certain sites deserves special attention.

3.3.1. CNS Metastases.

Brain metastases more often occur in elderly individuals with more advanced disease and have an overall poorer prognosis [53]. Surgical resection significantly improves median overall survival from four to 22 months in patients with 1 or more brain metastases [53]. Current guidelines recommend resection when one CNS lesion is present [54]. Radioiodine therapy and/or external beam radiotherapy (with steroids to minimize tumor swelling) should be considered after surgical resection [55]. If CNS lesions are not surgically resectable or the morbidity from surgery is unacceptable, whole brain radiotherapy for numerous lesions or gamma knife radiosurgery to selected lesions should be used in conjunction with radioiodine if the tumor concentrates iodine [56]. If radioiodine is to be used, prior radiotherapy and concomitant steroids should be strongly considered to decrease tumor swelling [57].

3.3.2. Bone Metastases.

Although bone lesions tend to concentrate radioiodine as well as lungs, there is complete resolution in less than 10% of the time. Metastases that cause pain or compression of spinal cord or other vital organs necessitate treatment. Symptoms from painful bone lesions or spinal-cord-compressing lesions may be relieved by surgical treatment. External beam radiation therapy (EBRT) or gamma knife radiosurgery has also been used successfully to render bone lesions pain-free. Arterial embolization has been used with successful reduction in pain and neurologic symptoms and can be used in conjunction with external beam radiation [58]. ^{131}I treatment may follow surgical resection of distant metastatic disease if the tumor takes up radioactive iodine. A recent study found that patients with solitary bony metastases treated with I131 and surgery had a better prognosis than those who did not [59].

Intravenous bisphosphonates (pamidronate or zoledronic acid) are prescribed for painful bony metastases with some success as well. Orita et al., retrospectively, examined 50 patients with bony metastases from DTC and found that those who had received monthly infusions of zoledronic acid had significantly fewer-skeletal related events (defined as fracture, spinal cord compression, and hypercalcemia) than those who did not receive this drug [60]. Whether this treatment slows progression of bone metastases is not known. The most common adverse event associated with intravenous bisphosphonates is a transient flu-like syndrome, usually associated with the first administration, with symptoms dissipating and disappearing with subsequent infusions. Osteonecrosis of the jaw is less common but serious adverse event associated with intravenous bisphosphonates.

3.4. Systemic Therapy.

Lack of RAI uptake by distant metastases confers a poor prognosis. For example, patients with no RAI uptake in the lungs have a 10-year survival rate of 25% compared with 76% in those whose lung metastases have RAI uptake [61]. Pulmonary metastases that do not take up radioactive iodine do not typically respond to that radionuclide therapy, and these patients are at high risk of death [62].

Most diagnostic scan-negative, thyroglobulin-positive patients who have disease seen on other imaging modalities are not rendered disease-free by repeat radioiodine treatments, although tumor burden may decrease [63]. No survival advantage nor decrease in morbidity has been seen with repeat radioactive iodine therapies. Repeated doses of radioactive iodine have been used in patients considered to have radioactive noniodine-avid, thyroglobulin-positive disease with little clinical benefit [64]. Although controversial, a single dose of 100–150 mCi of radioactive iodine therapy can be given to a patient with elevated thyroglobulin and negative diagnostic scan. A posttreatment scan should be done, and if negative, further radioactive iodine should be avoided.

Repeated radioiodine therapy has adverse events including xerostomia, nasolacrimal duct obstruction with epiphora, and secondary malignancies [37–42]. Further radioactive iodine therapy should generally be avoided in these patients, and the use of systemic agents should be considered [65].

Because metastatic differentiated thyroid cancer can be stable and quiescent for many years, only patients with progressive or symptomatic disease should be treated with other systemic treatments. Systemic therapy with targeted agents or cytotoxic chemotherapy is the usual treatment of choice for RAI-refractory, progressive distant metastatic disease.

Clinical trials should consider first-line therapy for those patients who do not take up radioactive iodine. If a clinical trial is not available or the patient is not suitable for one, then off-label use of targeted therapies such as pazopanib, sorafenib, sunitinib, or cytotoxic chemotherapy should be considered [54].

3.4.1. Cytotoxic Chemotherapy.

Traditional cytotoxic chemotherapies such as doxorubicin, taxol, and cisplatin are associated with a 25–37% partial response rate with rare complete remission [66–69]. Due to toxic side effects, short duration of responses, and low response rates, systemic cytotoxic chemotherapy is reserved for patients with rapidly progressive metastatic disease that is not suitable or nonresponsive to surgery, radioiodine, and external beam radiotherapy and those who cannot enter into clinical trials or use targeted agents (see below).

Systemic chemotherapy is used in certain cases of widespread progressive disease that is radioiodine resistant although available regimens have not been well studied and are not very effective to date. Doxorubicin is associated with a response rate of up to 40% for progressive differentiated cancers that do not respond to radioactive iodine [70, 71]. The recommended dosage is 60–75 mg/m^2 every 3 weeks. Combination therapies are also used, but data are limited because of the small number of patients in reported series. Doxorubicin, epirubicin, taxol, and cisplatin have all been used in various combinations; responses do not seem to be any better than single agent with increased toxicities [68, 69, 72]. Response rates vary from 25 to 37% with mostly partial responses. Doxorubicin has also been used as a radiation sensitizer with not much different results from radiation alone. Patients with advanced progressive radioiodine nonresponsive disease should be considered for participation in clinical trials.

3.4.2. Newer Targeted Therapies.

Newer approaches to thyroid carcinoma therapy include inhibition of the various metabolic pathways found to be altered in these cancerous cells. Prior to the discussion of the available and tried targeted therapies below, we briefly summarize the known aberrant pathways.

(1) Mutations and Promotion of Tumor Growth. Follicular cell tumorigenesis pathways have been key to the development of clinical trials testing novel therapies in the treatment of thyroid cancer. Mutations in either BRAF, RAS or RET/PTC rearrangements are present in most differentiated thyroid cancers [73]. Chromosomal rearrangement of the gene encoding the transmembrane tyrosine kinase receptors *ret* and *trk* is one identified early step in the development of these tumors. RET/PTC genetic alterations have been found in 40% and 60% of papillary carcinomas in adults and children, respectively, and are the most common

mutation found in the Chernobyl radiation-induced thyroid carcinomas [74–76].

Mutations and constitutive activation of the MAP kinase pathway have been of interest of late. BRAF (in papillary thyroid cancer) and RAS genes in the MAP kinase pathway normally code for growth and function in normal and tumor cells. BRAF mutations have been identified in approximately 45% or more of clinically evident papillary carcinomas and may behave more aggressively [77–79]. Activating mutations of RAS are more common in follicular variant PTC and follicular thyroid cancer [80] and may be a marker of more aggressive disease [81].

Other discoveries include the dependence of tumors on angiogenesis. Angiogenesis is important for tumor cell growth, promotion, and development of metastases [82]. Vascular endothelial growth factor (VEGF), an important proangiogenic factor, binds to VEGF receptors that in turn can further activate MAP kinase signaling and promote further tumor growth. VEGF receptors play a contributory role in the development and progression of thyroid cancer [73, 83]. VEGF expression is associated with higher risk of recurrence and shorter disease-free survival [84, 85]. Like in other tumors, epigenetic modifications of chromosomal DNA and histones, including the promoter gene of the sodium-iodine symporter, may also play an important role in promotion of tumor growth.

(2) Therapeutic Options and Clinical Trials. Patients with progressive or symptomatic metastatic thyroid cancer that is deemed nonradioiodine responsive should be considered for treatment on a clinical trial [5]. The recent identification of the molecular and cellular pathogenesis of both the development and progression of cancer has led to development of newer molecular-targeted therapies. Oncogenic mutations in the MAP kinase pathway (BRAF and RAS), as well as the importance of vascular endothelial growth factor receptors in thyroid cancer (mentioned above), have led to several clinical trials with small molecule inhibitors. These agents inhibit multiple kinases and can affect multiple signaling pathways. Tyrosine kinase inhibitors (TKIs) are orally administered and generally well tolerated. Immunomodulators, other oncogene inhibitors, and modulators of growth or apoptosis are all under investigation as well. Various clinical trials in the United States and Europe are recruiting differentiated thyroid cancer patients with radioiodine-negative progressive disease. The following are among the ones that have raised maximal interest and are summarized in Table 3.

(3) Commercially Available TKIs. (a) *Sorafenib.* Sorafenib is an oral, small molecule tyrosine kinase inhibitor that inhibits RET, BRAF, and VEGF receptors 2 and 3. It is currently approved in the United States for advanced renal cell carcinoma and unresectable hepatocellular carcinoma. Two phase II trials have been performed in patients with differentiated thyroid cancer that have both shown promise. In the larger, National Cancer Institute sponsored study with 58 patients with differentiated and anaplastic thyroid cancer (46 differentiated thyroid cancer patients evaluable

TABLE 3: Targeted therapies evaluated in clinical trials for thyroid cancer.

Drug	VEGFR1	VEGFR2	VEGFR3	RET	BRAF	Other	Response; PFS	Citation
Axitinib	X	X	X				31% PR; 18 mos (MTC included)	Cohen et al. [91, 99]
Motesanib	X	X	X	X			14% PR; 9 mos	Sherman et al. [97]
Sorafenib		X	X	X	X		13–32% PR; PFS 10–21 mos	Kloos et al. [86], Gupta-Abramson et al. [87], Cabanillas et al. [88]
Sunitinib	X	X	X	X			28% CR + PR; TTP 13 mos	Carr et al. [93]
Pazopanib	X	X	X	X			49% PR; PFS 12 mos	Bible et al. [94]
Lenvatinib	X	X	X	X		FGFR	50% PR; PFS 13 mos	Sherman et al. [105]
Cabozantinib	X	X		X		c-MET	53% PR; PFS n/a	Cabanillas et al. [101]

PR: partial response, SD: stable disease, TTP: time to progression, PFS: progression-free survival, n/a: not available, and mos: months.

for response). The partial response rate was 13%, and stable disease rate was 54% in patients with differentiated thyroid cancer; however, 6 patients who were deemed not assessable were excluded from this analysis [86]. A second phase II study reported partial remission in 7 of 22 (32%) patients with differentiated thyroid cancer [87]. With early data showing sorafenib to have promise in differentiated thyroid carcinoma (DTC) and sorafenib being a commercially available drug, many clinicians began using this drug in an off-label manner (not FDA approved for thyroid cancer). We recently reviewed our experience with off-label use of sorafenib in patients with DTC [88]. All patients had progressive nonradioactive iodine-avid disease to receive drug. Twenty percent of the patients developed a partial response, and 60% of patients developed stable disease achieving a clinical benefit rate of 80%. Progression-free survival was lengthened from four months predrug to 19 months. There was no difference in response based on BRAF mutational status in any of these studies thus far. A phase III international randomized controlled trial is underway currently evaluating sorafenib in progressive nonradioiodine-responsive metastatic differentiated thyroid cancer. This trial is randomized to placebo, and the primary endpoint is progression-free survival.

(b) *Sunitinib*. Sunitinib is another oral small molecule tyrosine kinase inhibitor that is FDA approved for the treatment of metastatic renal cell carcinoma. This drug inhibits RET, RET/PTC subtypes 1 and 3, and VEGFR [89]. Two patients with differentiated thyroid carcinoma treated with daily sunitinib for four weeks and two weeks holiday have had prolonged partial responses and decreases in SUV on PET scan [90]. An ongoing open-label phase II study showed a 13% partial response rate, and in another 68% percent of differentiated thyroid carcinoma patients, disease stabilization was seen [91]. A second phase II study has reported partial remission or disease stabilization in two of 12 patients thus far [92]. Other case reports have described prolonged partial responses [90]. The study by Carr et al. is the largest published trial to date using sunitinib in patients with metastatic PET-positive, RAI-refractory differentiated thyroid cancer. 28% of patients with differentiated thyroid

cancer achieved a response (complete or partial response) [93].

(c) *Pazopanib*. Pazopanib is a small molecule inhibitor of all VEGFR subtypes and PDGFR. It is approved in the United States for the treatment of advanced renal cell carcinoma. Mayo Clinic recently reported on 37 rapidly progressive DTC patients on a phase II single agent trial [94]. 49% of patients had partial responses with a starting dose of 800 mg. Progression-free survival was 12 months. This drug carries a black box warning due to severe and fatal hepatotoxicity observed in a renal cell carcinoma patient. Liver transaminase levels should be monitored closely with this drug.

(d) *Adverse Events Common to Sorafenib, Sunitinib, and Pazopanib*. Adverse events seen with these drugs are similar to those described with the treatment of advanced renal cell carcinoma and are summarized in Table 4. The most common ones include diarrhea, hand-foot syndrome, rash, hypertension, and fatigue. Skin changes have also been noted including keratoacanthomas and squamous cell carcinomas in about 5–11% of patients taking sorafenib. Due to the promise shown by these agents in differentiated thyroid carcinoma and the availability and tolerability of these drugs, sorafenib, sunitinib, and pazopanib have been added as treatment options for patients with progressive nonradioactive iodine-avid thyroid cancer who cannot be enrolled in a clinical trial [5]. Due to significant potential toxicity, only clinicians versed in the management of the side effects of these therapies should use these drugs in a permissible off-label manner.

(4) Clinical Trials with TKIs. (a) *Motesanib*. Motesanib is an oral tyrosine kinase inhibitor that inhibits VEGFRs 1, 2, and 3 [95]. It is currently not commercially available. A phase II trial was initiated based on responses in five patients with differentiated thyroid cancer in a phase I trial [96]. Patients with progressive differentiated thyroid cancer based on serial radiographic imaging in a six-month period were enrolled in this international phase II trial. 93 patients were enrolled, 14% had a partial response, and 35% of patients developed disease stabilization for 24 weeks [97]. One-third

TABLE 4: Adverse events associated with the commercially available TKIs used in thyroid cancer.

Adverse event	Sorafenib (%)		Sunitinib (%)		Pazopanib (%)	
	All grade	≥grade 3	All grade	≥grade 3	All grade	≥grade 3
Hypertension	17	4	30	12	40	4
CHF or LVEF decline	1.7	NR	13	3	<1%	NR
Proteinuria	NR	NR	NR	NR	9	<1
Hand-foot skin reaction	30	6	29	6	6	NR
Stomatitis	NR	NR	30	1	4	NR
Anorexia	16	<1	34	2	22	2
Weight loss	10	<1	12	<1	52	3.5
Diarrhea	43	2	61	9	52	3.5
AST elevation	NR	NR	56	2	53	7.5
ALT elevation	NR	NR	51	2.5	53	12
Fatigue	37	5	54	11	19	2
Hypothyroidism	NR	NR	14	2	7	NR
Arterial thromboembolism	2.9	NR	NR	NR	3	2
Hemorrhage/bleeding (all sites)	15	3	30	3	13	2

CHF: congestive heart failure; LVEF: left ventricular ejection fraction; AST: aspartate aminotransferase; ALT: alanine aminotransferase; NR: not reported. table adapted from [115].

of the patients were still on drug after 48 weeks. The median progression-free survival was 40 weeks. Tumors with BRAF mutations responded better than those without, despite the lack of BRAF inhibition by motesanib, suggesting that these BRAF-positive tumors may be more dependent on VEGF-mediated angiogenesis. The most common adverse events noted include fatigue, nausea, diarrhea, and hypertension. This trial also noted the unanticipated side effect of a 30% increase in levothyroxine requirement to maintain the purposeful TSH suppression; two-thirds of the patients developed a TSH outside of the range.

(b) *Axitinib.* Axitinib is an oral tyrosine kinase inhibitor that blocks VEGFRs and has been studied in thyroid cancer. It is not commercially available. A phase II, multicenter study was initiated based on the experience of five thyroid cancer patients in a phase I trial [98]. 31% of differentiated thyroid carcinoma patients had a partial response [99]. Many of the patients had been previously treated with various chemotherapeutic agents. Median progression-free survival for all histologic types of thyroid cancer was 18 months. The most common side effects seen in this trial include hypertension, stomatitis, fatigue, and diarrhea. A current trial is underway to evaluate axitinib's efficacy in doxorubicin-refractory metastatic thyroid cancer patients.

(c) *Other Therapeutic Agents.* A small molecule inhibitor of the epidermal growth factor receptor, gefitinib, has been looked at in advanced thyroid cancer but had no complete or partial responses [100]. With increased expression of c-MET described in PTC, cabozantinib (XL184), an oral small molecule inhibitor of various tyrosine kinases including C-MET and VEGFR2, is being studied in differentiated thyroid cancer [101–104]. Results presented at the American Thyroid Association (ATA) were very encouraging, with a partial response rate of 53% in a cohort of 15 DTC patients [101]. A phase 2 trial with lenvatinib (E7080) in 58 patients

with radioactive iodine refractory DTC showed 50% partial response and a progression-free survival of 13 months [105]. XL281, a small molecule inhibitor of BRAF kinases currently in a phase I trial, preliminarily shows five patients with papillary thyroid carcinomas with prolonged stable diseases. Two of these patients had V600E BRAF mutation [106]. Vemurafenib (also known as PLX4032, RO5185426, and RG7204), also a small molecule inhibitor of mutant BRAF kinase, has shown promise in thyroid cancer [107] and is currently being studied in patients with BRAF-mutated thyroid cancer in a phase II trial. An open-label phase II study in Kentucky examined the efficacy of thalidomide in progressive metastatic thyroid cancer of all histologies [108]. An 18% partial response rate with 32% stable disease as best response is described in the 28 evaluable patients of all thyroid histologies. Lenalidomide, a similar drug to thalidomide but less toxic, is being evaluated in a phase II open-label study in DTC patients currently [109]. Thus far, 39% of the patients developed a partial response and 50% in whom disease stabilized. Overall survival was shorter than in most trials with a median of 11 months.

(d) *Agents to Restore Radioactive Iodine Uptake.* Researchers have been searching for ways to restore loss of radioactive iodine to nonavid tumors. 13 cis-retinoic acid partially restored radioactive iodine uptake in poorly differentiated follicular thyroid cancer cells [110]. Many clinical trials using retinoid receptors and other drugs have been focused on this restoration of iodine avidity with little success. Bexarotene, a synthetic agonist of the retinoid X receptor, was evaluated in a phase II trial to attempt to restore radioiodine activity, followed by treatment. After six weeks of therapy, eight of 11 patients had partial restoration of iodine avidity, but there was not much tumor reduction [111]. Rosiglitazone, a peroxisomal proliferators-activated receptor-gamma agonist, was evaluated for restoration of radioiodine uptake [112].

After eight weeks of treatment, although four patients had iodine avidity, clinical response was lacking. Depsipeptide, a histone deacetylase inhibitor, was evaluated in a phase II trial of patients with nonradioiodine metastatic DTC [113]. Only one patient out of 14 showed improvement in radioiodine uptake, but significant cardiac toxicities were seen, including sudden death. The most encouraging of these studies was presented at the American Thyroid Association (ATA) in 2011, evaluating single-agent MEK1/2 inhibitor, selumetinib (AZD6244), in 17 patients who were RAI refractory. In 11 patients, RAI uptake was restored. Information on best response was available in 7 patients, 6 of whom had a partial response to RAI [114].

Other agents are under investigation in both phases I and II studies, including agents that inhibit the PI3kinase/aKt pathways, histone deacetylase inhibitors, and combinations of methylation inhibitors with histone deacetylase inhibitors.

4. Summary

Differentiated thyroid carcinoma that is nonradioiodine avid is difficult to detect and treat. Clinically dictated selected imaging including ultrasound of the neck, CT imaging of the chest, MRIs of the spine and brain, bone scan, and ^{18}FDG-PET-CT have all been useful in the detection of disease. Further radioactive iodine therapy in these patients tends to increase adverse events with minimal clinical benefit.

Recurrent neck disease is often treated with further surgery. In addition, patients may benefit from resection of specific symptomatic metastatic sites. Selected patients may benefit from external beam radiotherapy, radiofrequency ablation, or chemoembolization of other metastatic sites as well.

Patients with stable metastatic disease may be observed with thyroid hormone suppression therapy only. More advanced, progressive neck disease and progressive, distant metastatic disease require systemic treatment. Cytotoxic chemotherapy has limited response rates and significant toxicity and is therefore reserved for symptomatic progressive disease in a patient that cannot get on a clinical trial or tolerate antiangiogenic therapy. The advancement in understanding the molecular aberrations in thyroid cancer has led to an explosion of promising recent clinical trials. Targeted agents against the VEGF receptor and the MAP kinase pathway are amongst the most promising thus far. These agents have shown some of the most impressive responses and have fairly tolerable adverse effects.

Given our current knowledge and trial results, it remains difficult to choose the optimal therapy for selected patients. Many of the trials had varying entry criteria, many of which did not require progression. No trial thus far has overall survival as the primary endpoint, prolongation of this being the ultimate goal of patients. In addition, most patients eventually progress through these agents suggesting development of other pathways of resistance. Future trials will likely necessitate combination of therapy with minimal increased toxicity. Future trials may include agents that inhibit the PI3 kinase pathway in addition to the MAP kinase pathway or combination of cytotoxic chemotherapy with

targeted agents. The main goal of all these trials should be to prolong life with minimal decrease in quality of life.

Funding

N. L. Busaidy has grant funding from Bayer and Novartis; M. E. Cabanillas has grant funding from Eisai and Exelixis.

References

[1] A. Jemal, R. Siegel, E. Ward, Y. Hao, J. Xu, and M. J. Thun, "Cancer statistics, 2009," *CA Cancer Journal for Clinicians*, vol. 59, no. 4, pp. 225–249, 2009.

[2] J. Robbins, M. J. Merino, J. D. Boice et al., "Thyroid cancer: a lethal endocrine neoplasm," *Annals of Internal Medicine*, vol. 115, no. 2, pp. 133–147, 1991.

[3] F. D. Gilliland, W. C. Hunt, D. M. Morris, and C. R. Key, "Prognostic factors for thyroid carcinoma: a population-based study of 15,698 cases from the Surveillance, Epidemiology and End Results (SEER) program 1973–1991," *Cancer*, vol. 79, no. 3, pp. 564–573, 1997.

[4] A. Antonelli, P. Fallahi, S. M. Ferrari et al., "Dedifferentiated thyroid cancer: a therapeutic challenge," *Biomedicine and Pharmacotherapy*, vol. 62, no. 8, pp. 559–563, 2008.

[5] D. S. Cooper, G. M. Doherty, B. R. Haugen et al., "Revised American thyroid association management guidelines for patients with thyroid nodules and differentiated thyroid cancer," *Thyroid*, vol. 19, no. 11, pp. 1167–1214, 2009.

[6] A. Antonelli, P. Miccoli, M. Ferdeghini et al., "Role of neck ultrasonography in the follow-up of patients operated on for thyroid cancer," *Thyroid*, vol. 5, no. 1, pp. 25–28, 1995.

[7] M. Franceschi, Z. Kusić, D. Franceschi, L. Lukinac, and S. Rončević, "Thyroglobulin determination, neck ultrasonography and iodine-131 whole-body scintigraphy in differentiated thyroid carcinoma," *Journal of Nuclear Medicine*, vol. 37, no. 3, pp. 446–451, 1996.

[8] A. Frilling, R. Gorges, K. Tecklenborg et al., "Value of preoperative diagnostic modalities in patients with recurrent thyroid carcinoma," *Surgery*, vol. 128, no. 6, pp. 1067–1074, 2000.

[9] T. Uruno, A. Miyauchi, K. Shimizu et al., "Usefulness of thyroglobulin measurement in fine-needle aspiration biopsy specimens for diagnosing cervical lymph node metastasis in patients with papillary thyroid cancer," *World Journal of Surgery*, vol. 29, no. 4, pp. 483–485, 2005.

[10] A. Frasoldati, E. Toschi, M. Zini et al., "Role of thyroglobulin measurement in fine-needle aspiration biopsies of cervical lymph nodes in patients with differentiated thyroid cancer," *Thyroid*, vol. 9, no. 2, pp. 105–111, 1999.

[11] F. Pacini, L. Fugazzola, F. Lippi et al., "Detection of thyroglobulin in fine needle aspirates of nonthyroidal neck masses: a clue to the diagnosis of metastatic differentiated thyroid cancer," *The Journal of Clinical Endocrinology and Metabolism*, vol. 74, no. 6, pp. 1401–1404, 1992.

[12] L. Hooft, O. S. Hoekstra, W. Deville et al., "Diagnostic accuracy of 18F-fluorodeoxyglucose positron emission tomography in the follow-up of papillary or follicular thyroid cancer," *The Journal of Clinical Endocrinology and Metabolism*, vol. 86, no. 8, pp. 3779–3786, 2001.

[13] N. Khan, N. Oriuchi, T. Higuchi, H. Zhang, and K. Endo, "PET in the follow-up of differentiated thyroid cancer,"

British Journal of Radiology, vol. 76, no. 910, pp. 690–695, 2003.

[14] R. J. Robbins, Q. Wan, R. K. Grewal et al., "Real-time prognosis for metastatic thyroid carcinoma based on 2-[18F]fluoro-2-deoxy-D-glucose-positron emission tomography scanning," *The Journal of Clinical Endocrinology and Metabolism*, vol. 91, no. 2, pp. 498–505, 2006.

[15] D. Deandreis, A. Al Ghuzlan, S. Leboulleux et al., "Do histological, immunohistochemical, and metabolic (radioiodine and fluorodeoxyglucose uptakes) patterns of metastatic thyroid cancer correlate with patient outcome?" *Endocrine-Related Cancer*, vol. 18, no. 1, pp. 159–169, 2011.

[16] J. K. Chung, Y. So, J. S. Lee et al., "Value of FDG PET in papillary thyroid carcinoma with negative 131I whole-body scan," *Journal of Nuclear Medicine*, vol. 40, no. 6, pp. 986–992, 1999.

[17] N. S. Alnafisi, A. A. Driedger, G. Coates, D. J. Moote, and S. J. Raphael, "FDG PET of recurrent or metastatic 131I-negative papillary thyroid carcinoma," *Journal of Nuclear Medicine*, vol. 41, no. 6, pp. 1010–1015, 2000.

[18] W. Wang, S. M. Larson, M. Fazzari et al., "Prognostic value of [18F]fluorodeoxyglucose positron emission tomographic scanning in patients with thyroid cancer," *The Journal of Clinical Endocrinology and Metabolism*, vol. 85, no. 3, pp. 1107–1113, 2000.

[19] W. Wang, S. M. Larson, R. M. Tuttle et al., "Resistance of [18F]-fluorodeoxyglucose—avid metastatic thyroid cancer lesions to treatment with high-dose radioactive iodine," *Thyroid*, vol. 11, no. 12, pp. 1169–1175, 2001.

[20] U. Feine, R. Lietzenmayer, J. P. Hanke, J. Held, H. Wöhrle, and W. Müller-Schauenburg, "Fluorine-18-FDG and iodine-131-iodide uptake in thyroid cancer," *Journal of Nuclear Medicine*, vol. 37, no. 9, pp. 1468–1472, 1996.

[21] W. Wang, H. Macapinlac, S. M. Larson et al., "[18F]-2-fluoro-2-deoxy-D-glucose positron emission tomography localizes residual thyroid cancer in patients with negative diagnostic 131I whole body scans and elevated serum thyroglobulin levels," *The Journal of Clinical Endocrinology and Metabolism*, vol. 84, no. 7, pp. 2291–2302, 1999.

[22] A. D. Van Bruel, A. Maes, T. De Potter et al., "Clinical relevance of thyroid fluorodeoxyglucose-whole body positron emission tomography incidentaloma," *The Journal of Clinical Endocrinology and Metabolism*, vol. 87, no. 4, pp. 1517–1520, 2002.

[23] A. Shammas, B. Degirmenci, J. M. Mountz et al., "18F-FDG PET/CT in patients with suspected recurrent or metastatic well-differentiated thyroid cancer," *Journal of Nuclear Medicine*, vol. 48, no. 2, pp. 221–226, 2007.

[24] T. Petrich, A. R. Börner, D. Otto, M. Hofmann, and W. H. Knapp, "Influence of rhTSH on [18F]fluorodeoxyglucose uptake by differentiated thyroid carcinoma," *European Journal of Nuclear Medicine*, vol. 29, no. 5, pp. 641–647, 2002.

[25] F. Moog, R. Linke, N. Manthey et al., "Influence of thyroid-stimulating hormone levels on uptake of FDG in recurrent and metastatic differentiated thyroid carcinoma," *Journal of Nuclear Medicine*, vol. 41, no. 12, pp. 1989–1995, 2000.

[26] B. B. Chin, P. Patel, C. Cohade, M. Ewertz, R. Wahl, and P. Ladenson, "Recombinant human thyrotropin stimulation of fluoro-D-glucose positron emission tomography uptake in well-differentiated thyroid carcinoma," *The Journal of Clinical Endocrinology and Metabolism*, vol. 89, no. 1, pp. 91–95, 2004.

[27] S. Leboulleux, P. R. Schroeder, N. L. Busaidy et al., "Assessment of the incremental value of recombinant thyrotropin stimulation before 2-[18F]-fluoro-2—deoxy-D-glucose positron emission tomography/computed tomography imaging to localize residual differentiated thyroid cancer," *The Journal of Clinical Endocrinology and Metabolism*, vol. 94, no. 4, pp. 1310–1316, 2009.

[28] B. Schluter, K. H. Bohuslavizki, W. Beyer, M. Plotkin, R. Buchert, and M. Clausen, "Impact of FDG PET on patients with differentiated thyroid cancer who present with elevated thyroglobulin and negative 131I scan," *Journal of Nuclear Medicine*, vol. 42, pp. 71–76, 2011.

[29] B. O. Helal, P. Merlet, M. E. Toubert et al., "Clinical impact of 18F-FDG PET in thyroid carcinoma patients with elevated thyroglobulin levels and negative 131I scanning results after therapy," *Journal of Nuclear Medicine*, vol. 42, no. 10, pp. 1464–1469, 2001.

[30] L. A. Zimmer, B. McCook, C. Meltzer et al., "Combined positron emission tomography/computed tomography imaging of recurrent thyroid cancer," *Otolaryngology—Head and Neck Surgery*, vol. 128, no. 2, pp. 178–184, 2003.

[31] W. J. Simpson, T. Panzarella, J. S. Carruthers, M. K. Gospodarowicz, and S. B. Sutcliffe, "Papillary and follicular thyroid cancer: impact of treatment in 1578 patients," *International Journal of Radiation Oncology Biology Physics*, vol. 14, no. 6, pp. 1063–1075, 1988.

[32] N. A. Samaan, P. N. Schultz, T. P. Haynie, and N. G. Ordonez, "Pulmonary metastasis of differentiated thyroid carcinoma: treatment results in 101 patients," *The Journal of Clinical Endocrinology and Metabolism*, vol. 60, no. 2, pp. 376–380, 1985.

[33] J. J. Ruegemer, I. D. Hay, E. J. Bergstralh, J. J. Ryan, K. P. Offord, and C. A. Gorman, "Distant metastases in differentiated thyroid carcinoma: a multivariate analysis of prognostic variables," *The Journal of Clinical Endocrinology and Metabolism*, vol. 67, no. 3, pp. 501–508, 1988.

[34] M. Schlumberger, C. Challeton, F. de Vathaire et al., "Radioactive iodine treatment and external radiotherapy for lung and bone metastases from thyroid carcinoma," *Journal of Nuclear Medicine*, vol. 37, no. 4–6, pp. 598–605, 1996.

[35] E. L. Mazzaferri and R. T. Kloos, "Current approaches to primary therapy for papillary and follicular thyroid cancer," *The Journal of Clinical Endocrinology and Metabolism*, vol. 86, no. 4, pp. 1447–1463, 2001.

[36] R. T. Kloos and E. L. Mazzaferri, "A single recombinant human thyrotropin-stimulated serum thyroglobulin measurement predicts differentiated thyroid carcinoma metastases three to five years later," *The Journal of Clinical Endocrinology and Metabolism*, vol. 90, no. 9, pp. 5047–5057, 2005.

[37] A. M. Sawka, L. Thabane, L. Parlea et al., "Second primary malignancy risk after radioactive iodine treatment for thyroid cancer: a systematic review and meta-analysis," *Thyroid*, vol. 19, no. 5, pp. 451–457, 2009.

[38] T. R. Shepler, S. I. Sherman, M. M. Faustina, N. L. Busaidy, M. A. Ahmadi, and B. Esmaeli, "Nasolacrimal duct obstruction associated with radioactive iodine therapy for thyroid carcinoma," *Ophthalmic Plastic and Reconstructive Surgery*, vol. 19, no. 6, pp. 479–481, 2003.

[39] R. T. Kloos, V. Duvuuri, S. M. Jhiang, K. V. Cahill, J. A. Foster, and J. A. Burns, "Comment: nasolacrimal drainage system obstruction from radioactive iodine therapy for thyroid carcinoma," *The Journal of Clinical Endocrinology and Metabolism*, vol. 87, no. 12, pp. 5817–5820, 2002.

[40] R. Vassilopoulou-Sellin, L. Palmer, S. Taylor, and C. S. Cooksley, "Incidence of breast carcinoma in women with thyroid carcinoma," *Cancer*, vol. 85, no. 3, pp. 696–705, 1999.

[41] A. Y. Chen, L. Levy, H. Goepfert, B. W. Brown, M. R. Spitz, and R. Vassilopoulou-Sellin, "The development of breast carcinoma in women with thyroid carcinoma," *Cancer*, vol. 92, no. 2, pp. 225–231, 2001.

[42] F. de Vathaire, M. Schlumberger, M. J. Delisle et al., "Leukaemias and cancers following iodine-131 administration for thyroid cancer," *British Journal of Cancer*, vol. 75, no. 5, pp. 734–739, 1997.

[43] B. D. Lewis, I. D. Hay, J. W. Charboneau, B. McIver, C. C. Reading, and J. R. Goellner, "Percutaneous ethanol injection for treatment of cervical lymph node metastases in patients with papillary thyroid carcinoma," *American Journal of Roentgenology*, vol. 178, no. 3, pp. 699–704, 2002.

[44] S. Uchino, S. Noguchi, H. Yamashita, and S. Watanabe, "Modified radical neck dissection for differentiated thyroid cancer: operative technique," *World Journal of Surgery*, vol. 28, no. 12, pp. 1199–1203, 2004.

[45] N. Avenia, M. Ragusa, M. Monacelli et al., "Locally advanced thyroid cancer: therapeutic options," *Chirurgia Italiana*, vol. 56, no. 4, pp. 501–508, 2004.

[46] J. C. McCaffrey, "Evaluation and treatment of aerodigestive tract invasion by well- differentiated thyroid carcinoma," *Cancer Control*, vol. 7, no. 3, pp. 246–252, 2000.

[47] J. M. Czaja and T. V. McCaffrey, "The surgical management of laryngotracheal invasion by well- differentiated papillary thyroid carcinoma," *Archives of Otolaryngology—Head and Neck Surgery*, vol. 123, no. 5, pp. 484–490, 1997.

[48] T. J. Musholt, P. B. Musholt, M. Behrend, R. Raab, G. F. W. Scheumann, and J. Klempnauer, "Invasive differentiated thyroid carcinoma: tracheal resection and reconstruction procedures in the hands of the endocrine surgeon," *Surgery*, vol. 126, no. 6, pp. 1078–1088, 1999.

[49] R. W. Tsang, J. D. Brierley, W. J. Simpson, T. Panzarella, M. K. Gospodarowicz, and S. B. Sutcliffe, "The effects of surgery, radioiodine, and external radiation therapy on the clinical outcome of patients with differentiated thyroid carcinoma," *Cancer*, vol. 82, no. 2, pp. 375–388, 1998.

[50] J. Farahati, C. Reiners, M. Stuschke et al., "Differentiated thyroid cancer: impact of adjuvant external radiotherapy in patients with perithyroidal tumor infiltration (stage pT4)," *Cancer*, vol. 77, no. 1, pp. 172–180, 1996.

[51] D. L. Schwartz, M. J. Lobo, K. K. Ang et al., "Postoperative external beam radiotherapy for differentiated thyroid cancer: outcomes and morbidity with conformal treatment," *International Journal of Radiation Oncology Biology Physics*, vol. 74, no. 4, pp. 1083–1091, 2009.

[52] B. D. Rosenbluth, V. Serrano, L. Happersett et al., "Intensity-modulated radiation therapy for the treatment of nonanaplastic thyroid cancer," *International Journal of Radiation Oncology Biology Physics*, vol. 63, no. 5, pp. 1419–1426, 2005.

[53] A. C. Chiu, E. S. Delpassand, and S. I. Sherman, "Prognosis and treatment of brain metastases in thyroid carcinoma," *The Journal of Clinical Endocrinology and Metabolism*, vol. 82, no. 11, pp. 3637–3642, 1997.

[54] S. I. Sherman, R. M. Tuttle, R. T. Kloos et al., "Thyroid carcinoma: practice guidelines in oncology," *Journal of the National Comprehensive Cancer Network*, vol. 1, 2009.

[55] R. R. McWilliams, C. Giannini, I. D. Hay, J. L. Atkinson, S. L. Stafford, and J. C. Buckner, "Management of brain metastases from thyroid carcinoma: a study of 16 pathologically confirmed cases over 25 years," *Cancer*, vol. 98, no. 2, pp. 356–362, 2003.

[56] I. Y. Kim, D. Kondziolka, A. Niranjan, J. C. Flickinger, and L. D. Lunsford, "Gamma knife radiosurgery for metastatic brain tumors from thyroid cancer," *Journal of Neuro-Oncology*, vol. 93, no. 3, pp. 355–359, 2009.

[57] M. Luster, F. Lippi, B. Jarzab et al., "rhTSH-aided radioiodine ablation and treatment of differentiated thyroid carcinoma: a comprehensive review," *Endocrine-Related Cancer*, vol. 12, no. 1, pp. 49–64, 2005.

[58] C. F. A. Eustatia-Rutten, J. A. Romijn, M. J. Guijt et al., "Outcome of palliative embolization of bone metastases in differentiated thyroid carcinoma," *The Journal of Clinical Endocrinology and Metabolism*, vol. 88, no. 7, pp. 3184–3189, 2003.

[59] Z.-L. Qiu, H.-J. Song, Y.-H. Xu, and Q.-Y. Luo, "Efficacy and survival analysis of 131I therapy for bone metastases from differentiated thyroid cancer," *The Journal of Clinical Endocrinology and Metabolism*, vol. 96, no. 10, pp. 3078–3086, 2011.

[60] Y. Orita, I. Sugitani, K. Toda, J. Manabe, and Y. Fujimoto, "Zoledronic acid in the treatment of bone metastases from differentiated thyroid carcinoma," *Thyroid*, vol. 21, no. 1, pp. 31–35, 2011.

[61] G. Ronga, M. Filesi, T. Montesano et al., "Lung metastases from differentiated thyroid carcinoma. A 40 years' experience," *Quarterly Journal of Nuclear Medicine and Molecular Imaging*, vol. 48, no. 1, pp. 12–19, 2004.

[62] V. Fatourechi, I. D. Hay, H. Javedan, G. A. Wiseman, B. P. Mullan, and C. A. Gorman, "Lack of impact of radioiodine therapy in tg-positive, diagnostic whole-body scan-negative patients with follicular cell-derived thyroid cancer," *The Journal of Clinical Endocrinology and Metabolism*, vol. 87, no. 4, pp. 1521–1526, 2002.

[63] J. D. Pineda, T. Lee, K. Ain, J. C. Reynolds, and J. Robbins, "Iodine-131 therapy for thyroid cancer patients with elevated thyroglobulin and negative diagnostic scan," *The Journal of Clinical Endocrinology and Metabolism*, vol. 80, no. 5, pp. 1488–1492, 1995.

[64] F. Pacini, L. Agate, R. Elisei et al., "Outcome of differentiated thyroid cancer with detectable serum Tg and negative diagnostic 131I whole body scan: comparison of patients treated with high 131I activities versus untreated patients," *The Journal of Clinical Endocrinology and Metabolism*, vol. 86, no. 9, pp. 4092–4097, 2001.

[65] R. M. Tuttle, D. W. Ball, D. Byrd et al., "Thyroid carcinoma," *JNCCN*, vol. 8, no. 11, pp. 1228–1274, 2010.

[66] J. P. Droz, M. Schlumberger, P. Rougier, M. Ghosn, P. Gardet, and C. Parmentier, "Chemotherapy in metastatic nonanaplastic thyroid cancer: experience at the Institut Gustave-Roussy," *Tumori*, vol. 76, no. 5, pp. 480–483, 1990.

[67] S. Ahuja and H. Ernst, "Chemotherapy of thyroid carcinoma," *Journal of Endocrinological Investigation*, vol. 10, no. 3, pp. 303–310, 1987.

[68] F. Santini, V. Bottici, R. Elisei et al., "Cytotoxic effects of carboplatinum and epirubicin in the setting of an elevated serum thyrotropin for advanced poorly differentiated thyroid cancer," *The Journal of Clinical Endocrinology and Metabolism*, vol. 87, no. 9, pp. 4160–4165, 2002.

[69] B. R. Haugen, "Management of the patient with progressive radioiodine non-responsive disease," *Seminars in Surgical Oncology*, vol. 16, no. 1, pp. 34–41, 1999.

[70] J. A. Gottlieb and C. S. Hill Jr., "Chemotherapy of thyroid cancer with adriamycin. Experience with 30 patients," *The*

New England Journal of Medicine, vol. 290, no. 4, pp. 193–197, 1974.

[71] J. A. Gottlieb, C. S. Hill Jr., M. L. Ibanez, and R. L. Clark, "Chemotherapy of thyroid cancer. An evaluation of experience with 37 patients," *Cancer*, vol. 30, no. 3, pp. 848–853, 1972.

[72] K. B. Ain, M. J. Egorin, and P. A. DeSimone, "Treatment of anaplastic thyroid carcinoma with paclitaxel: phase 2 trial using ninety-six-hour infusion," *Thyroid*, vol. 10, no. 7, pp. 587–594, 2000.

[73] J. A. Fagin, "How thyroid tumors start and why it matters: kinase mutants as targets for solid cancer pharmacotherapy," *The Journal of Endocrinology*, vol. 183, no. 2, pp. 249–256, 2004.

[74] S. M. Jhiang, "The RET proto-oncogene in human cancers," *Oncogene*, vol. 19, no. 49, pp. 5590–5597, 2000.

[75] S. M. Jhiang, J. E. Sagartz, Q. Tong et al., "Targeted expression of the ret/PTC1 oncogene induces papillary thyroid carcinomas," *Endocrinology*, vol. 137, no. 1, pp. 375–378, 1996.

[76] C. Zafon, G. Obiols, J. Castellví et al., "Clinical significance of RET/PTC and p53 protein expression in sporadic papillary thyroid carcinoma," *Histopathology*, vol. 50, no. 2, pp. 225–231, 2007.

[77] C. Ugolini, R. Giannini, C. Lupi et al., "Presence of BRAF V600E in very early stages of papillary thyroid carcinoma," *Thyroid*, vol. 17, no. 5, pp. 381–388, 2007.

[78] T. Y. Kim, W. B. Kim, Y. S. Rhee et al., "The BRAF mutation is useful for prediction of clinical recurrence in low-risk patients with conventional papillary thyroid carcinoma," *Clinical Endocrinology*, vol. 65, no. 3, pp. 364–368, 2006.

[79] M. Xing, W. H. Westra, R. P. Tufano et al., "BRAF mutation predicts a poorer clinical prognosis for papillary thyroid cancer," *The Journal of Clinical Endocrinology and Metabolism*, vol. 90, no. 12, pp. 6373–6379, 2005.

[80] J. Fagin, "Molecular pathogenesis of tumors of thyroid follicular cells," in *Thyroid Cancer*, J. Fagin, Ed., Kluwer Academic, Boston, Mass, USA, 1998.

[81] G. Garcia-Rostan, H. Zhao, R. L. Camp et al., "ras Mutations are associated with aggressive tumor phenotypes and poor prognosis in thyroid cancer," *Journal of Clinical Oncology*, vol. 21, no. 17, pp. 3226–3235, 2003.

[82] P. Carmeliet, "Mechanisms of angiogenesis and arteriogenesis," *Nature Medicine*, vol. 6, no. 4, pp. 389–395, 2000.

[83] A. D. Laird and J. M. Cherrington, "Small molecule tyrosine kinase inhibitors: clinical development of anticancer agents," *Expert Opinion on Investigational Drugs*, vol. 12, no. 1, pp. 51–64, 2003.

[84] C. M. Lennard, A. Patel, J. Wilson et al., "Intensity of vascular endothelial growth factor expression is associated with increased risk of recurrence and decreased disease-free survival in papillary thyroid cancer," *Surgery*, vol. 129, no. 5, pp. 552–558, 2001.

[85] M. Klein, J. M. Vignaud, V. Hennequin et al., "Increased expression of the vascular endothelial growth factor is a pejorative prognosis marker in papillary thyroid carcinoma," *The Journal of Clinical Endocrinology and Metabolism*, vol. 86, no. 2, pp. 656–658, 2001.

[86] R. T. Kloos, M. D. Ringel, M. V. Knopp et al., "Phase II trial of sorafenib in metastatic thyroid cancer," *Journal of Clinical Oncology*, vol. 27, no. 10, pp. 1675–1684, 2009.

[87] V. Gupta-Abramson, A. B. Troxel, A. Nellore et al., "Phase II trial of sorafenib in advanced thyroid cancer," *Journal of Clinical Oncology*, vol. 26, no. 29, pp. 4714–4719, 2008.

[88] M. E. Cabanillas, S. G. Waguespack, Y. Bronstein et al., "Treatment with tyrosine kinase inhibitors for patients with differentiated thyroid cancer: the M. D. Anderson experience," *The Journal of Clinical Endocrinology and Metabolism*, vol. 95, no. 6, pp. 2588–2595, 2010.

[89] W. K. Dong, S. J. Young, S. J. Hye et al., "An orally administered multitarget tyrosine kinase inhibitor, SU11248, is a novel potent inhibitor of thyroid oncogenic RET/papillary thyroid cancer kinases," *The Journal of Clinical Endocrinology and Metabolism*, vol. 91, no. 10, pp. 4070–4076, 2006.

[90] S. J. Dawson, N. M. Conus, G. C. Toner et al., "Sustained clinical responses to tyrosine kinase inhibitor sunitinib in thyroid carcinoma," *Anti-Cancer Drugs*, vol. 19, no. 5, pp. 547–552, 2008.

[91] E. E. Cohen, B. M. Needles, K. J. Cullen et al., "Phase 2 study of sunitinib in refractory thyroid cancer," *Journal of Clinical Oncology*, vol. 26, article 6025, 2008.

[92] A. Ravaud, C. Fouchardiere, F. Courbon et al., "Sunitinib in patients with refractory advanced thyroid cancer: the THYSU phase II trial," *Journal of Clinical Oncology*, vol. 26, article 6025, 2008.

[93] L. L. Carr, D. A. Mankoff, B. H. Goulart et al., "Phase II study of daily sunitinib in FDG-PET-positive, iodine-refractory differentiated thyroid cancer and metastatic medullary carcinoma of the thyroid with functional imaging correlation," *Clinical Cancer Research*, vol. 16, no. 21, pp. 5260–5268, 2010.

[94] K. C. Bible, R. C. Smallridge, W. J. Maples et al., "Phase II trial of pazopanib in progressive, metastatic, iodine-insensitive differentiated thyroid cancers," *Journal of Clinical Oncology*, vol. 27, article 3521, 2009.

[95] A. Polverino, A. Coxon, C. Starnes et al., "AMG 706, an oral, multikinase inhibitor that selectively targets vascular endothelial growth factor, platelet-derived growth factor, and kit receptors, potently inhibits angiogenesis and induces regression in tumor xenografts," *Cancer Research*, vol. 66, no. 17, pp. 8715–8721, 2006.

[96] L. S. Rosen, R. Kurzrock, M. Mulay et al., "Safety, pharmacokinetics, and efficacy of AMG 706, an oral multikinase inhibitor, in patients with advanced solid tumors," *Journal of Clinical Oncology*, vol. 25, no. 17, pp. 2369–2376, 2007.

[97] S. I. Sherman, L. J. Wirth, J. P. Droz et al., "Motesanib diphosphate in progressive differentiated thyroid cancer," *The New England Journal of Medicine*, vol. 359, no. 1, pp. 31–42, 2008.

[98] H. S. Rugo, R. S. Herbst, G. Liu et al., "Phase I trial of the oral antiangiogenesis agent AG-013736 in patients with advanced solid tumors: pharmacokinetic and clinical results," *Journal of Clinical Oncology*, vol. 23, no. 24, pp. 5474–5483, 2005.

[99] E. E. W. Cohen, L. S. Rosen, E. E. Vokes et al., "Axitinib is an active treatment for all histologic subtypes of advanced thyroid cancer: results from a phase II study," *Journal of Clinical Oncology*, vol. 26, no. 29, pp. 4708–4713, 2008.

[100] N. A. Pennell, G. H. Daniels, R. I. Haddad et al., "A phase II study of gefitinib in patients with advanced thyroid cancer," *Thyroid*, vol. 18, no. 3, pp. 317–323, 2008.

[101] M. E. Cabanillas, M. S. Brose, D. A. Ramies, Y. Lee, D. Miles, and S. I. Sherman, "Anti-tumor activity observed in a cohort of patients with differentiated thyroid cancer in a phase 1 study of cabozantinib (XL184)," in *Proceedings of the 81st Annual Meeting of the American Thyroid Association*, abstract 0179, 2011.

[102] R. Mineo, A. Costantino, F. Frasca et al., "Activation of the Hepatocyte Growth Factor (HGF)-Met system in papillary thyroid cancer: biological effects of HGF in thyroid cancer

cells depend on Met expression levels," *Endocrinology*, vol. 145, no. 9, pp. 4355–4365, 2004.

[103] V. M. Wasenius, S. Hemmer, M. L. Karjalainen-Lindsberg, N. N. Nupponen, K. Franssila, and H. Joensuu, "MET receptor tyrosine kinase sequence alterations in differentiated thyroid carcinoma," *The American Journal of Surgical Pathology*, vol. 29, no. 4, pp. 544–549, 2005.

[104] R. Kurzrock, S. I. Sherman, D. S. Hong et al., "A Phase I study of XL184, a MET, VEGFR2, a RET kinase inhibitor orally administered to patients with advanced malignancies: including a subgroup of patients with medullary thyroid cancer (MTC)," in *Proceedings of the 20th EORTC-NCI-AACR Symposium on Molecular Targets and Cancer Therapeutics*, Geneva, Switzerland, 2008, abstract no. 379.

[105] S. Sherman, B. Jarzab, M. E. Cabanillas et al., "A phase II trial of the multitargeted kinase inhibitor E7080 in advanced radioiodine (RAI)-refractory differentiated thyroid cancer (DTC)," *Journal of Clinical Oncology*, vol. 29, 2011.

[106] G. K. Schwartz, S. Robertson, A. Shen et al., "A Phase i study of XL281, a potent and selective inhibitor of RAF kinases, administered orally to patients with advanced solid tumors," in *Proceedings of the 20th EORTC-NCI-AACR Symposium on Molecular Targets and Cancer Therapeutics*, Geneva, Switzerland, 2008, Abstract no. 383.

[107] K. T. Flaherty, I. Puzanov, K. B. Kim et al., "Inhibition of mutated, activated BRAF in metastatic melanoma," *The New England Journal of Medicine*, vol. 363, no. 9, pp. 809–819, 2010.

[108] K. B. Ain, C. Lee, and K. D. Williams, "Phase II trial of thalidomide for therapy of radioiodine-unresponsive and rapidly progressive thyroid carcinomas," *Thyroid*, vol. 17, no. 7, pp. 663–670, 2007.

[109] K. Ain, C. Lee, K. Holbrook, J. Dziba, and K. Williams, "Phase II study of lenalidomide in distantly metastatic, rapidly progressive, and radioiodine-unresponsive thyroid carcinomas: preliminary results," *Journal of Clinical Oncology*, vol. 26, 2008.

[110] A. J. Van Herle, M. L. Agatep, D. N. Padua et al., "Effects of 13 cis-retinoic acid on growth and differentiation of human follicular carcinoma cells (UCLA RO 82 W-1) in vitro," *The Journal of Clinical Endocrinology and Metabolism*, vol. 71, no. 3, pp. 755–763, 1990.

[111] Y. Y. Liu, M. P. Stokkel, A. M. Pereira et al., "Bexarotene increases uptake of radioiodide in metastases of differentiated thyroid carcinoma," *European Journal of Endocrinology*, vol. 154, no. 4, pp. 525–531, 2006.

[112] E. Kebebew, M. Peng, E. Reiff et al., "A phase II trial of rosiglitazone in patients with thyroglobulin-positive and radioiodine-negative differentiated thyroid cancer," *Surgery*, vol. 140, no. 6, pp. 960–967, 2006.

[113] Y. Su, R. Tuttle, M. Fury et al., "A phase II study of single agent depsipeptide (DEP) in patients (pts) wiht radioactive iodine (RAI)-refractory, metastatic, thyroid carcinoma: preliminary toxicity and efficacy experience," *Journal of Clinical Oncology*, vol. 24, 2006.

[114] L. Ho, R. K. Grewal, R. Leboeuf et al., "Reacquision of RAI uptake in RAI-refractory, metastatic thyroid cancers by pretreatment with the selective MEK inhibitor, selumetinib," in *Proceedings of the 81st Annual Meeting of the American Thyroid Association*, 2011.

[115] M. E. Cabanillas, M. I. Hu, J. B. Durand, and N. L. Busaidy, "Challenges associated with tyrosine kinase inhibitor therapy for metastatic thyroid cancer," *Journal of Thyroid Research*, vol. 2011, Article ID 985780, 9 pages, 2011.

19

Lymph Node Thyroglobulin Measurement in Diagnosis of Neck Metastases of Differentiated Thyroid Carcinoma

Luca Giovanella,[1,2] Luca Ceriani,[1] and Sergio Suriano[1]

[1] Department of Nuclear Medicine and Thyroid Unit, Oncology Institute of Southern Switzerland, Street Ospedale 12,
6500 Bellinzona, Switzerland
[2] Department of Clinical Chemistry and Laboratory Medicine, Ente Ospedaliero Cantonale, 6500 Bellinzona, Switzerland

Correspondence should be addressed to Luca Giovanella, luca.giovanella@eoc.ch

Academic Editor: Electron Kebebew

Aim. Enlarged cervical lymph nodes (LNs) in patients with thyroid cancer are usually assessed by fine-needle aspiration cytology (FNAC). Thyroglobulin (Tg) is frequently elevated in malignant FNAC needle wash specimens (FNAC-Tg). The objectives of the study were to (1) determine an appropriate diagnostic cut-off for FNAC-Tg levels (2) compare FNAC and FNAC-Tg results in a group of 108 patients affected by differentiated thyroid carcinoma (DTC). *Methods.* A total of 126 consecutive FNACs were performed on enlarged LNs and the final diagnosis was confirmed by surgical pathology examination or clinical follow-up. The best FNAC-Tg cut-off level was selected by receiver operating curve analysis, and diagnostic performances of FNAC and FNAC-Tg were compared. *Results.* The rate of FNAC samples adequate for cytological examination was 77% in contrast FNAC-Tg available in 100% of aspirates ($P < .01$). The sensitivity, specificity, and accuracy of FNAC were 71%, 80%, 74%, 100%, 80%, and 94%, respectively. The most appropriate cut-off value for the diagnosis of thyroid cancer metastatic LN was 1.1 ng/mL (sensitivity 100%, specificity 100%). *Conclusions.* The diagnostic performance of needle washout FNAC-Tg measurement with a cut-off of 1.1 ng/mL compared favorably with cytology in detecting DTC node metastases.

1. Introduction

The prognosis of patients who receive appropriate treatment for thyroid carcinoma is usually favourable, especially for differentiated thyroid carcinoma (DTC). However, although most patients have a long-term survival rate, 5% to 20% of patients will develop recurrence during the followup, primarily in the cervical lymph nodes (LNs) [1, 2]. These LNs metastases may be detected clinically, but now are most often discovered on ultrasonography (US) [3]. It is of great importance to differentiate accurately LN metastases from benign reactive lymph nodes in order to avoid unnecessary treatment, but also to treat metastatic patients without delay. As consequence, diagnostic procedures must offer good sensitivity, but also high negative predictive value. US criteria distinguishing benign from metastatic or suspicious LNs have been described but they lack accuracy [4]. US-guided fine needle cytology (FNAC) proved to be a reliable method in examining the neck in patients who were previously treated for thyroid cancer [5, 6]. However, sensitivity of FNAC is far from excellent, varying from 75% to 85%, and altered by high rate of nondiagnostic or false-negative samples. To improve the diagnostic yield of FNAC, several authors have proposed measurement of Tg in aspirates (FNAC-Tg), particularly in the cases involving small, partially cystic, lymph nodes [7–12]. On the basis of prior studies, an increased Tg level in the needle washout has been shown to directly reflect the status of metastatic lymph nodes in patients affected by differentiated thyroid carcinoma. However, controversies still persist concerning some issues. First, there are few studies to validate the benefit of FNAC-Tg over FNAC alone, and, second, cut-off values ranging from 0.9 to 39 ng/mL have been suggested for FNAC-Tg, depending on the method used for the measurement [7, 13–15]. As consequence, the exact place for FNAC-Tg in the management of DTC patients is still debated.

This study was then undertaken to (1) determine a diagnostic cut-off value for washout Tg in patients treated by total thyroidectomy for detecting recurrences, and (2) to compare the performance of the Tg cut-off value to US-guided FNAC for detecting DTC recurrences.

2. Materials and Methods

Our institutional review board approved our research study, and all subjects gave written informed consent.

2.1. Patients. Between January 2006 and February 2009 a total of 126 consecutive US-guided FNACs were performed on enlarged LNs. The samples were obtained from 108 patients (19 males, 89 females; age 42.7 ± 18.2 years; 91 patients with 1, 94 with 2, and 5 with 3 lesions, resp.). All patients had histologically confirmed primary DTC (papillary, $n = 99$, including two tall-cell variants; follicular, $n = 9$, including 2 Hürtle cells carcinomas). The primitive carcinoma was classified pT1 in 34 cases, pT2 in 43 cases, pT3 in 24 cases, and pT4 in 7 cases. Forty-five patients (42%) had LN metastases at diagnosis. All patients underwent (near) total thyroidectomy and subsequent radioiodine ablation (administered activity from 1.85 to 3.70 GBq). The US criteria for possible malignant infiltration of lymph nodes were rounded contour, irregular internal echogenicity, punctate calcifications, fluids components, and abnormal colour Doppler pattern. Patients with positive cytology and/or FNAC-Tg measurement ($n = 86$, 96 lesions) underwent surgery and, if necessary, further radioiodine treatments. The diagnosis was confirmed in all cases by surgical pathology examination. Patients with negative FNAC-Tg measurement and cytology ($n = 22$, 30 lesions) underwent further follow up by serial clinical examinations, serum Tg measurements, neck US, and, whenever necessary, additional imaging procedures (i.e., radioiodine scan, [18]FDG-PET/CT). No DTC recurrence was detected among these patients (follow up: mean 36 months, range 15–42 months).

2.2. US-Guided FNAC Procedure. All US-guided FNAC procedures were performed on supine patients with the neck hyperextended under continuous real-time US guidance with a high-resolution transducer (ACUSON ×150, Siemens, Erlangen, Germany). Each lesion was aspirated at least twice by a 21 G needle. The needle was inserted obliquely within the transducer plane of view, and moved back and forth through the nodule to compensate for patient movement and needle deflection. Gradual aspiration was applied by a 20 mL syringe connected to Cameco's device. Contents of needles were expelled onto glass slides and smeared with a second slide to spread fluid across the surface. Slides were fixed in 95% ethanol, papanicolaou stained to identify cellular details, and read by our cytopathologist. Following collection of cytology samples the needles were washed by 1 mL of normal saline in a plain serum tube (Vacutainer Systems, Plymouth, UK) and the washout directly sent to the laboratory [16]. Cytological examinations were performed by experienced cytopathologists and expressed as (1) positive: presence of epithelial cells with atypical

cytological characteristics, or with cytological features of papillary carcinoma; (2) negative: reactive lymphadenitis and absence of malignant cells; (3) inadequate or nondiagnostic: absence of cells or presence of blood cells.

2.3. Tg Measurement. Thyroglobulin was measured in fine-needle washouts using an immunoradiometric assay (IRMA) based on coated tubes with monoclonal antibodies directed against distinct epitopes of the molecule of Tg (DYNO test Tg-plus, BRAHMS Diagnostic GmbH, Berlin, Germany). With this measurement, analytic sensitivity, defined as the detectable minimum concentration different from zero (mean value + 2 standard deviation), and functional sensitivity, defined as the lowest value that was measured with the precision of a maximum 20% interassay variance, were 0.08 ng/mL and 0.2 ng/mL, respectively. We did not measure Tg antibodies (FNAC-TgAb) because the clinical performance of FNAC-Tg is unaffected by serum TgAb [17].

2.4. Data Analysis. Diagnostic performance (i.e., sensitivity, specificity, positive predictive value, negative predictive value, and accuracy) of FNAC and FNAC-Tg was evaluated by comparing the results of the two procedures to the status of the patients defined as follows: malignant lymph node from thyroid cancer was proved by histological examination of surgically resected LNs; benign lymph node was proved by negative histological examination of surgically respected LNs, or if disappearance or absence of evolution on imaging modalities was demonstrated at 12 months or more follow up.

The Chi-square (χ^2) test, performed with SAS version 9.1 for Windows (SAS Institute, Cary, NC, US) was employed to compare the diagnostic rate of FNAC and FNAC-Tg. The FNAC-Tg receiver operating characteristic curve was developed using MedCalc 6.1 software (MedCalc Software, Mariakerke, Belgium). The cut-off values which maximise the sum of sensitivity plus specificity were determined as the points in the upper left hand corner. A P value $< .05$ was considered to indicate statistical significance.

3. Results

Patients characteristics and cytological, pathological, and biochemical data are displayed in Table 1. Of the 126 lymph node lesions assessed for postoperative recurrences by US-guided FNAC and FNAC-Tg, 86 (68%) lesions were finally diagnosed as malignant and the remaining 40 (32%) lesions were diagnosed as benign LNs, respectively. The final diagnosis of the 86 malignant and 8 benign LN was established by surgical pathology; the remaining 32 benign lesions were diagnosed based on imaging follow up after at least 1 year. The time from thyroid ablation to US-FNAC was 19.5 ± 14.31 and 19.4 ± 13.76 months in patients with benign and malignant lesions, respectively (P not significant). Serum Tg levels were higher in patients with malignant lesions (median 4.20 ng/mL, range <0.2–27.10 ng/mL) than those with benign lesions (median .80 ng/mL, range <0.2–2.70 ng/mL; $P < .0001$). Serum TgAb were positive in 11

TABLE 1: Patients characteristics and cytological, pathological, and biochemical data.

| Patients | Histology | pTNM | Duration (months) | Tg (ng/mL) | TgAb (IU/mL) | Lesions | Sites | FNA | | Final diagnosis |
								Cytology	Tg (ng/mL)	
1	PTC	pT1N1Mx	6	1.0	<60	1	R II	ND	<0.2	B
2	PTC	pT1NxMx	15	4.6	<60	1	L III	Negative	435.2	M
3	PTC	pT1NxMx	18	1.7	<60	1	R IV	CTM	85.3	M
4	PTC	pT1NxMx	30	0.4	<60	1	R III	ND	<0.2	B
5	PTC	pT1N0Mx	6	3.1	<60	1	L II	ND	97.2	M
6	PTC	pT2N0Mx	19	9.1	<60	2	R IV, VI	CTM	118.5	M
7	PTC	pT2NxMx	47	<0.2	334	1	L IV	CTM	879.4	M
8	PTC	pT2N1Mx	6	0.9	78	1	VI	Negative	1.1	B
9	PTC	pT1N1Mx	9	9.8	<60	1	L II	ND	1348.6	M
10	PTC	pT2N0Mx	14	1.5	<60	1	L III	CTM	358.5	M
11	PTC	pT1NxMx	8	12.6	<60	3	R II	CTM	2387.4	M
12	PTC	pT2NxMx	16	9.7	<60	1	R III	CTM	875.9	M
13	PTC	pT1NxMx	9	6.3	<60	1	R II	CTM	958.6	M
14	PTC	pT1N0Mx	11	1.0	<60	1	L III	Negative	48.7	M
15	PTC	pT2N1Mx	39	9.5	<60	1	L IV	CTM	>3000	M
16	PTC	pT1NxMx	12	0.8	<60	1	L III	CTM	107.5	M
17	PTC	pT2NxMx	19	2.7	<60	3	R III-IV	ND, CTM	541.6	R III B, IV M
18	PTC	pT4N1Mx	6	1.6	<60	1	L III	CTM	31.8	M
19	PTC	pT1N1Mx	15	0.5	289	1	R IV	ND	<0.2	B
20	PTC	pT2N1Mx	3	2.3	<60	1	L III	ND	540.7	M
21	PTC	pT1NxMx	34	4.1	<60	1	L III	CTM	650.6	M
22	PTC	pT2N1Mx	8	<0.2	98	1	L II	ND	5.8	M
23	PTC	pT1NxMx	9	0.8	<60	2	R II, R III	CTM	87.5	M
24	PTC	pT4N0Mx	10	1.4	755	1	R II	CTM	196.4	M
25	PTC	pT2NxMx	21	11	<60	1	R III	ND	585.3	M
26	PTC	pT1NxMx	9	<0.2	<60	1	R III	Negative	<0.2	B
27	PTC	pT4N1M	12	1.1	160	1	L III	Negative	0.3	B
28	PTC	pT1N0Mx	23	5.3	<60	1	R III	CTM	784.2	M
29	PTC	pT2N1Mx	5	<0.2	>1000	1	R III	ND	<0.2	B
30	PTC	pT2N0Mx	22	4.9	<60	1	R III	CTM	641.5	M
31	PTC	pT1NxMx	36	0.3	367	1	R IV	Negative	<0.2	B
32	PTC	pT1NxMx	15	7.1	<60	1	R III	ND	665.4	M
33	PTC	pT2N0Mx	41	<0.2	<60	1	L II	Negative	<0.2	B
34	PTC	pT1NxMx	24	2.6	<60	1	R III	CTM	570.6	M
35	PTC	pT4N0Mx	31	1.4	>1000	3	L IV, VI	CTM	96.7	M
36	PTC	pT4N1M	12	27.1	<60	1	R II	CTM	2987.3	M
37	PTC	pT1N1Mx	54	6.8	<60	1	L III	CTM	875.6	M
38	PTC	pT2NxMx	12	<0.2	149	1	R IV	Negative	<0.2	B
39	PTC	pT2N0Mx	9	0.9	<60	1	R II	Negative	<0.2	B
40	PTC	pT1N0Mx	34	2.4	89	1	L III	ND	347.4	M
41	PTC	pT2NxMx	14	5.1	<60	1	L IV	ND	1655.7	M
42	PTC	pT4N1M	8	7.7	<60	1	L III	Negative	2076.5	M
43	PTC	pT1NxMx	61	1.1	<60	1	VI	Negative	<0.2	B
44	PTC	pT2N0Mx	22	1.0	<60	1	L II	CTM	90.6	M

TABLE 1: Continued.

Patients	Histology	pTNM	Duration (months)	Tg (ng/mL)	TgAb (IU/mL)	Lesions	Sites	FNA Cytology	FNA Tg (ng/mL)	Final diagnosis
45	PTC	pT2N1Mx	12	6.4	<60	2	R III-IV	CTM, ND	458.6	RIII M, IV B
46	PTC	pT1NxMx	45	0.6	<60	1	R IV	Negative	<0.2	B
47	PTC	pT4N0Mx	36	4.3	<60	1	R III	CTM	766.4	M
48	PTC	pT2NxMx	11	1.9	<60	1	L II	ND	306.5	M
49	PTC	pT3NxMx	18	7.0	<60	1	R III	CTM	955.6	M
50	PTC	pT2NxMx	10	1.2	<60	1	L III	Negative	<0.2	B
51	PTC	pT1N1Mx	12	3.9	<60	1	R III	CTM	564.7	M
52	PTC	pT3N0Mx	25	6.4	190	1	R III	ND	1078.6	M
53	PTC	pT2N1Mx	16	9.5	<60	1	L IV	CTM	759.4	M
54	PTC	pT1NxMx	9	0.6	<60	1	R III	Negative	<0.2	B
55	PTC	pT3N1Mx	60	<0.2	107	2	L II-III	CTM	137.5	M
56	PTC	pT1N0Mx	11	5.3	<60	1	R II	CTM	654.8	M
57	PTC	pT2N1Mx	18	1.1	860	1	L III	ND	<0.2	B
58	PTC	pT1NxMx	9	0.9	<60	1	R IV	Negative	<0.2	B
59	PTC	pT2NxMx	28	1.1	<60	1	R III	ND	99.6	M
60	PTC-TCV	pT3NxMx	13	4.6	<60	1	L II	CTM	436.8	M
61	PTC	pT1NxMx	2	2.7	<60	1	R II	CTM	194.5	M
62	PTC	pT3NxMx	7	21.9	<60	3	R III, L II	Neg., CTM	>3000	RIII B, LII M
63	PTC	pT1NxMx	18	1.1	<60	1	R III	CTM	27.4	M
64	PTC	pT3NxMx	10	3.5	<60	1	VI	CTM	147.4	M
65	PTC	pT2N0Mx	29	<0.2	>1000	1	R IV	Negative	<0.2	B
66	PTC	pT3N1Mx	6	5.6	<60	1	L III	CTM	<0.2	M
67	PTC	pT1N1Mx	11	2.1	<60	1	R III	ND	<0.2	M
68	PTC	pT3N0Mx	18	0.7	<60	1	R III	ND	<0.2	B
69	PTC	pT2N0Mx	23	1.7	<60	1	L IV	CTM	75.6	M
70	PTC	pT1NxMx	9	3.5	<60	1	L II	ND	72.6	M
71	PTC	pT3N0Mx	18	7.1	<60	2	R IV, VI	CTM	386.2	RIV B, VI M
72	PTC	pT1NxMx	7	1.8		1	L II	Negative	<0.2	B
73	PTC	pT2NxMx	11	3.6	<60	1	R III	ND	245.7	M
74	PTC	pT2NxMx	29	2.2	<60	2	L III-IV	CTM	67.4	IV M, III B
75	PTC	pT2N1Mx	14	5.7	<60	1	L II	CTM	198.7	M
76	PTC	pT1N0Mx	8	1.5	<60	1	R IV	CTM	26.1	M
77	PTC	pT2NxMx	10	2.1	<60	1	VI	CTM	59.7	M
78	PTC	pT1NxMx	18	0.7	<60	1	R IV	Negative	<0.2	B
79	PTC	pT3N1Mx	34	12.3	<60	1	R III	ND	678.4	M
80	PTC	pT1N1Mx	16	1.8	<60	1	L II	Negative	<0.2	B
81	PTC	pT2N0Mx	52	0.9	<60	1	R III	Negative	<0.2	B
82	PTC	pT2N1Mx	25	9.4	<60	1	L III	ND	563.6	M
83	PTC	pT1NxMx	9	4.1	<60	1	VI	CTM	64.7	M
84	PTC	pT2N1Mx	18	3.1	<60	1	R IV	CTM	116.4	M
85	PTC-TCV	pT2NxMx	20	15.5	<60	3	R IV-L III	CTM	432.9	M
86	PTC	pT3N0Mx	8	<0.2	56	1	VI	ND	<0.2	B
87	PTC	pT1N0Mx	31	2.9	<60	1	R IV	CTM	39.3	M
88	PTC	pT2NxMx	11	1.7	<60	1	R III	Negative	<0.2	B
89	PTC	pT2NxMx	54	6.5	<60	1	L IV	ND	467.7	M
90	PTC	pT1N1Mx	28	0.3	651	1	R II	Negative	<0.2	B
91	PTC	pT2NxMx	12	2.1	<60	1	L III	CTM	88.6	M

Carcinoma

139

TABLE 1: Continued.

Patients	Histology	pTNM	Duration (months)	Tg (ng/mL)	TgAb (IU/mL)	Lesions	Sites	FNA Cytology	FNA Tg (ng/mL)	Final diagnosis
92	PTC	pT3N0Mx	17	9.4	<60	2	R IV, VI	CTM	156.2	IV M, VI B
93	PTC	pT1NxMx	22	1.0	<60	1	L IV	Negative	<0.2	B
94	PTC	pT2N1Mx	9	4.3	<60	1	VI	Negative	53.8	M
95	PTC	pT2N0Mx	26	<0.2	<60	1	R IV	Negative	<0.2	B
96	PTC	pT1N0Mx	12	0.9	<60	1	R III	ND	2.7	M
97	PTC	pT2NxMx	17	8.1	<60	1	L II	ND	356.4	M
98	PTC	pT2NxMx	9	0.9	<60	1	R III	CTM	19.6	M
99	PTC	pT3N1Mx	12	1.1	<60	1	L III	ND	0.6	B
100	FTC	pT1N1Mx	45	4.9	<60	1	R III	CTM	117.5	M
101	FTC	pT3N0Mx	36	1.4	<60	1	R III	Negative	<0.2	B
102	FTC	pT2N1Mx	11	<0.2	>1000	2	R III-IV	Negative	<0.2	B
103	FTC (HC)	pT1NxMx	72	10.4	<60	1	R IV	ND	278.9	M
104	FTC	pT2N1Mx	11	0.7	<60	1	R III	Negative	<0.2	B
105	FTC	pT1N0Mx	18	2.1	<60	1	R IV	CTM	74.4	M
106	FTC (HC)	pT1N0Mx	6	1.9	<60	1	L III	Negative	0.8	B
107	FTC	pT2N1Mx	25	7.8	<60	1	R II	ND	116.4	M
108	FTC	pT1NxMx	19	4.6	<60	2	L II-III	CTM	89.5	M

FNA, fine-needle aspiration; PTC, papillary thyroid carcinoma; FTC, follicular thyroid carcinoma; TCV, tall-cell variant; HC Hürtle cell; R, right, L, left; duration, time from thyroid ablation to FNA; II-III-IV, upper, middle, lower neck lateral compartment, IV, central neck compartment.

TABLE 2: Diagnostic performance of FNAC cytology as compared to final diagnosis.

FNAC	Final diagnosis Malignant LNs ($n = 86$)	Benign LNs ($n = 40$)
Positive	61	0
Negative	4	32
Inadequate	21	8

TABLE 3: Diagnostic performance of FNAC-Tg as compared to final diagnosis.

	Malignant LNs ($n = 86$)	Benign LNs ($n = 40$)
FNAC-Tg >1.1 ng/mL	86	0
FNAC-Tg ≤1.1 ng/mL	0	40

TABLE 4: Figures of merits of FNAC cytology and FNAC Tg.

FNAC	Sensitivity	Specificity	PPV	NPV	Accuracy
Cytology	71%	80%	88%	56%	74%
Tg	100%	100%	100%	100%	100%

TABLE 5: Rate of positive FNAC-Tg values (i.e., >1.1 ng/mL) in patients with inadequate or misdiagnosed FNAC-cytology.

Final status	FNAC inadequate ($n = 29$)	FNAC false-negative ($n = 4$)
Malignant LNs ($n = 25$)	21/21	4/4
Benign LNs ($n = 8$)	0/8	—

of 40 patients with benign lesions and 7 of 67 patients with malignant lesions ($P < .001$). The rate of FNAC samples adequate for cytological examination was 77% (97 samples) in contrast FNAC-Tg available in 100% of aspirates ($P < .01$). As shown in Table 2 cytological examination correctly identified 61 malignant LNs, was negative in 4, and inadequate in 21. For benign LNs, FNAC was negative in 32 and inadequate in 8. It showed no false-positive results. Thus, sensitivity, specificity, positive predictive value (PPV), negative predictive value (NPV), and accuracy of FNAC were 71%, 80%, 88%, 56%, and 74%, respectively. The ROC curve analysis demonstrated that the most appropriate cut-off value for the diagnosis of thyroid cancer metastatic lesions was 1.1 ng/mL (sensitivity 100%, specificity 100%, PPV 100%, NPV 100%, accuracy 100%; Figure 1, Tables 3, and 4). Basing on this cut-off level, the FNAC-Tg results correctly concluded all 25 malignant (100%) and 8 benign (100%) cases with false-negative ($n = 4$) and nondiagnostic ($n = 29$) FNAC results, respectively (Table 5). The FNAC-Tg levels were significantly higher in malignant (median 513.8 ng/mL, range 1.7-> 3000 ng/mL) than benign (median <0.2 ng/mL, range <0.2–1.1 ng/mL) lesions, respectively ($P < .0000001$). Particularly, specimen Tg levels were undetectable (i.e., <0.2 ng/mL) in 36 cases and were 0.3, 0.6, 0.8, and 1.1 ng/mL in remaining 4 cases with benign lesions.

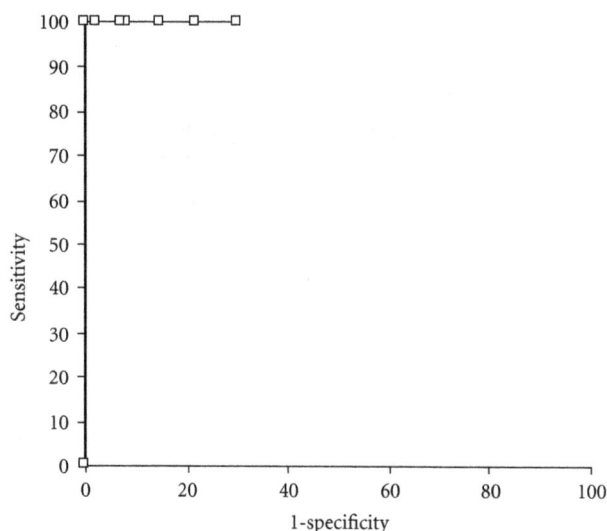

FIGURE 1: FNAC-Tg: ROC curve analysis.

4. Discussion

An accurate discrimination between metastatic and reactive LNs is essential in the management of thyroid cancer. Cytological examination of FNAC samples disclosed by US has been the most accurate method to diagnose a cervical LN. However, as showed also in our study, its sensitivity is negatively impacted by the rate of nondiagnostic samples although FNAC procedures are performed by US-experienced physicians and dedicated cytopathologists [5, 6, 15]. In the present study 23% of samples were nondiagnostic; this perfectly conforms with previously reported data [18]. Cystic metastasis and partial LN involvement comprise most of the inadequate/nondiagnostic FNAC-cytology cases and could be misinterpreted as a benign cervical cystic mass or branchial cleft cysts and could therefore delay the correct diagnosis and a further radical neck lymphadenectomy. The immunocytochemical Tg staining on FNAC samples from of neck nodes was previously evaluated in patients with DTC. Because an adequate FNAC sample is required, however, the practical impact of this technique is limited in clinical practice [19]. Recently, the FNAC-Tg measurement has been proposed to be a useful diagnostic technique in the management of patients with thyroid cancer. Because Tg is produced only by follicular thyrocyte-derived cells, measurement of Tg in FNAC specimens of nonthyroidal tissues enables the detection of persistence, recurrence, or metastasis of differentiated thyroid carcinoma. In our study FNAC-Tg analysis was more sensitive for detecting metastasis when compared with FNAC alone, and allows the accurate diagnosis in samples with inconclusive cytology. Our results perfectly conforms those recently reported by Bournaud and colleagues [18]. By contrast Tg could be determined in all aspirates and a sensitivity of 100% was achieved in our series, that is at the higher end of previously reported data (81%–100%) [7, 9, 14, 17, 18]. Although the performance of FNAC-Tg is well established, the Tg threshold value remains controversial. The Tg assays employed and methods for determining the cut-off value differed from one study to another, resulting in a large range, from 0.9 ng/mL to values as high as 39 ng/mL, proposed in the literature.

In our study the best Tg threshold was determined at 1.1 ng/mL by ROC curve analysis. Using a threshold of 1.1 ng/mL we observe neither false-positive results in nonmalignant LNs nor false-negative results in malignant LNs at final diagnosis. Additionally, FNAC-Tg results correctly classified as malignant 4 lesions that tested negatively in cytological examination. All in all, our results are in accordance with those of Snozek and colleagues that used a Tg assay with a functional sensitivity at 0.1 ng/mL and proposed a cut-off level of 1.00 ng/mL: basing on their results these authors suggested that FNAC-Tg should be substituted for FNAC in many cases [7]. Of importance, our samples were obtained in a population of well-differentiated thyroid carcinomas (i.e., only two Hürtle cell and two tall-cell variants among 108 DTC cases). Several authors reported, however, that FNAC-Tg levels could be undetectable in some types of thyroid cancers (i.e., poorly differentiated thyroid carcinomas) [13, 17]. This correspond to the fact that amount and intensity of Tg expression parallel with differentiation of the tumor and could produce false-negative results. As a consequence, caution is needed, and a combination of FNAC and FNAC-Tg should remain the standard, especially in patients harboring less differentiated thyroid carcinomas.

5. Conclusions

The diagnostic performance of needle washout FNAC-Tg measurement with a cut-off of 1.1 ng/mL compared favourably with cytology and allowed accurate diagnosis in all cases in whom cytology was nondiagnostic.

References

[1] L. Davies and H. G. Welch, "Increasing incidence of thyroid cancer in the United States, 1973–2002," *Journal of the American Medical Association*, vol. 295, no. 18, pp. 2164–2167, 2006.

[2] M. J. Schlumberger, "Papillary and follicular thyroid carcinoma," *The New England Journal of Medicine*, vol. 338, no. 5, pp. 297–306, 1998.

[3] N. A. Johnson and M. E. Tublin, "Postoperative surveillance of differentiated thyroid carcinoma: rationale, techniques, and controversies," *Radiology*, vol. 249, no. 2, pp. 429–444, 2008.

[4] A. Frasoldati and R. Valcavi, "Challenges in neck ultrasonography: lymphadenopathy and parathyroid glands," *Endocrine Practice*, vol. 10, no. 3, pp. 261–268, 2004.

[5] M. O. Bernier, C. Moisan, G. Mansour, A. Aurengo, F. Ménégaux, and L. Leenhardt, "Usefulness of fine needle aspiration cytology in the diagnosis of loco-regional recurrence of differentiated thyroid carcinoma," *European Journal of Surgical Oncology*, vol. 31, no. 3, pp. 288–293, 2005.

[6] G. W. Boland, M. J. Lee, P. R. Mueller, W. Mayo-Smith, S. L. Dawson, and J. F. Simeone, "Efficacy of sonographically

guided biopsy of thyroid masses and cervical lymph nodes," *American Journal of Roentgenology*, vol. 161, no. 5, pp. 1053–1056, 1993.

[7] C. L. H. Snozek, E. P. Chambers, C. C. Reading et al., "Serum thyroglobulin, high-resolution ultrasound, and lymph node thyroglobulin in diagnosis of differentiated thyroid carcinoma nodal metastases," *Journal of Clinical Endocrinology and Metabolism*, vol. 92, no. 11, pp. 4278–4281, 2007.

[8] S. J. Jeon, E. Kim, J. S. Park et al., "Diagnostic benefit of thyroglobulin measurement in fine-needle aspiration for diagnosing metastatic cervical lymph nodes from papillary thyroid cancer: correlations with US features," *Korean Journal of Radiology*, vol. 10, no. 2, pp. 106–111, 2009.

[9] M. J. Kim, E. K. Kim, B. M. Kim et al., "Thyroglobulin measurement in fine-needle aspirate washouts: the criteria for neck node dissection for patients with thyroid cancer," *Clinical Endocrinology*, vol. 70, no. 1, pp. 145–151, 2009.

[10] T. Uruno, A. Miyauchi, K. Shimizu et al., "Usefulness of thyroglobulin measurement in fine-needle aspiration biopsy specimens for diagnosing cervical lymph node metastasis in patients with papillary thyroid cancer," *World Journal of Surgery*, vol. 29, no. 4, pp. 483–485, 2005.

[11] Z. W. Baloch, J. E. Barroeta, J. Walsh et al., "Utility of thyroglobulin measurement in fine-needle aspiration biopsy specimens of lymph nodes in the diagnosis of recurrent thyroid carcinoma," *CytoJournal*, vol. 5, article 1, 2008.

[12] E. Sigstad, A. Heilo, E. Paus et al., "The usefulness of detecting thyroglobulin in fine-needle aspirates from patients with neck lesions using a sensitive thyroglobulin assay," *Diagnostic Cytopathology*, vol. 35, no. 12, pp. 761–767, 2007.

[13] A. L. Borel, R. Boizel, P. Faure et al., "Significance of low levels of thyroglobulin in fine needle aspirates from cervical lymph nodes of patients with a history of differentiated thyroid cancer," *European Journal of Endocrinology*, vol. 158, no. 5, pp. 691–698, 2008.

[14] N. Cunha, F. Rodrigues, F. Curado et al., "Thyroglobulin detection in fine-needle aspirates of cervical lymph nodes: a technique for the diagnosis of metastatic differentiated thyroid cancer," *European Journal of Endocrinology*, vol. 157, no. 1, pp. 101–107, 2007.

[15] A. Frasoldati, E. Toschi, M. Zini et al., "Role of thyroglobulin measurement in fine-needle aspiration biopsies of cervical lymph nodes in patients with differentiated thyroid cancer," *Thyroid*, vol. 9, no. 2, pp. 105–111, 1999.

[16] L. Giovanella, L. Ceriani, S. Suriano, and S. Crippa, "Thyroglobulin measurement on fine-needle washout fluids: influence of sample collection methods," *Diagnostic Cytopathology*, vol. 37, no. 1, pp. 42–44, 2009.

[17] F. Boi, G. Baghino, F. Atzeni, M. L. Lai, G. Faa, and S. Mariotti, "The diagnostic value for differentiated thyroid carcinoma metastases of thyroglobulin (Tg) measurement in washout fluid from fine-needle aspiration biopsy of neck lymph nodes is maintained in the presence of circulating anti-Tg antibodies," *Journal of Clinical Endocrinology and Metabolism*, vol. 91, no. 4, pp. 1364–1369, 2006.

[18] C. Bournaud, A. Charrié, C. Nozières et al., "Thyroglobulin measurement in fine-needle aspirates of lymph nodes in patients with differentiated thyroid cancer: a simple definition of the threshold value, with emphasis on potential pitfalls of the method," *Clinical Chemistry and Laboratory Medicine*, vol. 48, no. 8, pp. 1171–1177, 2010.

[19] T. Pisani, A. Vecchione, N. T. Sinopoli, A. Drusco, C. Valli, and M. R. Giovagnoli, "Cytological and immunocytochemical analysis of laterocervical lymph nodes in patients with previous thyroid carcinoma," *Anticancer Research*, vol. 19, no. 4, pp. 3527–3530, 1999.

20

The Evolving Role of Selenium in the Treatment of Graves' Disease and Ophthalmopathy

Leonidas H. Duntas

Endocrine Unit, Evgenidion Hospital, University of Athens, 20 Papadiamantopoulou Street, 11528 Athens, Greece

Correspondence should be addressed to Leonidas H. Duntas, ledunt@otenet.gr

Academic Editor: Juan Carlos Galofré

Graves' disease (GD) and ophthalmopathy (GO) are organ-specific autoimmune-inflammatory disorders characterized by a complex pathogenesis. The inflammatory process is dominated by an imbalance of the antioxidant-oxidant mechanism, increased production of radical oxygen species (ROS), and cytokines which sustain the autoimmune process and perpetuate the disease. Recently, selenium, which is a powerful antioxidant, has been successfully applied in patients with mild GO, slowing the progression of disease, decreasing the clinical activity score, and appreciably improving the quality of life. The mechanisms of selenium action are variable. The aim of this review is to summarize the actions of selenium in GD and GO. Selenium as selenocysteine is incorporated in selenoproteins, such as glutathione peroxidase which catalyzes the degradation of hydrogen peroxide and lipid hydroperoxide that are increasingly produced in hyperthyroidism. Moreover, selenium decreases the formation of proinflammatory cytokines, while it contributes, in synergy with antithyroid drugs, to stabilization of the autoimmune process in GD and alleviation of GO. It is now to be clarified whether enforced nutritional supplementation has the same results and whether prolonging selenium administration may have an impact on the prevention of disease.

1. Introduction

Observed and briefly described, though not published, by Parry in the late 1700s, Graves' disease (GD) was definitively identified and documented by Robert Graves in 1835 and classically described by von Basedow in 1840 [1–3]. GD is an autoimmune disease characterized by the activation of autoantibodies against the TSH receptor (TRAB), leading to excessive thyroid hormone production [4]. GD manifests, interalia, via thyrotoxicosis and extrathyroid involvement often entailing orbitopathy (GO) and, rarely, dermopathy (pretibial myxedema) and acropathy. Moreover, the TRAB, by stimulating cyclic adenosine monophosphate (AMP), cause proliferation and hyperplasia of the thyroid follicular cells resulting in enlargement of the gland, frequently the first sign of the disease, the swelling ranging from slight to marked [5]. Clinically, the thyroid is firm in consistency and tender in patients with a greatly enlarged goiter, while palpation lobulations are also commonly detected which can be mistaken for nodules.

No single gene has been pinpointed as causing GD, a disease which is most prevalent in women between the ages of 20 and 50 years. However, it has been associated with certain MHC Class II HLA alleles depending on the racial group, for example, HLA-DR3 in whites [4]. An association of GD with polymorphisms of the cytotoxic T-lymphocyte antigen 4 (CTLA-4) gene has also been established, suggesting a functional role of CTLA-4 in autoreactive T cells [4, 5].

A combination of genetic and environmental factors is responsible for the initiation of autoimmunity. Interactions between genetic and environmental factors are underscored by the existing associations linking age at diagnosis, goiter, disease severity, smoking, and family history [6]. In addition, iodine repletion in iodine-deficient areas is usually accompanied by an increased incidence of GD due to the Jod-Basedow phenomenon. Stress is also thought to be a significant factor precipitating GD in susceptible individuals [7], while smoking is well established as being linked to GO but not to GD [8].

Treatment modalities of GD consist of administration of antithyroid drugs, radioiodine therapy, or surgery. Radioiodine therapy, is favored only in USA, whereas antithyroid drugs, including methimazole, carbimazole, and propylthiouracil, comprise first choice treatment in the rest of the world. Nevertheless, according to a recent study examining the frequency of antithyroid drug prescription in USA, methimazole (MMI) has lately become the most frequently prescribed antithyroid drug, indicating a clear shift towards pharmacological treatment as the primary treatment option in GD [9]. Treatment should be planned for a period of at least 12 months, and patients are usually becoming euthyroid within this timeframe; nevertheless, the duration of the remission period is unpredictable, since the disease is marked by cycles of remission and relapse of variable duration [4].

Recently, evidence has emerged indicating that selenium administration could be effective and safe in patients with GD and with mild forms of GO [10].

The aim of this paper is to briefly evaluate the current knowledge concerning the pathogenesis of GD and GO and discuss the evolving role of selenium within the context of its potential as a therapeutic means of intervention in these disorders.

2. Pathogenesis of GD and GO

Hyperthyroidism is caused by the binding of TSH-stimulating antibodies to the TSH receptor, a G-protein-coupled receptor. However, the first step in this process is considered to be precipitation by environmental factors of an HLA-related organ-specific defect in suppressor T-lymphocyte function [5]. This leads to decreased suppression of thyroid-directed helper T-lymphocytes which, in the presence of dendritic cells and macrophages, produce the cytokines γ-interferon (IFNγ) and interleukin-1 (IL-1), subsequently differentiating B cells to plasma cells and generating TRAB. Concomitantly, IFNγ enhances the expression of HLA-DR antigens on the surface of thyroid cells (Figure 1). Thus, IFNγ modulates the autoimmune process and, by stimulating chemokine production by thyroid follicular cells, contributes to the maintenance of the autoimmune process [10]. The contribution of dendritic cells and B cells is apparently crucial for the initiation of disease since they express the costimulatory molecules, CD80 and CD86, that are key triggers for the reaction of T lymphocytes to thyroid cell presenting antigens [4]. TRAB stimulate the TSHR on the thyroid follicular cells, resulting in increased thyroid hormone production, which may further reduce the number and function of suppressor T lymphocytes and stimulate helper T lymphocyte, thus, perpetuating the cyclicity of disease [4, 5].

GO is a complex autoimmune disease. Whereas the cycle of GD consists of two components, immunological and hormonal, that perpetuate the process, the progression of GD to GO, and rarely to dermopathy, is likely to be a positive feedback cycle composed of three interrelated components: mechanical, immunological, and cellular [5]. Comprehensive reviews on the pathophysiology of GO have recently been published [11–14]. Briefly, the loss of tolerance of T cells to the TSHR, via as yet unknown mechanisms, ignites the autoimmune process. The TSHR is internalized and presented by antigen-presenting cells to helper T cells. Subsequently, the TRAB, which are secreted by activated B cells, recognize the TSHR on the fibroblasts

of the orbita, where they initiate the ocular changes [12, 13]. The fibroblasts have been recognized as target cells in GO. Orbital fibroblasts stimulated by IFNγ, tumor necrosis factor-α (TNF-α), growth factors and oxygen reactive species (ROS), secrete hyaluronic acid, and prostaglandin E$_2$, known mediators of inflammation, while a subgroup may differentiate into mature adipocytes presenting TSHR [13, 14]. The subsequent proliferation of adipocytes and fibroblasts results in increased synthesis of glycosaminoglycans (GAG), which causes edema of orbital structures, extraocular muscle enlargement, and adipose tissue expansion; these events are constituting the signs of disease [15].

Concerning the recent enquiry as to whether autoimmunity against IGF-1R is primarily involved in the pathogenesis of GO, it is likely that it is not specific but instead constitutes a secondary reaction of the autoimmune process [16]

The mechanisms promoting oxidative stress have also been implicated in the pathogenesis of GO. Hyperthyroidism increases oxidants and decreases antioxidants leading to oxidative stress, this process is dominated by the production of ROS which have long been recognized as intermediates of various essential biological redox reactions [17, 18]. The adverse effects induced by ROS have been suggested as being partly responsible for the tissue injury. Mitochondria are a major source of superoxide anion (O_2^-) and hydrogen peroxides (H_2O_2), while a number of intracellular enzymes, xanthine oxidase being the best known, are involved in oxidation reactions in which molecular oxygen (O_2) is reduced to O_2^- [19].

Ongoing autoimmunity may contribute to increased oxidative stress even in euthyroid GD patients, while patients who have relapsed present increased markers of oxidative stress [20]. Moreover, the content of 8-hydroxy 2'-deoxy-guanosine (8-OHdG), an important biomarker of oxidative DNA damage, was found significantly higher in orbital fibroblasts together with O_2^- and H_2O_2, underscoring the major role that ROS play in the pathogenesis of GO [21].

Recently, increased 11β-hydroxysteroid dehydrogenase (11β-HSD1) expression, induced by cytokines, was described in orbital adipose cells, a condition leading to elevated local generation of cortisol by 11β-HSD1, which may suppress cytokine synthesis and resolve the inflammation [22]. 11β-HSD1 activates cortisone to cortisol in peripheral and visceral adipose tissues. According to the authors, since failure to produce adequate levels of local glucocorticoids in the orbita may signify persistence of the disease, 11β-HSD1 could provide a new therapeutic target of disease [22].

3. Presentation and Treatment Novelties of GD and GO

TRAB levels in serum are pathognomonic for GD, predicting the course of disease and response to antithyroid treatment; they do not, on the other hand, predict the development of GO [23]. In conjunction with the high levels of TRAB, the risk of relapse is related to young age, male gender, and large goiter [24]. Tobacco smoking has been consistently linked to development or deterioration of GO [8, 25]. Since RAI

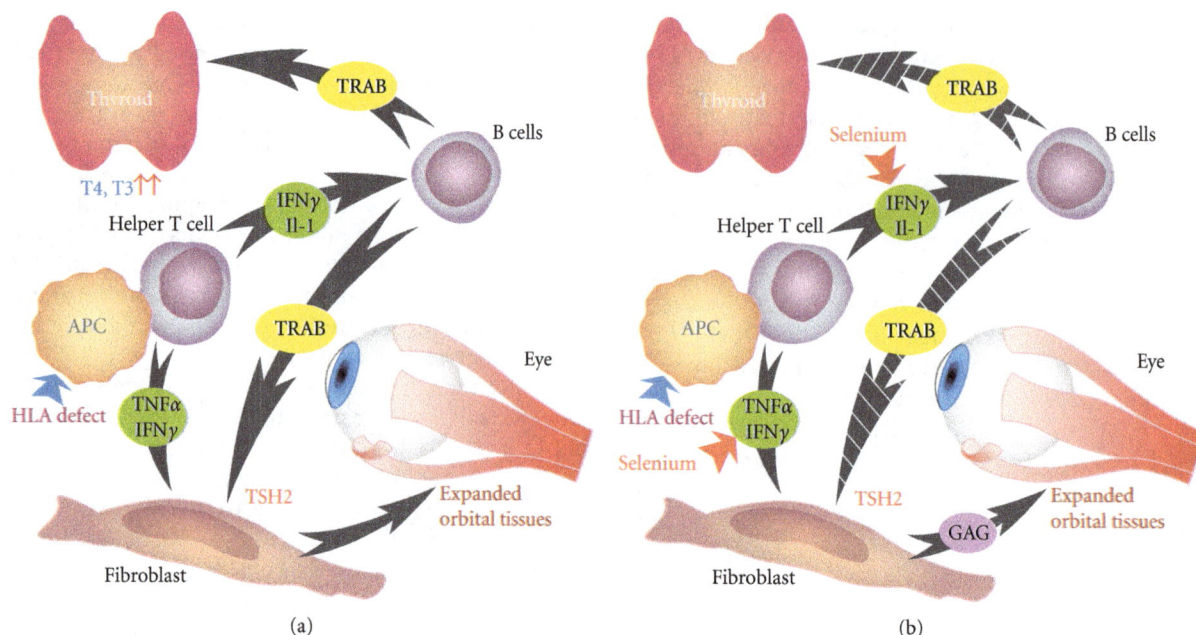

FIGURE 1: (a) Schematic presentation of the cascade of events in the pathogenesis of Graves' ophthalmopathy. Secretion of cytokines, such as IFN-γ and IL-2, by activated helper cells result in activation of B cells and secretion of TSH receptor antibodies. These bind to the TSH receptor in the orbital fibroblast and on the thyroid follicular cells, thereby, extending muscle enlargement resulting in oedema. (b) Selenium by suppressing cytokines production considerably attenuates the inflammation leading to alleviation of symptoms and signs. Abbreviations: HLA: human leukocyte antigen; APC: antigen presenting cell; IFN-γ: interferon-γ; IL-1: interleukin-1; TRAB: TSH-receptor antibodies; GAG: glycosaminoglycans.

treatment for GD is associated with a worsening of GO, patients, and particularly those who are smokers, should be administered oral steroids [26]. Interestingly, a recent study from Varese has suggested that steroid prophylaxis can be achieved by applying lower prednisone doses, that is, 0.2 mg/kg BW, than had previously been reported [27]. Moreover, RAI when applied for treatment for GD results more frequently in aggravation or appearance of GO than after antithyroid treatment [28]. Nevertheless, choice of the best treatment for hyperthyroidism in patients with active GO remains a dilemma [29]. In a recent prospective analysis of the data of 108 patients with Graves' hyperthyroidism and severe orbitopathy, it was reported that prolonged treatment applying partial block therapy with low-dose thionamides plus LT4, over a median duration of 80 months, led to euthyroidism and stabilized the orbitopathy [30]. Within this context, a retrospective study proposes block-replacement treatment of GD patients with GO as a feasible treatment option until the orbitopathy becomes inactive, and no further treatment is required [31].

Neither antithyroid drug treatment nor thyroidectomy has any impact on the course of GO, and treatment in the active phase is based on the clinical activity score (CAS) [32, 33]; introduced by Mourits et al. in 1989, the CAS remains a reliable and easily applied scoring system enabling the classification of patients into those with active or inactive disease [33].

Recently, rituximab, a CD-20 antibody which blocks the differentiation of B cells and potentially inhibits B-cells-mediated immunity, was applied with encouraging results

in patients with GO [34]. The compound was shown to improve GO without, however, affecting the TRAB levels [35]. Serum cytokine IL-6 levels did not change, while chemokine ligand 10 (CXCL10) increased at B-cell depletion.

Based on the knowledge of the crucial role of the oxidants in the pathogenesis of GD as well as in the development of GO, several studies have been conducted administrating antioxidants as the treatment modality in patients with GD and GO.

In a nonrandomized study, 82% of the 11 patients with active GO responded to antioxidant treatment with nicotinamide and allopurinol as compared to only 27% of the control group. Soft tissue inflammation parameters responded better than any other component of disease [36].

Supplementation with a mixture of antioxidants, including selenium, beta-carotene, and vitamins C and E, in addition to methimazole, in 29 patients with GD led to euthyroidism faster than in 28 patients taking only methimazole and who served as the control group [37]. Serum selenium levels as well as glutathione peroxidase activity were statistically significantly elevated in the supplemented patients, validating treatment with antioxidants, especially when this incorporated selenium.

In a more recent, randomized, double-blind, and placebo-controlled study recruiting 159 patients with mild GO, the effects of selenium administration for 6 months in the form of selenite were assessed versus an anti-inflammatory agent [10]. Selenium improved quality of life and significantly slowed the progression of GO, while it greatly decreased the CAS when compared with the pentoxifylline or placebo group. A 6-month followup confirmed the results of the 6-month treatment. The authors hypothesized a reversal of the disturbed antioxidant-oxidant balance in GD and GO although the exact mechanisms of selenium action are not elucidated.

In another study assessing the selenium levels in patients going into remission ($n = 24$) and relapses ($n = 59$), no statistically significant differences were detected between the two groups. However, patients in remission of GD had the highest (>120 μg/L) serum selenium levels, while it is of interest that TRAB levels and selenium were negatively correlated [38].

4. Mechanisms of Selenium Action in GD and GO

Selenium is vital for a wide range of biological processes; hence, the state of "selenostasis" is essential for wellbeing and human health [39]. The many biological and clinical benefits conferred by selenium are achieved by virtue of its remarkable antioxidative effects mediated mainly by the selenoproteins GPx and TRx reductase. TRx is a stress- and iodine-induced protein, possessing strong redox activities, and it has been postulated that it may be implicated in the regulation of T3 production in GD. It has been reported highly produced in GD and expressed in the thyroid follicular cells. Nevertheless, its precise role, though of considerable interest due to its characteristics, remains as yet unraveled [40].

The hypermetabolic state in acute GD, the intracellular ATP, and increased oxygen consumption lead to mitochondria dysfunction, which generates ROS and disrupts the oxidant and antioxidant balance, thereby, causing oxidative stress and tissue injury [41]. By activating GPxs, selenium ignites the "second line" of antioxidant defense, behind the enzymatic "first line" defense system composed of the superoxide dismutase (SOD) and catalase (CAT) [42]. Thus, SOD and CAT synthesize an efficient antioxidative mechanism capable of neutralizing the biologic effects of free radicals; when this mechanism is saturated, the "second line," regulated by selenium availability, is activated. Experimental studies in hyperthyroidism have documented an enhanced activity of the TRx and GPx systems, stimulated by the calcium phosphatidylinositol cascade which is usually activated in hyperthyroidism, as well as increased levels of SOD and of glutathione in erythrocytes [43, 44]. These findings provide evidence of an upregulation of the antioxidative and protective systems in acute GD, depending, however, on the duration and severity of the disease; these system(s) might become saturated, following which supplementation or nutritional intervention is required.

The induced oxidative stress enflames lipid peroxidation and activates various inflammatory pathways. ROS may stimulate the NF-κB pathway, a cornerstone of immune and inflammatory response, which has been associated with increased production of TNF-α and IL-6 cytokines [45]. Selenium inhibits NF-κB from binding to its gene promoters and consequently diminishes cytokine production and attenuates the inflammation; by contrast, selenium is likely not to interfere with the translocation of NF-κB and its subunits to the nucleus [46]. This could be one of the most important anti-inflammatory effects of selenium supplementation and thus be of potential benefit for patients suffering from GD and, especially, GO.

In GO, the balance of T helper (Th) 1/Th2 lymphocytes shifts to a prevalence of Th1 type CD4+, which plays a pivotal role in the development of disease [47]. Consequently, the ratio Th1/Th2 has been proposed as a biomarker of disease activity and as a target for specific immune therapy of GO. The subsequent overproduction of cytokines, such as TNF-α and IFNγ, sustains the inflammatory process. It is of interest that treatment with a mixture containing selenium-suppressed Th1 while upregulating Th2 [48]. Th1 predominate in eye muscles (EM) and IFN-γ, TNF-α, IL-1β, and IL-6 mRNA have been abundantly detected in EM in contrast to orbit fat where IL-4 and IL-10 mRNA, with significant variations within patients, were more frequently detected [49]. Thus, mediated by the suppression of Th1-like cytokines, selenium alleviates the soft tissue inflammation and improves eye motility.

ROS, such as H_2O_2, may also activate p38 mitogen-activated protein kinase (p38MAPK) and induce expression of high levels of cyclooxygenase (COX)-2; this reaction is depending on the severity of GO, in orbital fibroadipose tissues [50]. Recently, it has been shown that selenium was able to reduce H_2O_2-mediated expression of COX-2 in vascular endothelial cells by inhibiting the p38 MAPK pathway [51].

In summary, selenium influences the inflammatory process in GD and GO by inhibiting various pathways though its mechanism of action is not completely clarified. It is nonetheless possible that, in synergy with antithyroid drugs or immune modulators, selenium might offer an alternative therapeutic approach in patients with severe disease. It also remains to be established whether enforced nutritional supplementation has the same effects and whether long-term selenium administration in the form of selenomethionine or as nutritional intervention may have an impact on the incidence of relapse of GD and GO.

References

[1] C. H. Parry, *Collections from the Unpublished Medical Writings of the Late Caleb Hillier Parry*, vol. 2, Underwood, London, UK, 1982.

[2] R. Graves, "Newly observed affection of the thyroid: clinical lectures," *The London Medical and Surgical Journal*, vol. 7, pp. 516–517, 1835.

[3] K. von Basedow, "Exophthalmos durch Hypertrophie des Zellgewebes in der Augenhöhle," *Wochenschr Heilkunde*, vol. 6, pp. 197–204, 1840.

[4] A. P. Weetman, "Graves' disease," *The New England Journal of Medicine*, vol. 343, no. 17, pp. 1236–1248, 2000.

[5] R. Volpe, "Grave's disease. Pathogenesis," in *Werner and Ingbar's The Thyroid: A Fundamental and Clinical Text*,

L. E. Braverman and R. D. Utiger, Eds., pp. 648–657, J. B. Lippincott, Philadelphia, Pa, USA, 6th edition, 1986.

[6] N. Manji, J. D. Carr-Smith, K. Boelaert et al., "Influences of age, gender, smoking, and family history on autoimmune thyroid disease phenotype," *The Journal of Clinical Endocrinology & Metabolism*, vol. 91, no. 12, pp. 4873–4880, 2006.

[7] L. Chiovato and A. Pinchera, "Stressful life events and Graves' disease," *European Journal of Endocrinology*, vol. 134, no. 6, pp. 680–682, 1996.

[8] L. Bartalena, F. Bogazzi, M. L. Tanda, L. Manetti, E. Dell'Unto, and E. Martino, "Cigarette smoking and the thyroid," *European Journal of Endocrinology*, vol. 133, no. 5, pp. 507–512, 1995.

[9] A. B. Emiliano, L. Governale, M. Parks, and D. S. Cooper, "Shifts in propylthiouracil and methimazole prescribing practices: antithyroid drug use in the United States from 1991 to 2008," *The Journal of Clinical Endocrinology & Metabolism*, vol. 95, no. 5, pp. 2227–2233, 2010.

[10] C. Marcocci, G. J. Kahaly, G. E. Krassas et al., "Selenium and the course of mild Graves' orbitopathy," *The New England Journal of Medicine*, vol. 364, no. 20, pp. 1920–1931, 2011.

[11] M. Rotondi, E. Lazzeri, P. Romagnani, and M. Serio, "Role for interferon-γ inducible chemokines in endocrine autoimmunity: an expanding field," *Journal of Endocrinological Investigation*, vol. 26, no. 2, pp. 177–180, 2003.

[12] B. S. Prabhakar, R. S. Bahn, and T. J. Smith, "Current perspective on the pathogenesis of Graves' disease and ophthalmopathy," *Endocrine Reviews*, vol. 24, no. 6, pp. 802–835, 2003.

[13] R. S. Bahn, "Pathophysiology of Graves' ophthalmopathy: the cycle of disease," *The Journal of Clinical Endocrinology & Metabolism*, vol. 88, no. 5, pp. 1939–1946, 2003.

[14] T. J. Smith, "Pathogenesis of Graves' orbitopathy: a 2010 update," *Journal of Endocrinological Investigation*, vol. 33, no. 6, pp. 414–421, 2010.

[15] R.S. Bahn, "Mechanisms of disease-Graves' ophthalmopathy," *The New England Journal of Medicine*, vol. 362, pp. 726–738, 2010.

[16] W. M. Wiersinga, "Autoimmunity in Graves' ophthalmopathy: the result of an unfortunate marriage between TSH receptors and IGF-1 receptors?" *The Journal of Clinical Endocrinology & Metabolism*, vol. 96, no. 8, pp. 2386–2394, 2011.

[17] L. Bartalena, M. L. Tanda, E. Piantanida, and A. Lai, "Oxidative stress and Graves' ophthalmopathy: in vitro studies and therapeutic implications," *BioFactors*, vol. 19, no. 3-4, pp. 155–163, 2003.

[18] M. Aslan, N. Cosar, H. Celik et al., "Evaluation of oxidative status in patients with hyperthyroidism," *Endocrine*, vol. 40, no. 2, pp. 285–289, 2011.

[19] H. Kohler and H. Jenzer, "Interaction of lactoperoxidase with hydrogen peroxide. Formation of enzyme intermediates and generation of free radicals," *Free Radical Biology & Medicine*, vol. 6, no. 3, pp. 323–339, 1989.

[20] E. Ademoğlu, N. Özbey, Y. Erbil et al., "Determination of oxidative stress in thyroid tissue and plasma of patients with Graves' disease," *European Journal of Internal Medicine*, vol. 17, no. 8, pp. 545–550, 2006.

[21] C. C. Tsai, S. B. Wu, C. Y. Cheng et al., "Increased oxidative DNA damage, lipid peroxidation, and reactive oxygen species in cultured orbital fibroblasts from patients with Graves ophthalmopathy: evidence that oxidative stress has a role in this disorder," *Eye*, vol. 24, no. 9, pp. 1520–1525, 2010.

[22] J. W. Tomlinson, O. M. Durrani, I. J. Bujalska et al., "The role of 11β-hydroxysteroid dehydrogenase 1 in adipogenesis in thyroid-associated ophthalmopathy," *The Journal of Clinical Endocrinology & Metabolism*, vol. 95, no. 1, pp. 398–406, 2010.

[23] A. K. Eckstein, M. Plicht, H. Lax et al., "Thyrotropin receptor autoantibodies are independent risk factors for graves' ophthalmopathy and help to predict severity and outcome of the disease," *The Journal of Clinical Endocrinology & Metabolism*, vol. 91, no. 9, pp. 3464–3470, 2006.

[24] J. Orgiazzi and A. M. Madec, "Reduction of the risk of relapse after withdrawal of medical therapy for Graves' disease," *Thyroid*, vol. 12, no. 10, pp. 849–853, 2002.

[25] M. N. Stan and R. S. Bahn, "Risk factors for development or deterioration of Graves' ophthalmopathy," *Thyroid*, vol. 20, no. 7, pp. 777–783, 2010.

[26] L. Bartalena, C. Marcocci, F. Bogazzi, M. Panicucci, A. Lepri, and A. Pinchera, "Use of corticosteroids to prevent progression of Graves' ophthalmopathy after radioiodine therapy for hyperthyroidism," *The New England Journal of Medicine*, vol. 321, no. 20, pp. 1349–1352, 1989.

[27] A. Lai, L. Sassi, E. Compri et al., "Lower dose prednisone prevents radioiodine-associated exacerbation of initially mild or absent Graves' orbitopathy: a retrospective cohort study," *The Journal of Clinical Endocrinology & Metabolism*, vol. 95, no. 3, pp. 1333–1337, 2010.

[28] L. Bartalena, C. Marcocci, F. Bogazzi et al., "Relation between therapy for hyperthyroidism and the course of Graves' ophthalmopathy," *The New England Journal of Medicine*, vol. 338, no. 2, pp. 73–78, 1998.

[29] L. Bartalena, "The dilemma of how to manage Graves' hyperthyroidism in patients with associated orbitopathy," *The Journal of Clinical Endocrinology & Metabolism*, vol. 96, no. 3, pp. 592–599, 2011.

[30] P. Laurberg, D. C. Berman, S. Andersen, and I. B. Pedersen, "Sustained control of graves' hyperthyroidism during long-term low-dose antithyroid drug therapy of patients with severe graves' orbitopathy," *Thyroid*, vol. 21, no. 9, pp. 951–956, 2011.

[31] L. Elbers, M. Mourits, and W. Wiersinga, "Outcome of very long-term treatment with antithyroid drugs in Graves' hyperthyroidism associated with Graves' orbitopathy," *Thyroid*, vol. 21, no. 3, pp. 279–283, 2011.

[32] L. Bartalena, A. Pinchera, and C. Marcocci, "Management of graves' ophthalmopathy: reality and perspectives," *Endocrine Reviews*, vol. 21, no. 2, pp. 168–199, 2000.

[33] M. P. Mourits, L. Koornneef, W. M. Wiersinga, M. F. Prummel, A. Berghout, and R. van der Gaag, "Clinical criteria for the assessment of disease activity in Graves' ophthalmology: a novel approach," *British Journal of Ophthalmology*, vol. 73, no. 8, pp. 639–644, 1989.

[34] G. Vannucchi, I. Campi, M. Bonomi et al., "Rituximab treatment in patients with active Graves' orbitopathy: effects on proinflammatory and humoral immune reactions," *Clinical & Experimental Immunology*, vol. 161, no. 3, pp. 436–443, 2010.

[35] M. Salvi, G. Vannucchi, I. Campi, and P. Beck-Peccoz, "Rituximab in the treatment of thyroid eye disease: science fiction?" *Orbit*, vol. 28, no. 4, pp. 251–255, 2009.

[36] E. A. Bouzas, P. Karadimas, G. Mastorakos, and D. A. Koutras, "Antioxidant agents in the treatment of Graves' ophthalmopathy," *American Journal of Ophthalmology*, vol. 129, no. 5, pp. 618–622, 2000.

[37] V. B. Vrca, F. Skreb, I. Cepelak, Z. Romic, and L. Mayer, "Supplementation with antioxidants in the treatment of Graves' disease; the effect on glutathione peroxidase activity and concentration of selenium," *Clinica Chimica Acta*, vol. 341, no. 1-2, pp. 55–63, 2004.

[38] T. Wertenbruch, H. S. Willenberg, C. Sagert et al., "Serum selenium levels in patients with remission and relapse of Graves' disease," *Medicinal Chemistry*, vol. 3, no. 3, pp. 281–284, 2007.

[39] L. H. Duntas, "Selenium and the thyroid: a close-knit connection," *The Journal of Clinical Endocrinology & Metabolism*, vol. 95, no. 12, pp. 5180–5188, 2010.

[40] M. Kihara, K. Kontani, A. Yamauchi et al., "Expression of thioredoxin in patients with Graves' disease," *International Journal of Molecular Medicine*, vol. 15, no. 5, pp. 795–799, 2005.

[41] P. Venditti, S. Di Meo, and T. De Leo, "Effect of thyroid state on characteristics determining the susceptibility to oxidative stress of mitochondrial fractions from rat liver," *Cellular Physiology and Biochemistry*, vol. 6, no. 5, pp. 283–295, 1996.

[42] M. Abalovich, S. Llesuy, S. Gutierrez, and M. Repetto, "Peripheral parameters of oxidative stress in Graves' disease: the effects of methimazole and 131 iodine treatments," *Clinical Endocrinology*, vol. 59, no. 3, pp. 321–327, 2003.

[43] L. H. Duntas, "The role of selenium in thyroid autoimmunity and cancer," *Thyroid*, vol. 16, no. 5, pp. 455–460, 2006.

[44] A. Seven, O. Seymen, S. Hatemi, H. Hatemi, G. Yiğit, and G. Candan, "Antioxidant status in experimental hyperthyroidism: effect of vitamin E supplementation," *Clinica Chimica Acta*, vol. 256, no. 1, pp. 65–74, 1996.

[45] P. J. Barnes and M. Karin, "Nuclear factor-κB—a pivotal transcription factor in chronic inflammatory diseases," *The New England Journal of Medicine*, vol. 336, no. 15, pp. 1066–1071, 1997.

[46] F. Zhang, W. Yu, J. L. Hargrove et al., "Inhibition of TNF-α induced ICAM-1, VCAM-1 and E-selectin expression by selenium," *Atherosclerosis*, vol. 161, no. 2, pp. 381–386, 2002.

[47] N. Xia, S. Zhou, Y. Liang et al., "CD4+ T cells and the Th1/Th2 imbalance are implicated in the pathogenesis of Graves' ophthalmopathy," *International Journal of Molecular Medicine*, vol. 17, no. 5, pp. 911–916, 2006.

[48] Y. Chang, S. L. Piao, S. Gao, and D. M. Zheng, "Regulatory effects of micronutrient complex on the expression of Th1 and Th2 cytokines in diabetic C57BL mice," *Wei Sheng Yan Jiu*, vol. 34, no. 1, pp. 64–66, 2005.

[49] Y. Hiromatsu, D. Yang, T. Bednarczuk, I. Miyake, K. Nonaka, and Y. Inoue, "Cytokine profiles in eye muscle tissue and orbital fat tissue from patients with thyroid-associated ophthalmopathy," *The Journal of Clinical Endocrinology & Metabolism*, vol. 85, no. 3, pp. 1194–1199, 2000.

[50] Y. B. Li, J. Y. Han, W. Jiang, and J. Wang, "Selenium inhibits high glucose-induced cyclooxygenase-2 and P-selectin expression in vascular endothelial cells," *Molecular Biology Reports*, vol. 38, no. 4, pp. 2301–2306, 2011.

[51] E. B. Y. Konuk, O. Konuk, M. Misirlioglu, A. Menevse, and M. Unal, "Expression of cyclooxygenase-2 in orbital fibroadipose connective tissues of Graves' ophthalmopathy patients," *European Journal of Endocrinology*, vol. 155, no. 5, pp. 681–685, 2006.

21

Atypical Clinical Manifestations of Graves' Disease: An Analysis in Depth

Mohamed Osama Hegazi and Sherif Ahmed

Medical Department, Al Adan Hospital, P.O. Box 262, Hadiya 52853, Kuwait

Correspondence should be addressed to Mohamed Osama Hegazi, drosama02@gmail.com

Academic Editor: Juan C. Galofré

Over the past few decades, there has been an increase in the number of reports about newly recognized (atypical or unusual) manifestations of Graves' disease (GD), that are related to various body systems. One of these manifestations is sometimes the main presenting feature of GD. Some of the atypical manifestations are specifically related to GD, while others are also similarly seen in patients with other forms of hyperthyroidism. Lack of knowledge of the association between these findings and GD may lead to delay in diagnosis, misdiagnosis, or unnecessary investigations. The atypical clinical presentations of GD include anemia, vomiting, jaundice, and right heart failure. There is one type of anemia that is not explained by any of the known etiological factors and responds well to hyperthyroidism treatment. This type of anemia resembles anemia of chronic disease and may be termed GD anemia. Other forms of anemia that are associated with GD include pernicious anemia, iron deficiency anemia of celiac disease, and autoimmune hemolytic anemia. Vomiting has been reported as a presenting feature of Graves' disease. Some cases had the typical findings of hyperthyroidism initially masked, and the vomiting did not improve until hyperthyroidism has been detected and treated. Hyperthyroidism may present with jaundice, and on the other hand, deep jaundice may develop with the onset of overt hyperthyroidism in previously compensated chronic liver disease patients. Pulmonary hypertension is reported to be associated with GD and to respond to its treatment. GD-related pulmonary hypertension may be so severe to produce isolated right-sided heart failure that is occasionally found as the presenting manifestation of GD.

1. Introduction

Graves' disease (GD) accounts for up to 80% of hyperthyroidism cases and is estimated to affect 0.5% of the population [1]. It usually presents with the common well-known symptoms and signs (goiter, ophthalmopathy, weight loss, nervousness, tremors, palpitations, sweating, etc.) which are the distinctive features of the disease (Table 1). We can observe another group of manifestations, such as periodic paralysis, apathy, or psychosis, which are less common and less distinctive despite being well documented in relation to GD (Table 1). Over the past few decades, there has been an increase in the number of reports about newly recognized (atypical or unusual) manifestations of hyperthyroidism that are related to various body systems and may create a wide range of differential diagnosis [2, 3]. Most of these atypical manifestations are mainly reported in patients with GD

(Table 1), either due to a specific relation to the autoimmune thyroid disorder, or because GD accounts for the majority of hyperthyroidism cases. Occasionally, one of the atypical manifestations is the main presenting feature of GD [2]. Lack of knowledge of the association between these findings and GD may lead to delay in diagnosis, misdiagnosis, or unnecessary investigations.

The atypical manifestations of GD represent a wide spectrum of clinical and laboratory findings, and in this review we will focus on the clinical part of that spectrum. For example, while hematological manifestations of GD include thrombocytopenia, leucopenia, anemia, and pancytopenia; we will discuss anemia as the clinical presenting feature. Other atypical clinical presentations of GD that will be discussed here are vomiting, jaundice, and right heart failure. These manifestations can be attributed to a wide variety of hematological, gastrointestinal, and cardiopulmonary

TABLE 1: Manifestations of Graves' disease (GD).

Well recognized/common	Recognized/Less common	Unusual/atypical (estimated prevalence in GD patients)
Weight loss	Agitation/psychosis	Jaundice (mild hyperbilirubinemia in up to 30%)
Anxiety/nervousness	Apathy/depression	Vomiting (up to 44%)
Tremors	Confusion/delirium	Anemia (up to 33%)
Goiter	Myopathy	Pancytopenia
Tachyarrhythmia	Paraparesis or quadriparesis	Leukopenia/thrombocytopenia
Breathlessness	Abnormal liver function tests	Heart block
Left ventricular failure		Myocardial infarction
Increased bowel movements		Pulmonary hypertension (up to 43%)
Sweating		Right heart failure
Heat intolerance		Angioedema
Staring gaze/exophthalmos		Erythema annulare centrifugum

causes, and each of them represents a very common clinical condition.

2. Anemia

Anemia is not uncommonly found in association with GD. It has been found in 33% of GD patients [4], and was a presenting manifestation in up to 34% of cases with hyperthyroidism [5]. It is somewhat challenging to face anemia as the presenting manifestation of GD, especially when the typical clinical features of hyperthyroidism are subtle or overlooked. Regardless of the incidental association of GD with other forms of anemia (e.g., iron deficiency anemia, thalassemia, etc.), there are specific types of anemia that are directly or indirectly related to GD (Table 2). As an autoimmune disease, GD was found to be associated with other autoimmune diseases that include pernicious anemia, celiac disease, and autoimmune hemolytic anemia [6, 7]. Moreover, there is a certain type of anemia that occurs with Graves' disease and remains unexplained after excluding all other possible causes [4, 8]. Because of its clear relation to GD, and its cure following hyperthyroidism treatment, this type of anemia may be termed GD anemia [4].

2.1. Graves' Disease Anemia. In the study by Gianoukakis et al., GD anemia was found in 22% of GD patients [4]. In GD anemia the mean corpuscular volume (MCV) could be normal [8] or, probably more commonly, low [4, 9]. Generally the anemia that coexists with GD is observed to be mild and is commoner with severe disease [5] When GD anemia is microcytic, iron indices are normal and hereditary hemoglobinopathies are readily excluded [10]. Anemia may be the sole haematological abnormality, or it may be combined with thrombocytopenia, or leucopenia; and occasionally it may be present as a part of a GD-associated pancytopenia [9, 11, 12]. Erythropoietin levels are within normal reference ranges [4] and bone marrow, if examined, is hypercellular or, less commonly, normocellular; with normal iron stores [9, 13]. The exact pathogenesis of GD anemia remains unclear [8]; however an effect of

the excess thyroid hormones has been postulated [10]. The hypercellular marrow may indicate that erythropoiesis is enhanced due to hyperthyroidism, but in the same time it is ineffective, hence the finding of anemia with low MCV [10]. Hematologically, anemia in the presence of hypercellular marrow could be related to either organ sequestration such as observed in hypersplenism, an enhanced removal of circulating red blood cells by an immune or toxic mechanism, or a hemopoietic stem cell dysfunction such as myelodysplasia [9]. One or both of the latter 2 mechanisms could be responsible for the GD anemia, with myelodysplasia being the most widely accepted explanation [9, 10, 13]. The finding that thyroid-stimulating hormone (TSH) receptor antibodies nonspecifically attach to the surface of the red blood cells, may suggest an autoimmune basis for GD anemia [14]. However, the rare occurrence of GD anemia with hyperthyroid nodular goiter (toxic multinodular goiter and toxic adenoma) makes the effect of thyroid hormones on hemopoiesis a more likely explanation than the autoimmune mechanism [12, 13]. Generally, GD anemia resembles anemia of chronic disease in many aspects including red cell morphology, iron status, erythropoietin levels, and association with markers of inflammation [4]. GD anemia was observed to correct promptly with return to the euthyroid state following hyperthyroidism treatment [4, 9, 10, 12, 13]. Correction included normalisation of the haemoglobin concentration and also of the MCV [4, 9, 10]. This improvement was observed regardless of the mode of therapy of hyperthyroidism, with antithyroid drugs being the more commonly used agents in this regard [4, 9, 10, 13].

2.2. Pernicious Anemia. Pernicious anemia is a well-known form of the autoimmune diseases that may occur in association with GD [6, 7, 15]. In the study by Boelaert et al., the prevalence of pernicious anemia among patients with GD was 1.4% compared to 0.13% in the UK general population [7]. The finding of megaloblastic anemia (marked macrocytosis with hypersegmanted polymorphonuclear leukocytes) in the peripheral blood film of a GD patient should raise the suspicion of this association. Anemia may be associated with

TABLE 2: Types of Anemia Associated with Graves' disease (GD).

	MCV[¥]	Iron status[#]	Prevalence in GD patients	Response to GD treatment
GD Anemia	Low or normal	Normal or high	22%	Y
Pernicious Anemia	High	Normal	1.4%	N
Iron deficiency Anemia of Celiac Disease	Low	Low	0.9%	N
Autoimmune Hemolytic Anemia	Normal or high	Normal	Only single case reports	Y*

Y: Yes; N: No, [¥] mean corpuscular volume, [#] serum iron, serum ferritin, ±bone marrow iron stores, * may respond to thionamide drug therapy alone.

leukopenia or thrombocytopenia; or it could form a part of the pancytopenia of pernicious anemia [16]. The diagnostic workup is a straight forward one and includes checking serum vitamin B12 concentration, red cell or serum folate concentration (to rule out folate deficiency), anti-intrinsic factor antibody gastric parietal cell antibody and the Schilling test.

2.3. Iron Deficiency Anemia due to Celiac Disease. In general, the major cause of iron deficiency anemia (microcytic anemia with a low iron status) is blood loss, either overt or occult [17]. Lack of evidence of blood loss, or the refractoriness to treatment with oral iron may lead to the suspicion of celiac disease. In GD patients, the presence of an iron deficiency anemia may indicate an associated celiac disease, but of course it does not mean omitting blood loss as a common possible cause. In the study by Boelaert et al., the prevalence of celiac disease was 0.9% in GD patients compared to 0.047% in the general UK population [7]. Review of the literature also showed that asymptomatic cases of celiac disease were detected when patients with autoimmune thyroid disease (including GD) were screened by autoantibody testing and duodenal biopsy [18]. However, Sattar et al. stated that screening for celiac disease in patients with autoimmune thyroid disease may not be justified without comorbidities or symptoms [19]. When GD and celiac disease co-exist, it is not clear whether the treatment of one of them affects the course of the other, but it is interesting to mention that treatment with a gluten-free diet has been associated with improvement in the coexistent Hashimoto's hypothyroidism, with reduction of the required thyroxine doses an effect probably related to enhanced drug absorption [18].

2.4. Autoimmune Haemolytic Anemia. The association of GD with autoimmune haemolytic anemia has been described in single case reports in the English and non-English literatures [20–23]. It appears that autoimmune haemolytic anemia is much less commonly found in association with GD when compared with immune thrombocytopenia and pernicious anemia [24]. In some of the case reports, autoimmune haemolytic anemia was present as a part of Evans' syndrome (autoimmune haemolytic anemia and idiopathic thrombocytopenic purpura) in association with GD [25, 26]. In the study by Rajic et al., on 362 subjects with autoimmune haematological disorders, there was no evidence of simultaneous autoimmune thyroid disease in the subgroup of patients with autoimmune haemolytic anemia [24]. Ikeda et al. reported a case of Evans' syndrome in a patient with GD that was not hyperthyroid after treatment with radioiodine, and suggested that an underlying immunological mechanism could be responsible for the association [25]. In this regard it was very interesting to get an effective control of hemolysis with the use of an antithyroid drug alone (namely, propylthiouracil) that was observed in a case of autoimmune haemolytic anemia [20], and in another one with Evan's syndrome [26]. This finding might be related to the earlier observation that microsomal antibodies and TSH receptor antibodies decreased in parallel, while patients with GD were taking carbimazole, whereas no significant changes were observed during treatment with placebo or propranolol [27]. The changes in autoantibody levels during carbimazole treatment were independent of changes in serum thyroxine and could have been due to a direct effect of the drug on autoantibody synthesis [27].

3. Vomiting

Vomiting is one of the most common symptoms of gastrointestinal disease. Patients with GD may present mainly with gastrointestinal symptoms that include diarrhea, frequent defecation, dyspepsia, nausea, vomiting, and abdominal pain [28]. A special clinical situation arises when a thyrotoxic patient, who lacks the typical unique features of hyperthyroidism, presents with severe and persistent vomiting. In one of the earliest reports, Rosenthal et al. described 7 patients with thyrotoxic vomiting with a delay in the detection of hyperthyroidism of 8 & 17 months in two of the cases [29]. Lack of awareness about the association between vomiting and hyperthyroidism may lead to a more marked delay in the diagnosis; that was 7 years in one case report [30]. In a review of 25 newly diagnosed thyrotoxicosis cases 44% of subjects were complaining of vomiting [31]. The mechanism by which vomiting develops in hyperthyroid patients remains uncertain [32]. Researchers have documented increased levels of estrogens in patients of both sexes with thyrotoxicosis [32]. Estrogens may act as an emetic agent with individual variation in susceptibility between patients [32]. Another postulated mechanism is through an increase in beta adrenergic activity due to an increased number of beta adrenergic receptors in hyperthyroid patients [32]. This mechanism has been concluded from the finding of increased adrenergic activity in hyperthyroidism [33], and from the observation that starting treatment with beta blockers ameliorates the vomiting in some cases [32]. However, such an explanation may be debated, as vomiting is more likely to be linked to hypo-, rather than hyper-adrenalism. In addition, the beneficial effect of beta blockers could be due to the reduced thyroid hormone activity (reduced T3 concentration) and not due to a decrease in beta adrenergic activity. Another possible mechanism is through the effect of excess thyroid hormones on gastric motility. Thyroid hormones are thought to decrease gastric emptying secondary to a malfunction of the pyloric sphincter [32]. In a study on 23 patients with hyperthyroidism, 50% had delayed gastric emptying [34]. In another study, a slight but a statistically significant increase in the rate of gastric emptying occurred in patients after restoration of euthyroidism as compared with healthy control subjects [35]. In almost all reports, thyrotoxic vomiting showed an excellent improvement either within several days after the initiation of antithyroid treatment, or in temporal relation with the return to the euthyroid state [29, 30, 32].

3.1. Hyperthyroidism with Vomiting in Pregnancy. Vomiting is common in pregnancy and pregnant women are frequently checked for thyroid disorders [36, 37]. Hyperemesis gravidarum (HG) is known to be associated with mild transient hyperthyroidism probably due to the thyroid stimulating effect of human chorionic gondotropin [36–39]. On the other hand, frank hyperthyroidism is not infrequently discovered for the first time during pregnancy with GD being the most common cause [36, 40, 41]. Moreover, hyperthyroidism occurs in pregnancy with clinical presentation similar to HG and pregnancy itself [36, 41].

A common, challenging scenario develops when a pregnant lady gets severe vomiting together with a biochemical evidence of hyperthyroidism. Here she could be having either transient hyperthyroidism that is associated with HG, or overt hyperthyroidism that manifests with vomiting. It is important to differentiate between the two conditions (Table 3) because transient hyperthyroidism with HG is usually mild, self-limited, and requires no treatment [36, 37]; while frank hyperthyroidism (due to GD in 90% of cases) confers high maternal and fetal morbidity and mortality, and needs to be early detected and treated [36, 40, 41]. The presence of marked tachycardia, tremors, muscle weakness, and ophthalmopathy make the diagnosis of frank hyperthyroidism more likely (Table 3). Goiter especially if associated with a thyroid bruit may point to GD, but one should bear in mind that the thyroid gland may physiologically enlarge during normal pregnancy [41]. The presence of severe vomiting makes HG the likely diagnosis only with the exception of the unusual situation when vomiting is the main presenting symptom of thyrotoxicosis. Biochemically, transient hyperthyroidism of HG usually shows a picture of subclinical hyperthyroidism (Low TSH and normal free T4). The diagnosis of overt hyperthyroidism in pregnant women should be based primarily on a serum TSH value <0.01 mU/L and also a high serum-free T4 value [42]. Free T3 measurements may be useful in women with significantly suppressed serum TSH concentrations and normal or minimally elevated free T4 values [42]. Thyroid

Table 3: Comparison between Graves' disease hyperthyroidism (GD) and Transient hyperthyroidism of hyperemesis Gravidarum (THHG).

	GD	THHG
Hyperthyroidism symptoms[1]	Y	N
Ophthalmopathy	Y	N
Goiter	Y[2]	N[3]
Significant weight loss	Y	N[4]
Severe vomiting	N[5]	Y
TSH	Low (usually <0.01 mU/L)	Low (usually not <0.01 mU/L)
free T4	High (significant rise)	Normal (or mild rise)
Free T3	High	Normal
Persistence >1st trimester	Y	N
Treatment required	Y	N

Y: Yes; N: No, [1]tremors, marked tachycardia, muscle weakness. [2]especially with a bruit. [3]Thyroid gland may enlarge during normal pregnancy. [4]may be 5% or more in severe cases of HG. [5]Rarely severe vomiting is a hyperthyroidism feature.

peroxidase antibodies are markers of autoimmune thyroid disease in general and will not differentiate as they are found in a considerable percentage of pregnant women. TSH receptor antibodies may help to indicate that GD is the cause of the overt hyperthyroidism. Finally, if the clinical and/or the biochemical hyperthyroidism persist beyond the first trimester, causes of hyperthyroidism other than HG should be actively sought, putting in mind that some 10% of women with HG may continue to have symptoms throughout pregnancy [40].

4. Jaundice

The spectrum of liver affection in GD extends from asymptomatic biochemical abnormality to frank hepatitis [3, 43]. In the vast majority of cases it is only the biochemical abnormality that attracts the physician rather than the clinically obvious liver disease [3, 43, 44]. Liver function derangement in hyperthyroid patients can be mainly subdivided into either transaminases elevations (hepatocellular pattern), or intrahepatic cholestasis [3, 43, 45]. In a study by Gürlek et al., at least one liver function test abnormality was found in 60.5% of hyperthyroid patients [44]. Elevations of alkaline phosphatase, alanine aminotransferase, and gamma-glutamyl transpeptidase levels were observed in 44%, 23%, and 14% of the patients, respectively [44]. The mechanism of hepatic injury appears to be relative hypoxia in the perivenular regions, due to an increase in hepatic oxygen demand without an appropriate increase in hepatic blood flow [46]. One theory suggests that the liver is damaged by the systemic effects of excess thyroid hormones [47]. The hypermetabolic state makes the liver more susceptible to injury, and, in addition, thyroid hormones might also have a direct toxic effect on hepatic tissue [47]. In almost all the reported cases, the relation of the intrahepatic cholestasis to hyperthyroidism was documented when the jaundice has resolved with hyperthyroidism treatment, and after excluding all other possible causes of cholestasis [45–47]. Histologically, there are mild lobular inflammatory cellular infiltrates in addition to centrilobular intrahepatic cholestasis [46]. In a case series analysis by Fong et al. the liver histology changes due to hyperthyroidism were not characteristic and nonspecific [48].

Jaundice due to intrahepatic cholestasis may be a prominent symptom in GD patients, and very occasionally it is the presenting manifestation of thyrotoxicosis [44, 48]. Very high-serum bilirubin levels (up to 581 μmol/L) were occasionally noted in patients with hyperthyroidism [45, 47, 48].

The relation of jaundice to GD (or hyperthyroidism in general) can be presented in three clinical scenarios. GD may be the underlying cause of jaundice that develops in a previously healthy subject [47, 49]. The presentation of GD for the first time with jaundice may lead to unnecessary investigations and a delay in management [47]. It is prudent to look carefully for clinical stigmata of thyroid dysfunction, and to consider checking thyroid hormone levels while investigating patients with jaundice of unknown cause. The second clinical scenario develops when a patient with a preexisting chronic liver disease gets deterioration of his liver function tests with deep jaundice. Numerous possibilities are usually considered in this situation including a complicating hepatocellular carcinoma, viral reactivation or superinfection, sepsis, and drug side effects. In this setting, hyperthyroidism should not be omitted as a possible cause. Hegazi et al. reported a case of deep jaundice caused by hyperthyroidism due to a toxic adenoma in a patient with hepatitis B cirrhosis, with return of serum bilirubin to baseline level after treatment with radio-iodine [45]. Thompson et al. reported a patient with primary biliary cirrhosis who had dramatic deterioration of liver functions with jaundice due to the development of GD [50]. The patient's jaundice entirely reversed with treatment of the hyperthyroidism [50]. Thirdly, when a GD patient develops jaundice, a list of possible causes should be considered. These include, an unrelated biliary or hepatic disease [48, 51], an autoimmune liver disease that is known to be associated with GD [46], hepatic congestion due to concomitant congestive cardiac failure [48], hepatic manifestations of hyperthyroidism [47, 49], and hepatotoxic side effects of antithyroid drugs [52]. In the analysis made by Fong et al., severe liver test abnormalities, including deep jaundice occurred in patients with hyperthyroidism alone and with hyperthyroidism with congestive cardiac failure [48]. Drug-induced hepatotoxicity should be considered in those who present with hepatic dysfunction after initiation of thionamide therapy [46, 53].

Treatment of a hyperthyroid patient with jaundice needs to be considered and therefore, it will be discussed here. Review of the literature showed that treatment options other than thionamide drugs might have been preferably used in cases of jaundice and hyperthyroidism. In many of the cases the mode of antithyroid therapy was radio-iodine [45, 54], or thyroidectomy [51, 55]. Antithyroid drugs have hepatotoxic side effects in 0.5% of cases with

methimazole and carbimazole mainly producing cholestasis, and propylthiouracil mainly causing hepatocellular damage [52]. These side effects are idiosyncratic rather than dose related [46]. Methimazole therapy may deteriorate a GD-related cholestatic jaundice [53]. However, it has been reported that carbimazole and methimazole were successfully used in restoring euthyroidism as well as ameliorating the hyperthyroidism-related jaundice [47, 56].

In the absence of another evidence of liver disease, and when jaundice is purely due to the hyperthyroidism, thionamide drugs may be used with monitoring of serum bilirubin and liver function tests. In patients with acute or chronic liver disease who develop GD that aggravates their jaundice, the small probability of hepatotoxic side effects of thionamide drugs may carry the risk of inducing fulminating hepatic failure [51], so that alternative GD treatment options are preferred.

5. Right Heart Failure

Thyroid hormone effects on the cardiovascular system include increased resting heart rate, left ventricular contractility, blood volume, and decreased systemic vascular resistance [57, 58]. Cardiac contractility is enhanced and cardiac output may be increased by 50% to-300% over that of normal subjects [57, 58]. The well-recognized cardiovascular manifestations of hyperthyroidism include palpitations, tachycardia, exercise intolerance, dyspnea on exertion, widened pulse pressure, and atrial fibrillation [57, 58]. In spite of the increased cardiac output and contractility, the left ventricular failure that may occur in severe and chronic cases of hyperthyroidism could be explained by a tachycardia-related left ventricular dysfunction, and/or a thyrotoxic cardiomyopathy [57, 58]. The higher prevalence of hyperthyroid heart failure in older age groups signifies the contribution of other cardiovascular comorbidities that include hypertension and coronary artery disease [57].

In addition to the well-known presentations, a variety of unusual cardiovascular manifestations are increasingly being reported in association with hyperthyroidism. These include pulmonary arterial hypertension (PH) [59, 60], right heart failure [61, 62], myocardial infarction [63], and heart block [64]. Clinically, isolated right-sided heart failure may be the presenting feature of GD.

In an echocardiographic study by Marvisi et al., mild PH was found in 43% of the 114 hyperthyroid patients and in none of the healthy control group [59]. In another study by Mercé et al., there was a high prevalence of PH in hyperthyroid patients [60]. Additional studies [65], case series [66], and case reports [61] have shown similar findings. The pathophysiologic link between thyroid disease and PH remains unclear [67]. Possible explanations include immune-mediated endothelial damage or dysfunction, increased cardiac output resulting in endothelial injury, and increased metabolism of intrinsic pulmonary vasodilator substances [60]. Review of the literature reveals some support for the immune-mediated mechanism [68, 69]. In a review by Biondi and kahaly, PH was more linked to GD than to other causes of hyperthyroidism [68]; and in a study by Chu et al., there was a high prevalence of autoimmune thyroid disease in patients with PH [69]. However, in a study by Armigliato et al., the immune mechanism has been questioned because 52% of hyperthyroid subjects with PH did not have evidence of autoimmune thyroid disease [70]. Also in the study by Mercé et al., pulmonary hypertension did not correlate with the cause of hyperthyroidism [60]. Furthermore, Marvisi et al. found no statistical difference in thyroid antibody levels between the hyperthyroid study group and the euthyroid control group and stated that PH could be due to a direct influence of thyroid hormones on pulmonary vasculature [59]. We tend to believe that an effect of excess thyroid hormones may be responsible for the development of PH, especially with the finding of PH also in patients with hyperthyroid nodular goiter.

In spite of the observation that PH was mild in most of the studied hyperthyroid patients [58], cases of severe PH leading to right-sided heart failure are increasingly being recognized [71]. GD occasionally presents with frank isolated right heart failure due to the severe PH [61, 72, 73]. All other possible causes of right ventricular failure including left-sided systolic and/or diastolic dysfunctions have been excluded in reported cases [61]. PH as well as right heart failure showed improvement after the treatment of the concomitant hyperthyroidism [58, 61, 71, 73]. It may take several months for the pulmonary artery pressure to normalize following the initiation of antithyroid treatment [61, 66]. In one case report, the severe pulmonary hypertension has dropped to a near-normal value, only after 14 months from initiation of carbimazole therapy, in spite of a long period of clinical and biochemical euthyroidism [61].

6. Conclusions and Recommendations

The unusual manifestations of GD are diverse and affect various body systems. They include hematological, cardiovascular, gastrointestinal, hepatic, and dermatological manifestations (Table 1). Reports of other less frequent or rare presentations like venous thromboembolism [74] and cerebral vasculitis [75] may need further support and documentation. One or more of the unusual manifestations may be the main presenting feature of GD. Awareness about the relation of these presentations to GD or hyperthyroidism is essential to avoid wrong diagnosis and unnecessary investigations.

The mechanism remains uncertain in the majority of the atypical manifestations. However, a good response to hyperthyroidism treatment is almost guaranteed. The response to hyperthyroidism treatment is either rapid or quite delayed. In the case of vomiting the response occurs within days, however, in the case of right heart failure the improvement occurs within several months from starting the treatment. The excellent recovery that occurs in response to the restoration of euthyroidism makes the effect of excess thyroid hormones the likely underlying mechanism in most of the cases. With the exception of the autoimmune conditions that are associated with GD, the occurrence of the atypical manifestations also in patients with hyperthyroid nodular goiter stands against an autoimmune basis of pathogenesis.

Such atypical presentations appear to affect significant percentages of GD patients; however, most of the studies conducted in this respect were small. For instance, vomiting was a symptom in 44% of 25 thyrotoxic patients [31], and alkaline phosphatase was raised in 44% of 43 hyperthyroid patients [44]. Larger studies to further evaluate the prevalence of each of the atypical features in GD patients are needed to confirm that some of these findings are not unusual, but are rather under-recognized. The widespread hyperthyroidism manifestations that influence all body systems make us believe that the thyroid hormone effects on various body tissues are not yet fully unveiled.

References

[1] G. A. Brent, "Clinical practice. Graves' disease," *The New England Journal of Medicine*, vol. 358, no. 24, pp. 2594–2605, 2008.

[2] E. A. Boxall, R. W. Lauener, and H. W. Mcintosh, "Atypical manifestations of hyperthyroidism," *Canadian Medical Association Journal*, vol. 91, pp. 204–211, 1964.

[3] M. O. Hegazi and M. R. El-sonbaty, "Unusual presentations of hyperthyroidism," in *Handbook of Hyperthyroidism: Etiology, Diagnosis and Treatment*, L. Mertens and J. Bogaert, Eds., pp. 265–270, Nova Publishers, 2011.

[4] A. G. Gianoukakis, M. J. Leigh, P. Richards et al., "Characterization of the anaemia associated with Graves' disease," *Clinical Endocrinology*, vol. 70, no. 5, pp. 781–787, 2009.

[5] M. Klein, G. Weryha, P. Kaminsky, M. Duc, and J. Leclère, "Hematological manifestations of hyperthyroidism," *Annales de Medecine Interne*, vol. 144, no. 2, pp. 127–135, 1993.

[6] E. Biró, Z. Szekanecz, L. Czirják et al., "Association of systemic and thyroid autoimmune diseases," *Clinical Rheumatology*, vol. 25, no. 2, pp. 240–245, 2006.

[7] K. Boelaert, P. R. Newby, M. J. Simmonds et al., "Prevalence and relative risk of other autoimmune diseases in subjects with autoimmune thyroid disease," *American Journal of Medicine*, vol. 123, no. 2, pp. 183.e1–183.e9, 2010.

[8] D. Barth and J. V. Hirschmann, "Anemia of endocrine disorders," in *Wintrobe's Atlas of Clinical Hematology*, D. C. Tkachuk and J. V. Hirschmann, Eds., p. 6, Lippincott Williams & Wilkins, 2007.

[9] M. Hegazi, R. Kumar, Z. Bitar, and E. Ibrahim, "Pancytopenia related to Graves' disease," *Annals of Saudi Medicine*, vol. 28, no. 1, pp. 48–49, 2008.

[10] M. S. Akasheh, "Graves' disease mimicking β-thalassaemia trait," *Postgraduate Medical Journal*, vol. 70, no. 822, pp. 300–301, 1994.

[11] B. Shaw and A. B. Mehta, "Pancytopenia responding to treatment of hyperthyroidism: a clinical case and review of the literature," *Clinical and Laboratory Haematology*, vol. 24, no. 6, pp. 385–387, 2002.

[12] M. Duquenne, D. Lakomsky, J. C. Humbert, S. Hadjadj, G. Weryha, and J. Leclère, "Resolutive pancytopenia with effective treatment of hyperthyroidism," *Presse Medicale*, vol. 24, no. 17, pp. 807–810, 1995.

[13] R. Akoum, S. Michel, T. Wafic et al., "Myelodysplastic syndrome and pancytopenia responding to treatment of hyperthyroidism: peripheral blood and bone marrow analysis before and after antihormonal treatment," *Journal of Cancer Research and Therapeutics*, vol. 3, no. 1, pp. 43–46, 2007.

[14] A. Sato, M. Zakarija, and J. M. McKenzie, "Characteristics of thyrotropin binding to bovine thyroid plasma membranes and the influence of human IgG," *Endocrine Research Communications*, vol. 4, no. 2, pp. 95–113, 1977.

[15] B. H. Toh, I. R. van Driel, and P. A. Gleeson, "Mechanisms of disease: pernicious anemia," *The New England Journal of Medicine*, vol. 337, no. 20, pp. 1441–1448, 1997.

[16] R. W. Burns and T. W. Burns, "Pancytopenia due to vitamin B12 deficiency associated with Graves' disease," *Missouri Medicine*, vol. 93, no. 7, pp. 368–372, 1996.

[17] J. D. Cook and B. S. Skikne, "Iron deficiency: definition and diagnosis," *Journal of Internal Medicine*, vol. 226, no. 5, pp. 349–355, 1989.

[18] C. L. Ch'ng, M. K. Jones, and J. G. Kingham, "Celiac disease and autoimmune thyroid disease," *Clinical Medicine and Research*, vol. 5, no. 3, pp. 184–192, 2007.

[19] N. Sattar, F. Lazare, M. Kacer et al., "Celiac disease in children, adolescents, and young adults with autoimmune thyroid disease," *Journal of Pediatrics*, vol. 158, pp. 272–275, 2011.

[20] T. Ogihara, H. Katoh, H. Yoshitake, S. Iyori, and I. Saito, "Hyperthyroidism associated with autoimmune hemolytic anemia and periodic paralysis: a report of a case in which anti-hyperthyroid therapy alone was effective against hemolysis," *Japanese Journal of Medicine*, vol. 26, no. 3, pp. 401–403, 1987.

[21] D. O'Brien, D. J. Lyons, and J. F. Fielding, "A case of Graves' disease associated with autoimmune haemolytic anaemia," *Irish Journal of Medical Science*, vol. 158, no. 6, p. 155, 1989.

[22] M. Mukai, A. Sagawa, I. Watanabe et al., "A case of autoimmune hemolytic anemia associated with Graves' disease," *Nihon Naika Gakkai zasshi Journal*, vol. 75, no. 5, pp. 644–649, 1986.

[23] A. B. Andrusenko, T. S. Kamynina, and O. P. Bogatyrev, "Cushing's syndrome associated with toxic goiter and autoimmune hemolytic anemia," *Sovetskaya Meditsina*, no. 8, pp. 115–116, 1990.

[24] M. Rajic, S. Djurica, D. P. Milosevic, and N. Markovic, "Autoimmune haemopoietic disturbances simultaneous with autoimmune thyroid diseases," *Srpski Arhiv za Celokupno Lekarstvo*, vol. 133, pp. 52–54, 2005.

[25] K. Ikeda, Y. Maruyama, M. Yokoyama et al., "Association of Graves' disease with Evan's syndrome in a patient with IgA nephropathy," *Internal Medicine*, vol. 40, no. 10, pp. 1004–1010, 2001.

[26] T. Ushiki, M. Masuko, K. Nikkuni et al., "Successful remission of Evans syndrome associated with Graves' disease by using propylthiouracil monotherapy," *Internal Medicine*, vol. 50, pp. 621–625, 2011.

[27] A. M. McGregor, M. M. Petersen, S. M. McLachlan, P. Rooke, B. R. Smith, and R. Hall, "Carbimazole and the autoimmune response in Graves' disease," *The New England Journal of Medicine*, vol. 303, no. 6, pp. 302–307, 1980.

[28] E. C. Ebert, "The thyroid and the gut," *Journal of Clinical Gastroenterology*, vol. 44, no. 6, pp. 402–406, 2010.

[29] F. D. Rosenthal, C. Jones, and S. I. Lewis, "Thyrotoxic vomiting," *British Medical Journal*, vol. 2, no. 6029, pp. 209–211, 1976.

[30] L. Y. Chen, B. Zhou, Z. W. Chen, and L. Z. Fang, "Recurrent severe vomiting due to hyperthyroidism," *Journal of Zhejiang University Science B*, vol. 11, no. 3, pp. 218–220, 2010.

[31] M. B. Harper, "Vomiting, nausea, and abdominal pain: unrecognized symptoms of thyrotoxicosis," *Journal of Family Practice*, vol. 29, no. 4, pp. 382–386, 1989.

[32] S. Shim, H. S. Ryu, H. J. Oh, and Y. S. Kim, "Thyrotoxic vomiting: a case report and possible mechanisms," *Journal of Neurogastroenterology and Motility*, vol. 16, pp. 428–432, 2010.

[33] J. P. Bilezikian and J. N. Loeb, "The influence of hyperthyroidism and hypothyroidism on α- and β-adrenergic receptor systems and adrenergic responsiveness," *Endocrine Reviews*, vol. 4, no. 4, pp. 378–388, 1983.

[34] B. Pfaffenbach, R. J. Adamek, D. Hagelmann, J. Schaffstein, and M. Wegener, "Effect of hyperthyroidism on antral myoelectrical activity, gastric emptying and dyspepsia in man," *Hepato-Gastroenterology*, vol. 44, no. 17, pp. 1500–1508, 1997.

[35] K. Jonderko, G. Jonderko, C. Marcisz, and T. Golab, "Gastric emptying in hyperthyroidism," *American Journal of Gastroenterology*, vol. 92, no. 5, pp. 835–838, 1997.

[36] D. M. Neale, A. C. Cootauco, and G. Burrow, "Thyroid disease in pregnancy," *Clinics in Perinatology*, vol. 34, no. 4, pp. 543–557, 2007.

[37] T. J. Caffrey, "Transient hyperthyroidism of hyperemesis gravidarum: a sheep in wolf's clothing," *Journal of the American Board of Family Practice*, vol. 13, no. 1, pp. 35–38, 2000.

[38] J. E. Haddow, M. R. McClain, G. Lambert-Messerlian et al., "Variability in thyroid-stimulating hormone suppression by human chronic gonadotropin during early pregnancy," *Journal of Clinical Endocrinology and Metabolism*, vol. 93, no. 9, pp. 3341–3347, 2008.

[39] T. M. Goodwin, M. Montoro, J. H. Mestman, A. E. Pekary, and J. M. Hershman, "The role of chorionic gonadotropin in transient hyperthyroidism of hyperemesis gravidarum," *Journal of Clinical Endocrinology and Metabolism*, vol. 75, no. 5, pp. 1333–1337, 1992.

[40] A. T. Luetic and B. Miskovic, "Is hyperthyroidism underestimated in pregnancy and misdiagnosed as hyperemesis gravidarum?" *Medical Hypotheses*, vol. 75, no. 4, pp. 383–386, 2010.

[41] J. C. Galofre and T. F. Davies, "Autoimmune thyroid disease in pregnancy: a review," *Journal of Women's Health*, vol. 18, no. 11, pp. 1847–1856, 2009.

[42] American College of Obstetricians and Gynecologists, "ACOG practice bulletin. Clinical management guidelines for obstetrician-gynecologists. Number 37, August 2002. (replaces practice bulletin number 32, November 2001). Thyroid disease in pregnancy," *Obstet Gynecol*, vol. 100, pp. 387–396, 2002.

[43] A. Maheshwari and P. J. Thuluvath, "Endocrine diseases and the liver," *Clinics in Liver Disease*, vol. 15, no. 1, pp. 55–67, 2011.

[44] A. Gürlek, V. Cobankara, and M. Bayraktar, "Liver tests in hyperthyroidism: effect of antithyroid therapy," *Journal of Clinical Gastroenterology*, vol. 24, no. 3, pp. 180–183, 1997.

[45] M. O. Hegazi, A. Marafie, and M. Alajmi, "Thyrotoxicosis-associated cholestasis in a patient with hepatitis B cirrhosis," *Turkish Journal of Endocrinology and Metabolism*, vol. 12, pp. 99–100, 2008.

[46] R. Malik and H. Hodgson, "The relationship between the thyroid gland and the liver," *QJM*, vol. 95, no. 9, pp. 559–569, 2002.

[47] P. J. Owen, A. Baghomian, J. H. Lazarus, and A. J. Godkin, "An unusual cause of jaundice," *British Medical Journal*, vol. 335, no. 7623, pp. 773–774, 2007.

[48] T. L. Fong, J. G. McHutchison, and T. B. Reynolds, "Hyperthyroidism and hepatic dysfunction: a case series analysis," *Journal of Clinical Gastroenterology*, vol. 14, no. 3, pp. 240–244, 1992.

[49] S. C. Barnes, J. M. Wicking, and J. D. Johnston, "Graves' disease presenting with cholestatic jaundice," *Annals of Clinical Biochemistry*, vol. 36, no. 5, pp. 677–679, 1999.

[50] N. P. Thompson, S. Leader, C. P. Jamieson, W. R. Burnham, and A. K. Burroughs, "Reversible jaundice in primary biliary cirrhosis due to hyperthyroidism," *Gastroenterology*, vol. 106, no. 5, pp. 1342–1343, 1994.

[51] M. Enghofer, K. Badenhoop, S. Zeuzem et al., "Fulminant hepatitis A in a patient with severe hyperthyroidism: rapid recovery from hepatic coma after plasmapheresis and total thyroidectomy," *Journal of Clinical Endocrinology and Metabolism*, vol. 85, no. 5, pp. 1765–1769, 2000.

[52] D. S. Cooper, "Hyperthyroidism," *The Lancet*, vol. 362, no. 9382, pp. 459–468, 2003.

[53] M. Majeed and A. Babu, "Cholestasis secondary to hyperthyroidism made worse by methimazole," *American Journal of the Medical Sciences*, vol. 332, no. 1, pp. 51–53, 2006.

[54] M. Chawla and C. S. Bal, "Four cases of coexistent thyrotoxicosis and jaundice: results of radioiodine treatment and a brief review," *Thyroid*, vol. 18, no. 3, pp. 289–292, 2008.

[55] K. Hull, R. Horenstein, R. Naglieri, K. Munir, M. Ghany, and F. S. Celi, "Two cases of thyroid storm-associated cholestatic jaundice," *Endocrine Practice*, vol. 13, no. 5, pp. 476–480, 2007.

[56] H. Ichikawa, H. Ebinuma, S. Tada et al., "A case of severe cholestatic jaundice with hyperthyroidism successfully treated with methimazole," *Clinical Journal of Gastroenterology*, vol. 2, no. 4, pp. 315–319, 2009.

[57] I. Klein and S. Danzi, "Thyroid disease and the heart," *Circulation*, vol. 116, no. 15, pp. 1725–1735, 2007.

[58] I. Klein and K. Ojamaa, "Thyroid hormone and the cardiovascular system," *The New England Journal of Medicine*, vol. 344, no. 7, pp. 501–509, 2001.

[59] M. Marvisi, P. Zambrelli, M. Brianti, G. Civardi, R. Lampugnani, and R. Delsignore, "Pulmonary hypertension is frequent in hyperthyroidism and normalizes after therapy," *European Journal of Internal Medicine*, vol. 17, no. 4, pp. 267–271, 2006.

[60] J. Mercé, S. Ferrás, C. Oltra et al., "Cardiovascular abnormalities in hyperthyroidism: a prospective Doppler echocardiographic study," *American Journal of Medicine*, vol. 118, no. 2, pp. 126–131, 2005.

[61] M. O. Hegazi, A. El Sayed, and H. El Ghoussein, "Pulmonary hypertension responding to hyperthyroidism treatment," *Respirology*, vol. 13, no. 6, pp. 923–925, 2008.

[62] Y. Paran, A. Nimrod, Y. Goldin, and D. Justo, "Pulmonary hypertension and predominant right heart failure in thyrotoxicosis," *Resuscitation*, vol. 69, no. 2, pp. 339–341, 2006.

[63] R. Patel, G. Peterson, A. Rohatgi et al., "Hyperthyroidism-associated coronary vasospasm with myocardial infarction and subsequent euthyroid angina," *Thyroid*, vol. 18, no. 2, pp. 273–276, 2008.

[64] J. A. Dave and I. L. Ross, "Complete heart block in a patient with Graves' disease," *Thyroid*, vol. 18, no. 12, pp. 1329–1331, 2008.

[65] A. Yazar, O. Döven, S. Atis et al., "Systolic pulmonary artery pressure and serum uric acid levels in patients with hyperthyroidism," *Archives of Medical Research*, vol. 34, no. 1, pp. 35–40, 2003.

[66] A. Soroush-Yari, S. Burstein, G. W. Hoo, and S. M. Santiago, "Pulmonary hypertension in men with thyrotoxicosis," *Respiration*, vol. 72, no. 1, pp. 90–94, 2005.

[67] J. H. Li, R. E. Safford, J. F. Aduen, M. G. Heckman, J. E. Crook, and C. D. Burger, "Pulmonary hypertension and thyroid disease," *Chest*, vol. 132, no. 3, pp. 793–797, 2007.

[68] B. Biondi and G. J. Kahaly, "Cardiovascular involvement in patients with different causes of hyperthyroidism," *Nature Reviews Endocrinology*, vol. 6, no. 8, pp. 431–443, 2010.

[69] J. W. Chu, P. N. Kao, J. L. Faul, and R. L. Doyle, "High prevalence of autoimmune thyroid disease in pulmonary arterial hypertension," *Chest*, vol. 122, no. 5, pp. 1668–1673, 2002.

[70] M. Armigliato, R. Paolini, S. Aggio et al., "Hyperthyroidism as a cause of pulmonary arterial hypertension: a prospective study," *Angiology*, vol. 57, no. 5, pp. 600–606, 2006.

[71] P. Dahl, S. Danzi, and I. Klein, "Thyrotoxic cardiac disease," *Current Heart Failure Reports*, vol. 5, no. 3, pp. 170–176, 2008.

[72] T. E. Whitner, C. J. Hudson, T. D. Smith, and L. Littmann, "Hyperthyroidism: presenting as isolated tricuspid regurgitation and right heart failure," *Texas Heart Institute Journal*, vol. 32, no. 2, pp. 244–245, 2005.

[73] H. F. Lozano and C. N. Sharma, "Reversible pulmonary hypertension, tricuspid regurgitation and right-sided heart failure associated with hyperthyroidism: case report and review of the literature," *Cardiology in Review*, vol. 12, no. 6, pp. 299–305, 2004.

[74] M. Franchini, G. Lippi, and G. Targher, "Hyperthyroidism and venous thrombosis: a casual or causal association? A systematic literature review," *Clinical and Applied Thrombosis/Hemostasis*, vol. 17, no. 4, pp. 387–392, 2010.

[75] M. S. Rocha, S. M. Brucki, and A. C. Ferraz, "Cerebral vasculitis and basedow-graves disease: report of two cases," *Arquivos de Neuropsiquiatria*, vol. 59, no. 4, pp. 948–953, 2001.

22

Iodine Intake and Thyroid Function in Pregnant Women in a Private Clinical Practice in Northwestern Sydney before Mandatory Fortification of Bread with Iodised Salt

Norman Blumenthal,[1] Karen Byth,[2] and Creswell J. Eastman[3, 4]

[1] Department of Obstetrics and Gynaecology, Blacktown Hospital and Norwest Private Hospital, 9 Norbrik Drive, Bella Vista 2153, Sydney, NSW, Australia
[2] NHMRC Clinical Trials Centre, Faculty of Medicine, 92 Parramatta Road, Camperdown, Sydney, NSW 2050, Australia
[3] International Council for Control of Iodine Deficiency Disorders, Sydney Medical School, University of Sydney, Sydney, NSW, Australia
[4] Sydney Thyroid Clinic, Westmead Specialist Centre, Suite 8, 16-18 Mons Road Westmead, NSW 2145, Australia

Correspondence should be addressed to Creswell J. Eastman, eastcje@ozemail.com.au

Academic Editor: Elizabeth N. Pearce

Aim. The primary objective of the study was to assess the iodine nutritional status, and its effect on thyroid function, of pregnant women in a private obstetrical practice in Sydney. *Methods.* It was a cross-sectional study undertaken between November 2007 and March 2009. Blood samples were taken from 367 women at their first antenatal visit between 7 and 11 weeks gestation for measurement of thyroid stimulating hormone (TSH) and free thyroxine (FT4) levels and spot urine samples for urinary iodine excretion were taken at the same time as blood collection. *Results.* The median urinary iodine concentration (UIC) for all women was 81 μg/l (interquartile range 41–169 μg/l). 71.9% of the women exhibited a UIC of <150 μg/l. 26% of the women had a UIC <50 μg/l, and 12% had a UIC <20 μg/l. The only detectable influences on UIC were daily milk intake and pregnancy supplements. There was no statistically significant association between UIC and thyroid function and no evidence for an effect of iodine intake on thyroid function. *Conclusions.* There is a high prevalence of mild to moderate iodine deficiency in women in Western Sydney but no evidence for a significant adverse effect on thyroid function. The 6.5% prevalence of subclinical hypothyroidism is unlikely to be due to iodine deficiency.

1. Introduction

Iodine deficiency has been well documented in many parts of the developing world and surprisingly it has reemerged in Australia despite various programs to reduce its incidence [1, 2]. Urinary iodine levels, which are used as a measure of dietary iodine intake, have declined over the past decade, and Australia is now defined by the World Health Organization (WHO) criteria as a mildly iodine-deficient country [3]. The physiological importance of iodine is its central role in maintaining normal thyroid function. Inadequate iodine supply to the thyroid gland will result in decreased thyroid hormone synthesis and enlargement of the gland. During pregnancy iodine intake needs to be increased to meet the demands upon the thyroid gland to boost thyroid hormone production by up to 50% more than preconception requirements, to ensure a supply of thyroxine and iodine to the foetus and to compensate for increased renal iodide clearance [4]

Iodine deficiency in an asymptomatic young female population may have a negative impact on thyroid function and neonatal outcome, as infants born in areas of moderate to-severe iodine deficiency suffer from a variety of neurodevelopmental disorders caused by irreversible brain damage in utero [5, 6], but adverse effects from mild maternal iodine-deficiency remain less certain. The incidence of neonatal hypothyroidism is also increased in an iodine deficient population, and there is evidence to suggest that severe

TABLE 1: Summary statistics for the 367 patients studied.

Mean age (SD) years	32.0 yrs	(4.3) yrs
Parity	n	(%)
Primiparas	145	(40%)
Multiparas	222	(60%)
Highest level education		
School certificate	92	(25%)
Higher school certificate	100	(27%)
Tertiary	175	(48%)
Ethnicity		
Australian born	294	(79.3%)
European	13	(3.5%)
Asian	9	(2.5%)
Filipino	4	(1.1%)
Other	45	(12.3%)
Not available	5	(1.4%)

iodine deficiency may increase rates of miscarriage and stillbirths [6].

There is an increasing body of information confirming a high prevalence of mild-to-moderate iodine deficiency in pregnant women in the Australian State of New South Wales (NSW), Victoria, and Tasmania, as evidenced by reduced median urinary iodine concentrations in a number of sporadic studies. [3, 7–11]. None of these studies in pregnant women have examined thyroid function or thyroid volume so it is unknown if iodine deficiency documented in pregnant Australian women has any significant adverse effect on thyroid function.

The aim of this study was to assess the iodine nutritional status, and its effect on thyroid function, in pregnant women in a private obstetrical practice in metropolitan Sydney. We also wanted to determine if there was an association between urinary iodine concentration, the intake of specific iodine-rich foods, and the use of vitamin and mineral supplements taken by the pregnant women. Analysis of supplements was not undertaken to confirm iodine content reported on the label.

2. Materials and Methods

2.1. Participants and Setting. This study was performed in a private practice setting in North Western Sydney between November 2007 and February 2009, where 367 new consecutive antenatal patients were reviewed in their first trimester. At the time of initial booking with the private clinic, between 7 and 11 weeks gestation, routine antenatal investigations were performed. At the same time thyroid function tests, thyroid antibodies, and urinary iodine concentrations were measured. The patients answered questions in relation to their dietary habits, vitamin and mineral supplementation, and family history of thyroid disease. The personal details of the participants are given in Table 1. All women consented to have their blood and urine samples assessed for this study and freely provided the historical information. Women with known thyroid disease were excluded from the study. The

study has been approved by the Ethics Committee of the Sydney West Area Health Service.

2.2. Urinary Iodine Concentration (UIC), Serum-Free T4, Free T3, and Thyroid-Stimulating Hormone (TSH) Measurements. Iodine concentrations were measured on spot samples of urine by inductively coupled plasma mass spectrometry (ICPMS) in Laverty pathology laboratories in Sydney. Analytical details of the ICPMS method have previously been published (3). Serum TSH concentrations were measured by a chemiluminescent immunoassay on the ADVIA Centaur platform (Bayer Health Care). Serum-free T3 and T4 concentrations were also measured on the ADVIA Centaur platform by a chemiluminescent immunoassay method. For serum TSH the detection limit was 0.01 mIU/L, and intraassay coefficients of variation (CV) were 2.48 and 2.44% at TSH concentrations of 0.74 mIU/L and 5.65 mIU/L, respectively. Between assay % CV varied from 3.2 to 5.9%. The intraassay and inter-assay CVs for FT4 at 13.9 pmol/L were 2.31% and 3.03%, respectively. Reference intervals provided by the laboratory for serum TSH, FT4, and FT3 in euthyroid adults were from 0.5 to 4.5 mIU/L, 10 to 20 pmol/L, and 3.5 to 6.0 pmol/L, respectively. This laboratory did not provide a specific reference range for pregnancy.

2.3. Questionnaire. All patients were asked to state their parity, level of education and ethnicity. A personal history or family history of thyroid dysfunction was obtained, and dietary questions were asked in relation to servings of milk and dairy products per day and portions of fish per week over the preceding weeks of the pregnancy. The use of iodised or noniodised salt was determined and also the use (if any) of vitamin and mineral supplementation, including the brands used.

2.4. Statistical Analysis. The statistical software package SPSS Version 17 was used to analyse the data. Two-tailed tests with a significance level of 5% were used throughout. Chi-squared or Fisher's exact tests, as appropriate, were used to test for association between categorical variables. The Mann-Whitney test or Kruskal-Wallis nonparametric analysis of variance were used to test for differences in the distribution of continuous variables by group. Spearman rank correlation (r) was used to quantify the degree of association between continuous and ordered categorical variables.

3. Results

3.1. Urinary Iodine. The median urinary iodine concentration (UIC) for all women (n = 367) was 81 µg/L with an interquartile range of 41 to 169 µg/L. A histogram illustrates the distribution of UIC in Figure 1. By conventional WHO UIC standards for a nonpregnant, nonlactating adult population (12), 58% of the women in this study were iodine deficient, comprising 26% with UIC < 50–100 µg/L,, 20% with a UIC 20–49 µg/L, and 12% <20 µg/L. By current WHO standards for pregnant women, 71.9% of the women were iodine deficient having a UIC of

TABLE 2: Median and quartiles for UIC by subgroup and P value for test of homogeneity across subgroups.

Variable	Values taken	(Percent)	Median	Percentile 25	Percentile 75	P value
Parity	Primiparas	(40%)	85	41	175	0.736
	Multiparas	(60%)	80	41	161	
Education	School certificate	(25%)	105	52	231	
	Higher school certificate	(27%)	64	33	117	0.002
	Tertiary	(48%)	86	42	166	
Ethnicity	Australian	(79.3%)	78	41	156	
	European	(3.5%)	81	39	178	
	Asian	(2.5%)	80	44	185	0.582
	Filipino	(1.1%)	94	41	177	
	Other	(12.3%)	114	56	180	
History of thyroid disease	Familial and patient	(2.2%)	91	51	183	
	Familial	(14.9%)	90	43	226	0.351
	Patient	(3.3%)	106	72	244	
	Nil	(79.6%)	79	39	156	
Vitamin supplements	Nil	(28.3%)	69	38	136	
	Elevit	(31.9%)	71	39	120	
	Fefol	(0.3%)	32	32	32	<0.001
	Blackmores (iodine 150 μg)	(27.8%)	123	61	226	
	Fabfol (iodine 150 μg)	(4.7%)	60	31	78	
	Other	(6.9%)	123	59	260	
Vitamin supplement containing iodine	No	(67.5%)	72	39	141	0.001
	Yes	(32.5%)	115	48	213	
Iodised salt	No	(78.6%)	81	39	162	0.396
	Yes	(21.4%)	81	47	185	
Milk (grouped)	Nil	(13.0%)	71	39	180	
	<1 serve/day	(23.8%)	77	31	126	0.035
	1 serve/day	(42.3%)	75	45	155	
	>1 serve/day	(21.0%)	105	59	208	
Dairy (grouped)	Nil	(19.1%)	101	47	273	
	<1 serve/day	(22.2%)	76	41	154	0.078
	1 serve/day	(40.7%)	78	34	149	
	>1 serve/day	(18.0%)	87	42	129	
Fish (grouped)	Nil	(29.8%)	72	41	159	
	<1 serve/day	(15.2%)	83	51	120	0.764
	1 serve/day	(39.1%)	89	38	193	
	>1 serve/day	(16.0%)	87	47	179	
Overall		$N = 367$	81	41	169	

less than 150 μg/L (13). Table 2 sets out the median and interquartile range of UIC by subgroup. There was a statistically significant association between UIC and vitamin supplement ($P < 0.001$). Supplements, during the period of the study, known to contain iodine include Blackmores and Fabfol preparations. In particular, the median UIC of those not taking an iodine supplement was 72 μg/L (IQR 39 to 141), compared with 115 μg/L (from IQR 48 to 213) for those taking a supplement containing iodine ($P = 0.001$). There was no statistically significant association between UIC and parity, ethnicity, and history of thyroid disease. Although there was a significant association between UIC and educational level ($P = 0.002$), there was no significant

rank correlation between UIC and increasing educational level ($r = -0.054$, $P = 0.307$). With respect to diet, there was no significant association between UIC, use of iodised salt, dairy or seafood intake. However, there was a significant association between UIC and milk intake ($P = 0.035$).

3.2. Serum TSH and FT4 Concentrations.

Table 3 sets out the mean (SD), median, 2.5th, and 97.5th percentiles for the distributions of UIC, TSH and Free T4 concentrations. The distributions for TSH, and Free T4 are illustrated in Figure 2. The mean TSH level was 1.17 mIU/L ±1.11 (SD),

TABLE 3: Mean, SD, median, 2.5th, and 97.5th percentiles for TSH, Free T4, and UI concentrations.

	Mean	Standard deviation	Median	Percentile 2.5	Percentile 97.5
TSH (mIU/L)	1.17	(1.11)	0.98	0.03	3.40
T4 (pmol/L)	15.4	(2.7)	15.0	10.0	20.5
Urinary iodine (μg/L)	134.4	(190.0)	81.0	9.2	508.0

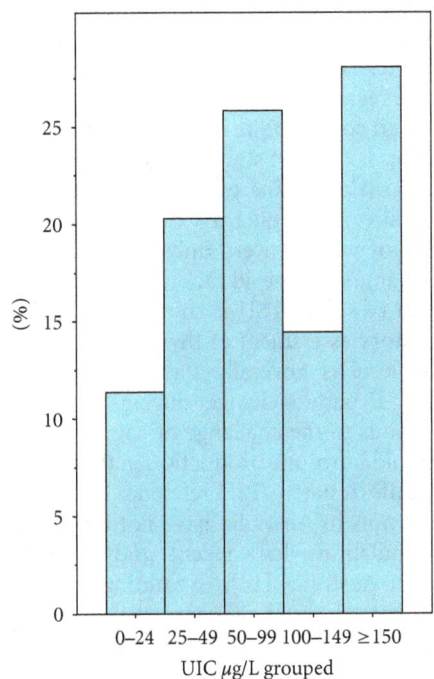

(a)

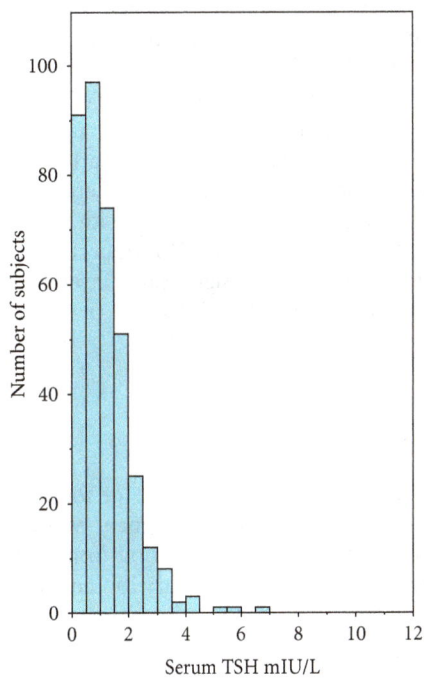

(b)

FIGURE 1: Frequency distribution of UIC in all women.

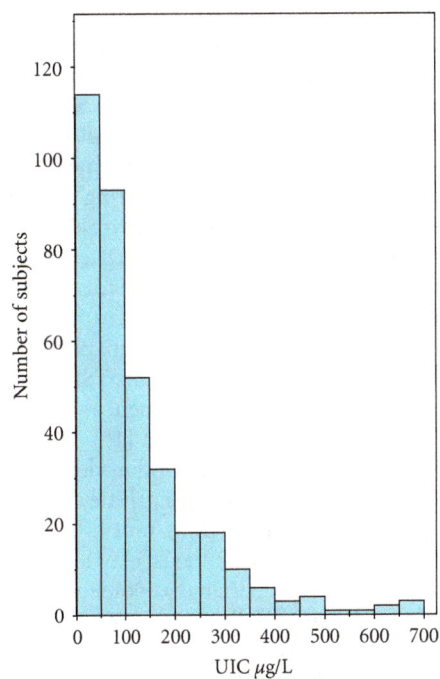

(a)

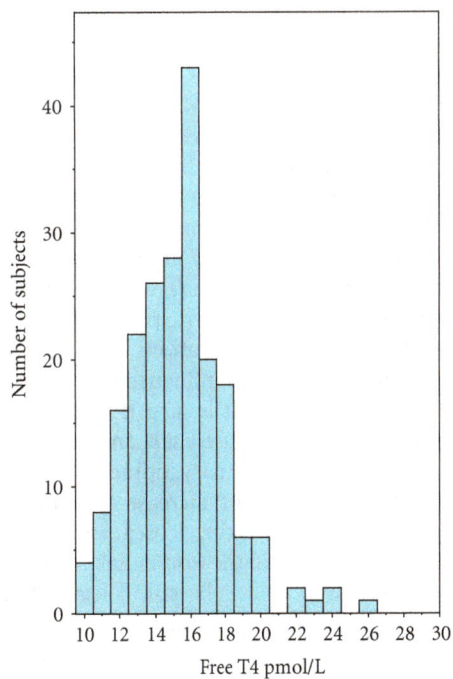

(b)

FIGURE 2: Frequency distributions of serum TSH and Free T4 concentrations.

and median TSH level was 1.19 mIU/L. 6.5% of the women had a serum TSH >2.5 mIU/L.

There was no significant association between serum TSH and UIC levels ($r = 0.049$, $P = 0.352$), nor between Free T4 and UIC levels ($r = 0.039$, $P = 0.586$). Considering UIC, TSH and Free T4 concentrations as continuous variables, there was no statistically significant association between UIC and either TSH and Free T4 (Spearman rank correlations; 0.049, $P = 0.352$ and 0.039, $P = 0.586$, resp.). When UIC levels are grouped into categories of <50 μg/L, 50–99 μg/L and >100 μg/L, there is no statistically significant evidence of differences in TSH levels or Free T4 levels between these UIC groups (Kruskal Wallis nonparametric ANOVA, $P = 0.246$ and $P = 0.586$, resp.). Similarly, there was no significant evidence of differences in TSH and Free T4 levels in those with UIC <50 μg/L compared with those with UIC >100 μg/L, $P = 0.312$, and $P = 0.514$, respectively.

However, there was a significant inverse association between serum TSH and Free T4 levels ($r = -0.490$, $P < 0.001$).

4. Discussion

There was a high overall prevalence of iodine deficiency of 72%, in our population of pregnant women resident in Western Sydney, with 32% suffering from moderate-to-severe deficiency. The median urinary iodine level of 81 μg/L was similar to the level we found in a pregnant population in Sydney approximately 10 years ago indicating that the situation has not improved despite publicity in the medical and lay press about iodine deficiency [7]. Similar reports of iodine deficiency have come from Victoria and Tasmania where the degree of iodine deficiency in pregnant women may be even worse than NSW [9, 11]. Extrapolating from the urinary iodine excretion to calculate daily intake [6], it is evident that these pregnant women are only taking, on average, a little more than half (132 μg) the recommended daily intake (RDI for pregnancy of 250 μg per day [12].

While we are not certain how much reliance one can put on self-reported food and mineral supplement intakes without specific quantitative data, there were some interesting associations between what the participants reported and the measurement of iodine concentrations in their urine. The only food group appearing to influence the urinary iodine level was the intake of milk. It is surprising that other rich sources of iodine such as iodised salt and regular seafood intake did not influence the urinary iodine level. By contrast, there was a highly significant increase in urinary iodine levels in women who were taking a pregnancy supplement. However, the median UIC in the women taking supplements was 115 μg/L, still well below the cutoff level of 150 μg/L, consistent with the RDI for pregnancy of 250 μg per day. It is clear that many of the popular pregnancy supplements either do not contain any iodine, or the amounts are less than what is required to optimise iodine intake for pregnant women. In a recent study Charlton et al. found a median UIC of 87.5 μg/L in a small sample of women attending an antenatal clinic in Wollongong [13]. 59% of the women were taking

a pregnancy supplement of which 35% contained iodine. Their findings were similar to ours in that the median UIC in the women taking a pregnancy supplement was significantly increased to 139 μg/L, but still below the recommended level of 150 μg/L. As we have not analysed the iodine content of the supplements taken by our patients we have been unable to verify the quality of these products.

The shortcomings of the study are firstly that it comprised a relatively homogeneous population of women most of whom were well educated and able to afford private obstetric care. In addition the data obtained by questionnaire regarding food intakes and supplements relied upon recall and could not be independently verified. To our knowledge this is the first study of a pregnant population in Australia measuring iodine excretion levels and examining possible negative consequences on thyroid function. As the majority of women were only mildly iodine-deficient significant changes in thyroid function were not anticipated. Measurement of serum TSH is considered the first line test in the laboratory assessment of thyroid function. While the serum TSH level is normally stable in euthyroid adults, it undergoes dynamic change during pregnancy as the thyroid responds to the challenge of having to dramatically increase thyroid hormone production in the first and second trimesters. Unfortunately, TSH reference ranges provided by most laboratories in Australia have not been derived from pregnant populations. In a recent study by Gilbert et al. from Western Australia [14], examining thyroid function during the first trimester of pregnancy in a large sample (excluding women with positive thyroid autoantibodies), they reported a reference range for serum TSH of 0.4 to 4.0 mIU/L and for serum Free T4 of 9.0 to 19 pmol/L. They did not assess iodine nutritional status of their population. Our data, which does not exclude women with positive thyroid autoantibodies, provide similar results with a 2.5 to 97.5 percentile range for serum TSH and Free T4 of 0.03 to 3.4 mIU/L, and 10.0 to 20.5 pmol/L, respectively. Thus, despite the presence of mild iodine deficiency in our pregnant population, it is reassuring that we could not find any evidence for disturbed thyroid function as a consequence of the iodine deficiency. Of course this does not exclude an effect on the thyroid that may be detected by more sensitive measures such as serum thyroglobulin and thyroid volume changes during pregnancy. The fact that 6.5% of the women studied had serum TSH levels greater than 2.5 mIU/L identifies these women as suffering from gestational subclinical hypothyroidism [15]

In summary, mild-to-moderate iodine deficiency is common in pregnant women attending a private obstetrical practice in Western Sydney, but there is no evidence of adverse effects in thyroid function from the level of iodine deficiency in the population studied. Urinary iodine excretion levels have not changed substantially over the past decade despite attempts to improve iodine nutrition in the population at risk [16]. Since this study was completed, it has been mandatory in Australia to replace all salt used in bread making with iodised salt [17]. It is estimated that this strategy would increase mean iodine intake by 46 ug/day and reduce the proportion of nonpregnant women with inadequate intakes from 59% to 9%, but most pregnant women will remain iodine deficient. Iodine supplementation has been recommended as one of the means to achieve improved iodine nutrition in pregnant Australian women [18]. The estimated daily iodine supplement required to provide sufficient iodine intake for pregnant and breastfeeding women has been calculated to be in the range of 100–150 ug/day [19].

Acknowledgment

The authors thank Laverty Pathology for providing the laboratory estimations on this patient population.

References

[1] C. J. Eastman, "Where has all our iodine gone? The possible re-emergence of iodine deficiency in Australia needs to be investigated in national surveys," *Medical Journal of Australia*, vol. 171, no. 9, pp. 455–456, 1999.

[2] C. J. Eastman, "Iodine supplementation: the benefits for pregnant and lactating women in Australia and New Zealand," *Royal Australian and New Zealand College of Obstetricians and Gynaecologists O & G Magazine*, vol. 7, pp. 65–66, 2005.

[3] M. Li, C. J. Eastman, K. V. Waite et al., "Are Australian children iodine deficient? Results of the Australian National Iodine Nutrition Study," *Medical Journal of Australia*, vol. 184, no. 4, pp. 165–169, 2006.

[4] D. Glinoer, "The importance of iodine nutrition during pregnancy," *Public Health Nutrition*, vol. 10, no. 12 A, pp. 1542–1546, 2007.

[5] M. Qian, D. Wang, W. E. Watkins et al., "The effects of iodine on intelligence in children: a meta-analysis of studies conducted in China," *Asia Pacific Journal of Clinical Nutrition*, vol. 14, no. 1, pp. 32–42, 2005.

[6] M. B. Zimmermann, P. L. Jooste, and C. S. Pandav, "Iodine-deficiency disorders," *The Lancet*, vol. 372, no. 9645, pp. 1251–1262, 2008.

[7] M. Li, "Re-emergence of iodine deficiency in Australia," *Asia Pacific Journal of Clinical Nutrition*, vol. 10, no. 3, pp. 200–203, 2001.

[8] J. E. Gunton, G. Hams, M. Fiegert, and A. McElduff, "Iodine deficiency in ambulatory participants at a Sydney teaching hospital: is Australia truly iodine replete?" *Medical Journal of Australia*, vol. 171, no. 9, pp. 467–470, 1999.

[9] M. A. Hamrosi, E. M. Wallace, and M. D. Riley, "Iodine status in pregnant women living in Melbourne differs by ethnic group," *Asia Pacific Journal of Clinical Nutrition*, vol. 14, no. 1, pp. 27–31, 2005.

[10] C. A. Travers, K. Guttikonda, C. A. Norton et al., "Iodine status in pregnant women and their newborns: are our babies at risk of iodine deficiency?" *Medical Journal of Australia*, vol. 184, no. 12, pp. 617–620, 2006.

[11] J. A. Seal, Z. Doyle, J. R. Burgess, R. Taylor, and A. R. Cameron, "Iodine status of Tasmanians following voluntary fortification of bread with iodine," *Medical Journal of Australia*, vol. 186, pp. 69–71, 2007.

[12] M. Andersson, B. De Benoist, F. Delange, and J. Zupan, "Prevention and control of iodine deficiency in pregnant and lactating women and in children less than 2-years-old: conclusions and recommendations of the Technical Consultation," *Public Health Nutrition*, vol. 10, no. 12 A, pp. 1606–1611, 2007.

[13] K. E. Charlton, L. Gemming, H. Yeatman, and G. Ma, "Sub-optimal iodine status of Australian pregnant women reflects poor knowledge and practices related to iodine nutrition," *Nutrition*, vol. 26, no. 10, pp. 963–968, 2010.

[14] R. M. Gilbert, N. C. Hadlow, J. P. Walsh et al., "Assessment of thyroid function during pregnancy: first-trimester (weeks 9–13) reference intervals derived from Western Australian women," *Medical Journal of Australia*, vol. 189, no. 5, pp. 250–253, 2008.

[15] C. J. Eastman, "Screening for thyroid disease and iodine deficiency," *Pathology*, vol. 44, pp. 153–159, 2012.

[16] M. Li, S. Chapman, K. Agho, and C. J. Eastman, "Can even minimal news coverage influence consumer health-related behaviour? A case study of iodized salt sales, Australia," *Health Education Research*, vol. 23, no. 3, pp. 543–548, 2008.

[17] Food Standards Australia and New Zealand, "Proposal P1003. Mandatory iodine fortification for Australia," Canberra: FSANZ, 2008, http://www.foodstandards.gov.au/_srcfiles /AppR_P1003_Mandatory_Iodine_Fortification_Aust%20 APPR.pdf.

[18] G. Gallego, S. Goodall, and C. J. Eastman, "Iodine deficiency in Australia: is iodine supplementation for pregnant and lactating women warranted?" *Medical Journal of Australia*, vol. 192, no. 8, pp. 461–463, 2010.

[19] D. E. M. Mackerras and C. J. Eastman, "Estimating the iodine supplementation level to recommend for pregnant and breastfeeding women in Australia," *Medical Journal of Australia*, vol. 197, pp. 238–242, 2012.

23

Proteomic Profiling of Thyroid Papillary Carcinoma

Yoshiyuki Ban,[1] Gou Yamamoto,[2] Michiya Takada,[1] Shigeo Hayashi,[2] Yoshio Ban,[3] Kazuo Shimizu,[4] Haruki Akasu,[4] Takehito Igarashi,[4] Yasuhiko Bando,[5] Tetsuhiko Tachikawa,[2, 6] and Tsutomu Hirano[1]

[1] *Division of Diabetes, Metabolism and Endocrinology, Department of Medicine, Showa University School of Medicine, 1-5-8 Hatanodai, Shinagawa-ku, Tokyo 142-8666, Japan*
[2] *Department of Oral Pathology and Diagnosis, School of Dentistry, Showa University, 1-5-8 Hatanodai, Shinagawa-ku, Tokyo 142-8555, Japan*
[3] *Ban Thyroid Clinic, 2-11-16 Jiyugaoka, Megro-ku, Tokyo 152-0035, Japan*
[4] *Division of Endocrine Surgery, Department of Surgery, Nippon Medical School, 1-1-5 Sendagi, Bunkyo-ku, Tokyo 113-8602, Japan*
[5] *Biosys Technologies, Inc., 2-13-18 Nakane, Meguro-ku, Tokyo 152-0031, Japan*
[6] *Comprehensive Research Center of Oral Cancer, Showa University, 1-5-8 Hatanodai, Shinagawa-ku, Tokyo 142-8555, Japan*

Correspondence should be addressed to Yoshiyuki Ban, yshyban@yahoo.co.jp

Academic Editor: Fausto Bogazzi

Papillary thyroid carcinoma (PTC) is the most common endocrine malignancy. We performed shotgun liquid chromatography (LC)/tandem mass spectrometry (MS/MS) analysis on pooled protein extracts from patients with PTC and compared the results with those from normal thyroid tissue validated by real-time (RT) PCR and immunohistochemistry (IHC). We detected 524 types of protein in PTC and 432 in normal thyroid gland. Among these proteins, 145 were specific to PTC and 53 were specific to normal thyroid gland. We have also identified two important new markers, nephronectin (NPNT) and malectin (MLEC). Reproducibility was confirmed with several known markers, but the one of two new candidate markers such as MLEC did not show large variations in expression levels. Furthermore, IHC confirmed the overexpression of both those markers in PTCs compared with normal surrounding tissues. Our protein data suggest that NPNT and MLEC could be a characteristic marker for PTC.

1. Introduction

Papillary thyroid carcinoma (PTC) is the most common form of the follicular-cell-derived carcinomas and comprises three quarters of all newly diagnosed thyroid cancers [1]. PTC is derived from the follicular cells. These cells tend to concentrate iodine and secrete thyroglobulin. As a result, surveillance and detection of recurrence can be relatively straightforward. The prognosis for PTC is usually excellent (reviewed in [2]).

Over the past 10–15 years, several candidate genes have been studied in the development of different types of thyroid cancer (e.g., TSH receptor, RET/PTC, Ras, BRAF, and p53) [3–5]. These genes have been evaluated in thyroid cancer based on what was known or other cancers or based on what was expected from normal cell signaling (protooncogenes). Recent studies using gene array technology have attempted to use a hypothesis-generating approach to understand thyroid neoplasms [6–8], but these studies rely on mRNA differences that may not be related to significant biologic processes. mRNA differences do not necessarily reflect differences at the protein level, and these RNA-based studies fail to identify protein variants and posttranslational modifications that affect the tumor biology.

Proteomics is the name given to a set of analytical strategies that can simultaneously identify and quantify thousands of protein components in a biological sample [9]. There is, however, no single approach that optimally meets this demanding objective; instead, several complementary technologies have emerged, each offering distinctive strengths

TABLE 1: Clinical details of analyzed tissue samples.

No.	Age (yr)	Gender	Possible PTC-subtype	Proteomics	RT-PCR	IHC
1	49	F	Common type	+	+	+
2	41	F	Common type	+	+	+
3	28	F	Common type	+	+	+
4	43	F	Common type	−	+	+

F: Female; PTC: papillary thyroid cancer; IHC: Immunohistochemistry; −: not tested.

and weaknesses. These approaches are now facilitating new biomarker discoveries in many areas of medicine. Studies of the thyrocyte and thyroid cancer cell proteome are in their infancy compared with studies of the genome and transcriptome [9].

We employed nanoflow liquid chromatography and mass spectrometry, followed by protein identification by tandem mass spectrometry (LC/MS/MS) to gain a better understanding of thyroid cancer and the unique alterations that are characteristic of PTC. This technique provides an accurate quantitative comparison of two groups of samples, allowing the identification of proteins whose levels differ significantly between the two conditions. Using this approach, we have identified novel differentially expressed proteins that may provide insights into diagnosis, prognosis, and therapeutic targets for patients with thyroid neoplasms, as well as into the underlying pathophysiology of thyroid tumor development and progression.

2. Materials and Methods

2.1. Ethics Statement.
The research protocol was approved by the Ethic Committee of the Showa University Hospital, and each subject signed the informed consent form approved by the Institutional Review Board at the Showa University Hospital.

2.2. Thyroid Tissue Samples.
Tumor and matched normal thyroid tissue was collected from four patients undergoing surgery for PTC. Specimens (100–500 mg) from each patient, verified by histopathology, were snap frozen after confirmation of tissue type. Tissue samples were collected from women aged 28–49 years with no evidence of chronic lymphocytic thyroiditis in an attempt to minimize differences due to gender, menopausal status, and autoimmune thyroid disease. Unaffected (normal) thyroid tissue was defined as tissue adjacent to the site of the lesion with no histologic signs of abnormal pathology. Normal tissue was collected from each patient undergoing surgery for PTC so that the biologic variability in protein expression in a region proximate to pathology could be assessed. All cases were analyzed by real-time (RT) PCR analysis and immunohistochemistry (IHC), while LC/MS/MS was applied on 3 out of 4 cases. The clinical details of patients are summarized in Table 1.

2.3. Peptide Extraction for LC/MS/MS Analysis.
Proteins from samples for LC/MS/MS were extracted using $10\,\mu L$ of 8 M Urea solution with an ultrasonic homogenizer. After homogenization, $90\,\mu L$ of 90% 100 mM Ammonium Bicarbonate Buffer (ABB: pH 8.0)/10% Acetonitrile were added, followed by addition of $4\,\mu L$ of 100 mM dithiothreitol in ABB. Samples were incubated at 37°C for 60 min and were cooled at room temperature. Next, $10\,\mu L$ of 100 mM iodoacetamide in ABB was added, and samples were incubated at 37°C for 30 min in the dark. Finally, proteins in the samples were digested with trypsin (15–18 units) by overnight incubation at 37°C. After extraction, all samples were stored at −20°C until LC/MS/MS analysis.

2.4. Shotgun Liquid Chromatography (LC)/Tandem Mass Spectrometry (MS/MS).
Peptide-mixture samples processed from each tissue were used for nanoflow reverse phase liquid chromatography followed by tandem MS, using an LTQ linear ion-trap mass spectrometer (Thermo Fischer, San Jose, CA). The capillary reverse phase HPLC-MS/MS system (ZAPLOUS System; AMR, Tokyo, Japan) was composed of a Paradigm MS4 dual solvent delivery system (Michrom BioResources, Auburn, CA), an HTC PAL autosampler (CTC Analytics, Zwingen, Switzerland), and Finnigan LTQ linear ion-trap mass spectrometers (ITMS; Thermo Fischer, San Jose, CA) equipped with an XYZ nanoelectrospray ionization (NSI) source (AMR, Tokyo, Japan).

All samples were evaporated, and peptides were redissolved with MS-grade water containing 0.1% trifluoroacetic acid and 2% acetonitrile (solvent A). Aliquots of $10\,\mu L$ (equivalent to $1\,\mu g$ of protein) were automatically injected into a peptide Cap-trap column (Michrom BioResources) attached to an injector valve for desalinating and concentrating peptides. After washing the trap with solvent A, peptides were loaded onto a separation capillary reverse phase column (Mono Cap 150 × 0.2 mm; GL Sciences, Tokyo, Japan) by switching the valve. The eluents used were: A, 98% H_2O/2% acetonitrile/0.1% formic acid; B, 10% H_2O/90% acetonitrile/0.1% formic acid. The column was developed at a flow rate of approximately $1\,\mu L$/min with the concentration gradient of acetonitrile, as follows: first, from 5% B to 55% B in 100 min, then from 55% B to 95% B in 1 min, maintenance at 95% B for 9 min, then from 95% B to 5% B in 3 min, and finally reequilibration with 5% B for 15 min.

Effluents were introduced into the mass spectrometer via the NSI interface, which had a separation column outlet connected directly with an NSI needle (150-μm OD/20-μm ID FortisTip; OmniSeparo-TJ, Hyogo, Japan). ESI voltage was 2.0 kV, and the transfer capillary of the LTQ inlet was heated at 200°C. No sheath or auxiliary gas was used. The mass spectrometer was operated in a z range of 450–1800 in a data-dependent acquisition mode, in which detecting the most abundant ions at a retention time automatically acquires MS/MS scans for those ions under the control of Xcalibur software (Thermo Fischer) with an isolation width of m/z 2.0 and a collisional activation amplitude of 35%. Full-scan MS used enhanced/centroid mode, and sequential MS/MS used normal/centroid mode, with dynamic exclusion capability, which allows sequential acquisition of MS/MS of abundant ions in the order of their intensities with an exclusion duration of 1.0 min and exclusion mass widths of −1 and +2 Da. The trapping time was 50 ms using auto gain control.

All MS/MS spectral data were searched against the SwissProt 57.3 Homo sapiens database (468,851 entries) using Mascot (version 2.1.04, Matrix Science, London, UK), in which the peptide and fragment mass tolerances were 2.0 Da and 0.8 Da, respectively. For variable peptide modifications, methionine oxidation and carbamidomethyl (Cys) were taken into account. A P value less than 0.05 was considered to indicate a statistically significant difference, and the expected score cut-off was 0.05. Reported results were obtained from triplicate LC-MS runs for each sample with all peptide hits included. Unique peptides and proteins were determined by following proteomics guidelines. Relative abundances of identified proteins were also obtained using the normalized spectral abundance factor (NSAF) introduced by Kawamura et al. and Zybailov et al. [10, 11].

2.5. Laser Microdissection and Semiquantitative Real-Time PCR. Tumor cells of PTC and follicular epithelium of normal thyroid tissue (periphery of PTC area) were collected from frozen sections by laser microdissection. Total RNA was extracted from each population of laser-microdissected cells using an RNeasy Plus Micro kit (QIAGEN, Valencia, CA) according to the manufacturer's instructions. Reverse transcription was carried out in 20-μL volumes using a High Capacity RNA to cDNA MasterMix (Applied Biosystems, Carlsbad, CA).

PCR was performed using an ABI PRISM 7500 Sequence Detection System (Applied Biosystems), and analysis was carried out using the sequence detection software supplied with the instrument. Each reaction mixture contained 10 μL of TaqMan Gene Expression Master Mix (Applied Biosystems), 1 μL of TaqMan Gene Expression Assay primer (Applied Biosystems), and 2 μL of template cDNA supplemented with RNase-free water to a final volume of 20 μL. Primers were positioned to span exon-intron boundaries, reducing the risk of detecting genomic DNA. Each PCR consisted of 10 min at 95°C for enzyme activation, followed by 50 cycles of denaturation at 95°C for 15 s and annealing/extension at 60°C for 1 min. Negative control (RNA with no reverse transcription) was included to control for DNA contamination. The housekeeping gene glyceradehyde-3-phosphate dehydrogenase (GAPDH: Assay ID Hs99999905_m1) was used as an endogenous control. Expression values of nephronectin (NPNT) (Assay ID Hs00405900_m1) and malectin (MLEC) (Assay ID Hs00207082_m1) were normalized against the GAPDH values for each sample. Each sample was run in triplicate, and the means were used in semiquantitative analysis.

2.6. Immunohistochemical Study. Immunohistochemical analysis using the DAKO EnVision system (DAKO, Carpinteria, CA) was performed. Each sample was studied using H-E staining and immunohistochemical staining. Frozen sections were fixed for 30 min in 4% paraformaldehyde and

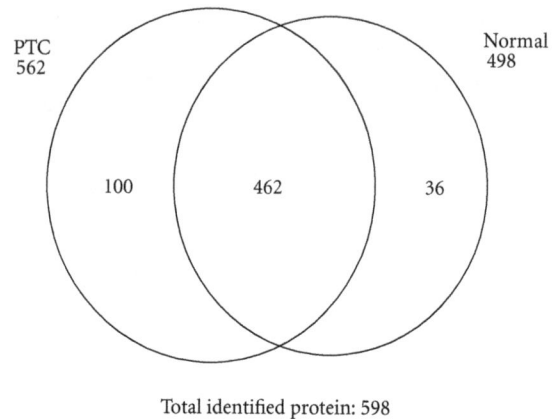

FIGURE 1: Venn diagram of identified proteins. In PTC, 562 proteins were identified, and 498 were identified in normal thyroid tissue, with 462 proteins being common to both PTC and normal thyroid tissue. The total number of identified proteins was 598 (Normal; normal thyroid tissue; PTC; Papillary thyroid carcinoma).

were washed with phosphate-buffered solution (PBS, pH 7.4) three times for 3 min each. Blocking reagent (DAKO) was then applied at room temperature for 10 min in order to prevent nonspecific binding of antibodies, and sections were washed in PBS three times for 3 min each. In this study, anti-MLEC rabbit polyclonal (Sigma-Aldrich Inc., St. Louis, MO) and Anti-POEM/NPNT rabbit polyclonal (Trans Genic Inc., Kobe, Japan) antibodies were used. Antibodies were diluted 200× and were dropped onto sections for 60 min at room temperature. Sections were incubated with polymer reagent (DAKO EnVision) for 30 min. After washing with PBS, sections were incubated with 3,3′-diaminobenzidine tetrahydrochloride (DAKO) for 1-2 min. Finally, sections were washed with distilled water, counterstained with hematoxylin for 1 min, washed with tap water and ethanol, and covered with cover slips.

2.7. Statistical Analysis. All values are expressed as means ± SD. The statistical significance of differences between groups was analyzed by unpaired Student's t-test. A P value of less than 0.05 was considered to be statistically significant.

3. Results

3.1. Protein Identification by LC/MS/MS. Protein identification results for triplicate injections were merged and proteins detected twice or more were studied. In PTC and normal thyroid tissue, the numbers of proteins were 562 and 498, respectively, and 462 proteins were common to both. Thus, 100 proteins were unique to PTC, and 36 to normal thyroid tissue (Figure 1). Among the identified proteins in both tissue types, several known markers and two new markers (NPNT and MLEC), with large numbers of NSAF, are shown in Figure 2. Previous studies indicated that Keratin 19 (K1C19) and Dipeptidyl peptidase 4 (DPP4) were strongly expressed in PTC, and Fatty acid-binding protein 4 (FABP4) was strongly expressed in normal thyroid tissues

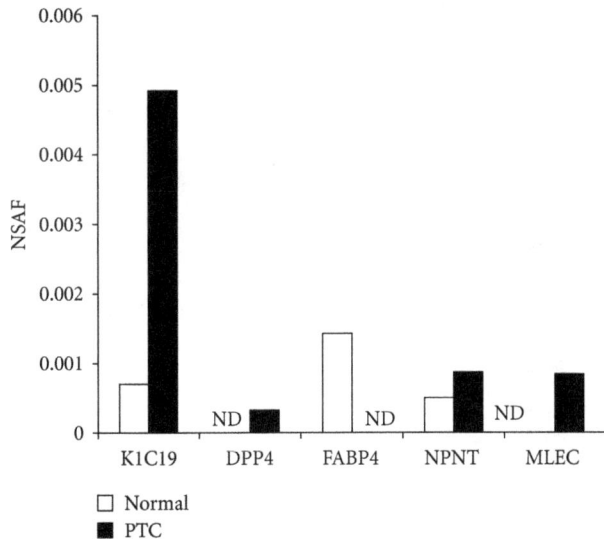

FIGURE 2: Comparison of NSAF in the identified proteins in PTC tissues ($n = 3$) with NSAF in normal thyroid tissues ($n = 3$). Similar to previous reports, Keratin 19 (K1C19) and Dipeptidyl peptidase 4 (DPP4) were strongly expressed in PTC, and Fatty acid-binding protein 4 (FABP4) was strongly expressed in normal thyroid tissues. NPNT and MLEC were discovered as strongly expressed candidate markers in PTC (Normal: normal thyroid tissue, PTC: Papillary thyroid carcinoma, ND: not detectable).

[12]. These observations suggest that our results reflect characteristics unique to each type of membrane, as well as common features between the three. As shown in Figure 2, two new candidate markers, NPNT and MLEC, were strongly expressed in PTC.

3.2. Gene Expression of NPNT and MLEC in PTC and Normal Thyroid Tissues. In order to confirm the validity of the LC/MS/MS results, semiquantitative real-time PCR was performed with a set of human-specific primers and template cDNA generated by reverse transcription. Similarly to the LC/MS/MS results and previous reports, the levels of K1C19 and DPP4 expression in the PTC were significantly higher than in normal thyroid tissue, while FABP4 levels were lower (Figure 3). With regard to new candidate markers, although the levels of NPNT expression were significantly higher in PTC, there were no significant differences in MLEC expression (Figure 4).

3.3. Immunohistochemical Analysis of NPNT and MLEC in PTC and Normal Thyroid Tissues. The distribution of NPNT and MLEC protein expression in normal thyroid tissue and PTC was examined by immunohistochemical analysis. Few positive reactions for NPNT and MLEC were observed in the follicular epithelium (surrounding tumor); on the other hand, carcinoma cells were strongly stained (Figure 5). Particularly for MLEC, no significant differences in gene expression were observed between normal thyroid tissue and PTC; nevertheless, the protein localization was clearly different.

4. Discussion

MS-based proteome analysis of frozen tissue sections has identified thousands of unique proteins in various histological tissue samples. The results presented herein demonstrate that a protein solubilization methodology allows global proteomic investigation of tissues. In the present study using our proteome platform, we identified two new markers for PTC, NPNT and MLEC, as well as several known markers, such as KRT19 and DPP4, with significantly increased expression in tissue samples from PTC.

PreOsteoblast EGF-like repeat protein with MAM domain (NPNT) was originally identified in developing mouse organs, particularly at epithelial-mesenchymal interfaces in tissues undergoing morphogenesis [13, 14]. The protein was determined to be associated with cells or with the extracellular matrix but was not found in culture medium, leading to the hypothesis that NPNT is a matrix protein binding to the cell surface. This agrees with an arg-gly-asp binding domain and an integrin binding site found in the amino acid sequence, as well as with a study showing that integrin α-8 β-1 binds to NPNT [14]. Binding to other integrin molecules has not specifically been observed to date. In a recent study by Eckhardt et al., NPNT was first suggested to be involved in cancer [15]. They applied a genomic analysis to cell lines derived from a spontaneous breast cancer model in mice, and NPNT expression was shown to be related to metastasis. In breast cancer, strong NPNT expression was found in the tumor epithelium of high-metastasis tumors.

MLEC is a novel carbohydrate-binding protein in the endoplasmic reticulum (ER) and is a candidate player in the early steps of protein N-glycosylation [16]. The recent discovery of MLEC, an ER-resident protein that binds oligosaccharides displaying terminal glucose residues with a strong preference for di-glycosylated residues in vitro [16–18], led to speculation on the possible involvement of this lectin in the calnexin chaperone system and in glycoprotein quality control in the mammalian ER [19, 20]. Recently, Galli et al. [21] showed that MLEC is an ER stress-induced type I membrane protein that is associated with newly synthesized glycoproteins in living cells. Analysis of the influenza virus HA revealed that calnexin and MLEC have distinct kinetics in association with newly synthesized polypeptides and that MLEC is preferentially associated with misfolded HA conformers [21]. Changes in the intraluminal levels in MLEC did not affect the function of the calnexin chaperone system or the maturation of HA, an obligate calnexin substrate [21]. It is, therefore, unlikely that MLEC participates in the calnexin chaperone system [21].

There are three main limitations to the present study. The first involves the intrinsic limitations of LC/MS in the analysis of complex protein mixtures. Proteins of very high or low molecular mass are frequently eliminated from analysis by the electrophoresis procedure itself. Conversely, even after depletion of very abundant proteins, both detection by LC and identification by MS are limited by the abundance of the proteins in the mixture, and minor components will always escape analysis. Therefore, candidates proteins at

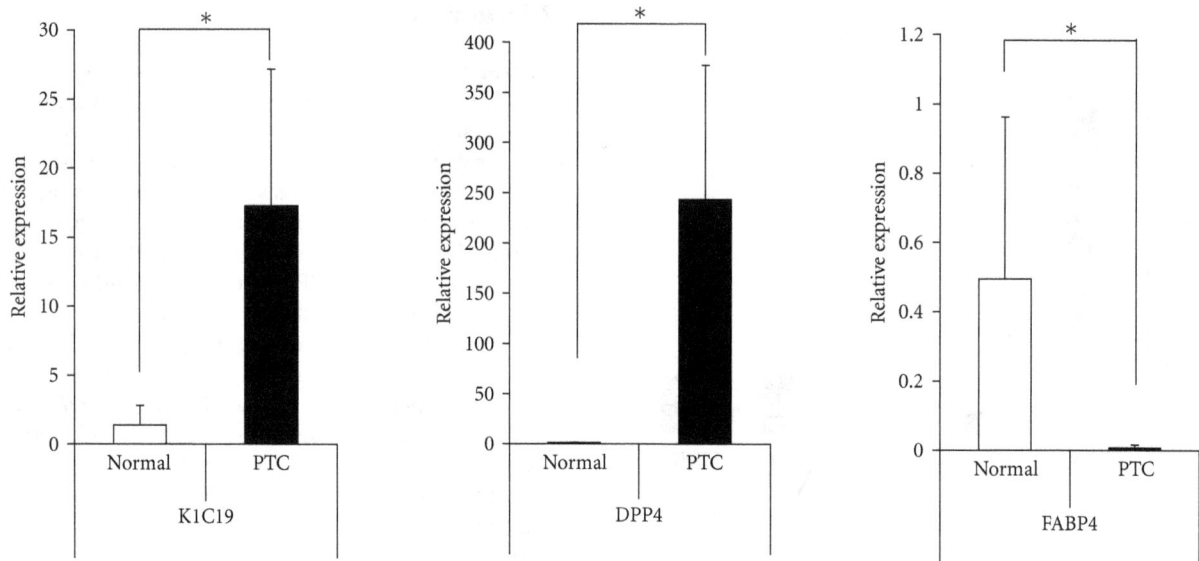

FIGURE 3: Gene expression of previously known markers (K1C19, DPP4, and FABP4) in normal thyroid tissue and PTC. Gene expression levels of K1C19 and DPP4 were significantly higher in PTC when compared with normal thyroid tissue. In contrast, FABP4 expression was lower (Normal: normal thyroid tissue, PTC: Papillary thyroid carcinoma, *P < 0.05, Bar: 1 SD).

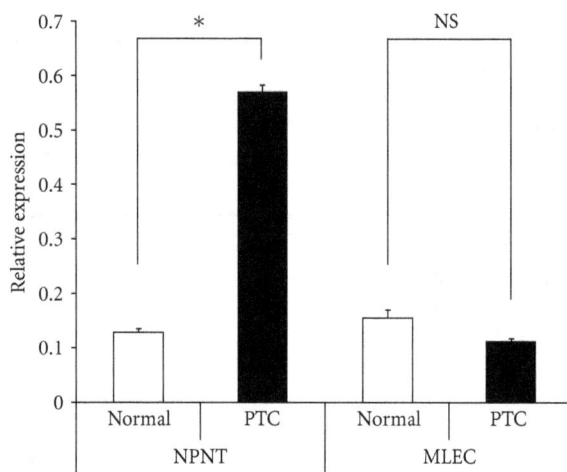

FIGURE 4: Gene expression of new candidate markers (NPNT and MLEC) in normal thyroid tissue and PTC. Gene expression of NPNT was significantly higher in PTC when compared with normal thyroid tissue. However, expression of MLEC showed no significant differences (Normal: normal thyroid tissue, PTC: Papillary thyroid carcinoma, *P < 0.05, NS: not significant, Bar: 1 SD).

group. The observed differences by LC/MS were further validated by RT-PCR analysis of samples from different patients, which confirmed the observed differences with good quantitative agreement. Therefore, although additional differentially expressed proteins could probably be identified by analyzing a larger set of samples, those reported herein would likely also be found. Another limitation is that our data does not demonstrate whether NPNT and MLEC cause PTC, or are simply over-expressed due to tissue proliferation in PTC. Moreover, apparently contrasting data (proteomic analysis and IHC on one side, gene expression on the other side) for malectin are shown, while for nephronectin they are all concordant. This discrepancy may be due to protein variants or posttranslational modifications that affect the tumor biology. Further studies are necessary in order to elucidate whether NPNT and malectin play a role in the etiology of PTC.

5. Conclusions

Recent advances in proteomic technologies are increasingly being applied to the study of clinical samples in the search for diagnostic biomarkers and therapeutic targets. Herein, we demonstrated that the powerful combination of LC/MS/MS and frozen tissue samples, for which matching clinicopathological information is available, is beginning to show promise as a research tool. Using this method, we may thus be able to identify new markers that cannot be distinguished on gene expression analysis. Although the number of samples included in this study was low, these data suggest that NPNT and MLEC are characteristic markers and therapeutic targets for PTC.

picogram levels cannot be identified. The second limitation pertains to the rigorous selection of membrane samples, which does not allow the inclusion of an ample set of samples and may consequently impede the consideration of other candidate proteins existing in the tissues of PTC patients. However, although the number of samples included in this study was low, the selection process enabled us to minimize the dispersion of the measurements in each

Normal   PTC

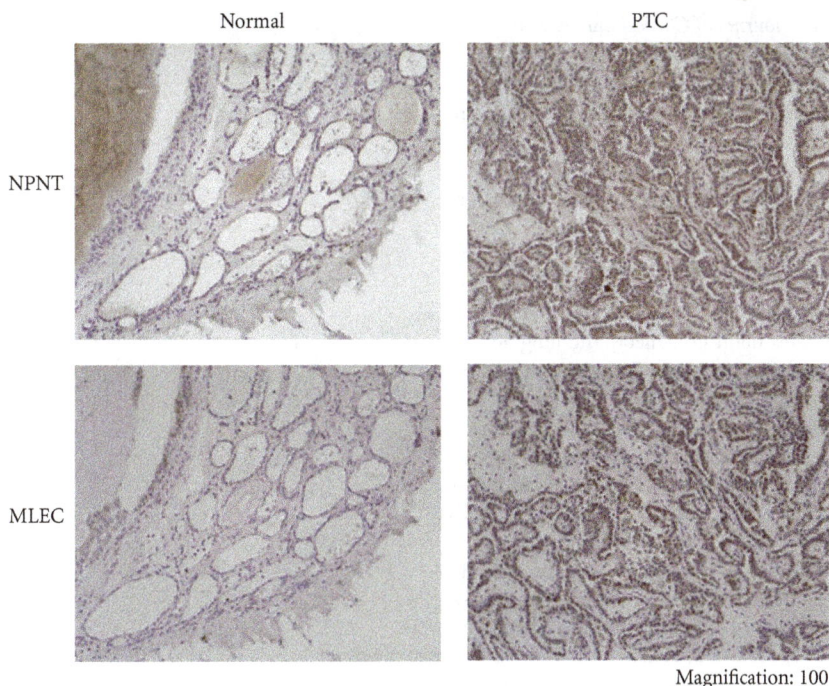

Magnification: 100

FIGURE 5: Immunohistochemical localization of NPNT and MLEC in normal thyroid tissue and PTC. Only weak staining of NPNT and MLEC were observed in follicular epithelium of normal thyroid tissue (surrounding tumor). In PTC, strong staining was seen with both antibodies (Normal: normal thyroid tissue, PTC: Papillary thyroid carcinoma).

Abbreviations

PTC: Papillary thyroid carcinoma
LC/MS/MS: Shotgun liquid chromatography/tandem
            mass spectrometry
RT-PCR: Real-time PCR
IHC: Immunohistochemistry
NPNT: Nephronectin
MLEC: Malectin
NSAF: Normalized spectral abundance factor
GAPDH: Glyceradehyde-3-phosphate
            dehydrogenase.

Acknowledgments

This work was supported by a Showa University Grant-in-aid for Innovative Collaborative Research Projects (to Y. Ban), a grant from the Showa University School of Medicine Alumni Association (to Y. Ban), a grant from the Yamaguchi Endocrine Research Association (to Y. Ban), The Project to Establish Strategic Research Center (to T. Tachikawa), and a Grant-in-Aid for Young Scientists (B) (to G. Yamamoto) from the Ministry of Education, Culture, Sports, Science and Technology, Japan. The funders had no role in study design, data collection and analysis, decision to publish, or preparation of the paper. No additional external funding received for this study.

References

[1] S. A. Hundahl, I. D. Fleming, A. M. Fremgen, and H. R. Menck, "A National Cancer Data Base report on 53,856 cases of thyroid carcinoma treated in the U.S., 1985–1995," Cancer, vol. 83, no. 12, pp. 2638–2648, 1998.

[2] J. M. Gasent Blesa, E. Grande Pulido, M. Provencio Pulla et al., "Old and new insights in the treatment of thyroid carcinoma," Journal of Thyroid Research, vol. 2010, Article ID 279468, 16 pages, 2010.

[3] J. A. Fagin, "Genetic basis of endocrine disease 3: molecular defects in thyroid gland neoplasia," Journal of Clinical Endocrinology and Metabolism, vol. 75, no. 6, pp. 1398–1400, 1992.

[4] E. T. Kimura, M. N. Nikiforova, Z. Zhu, J. A. Knauf, Y. E. Nikiforov, and J. A. Fagin, "High prevalence of BRAF mutations in thyroid cancer: genetic evidence for constitutive activation of the RET/PTC-RAS-BRAF signaling pathway in papillary thyroid carcinoma," Cancer Research, vol. 63, no. 7, pp. 1454–1457, 2003.

[5] J. A. Fagin, "Challenging dogma in thyroid cancer molecular genetics—role of RET/PTC and BRAF in tumor initiation," Journal of Clinical Endocrinology and Metabolism, vol. 89, no. 9, pp. 4264–4266, 2004.

[6] C. Mazzanti, M. A. Zeiger, N. Costourous et al., "Using Gene Expression Profiling to Differentiate Benign versus Malignant Thyroid Tumors," Cancer Research, vol. 64, no. 8, pp. 2898–2903, 2004.

[7] D. J. Finley, N. Arora, B. Zhu, L. Gallagher, and T. J. Fahey, "Molecular profiling distinguishes papillary carcinoma from

benign thyroid nodules," *Journal of Clinical Endocrinology and Metabolism*, vol. 89, no. 7, pp. 3214–3223, 2004.

[8] J. M. Cerutti, R. Delcelo, M. J. Amadei et al., "A preoperative diagnostic test that distinguishes benign from malignant thyroid carcinoma based on gene expression," *Journal of Clinical Investigation*, vol. 113, no. 8, pp. 1234–1242, 2004.

[9] B. R. Haugen and M. W. Duncan, "Applications of proteomics to thyroid neoplasms: are we there yet? " *Thyroid*, vol. 20, no. 10, pp. 1051–1052, 2010.

[10] T. Kawamura, M. Nomura, H. Tojo et al., "Proteomic analysis of laser-microdissected paraffin-embedded tissues: (1) Stage-related protein candidates upon non-metastatic lung adeno-carcinoma," *Journal of Proteomics*, vol. 73, no. 6, pp. 1089–1099, 2010.

[11] B. Zybailov, M. K. Coleman, L. Florens, and M. P. Washburn, "Correlation of relative abundance ratios derived from peptide ion chromatograms and spectrum counting for quantitative proteomic analysis using stable isotope labeling," *Analytical Chemistry*, vol. 77, no. 19, pp. 6218–6224, 2005.

[12] M. Eszlinger, K. Krohn, A. Kukulska, B. Jarzab, and R. Paschke, "Perspectives and limitations of microarray-based gene expression profiling of thyroid tumors," *Endocrine Reviews*, vol. 28, no. 3, pp. 322–338, 2007.

[13] N. Morimura, Y. Tezuka, N. Watanabe et al., "Molecular clon-ing of NPNT: a novel adhesion molecule that interacts with $\alpha 8\beta$ integrin," *The Journal of Biological Chemistry*, vol. 276, no. 45, pp. 42172–42181, 2001.

[14] R. Brandenberger, A. Schmidt, J. Linton et al., "Identification and characterization of a novel extracellular matrix protein nephronectin that is associated with integrin $\alpha 8\beta 1$ in the embryonic kidney," *Journal of Cell Biology*, vol. 154, no. 2, pp. 447–458, 2001.

[15] B. L. Eckhardt, B. S. Parker, R. K. van Laar et al., "Genomic analysis of a spontaneous model of breast cancer metastasis to bone reveals a role for the extracellular matrix," *Molecular Cancer Research*, vol. 3, no. 1, pp. 1–13, 2005.

[16] T. Schallus, C. Jaeckh, K. Fehér et al., "Malectin: a novel carbohydrate-binding protein of the endoplasmic reticulum and a candidate player in the early steps of protein N-glycosylation," *Molecular Biology of the Cell*, vol. 19, no. 8, pp. 3404–3414, 2008.

[17] L. N. Muller, C. Muhle-Goll, and M. B. Biskup, "The Glc_2Man_2-fragment of the N-glycan precursor—a novel lig-and for the glycan-binding protein malectin?" *Organic and Biomolecular Chemistry*, vol. 8, no. 14, pp. 3294–3299, 2010.

[18] T. Schallus, K. Feher, U. Sternberg, V. Rybin, and C. Muhle-Goll, "Analysis of the specific interactions between the lectin domain of malectin and diglucosides," *Glycobiology*, vol. 20, no. 8, pp. 1010–1020, 2010.

[19] M. Aebi, R. Bernasconi, S. Clerc, and M. Molinari, "N-glycan structures: recognition and processing in the ER," *Trends in Biochemical Sciences*, vol. 35, no. 2, pp. 74–82, 2010.

[20] G. Z. Lederkremer, "Glycoprotein folding, quality control and ER-associated degradation," *Current Opinion in Structural Biology*, vol. 19, no. 5, pp. 515–523, 2009.

[21] C. Galli, R. Bernasconi, T. Soldà, V. Calanca, and M. Molinari, "Malectin participates in a backup glycoprotein quality con-trol pathway in the mammalian ER," *PLoS ONE*, vol. 6, no. 1, article e16304, 2011.

24

Medullary Thyroid Carcinoma: Molecular Signaling Pathways and Emerging Therapies

Karen Gómez,[1] **Jeena Varghese,**[2] **and Camilo Jiménez**[2]

[1] *Department of Endocrinology, Hospital San Juan de Dios, Avenida 14, Calles 6 Y 7 Paseo Colon, 1475-1000 San José, Costa Rica*
[2] *Department of Endocrine Neoplasia and Hormonal Disorders, Unit 1461, The University of Texas MD Anderson Cancer Center, 1515 Holcombe Boulevard, Houston, TX 77030, USA*

Correspondence should be addressed to Camilo Jiménez, cjimenez@mdanderson.org

Academic Editor: Ana O. Hoff

Research on medullary thyroid carcinoma (MTC) over the last 55 years has led to a good understanding of the genetic defects and altered molecular pathways associated with its development. Currently, with the use of genetic testing, patients at high risk for MTC can be identified before the disease develops and offered prophylactic treatment. In cases of localized neck disease, surgery can be curative. However, once MTC has spread beyond the neck, systemic therapy may be necessary. Conventional chemotherapy has been shown to be ineffective; however, multikinase inhibitors have shown promise in stabilizing disease, and this year will probably see the approval of a drug (Vandetanib) for advanced unresectable or metastatic disease, which represents a new chapter in the history of MTC. In this paper, we explore newly understood molecular pathways and the most promising emerging therapies that may change the management of MTC.

1. Introduction

Medullary thyroid carcinoma (MTC) is a neuroendocrine tumor derived from parafollicular cells of the thyroid gland [1]. MTC represents less than 3% of thyroid carcinomas in the United States [2]. The first description of its major histological features and characterization as a separate entity was done in 1959 by Hazard et al. [3]. It was then rapidly recognized that this carcinoma had distinctive clinical features, in that MTC was found to be associated with pheochromocytomas and other tumors, an association now known as multiple endocrine neoplasia type 2 (MEN2) [4]. The identification of familial cases led to the conclusion that many MTCs were probably hereditary [5]. In 1966, MTC was found to arise from the calcitonin-secreting parafollicular cells [6]. Subsequently, calcitonin provocation tests with calcium and/or pentagastrin were used to identify individuals susceptible to familial MTC, and those individuals were offered prophylactic thyroidectomy [7].

Activating mutations of the *Rearranged during Transfection (RET)* proto-oncogene were described for the first time in patients with familial forms of MTC in 1993 [8, 9].

Since then, several germline *RET* proto-oncogene mutations have been found in almost 100% of hereditary MTCs. Additionally, somatic *RET* proto-oncogene mutations have been found in approximately 40% of patients with sporadic MTC [10, 11]. These discoveries created new paradigms for the management of MTC: (1) the identification of germline *RET* proto-oncogene mutation carriers would allow the removal of the thyroid cells at risk for transformation early in life (this paradigm is perhaps the most perfect example of primary cancer prevention in humans to date), (2) the identification of several hidden familial medullary thyroid cancers [12], and (3) the abnormally activated *RET* gene might become a target to treat patients with advanced sporadic and hereditary MTC. Our goal in this paper is to describe the molecular pathways associated with MTC tumorigenesis and emerging therapies against this disease (Figure 1).

2. MTC and the *RET* Proto-Oncogene

Autonomous cell growth is the defining feature of all benign or malignant tumors. Malignant neoplasms have

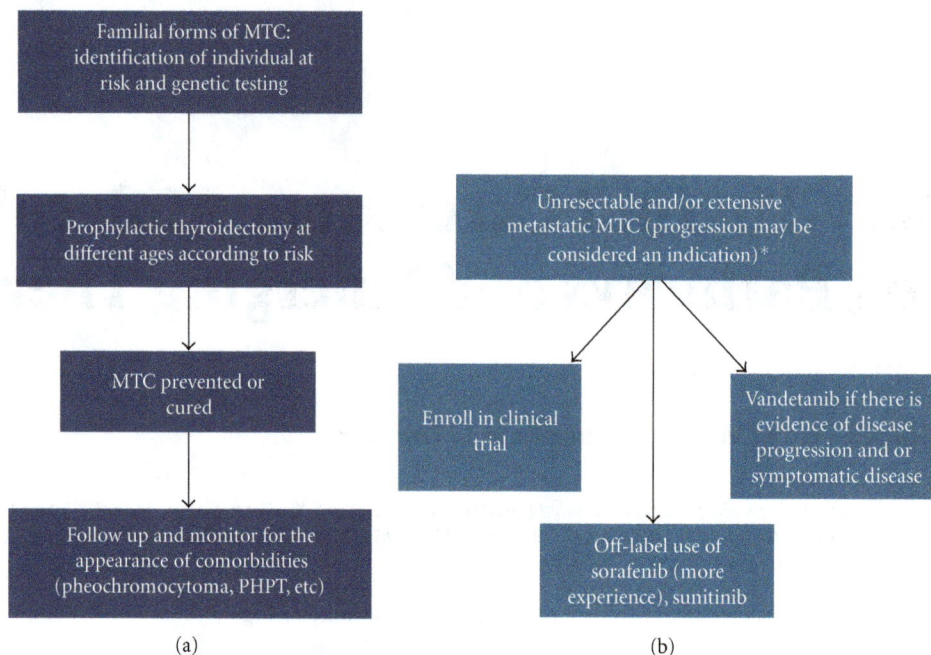

FIGURE 1: From prevention of MTC to treatment of incurable disease. Ideal approach to familial forms of MTC (a) versus treatment options in unresectable and/or extensive metastatic disease and/or progression. (b) *Every patient should be evaluated in an individual basis, and the decision to treat as well as the indication is not always clear cut as one must take into consideration quality of life issues and adverse events associated with treatment.

the capacity to invade the surrounding normal tissue and metastasize to distant sites. Molecules that are responsible for growth and other fundamental cell functions are frequently mutated in cancers. An example of such molecules is the tyrosine kinase (TK) receptors (Figure 2). TK receptors are membrane-spanning proteins with large N-terminal extracellular domains that act as ligand-binding sites and intracellular domains that catalyze the transfer of the γ phosphate of adenosine-5'-triphosphate (ATP) to hydroxyl groups of tyrosines of target proteins. TKs control a wide range of fundamental processes of cells such as the cell cycle, proliferation, angiogenesis, differentiation, motility, apoptosis, and survival.

The *RET* proto-oncogene is located in chromosome 10q11.2 [13]. The gene has 21 exons [14] and codes for a receptor TK [15]. The RET receptor is a transmembrane protein constituted by extracellular, transmembrane, and cytoplasmatic domains. The extracellular domain has a stretch of approximately 100 amino acids that are similar to members of the cadherin family of Ca^{2+} dependent cell adhesion molecules [16]. The binding of calcium to this cadherin-like domain is needed for conformational changes necessary for the interaction with different glial cell line-derived neurotrophic factor ligand family members (GDNF, neurturin, artemin, and persephin) [17]. These ligands in conjunction with a ligand-specific coreceptor (GFRα 1–4) activate RET [18]. These ligands or coreceptors are not always needed for RET activation [19]. Following RET activation, specific tyrosine residues are phosphorylated. These residues serve as docking sites for adaptor proteins that

link the receptor to the main signal transduction pathways. Different activated sites trigger the activation of different pathways. For instance, tyrosine 1015 is a binding site for phospholipase C that activates protein kinase C (PKC). Other examples are given by the phosphorylated γ tyrosine 981 which is responsible for Src activation upon RET engagement [20] and the phosphorylation of tyrosine 1062, several adaptor or effector proteins are recruited including Shc, FRS2, Dok family proteins, insulin receptor substrate 2, and Enigma [21]. Then, various pathways that regulate cell survival, differentiation, proliferation, and chemotaxis [20] are activated, including RAS-extracellular signal-regulated kinase (ERK), phosphatidylinositol 3-kinase (PI3K)-Akt, p58 mitogen-activated protein kinase (MAPK), and Jun N-terminal kinase (JNK) [22] (Figure 3).

Mutated *RET* is expressed in derivatives of neural crest cells, including hereditary and sporadic MTC and pheochromocytoma [23]. These mutations are referred to as gain-of-function, because they lead to either a constitutively active TK or decreased specificity of the TK for its substrate [24].

3. *RET* Genotype-Phenotype Correlations

3.1. Sporadic MTC. Sporadic MTC constitutes 65% to 75% of MTC cases [25]. The most frequent clinical presentation is that of a thyroid nodule. Up to 75% of patients with palpable MTC have nodal metastases in the central and ipsilateral neck compartments, and 47% of patients with palpable MTC have nodal metastases in the contralateral neck [26]. Distant metastases frequently occur in the liver, lungs, and bones.

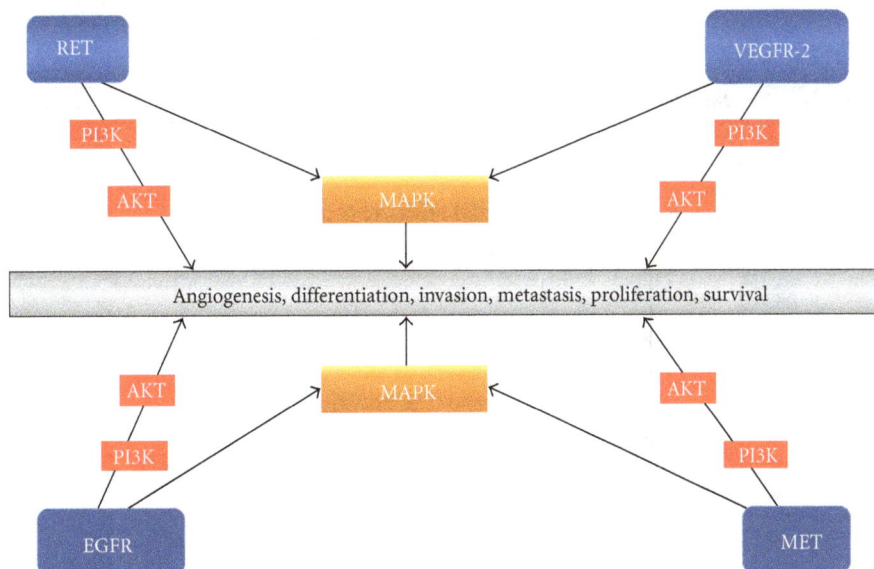

FIGURE 2: Simplified schematic representation of some of the TKs and pathways involved in MTC carcinogenesis as well normal physiology. These TKs represent important targets of TKIs. Written in the gray box are the consequences of the activation of multiple pathways and not of any one in particular.

Somatic mutations occur in 30% to 40% of cases [10, 11]. Exon 16, codon 918 ATG → ACG mutation is the most common somatic mutation in sporadic MTC [27]. This mutation is associated with larger tumors and a more advanced disease stage at diagnosis [11].

3.2. Hereditary MTC. Hereditary MTC constitutes 25% to 35% of MTC cases [25]. Hereditary MTC is preceded by C-cell hyperplasia and is usually bilateral and multicentric [28]. Hereditary forms of MTC are caused by germline *RET* proto-oncogene mutations and occurs as part of the MEN2 syndromes. MEN2A is characterized by MTC in almost 100% of gene carriers, pheochromocytomas, and parathyroid tumors. The most common mutations in MEN2A occur in one of six cysteine residues (codons 609, 611, 618, 620, 630, and 634) in the RET extracellular domain. The most frequently mutated residue found in patients with MEN2A is cysteine 634, in which removal of one-half of an intramolecular disulfide bond allows formation of an intermolecular disulfide bond with a second mutant molecule, thus leading to constitutive receptor dimerization [29]. PI3K-Akt and MAPK pathways have been implicated in MEN2A [30].

There are three variants of the syndrome: (1) MEN2A with Hirschsprung disease, (2) MEN2A associated with cutaneous lichen amyloidosis, and (3) familial MTC, in which MTC is the only manifestation. Familial MTC *RET*-mutation affects the extracellular cysteine-rich region and the TK domain. This variant tends to be the least aggressive form of hereditary MTC.

MEN2B is the most distinctive and aggressive MEN2 syndrome. The most common mutations associated with MEN2B are M918T and A883F. These mutations, unlike MEN2A, are in the TK domain and lead to an activated monomeric form, thus altering substrate specificity [29]. The PI3K/Akt cascade has been shown to be important in the pathogenesis of MEN2B in cell lines [31].

4. TK Receptors Other Than RET Involved in MTC Tumorigenesis

4.1. Epidermal Growth Factor Receptor. The epidermal growth factor receptor (EGFR/HER-1/erbB1) is a TK receptor. It is one of four homologous transmembrane receptors (the others are HER-2/erbB-2, HER-3/erbB-3, and HER-4/erbB-4) that mediate the actions of different growth factors, such as epidermal growth factor, transforming growth factor-α, and neuregulins [32]. The binding of ligands to these receptors induces EGFR homo- and/heterodimer formation, kinase domain activation, and phosphorylation of specific tyrosine residue that serve as docking sites for molecules that lead to the activation of several cascades, including the MAPK and PI3K pathways [33].

EGFR oncogenic activation can occur due to several mechanisms: excess ligand or receptor expression, activating mutations, failure of inactivation, or transactivation through receptor dimerization [34]. To date, two major types of EGFR-targeting agents exists monoclonal antibodies and small-molecule ATP-competitive TK inhibitors (TKIs) [35, 36]. PKI166, a potent EGFR kinase inhibitor, also decreases RET autophosphorylation and signaling in cell extracts despite lacking an effect on RET kinase activity. PKI166 was tested in clinical trial in patients with MTC amongst others. However, due to liver toxicities the development of this drug was halted [37]. AEE788, another EGFR kinase inhibitor, inhibits RET-induced growth at concentrations below its half maximal inhibitory concentration (IC50) [38]. However, AEE788 does not have any active clinical trials

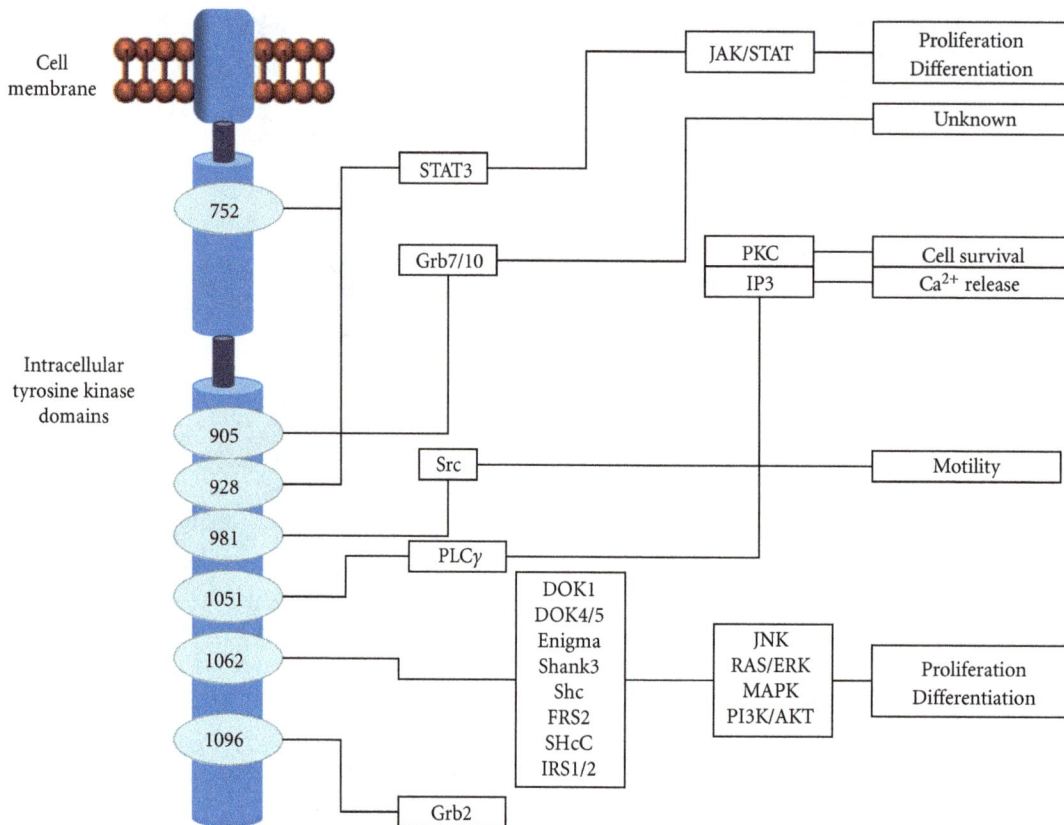

FIGURE 3: A summary of the signaling pathway mediated by RET.

in MTC patients. A study of 153 primary and metastatic MTC samples revealed that although *EGFR* mutations were rare, EGFR expression was higher in metastatic sites than in primary tumor sites [39]. MTC samples associated with *RET* 883 and 918 mutations had a significantly lower number of EGFR polysomes and a tendency toward less EGFR immunopositivity compared with samples associated with other *RET* mutations. Therefore, it is speculated that the most aggressive *RET* mutations are less dependent on EGFR activation, thereby explaining why EGFR inhibitors are less effective in codon 918-mutated cell lines than in codon 634-mutated cell lines.

4.2. Vascular Endothelial Growth Factor. The vascular endothelial growth factor (VEGF) family of growth factors stimulates angiogenesis, endothelial cell proliferation, migration, survival, and vascular permeability by various TK receptors: VEGFR-1, VEGFR-2, and VEGFR-3 [40]. There are several ligands for VEGFRs: VEGF-A (VEGF) binds to both VEGFR-1 and VEGFR-2; VEGF-B and placenta growth factor bind to only VEGFR-1; and VEGF-C and VEGF-D are specific ligands for VEGFR-3 [41].

Angiogenesis is one of the essential alterations in cell physiology that predispose to malignancy in many tumors, and it is fundamental in tumor growth and metastasis. Many molecules have been implicated as positive regulators of angiogenesis, including VEGF, hepatocyte growth factor, interleukin-8, and platelet-derived growth factor (PDGF).

The major mediator of tumor angiogenesis is VEGF, which signals mainly through VEGFR-2. Activation of this receptor leads to a cascade of different pathways, including PLC γ-PKC-Raf-MEK-MAPK and PI3K-Akt [42]. Lymphangiogenesis is also involved in tumor biology, and since lymphatic vessels arise from blood vessels, some of the angiogenic mechanisms are also used in this process. VEGF-C and VEGF-D stimulate both angiogenesis and lymphangiogenesis and link both processes [43]. VEGFR-3 is expressed mainly in lymphatic endothelial cells and is thought to be primarily involved in lymphangiogenesis.

MTC has at least twofold expression when compared with normal thyroid tissue of VEGF and VEGF-R2 [44]. There is also an up to 20-fold increased expression of VEGF-C and VEGF-R3 in metastatic MTC [45]. Overexpression and activation of VEGFR-2 in MTC correlate with metastasis [39].

4.3. c-MET. The *c-met (MET)* proto-oncogene codes for the TK receptor of the hepatocyte growth factor [46]. *MET* is an important factor in tumorigenesis. Deregulated activation of MET confers unrestricted proliferative, antiapoptotic, cell motility/migration, invasive, metastatic, and angiogenenic properties to cancer cells [47]. Silencing the endogenous *MET* proto-oncogene, which is overexpressed in tumor cells, has been proven to impair the invasive growth in vitro, to decrease the generation of metastases in vivo, and to promote the regression of already established metastases [48].

TABLE 1: Some of the TKIs currently used for the treatment of MTC in clinical trials and off-label.

Drug	Oral daily dose	Major targets
Vandetanib	100–300 mg	VEGFR-1, VEGFR-2, VEGFR-3, RET, EGFR
Sorafenib	400–800 mg	RET, VEGFR-2, VEGFR-3, Flt-3, PDGFRβ, KIT, RAF-1
Sunitinib	37.5 mg every day 50 mg daily 4 weeks on 2 weeks off	VEGFR-2, PDGFRβ, KIT, RET
Cabozantinib (XL184)	125–175 mg/day	MET, VEGFR-2, RET, KIT, Flt-3, Tie-2
E7080	24 mg	VEGFR-2, VEGFR-3, VEGFR-1, KIT, FGFR1, PDGFR, EGFR

MET and hepatocyte growth factor coexpression has been seen in a subset of MTC tumors and is associated with multifocality in MTC [49].

5. Targeted Therapy

Different TKs and pathways are abnormally activated in MTC cells. Inhibiting only one receptor may induce other TKs compensatory activation [50]. Therefore, simultaneous inhibition of different activated TKs may be the best way to approach MTC (Table 1) [51]. To date, systemic targeted therapy for MTC has been administered in the context of clinical trials or has consisted of off-label use of drugs approved for other solid tumors. In this section, we review the most promising TK inhibitors against MTC.

5.1. Vandetanib. Vandetanib is a 4-anilinoquinazoline that is available as an oral daily agent. It inhibits VEGFR-2, VEGFR-3, RET, and to a lesser extent EGFR and VEGFR-1 [52]. The 4-anilinoquinazoline docks to the ATP binding pocket of RET kinase, inhibiting it [53].

At pharmacologically relevant doses, vandetanib inhibits tumor cell proliferation, survival, and angiogenesis without leading to direct cytotoxic effects on tumor or endothelial cells [52]. In 2002, vandetanib was shown to inhibit the kinase activity of NIH-RET/C634R (MEN2A) and NIH-RET/M918T (MEN2B) oncoproteins in vitro and to inhibit RET/MEN2B phosphorylation and RET/MEN2B-dependent MAPK activation in vivo in NIH-RET/MEN2B [54]. Two years later, a panel of point mutations targeting the RET kinase domain in MEN2 and sporadic MTC was screened for susceptibility to vandetanib. Most of the mutant oncoproteins (RET/E768D, RET/L790F, RET/Y791F, RET/S891A, and RET/A883F) were sensitive to vandetanib, while mutations substituting valine 804 either to leucine or to methionine (as occur in some cases of MEN2A) rendered the RET kinase significantly resistant. This is probably due to steric hindrance, because the Val804Gly mutation increased the sensitivity of RET to vandetanib [55]. Mice carrying a *RET* C634R mutation from a sporadic human MTC treated with vandetanib had inhibition of tumor growth [56].

Inhibition of other kinases seems to be very important, too. MTC metastases express more EGFR and VEGFR-2 than primary tumor sites. Both EGFR and VEGFR-2 have been shown to be phosphorylated in TT and MZ-CRC-1 cells

and inhibited by vandetanib. Yet, in the presence of active RET, neither plays a prominent role in TT cell proliferation. However, when RET activity is inhibited, overstimulation of EGFR is able to partially replace RET through a partial rescue of the MAPK pathway. In such scenario, the inhibition of EGFR by vandetanib was shown to prevent this rescue of the MAPK pathway. These data support the idea that dual inhibition of RET and EGFR is important, as it may overcome the risk of MTC cells' escaping from RET blockade through compensatory overstimulation of EGFR [50].

In phase I clinical studies of patients with solid tumors (not including MTC) [57], doses of vandetanib up to 300 mg/day were well tolerated, and adverse effects were generally mild and controlled with either dose adjustments or symptomatic therapy. The most common adverse events were rash, diarrhea, fatigue, asymptomatic QTc prolongation, proteinuria, and hypertension. Since QT prolongation was note as an adverse event, patients should have EKG and electrolytes at baseline and at regular intervals during the course of treatment.

In a phase II study, 30 adult patients with unresectable, locally advanced, or metastatic hereditary MTC received 300 mg/day of vandetanib [58]. The primary endpoint was the objective response rate (ORR) according to the 2000 Response Evaluation Criteria in Solid Tumors (RECIST) guidelines [59]. Objective partial responses (PRs) were observed in 20% of patients, and the median duration of PR was 10.2 months. Additionally, 53% of patients had stable disease (SD) for a median of 24 weeks. In another trial of vandetanib at 100 mg/day (or up to 300 mg/day in cases with disease progression), patients with similar disease characteristics achieved similar results (ORR 68%) [60]. Both trials showed a ≥50% reduction in calcitonin and carcinoembryonic antigen levels from baseline. However, the reduction in calcitonin levels did not correlate with the degree of tumor growth inhibition. It seems that RET activity is required for ligand-induced calcitonin gene expression [61]. In that sense, carcinoembryonic antigen levels may be a better marker of tumor response to vandetanib. Of interest, there was no apparent association between specific *RET* germline mutations and response to treatment (no patients with 804 *RET* mutation were included). Other phase I and II studies are ongoing to determine the effectiveness of vandetanib in sporadic MTC and its safety and efficacy in children and adolescents. (http://www.ClinicalTrials.gov/).

Data on vandetanib have been presented to the United States Food and Drug Administration (FDA), including results from the largest randomized, double-blind, placebo-controlled trial, which was conducted in 331 patients with advanced unresectable or metastatic MTC, "Study D4200C00058". This trial showed that median progression-free survival (PFS) was 11 months longer in the group randomly assigned to vandetanib and 45% had an ORR. As the drug seems to be effective in stabilizing symptomatic and/or progressive disease, it will likely become the first FDA-approved drug for MTC.

Nuclear factor κB (NF-κB) activation can block cell-death pathways and contribute to the oncogenic state by driving proliferation, enhancing cell survival, and promoting angiogenesis and metastasis. NF-κB has a high baseline activity in MTC cell lines through RET-induced phosphorylation, ubiquitination, and proteosomal degradation of inhibitors of NF-kB (IkB), which allows NF-κB to enter the nucleus and bind to the DNA [62]. Bortezomib inhibits proteosome-mediated IkB degradation in MTC cells, resulting in its accumulation and thus preventing NF-κB translocation to the nucleus [63], thereby leading to apoptosis. A phase I/II trial of the combination of vandetanib plus bortezomib is currently recruiting patients (http://www.ClinicalTrials.gov/). Patients with MTC will participate in the phase II study.

5.2. Sorafenib. Sorafenib is a small TKI that targets RET, VEGFR-2, VEGFR-3, Flt3, PDGFR-β, KIT, and the RAF family serine/threonine kinases RAF-1 and BRAF. It inhibits the growth of RET-driven tumors by a combination of activities that target RET-dependent thyroid cancer cell proliferation and VEGF-dependent tumor angiogenesis. In vitro, sorafenib inhibits RET signaling and the growth of *RET*-transfected fibroblasts and human thyroid cancer cells that harbor *RET/PTC* and *RET/MEN2* oncogenes. Sorafenib action is mainly cytostatic, but the drug also exerts a proapoptotic effect. Sorafenib has been shown to significantly reduce tumor growth in nude mice with xenograft tumors derived from MTC cell lines [64]. Sorafenib has been investigated in four phase I trials with different doses and administration schedules. A dose of 400 mg orally twice daily was found to be safe and generally well tolerated, and the most frequently reported drug-related adverse events were fatigue, anorexia, diarrhea, rash/desquamation, and hand-foot syndrome. Hand-foot syndrome is characterized by painful erythematous lesions that affect the palmo-plantar surface. It is the most common reported adverse effect in patients taking the multikinase inhibitors like sorafenib and sunitinib. The lesions are pronounced on the pressure points on the palms and the soles but can also affect the margins of the feet and skin between fingers and toes. These lesions are not life threatening but significantly impair the quality of life requiring dose reduction or even discontinuation of the drug [65].Severe hematological, cardiovascular, hepatic, and renal toxic effects were not reported. Treatment-related hypertension was reported in 5% to 11% of patients in all four phase I trials. Sorafenib demonstrated evidence of antitumor activity by inducing disease stabilization in patients with refractory tumors, a finding that was consistent

with the results of preclinical studies [66]. No patients with thyroid cancer were included in the phase I study. Because of the role of *RET* signaling in MTC and the antitumor activity exhibited by sorafenib in preclinical and in vitro studies, MTC was recognized as a potential target for sorafenib. In a small 2007 pilot study that included five patients with metastatic MTC with excessive calcitonin secretion, calcitonin secretion was decreased by >50% in all patients after 3 months of treatment, and all patients were free of calcitonin-related symptoms. After 6 months of therapy, one patient had a complete response (CR), and patient had a PR [67]. Sorafenib was administered orally at a dose of 400 mg twice daily continuously in a larger, open-label phase II study in patients with histologically confirmed metastatic or locally advanced MTC. Patients were monitored regularly with physical examination and biochemical and radiologic testing. In the event of any significant drug-related adverse event, the drug was withheld and restarted at a lower dose of 400 to 600 mg/day with dose re-escalation as tolerated. The median duration of therapy with sorafenib was 15 months. ORR was assessed using RECIST version 1.0. Of the 15 evaluable patients in this study, all showed some degree of tumor shrinkage. One patient achieved PR; 14 patients had SD, eight of whom had SD ≥15 months; and one patient had clinically progressive disease. Most patients had decreased calcitonin levels 2 months after treatment initiation, but they did not correlate with the degree or duration of response as assessed using RECIST [68]. Sorafenib has been approved by the FDA for treatment of renal cell and hepatocellular carcinoma. Therefore, sorafenib is an option for patients with advanced MTC who are not eligible for clinical trials [69].

5.3. Tipifarnib. Tipifarnib inhibits farnesylation of RAS and other proteins. Farnesylation is a type of lipid modification that is critical for the biological functionality including several signal transduction proteins. Farnesyltransferase inhibitors target multiple pathways, including the RAS pathway, and are among the first systematically investigated drugs in oncogene-targeted therapy. *RAS* genes encode proteins involved in cell proliferation, differentiation, and adhesion and apoptosis regulation. At least three associated genes (*H-RAS*, *K-RAS*, and *N-RAS*) are present in mammalian cells. Of all human tumors, 30% might have a mutated *RAS* isoform. Thyroid cancer has mutations in all three *RAS* genes. In in vitro studies, tipifarnib inhibited the growth of several human tumor cell lines, and in in vivo studies, tipifarnib was shown to inhibit colon and pancreatic cancer xenografts in a dose-dependent manner. The antitumor effects were mainly due to decreased cell proliferation, antiangiogenesis, and apoptosis. A phase I trial of tipifarnib in combination with sorafenib in patients with advanced malignancies included 15 patients with thyroid cancer, eight of whom had MTC. Three of the six patients who reached first restaging had PRs, whereas the others had some minor regressions and hence SD lasting from 12 to 16 months. The most common side effects reported were rash, hyperglycemia, and diarrhea. *RET* mutational analysis in these six patients revealed *RET* mutations; thus, it is unclear whether the response to sorafenib and tipifarnib was entirely due to *RET* inhibition by sorafenib [70]. In a previously reported case, the rate of response rate to combination therapy was higher than that reported for sorafenib alone. It should be noted that the *RET* pathway is complex and the RET kinase can activate a cascade of signaling pathways. Tipifarnib can also affect various other pathways, including Akt and MAP/ERK, and may have acted synergistically to produce the clinical response [71]. The FDA has not approved tipifarnib because of its inferior outcomes in phase III trials in patients with other malignancies [72]. However, the data from trials of thyroid cancer so far seem encouraging, and studies combining various oncogene-targeted therapies are needed.

Preclinical studies have shown that activating *RET* mutations in V804 (V804L and V804M) causes resistance to various structural classes, including vandetanib. Mutations in V804 slightly affect RET susceptibility to sorafenib, thus indicating that a structurally different inhibitor may be used to overcome the mutational resistance to a particular TKI [73]. This might be clinically significant as a recent study showed RET V804M (19.6%) is a prevalent cause of hereditary MTC [74].

5.4. Sunitinib. Sunitinib is a derivative of indolinone and inhibits the activity of many TKs, including VEGFR, PDGFR, KIT, and RET. Sunitinib exerts antitumor activity by affecting cell proliferation and survival in cancers in which these receptors are involved [75]. Its inhibitory effect on VEGF and RET makes this drug a rational choice for treating MTC. In a phase II study of sunitinib in patients with progressive thyroid cancer that included six patients with MTC, disease stabilization was seen in five of the six patients (83%) [76]. Results from another phase II study that included only patients with progressive MTC also showed responses. Among the 23 patients evaluated, eight (35%) achieved PR, with a median response duration of 37 weeks, and 13 (57%) had SD, with a median response duration of 32 weeks [77]. A trial using a lower dose of 37.5 mg/day in a continuous manner included six patients with MTC. Three of the six patients had an objective response [78]. The most common drug-related adverse events were fatigue, diarrhea, palmar-plantar erythrodysesthesia, neutropenia, and hypertension. Sunitinib has been approved by the FDA as the treatment of renal cell carcinoma and is therefore available for use in selected patients with MTC not enrolled in a clinical trial [69].

5.5. Cabozantinib (XL184). Cabozantinib (XL184) is a small molecule that inhibits MET, VEGFR-2, RET, KIT, Flt-3, and Tie-2 [79]. In the context of MTC, preclinical data have demonstrated that XL184 can inhibit the proliferation of cells harboring activated *RET*. In 2009, results of a phase I trial that included 37 patients with MTC revealed that 44% of patients achieved at least 30% reduction in tumor size, and 29% of patients confirmed PR. There was no correlation between *RET* mutation status (either germline or somatic) and tumor response [80]. Side effects included fatigue, diarrhea, appetite loss, weight loss, hair hypopigmentation, and hypertension. Other effects, such as elevated

aspartate aminotransferase, alanine aminotransferase, lipase elevations, palmar/plantar erythema, and mucositis, were dose dependent. Because of the noted antitumor effects of XL184, a phase III clinical trial called the "Efficacy of XL184 in Advanced Medullary Thyroid Cancer (EXAM)" is recruiting patients (http://www.ClinicalTrials.gov/). The purpose of the study is to evaluate PFS with XL184 compared to PFS with placebo in subjects with unresectable, locally advanced, or metastatic MTC.

Recently, in addition to giving XL184 a generic drug name, FDA had granted XL184 an orphan drug designation for treatment of follicular, medullary, and anaplastic thyroid carcinoma, and metastatic or locally advanced papillary thyroid cancer.

5.6. E7080. E7080 inhibits VEGFR-1, VEGFR-2, VEGFR-3, KIT, FGFR1, PDGFR, and to a lesser extent EGFR. This drug has been shown to be a potent inhibitor of in vitro angiogenesis in human small cell lung cancer via inhibition of VEGF/VEGF-2 and the stem cell factor/KIT signaling pathways. Via dual inhibition of VEGFR-2 and VEGFR-3, E7080 has also been shown to decrease lymphatic vessel density in the primary tumors of VEGFC-overexpressing MDA-MB-231 mammary fat pad xenograft models as well as within the metastatic nodules in the lymph nodes of nude mice [81].

In phase I trials, E7080 caused hypertension and proteinuria, which were the major dose-limiting toxic effects [82]. Other observed adverse events included thrombosis, tachycardia, febrile neutropenia, and thrombocytopenia.

A phase II trial to evaluate the safety and efficacy of oral E7080 in medullary and iodine-131-refractory, unresectable differentiated thyroid cancers is ongoing (http://www.clinicaltrials.gov/). The primary purpose of the trial is to determine the effect of E7080 on the objective tumor response rate according to RECIST.

5.7. Pazopanib. Pazopanib is an oral multikinase inhibitor. In vitro studies have shown that it is a potent inhibitor of VEGFR-1, VEGFR-2, VEGFR-3, PDGFR-α and $-\beta$, and KIT [83]. The antineoplastic activity of pazopanib is primarily due to its effect on the angiogenic pathways. Phase II studies of pazopanib for MTC are ongoing [84].

6. Conclusion

Research on MTC over the last 55 years has led to a good understanding of the genetic defects and altered molecular pathways associated with its development. Subsequently, promising targeted therapies have been developed for progressive and advanced MTC. Multikinase inhibitors have shown good results in terms of stabilizing disease, and this year will probably see the approval of a drug for advanced unresectable or metastatic MTC, which would represent a new chapter in the history of this disease. The challenge for the years to come is to discover more effective ways to target multiple key pathological pathways as well as the identification of the individuals who will benefit the most.

Acknowledgments

This research is supported in part by the National Institutes of Health through MD Anderson's Cancer Center Support Grant CA016672. K. Gómez and J. Varghese equally contributed to this work and should be rewarded as joint first authors.

References

[1] R. A. DeLellis, R. Lloyd, P. U. Heitz, and C. Eng, *WHO Classification of Tumours, Pathology and Genetics of Tumours of Endocrine Organs*, IARC Press, Lyon, France, 2004.

[2] L. Davies and H. G. Welch, "Increasing incidence of thyroid cancer in the United States, 1973–2002," *Journal of the American Medical Association*, vol. 295, no. 18, pp. 2164–2167, 2006.

[3] J. B. Hazard, W. A. Hawk, and G. Crile Jr., "Medullary (solid) carcinoma of the thyroid: a clinicopathologic entity," *Journal of Clinical Endocrinology & Metabolism*, vol. 19, no. 1, pp. 152–161, 1959.

[4] J. H. Sipple, "The association of pheochromocytoma with carcinoma of the thyroid gland," *The American Journal of Medicine*, vol. 31, no. 1, pp. 163–166, 1961.

[5] E. D. Williams, C. L. Brown, and I. Doniach, "Pathological and clinical findings in a series of 67 cases of medullary carcinoma of the thyroid," *Journal of Clinical Pathology*, vol. 19, no. 2, pp. 103–113, 1966.

[6] E. D. Williams, "Histogenesis of medullary carcinoma of the thyroid," *Journal of Clinical Pathology*, vol. 19, no. 2, pp. 114–118, 1966.

[7] K. Graze, I. J. Spiler, A. H. Tashjian Jr. et al., "Natural history of familial medullary thyroid carcinoma. Effect of a program for early diagnosis," *New England Journal of Medicine*, vol. 299, no. 18, pp. 980–985, 1978.

[8] H. Donis-Keller, S. Dou, D. Chi et al., "Mutations in the RET proto-oncogene are associated with MEN 2A and FMTC," *Human Molecular Genetics*, vol. 2, no. 7, pp. 851–856, 1993.

[9] L. M. Mulligan, J. B. J. Kwok, C. S. Healey et al., "Germ-line mutations of the RET proto-oncogene in multiple endocrine neoplasia type 2A," *Nature*, vol. 363, no. 6428, pp. 458–460, 1993.

[10] S. Dvořáká, E. Václavíková, V. Sýkorová et al., "New multiple somatic mutations in the RET proto-oncogene associated with a sporadic medullary thyroid carcinoma," *Thyroid*, vol. 16, no. 3, pp. 311–316, 2006.

[11] R. Elisei, B. Cosci, C. Romei et al., "Prognostic significance of somatic RET oncogene mutations in sporadic medullary thyroid cancer: a 10-year follow-up study," *Journal of Clinical Endocrinology and Metabolism*, vol. 93, no. 3, pp. 682–687, 2008.

[12] C. Romei, B. Cosci, G. Renzini et al., "RET genetic screening of sporadic medullary thyroid cancer (MTC) allows the preclinical diagnosis of unsuspected gene carriers and the identification of a relevant percentage of hidden familial MTC (FMTC)," *Clinical Endocrinology*, vol. 74, no. 2, pp. 241–247, 2011.

[13] E. Gardner, L. Papi, D. F. Easton et al., "Genetic linkage studies map the multiple endocrine neoplasia type 2 loci to a small interval on chromosome 10q11.2," *Human Molecular Genetics*, vol. 2, no. 3, pp. 241–246, 1993.

[14] B. Pasini, R. M. W. Hofstra, L. Yin et al., "The physical map of the human RET proto-oncogene," *Oncogene*, vol. 11, no. 9, pp. 1737–1743, 1995.

[15] M. Takahashi, Y. Buma, T. Iwamoto, Y. Inaguma, H. Ikeda, and H. Hiai, "Cloning and expression of the ret proto-oncogene encoding a tyrosine kinase with two potential transmembrane domains," *Oncogene*, vol. 3, no. 5, pp. 571–578, 1988.

[16] T. Iwamoto, M. Taniguchi, N. Asai, K. Ohkusu, I. Nakashima, and M. Takahashi, "cDNA cloning of mouse ret proto-oncogene and its sequence similarity to the cadherin super-family," *Oncogene*, vol. 8, no. 4, pp. 1087–1091, 1993.

[17] J. Anders, S. Kjær, and C. F. Ibáñez, "Molecular modeling of the extracellular domain of the RET receptor tyrosine kinase reveals multiple cadherin-like domains and a calcium-binding site," *Journal of Biological Chemistry*, vol. 276, no. 38, pp. 35808–35817, 2001.

[18] M. S. Airaksinen and M. Saarma, "The GDNF family: signalling, biological functions and therapeutic value," *Nature Reviews Neuroscience*, vol. 3, no. 5, pp. 383–394, 2002.

[19] B. A. Tsui-Pierchala, J. Milbrandt, and E. M. Johnson Jr., "NGF utilizes c-Ret via a novel GFL-independent, inter-RTK signaling mechanism to maintain the trophic status of mature sympathetic neurons," *Neuron*, vol. 33, no. 2, pp. 261–273, 2002.

[20] J. W. B. De Groot, T. P. Links, J. T. M. Plukker, C. J. M. Lips, and R. M. W. Hofstra, "RET as a diagnostic and therapeutic target in sporadic and hereditary endocrine tumors," *Endocrine Reviews*, vol. 27, no. 5, pp. 535–560, 2006.

[21] M. Takahashi, "The GDNF/RET signaling pathway and human diseases," *Cytokine and Growth Factor Reviews*, vol. 12, no. 4, pp. 361–373, 2001.

[22] M. Ichihara, Y. Murakumo, and M. Takahashi, "RET and neuroendocrine tumors," *Cancer Letters*, vol. 204, no. 2, pp. 197–211, 2004.

[23] C. Eng, "Seminars in medicine of the Beth Israel Hospital, Boston: the RET proto- oncogene in multiple endocrine neoplasia type 2 and Hirschsprung's disease," *New England Journal of Medicine*, vol. 335, no. 13, pp. 943–951, 1996.

[24] K. M. Zbuk and C. Eng, "Cancer phenomics: RET and PTEN as illustrative models," *Nature Reviews Cancer*, vol. 7, no. 1, pp. 35–45, 2007.

[25] C. Jiménez, M. I.-N. Hu, and R. F. Gagel, "Management of medullary thyroid carcinoma," *Endocrinology and Metabolism Clinics of North America*, vol. 37, no. 2, pp. 481–496, 2008.

[26] J. F. Moley and M. K. DeBenedetti, "Patterns of nodal metastases in palpable medullary thyroid carcinoma: recommendations for extent of node dissection," *Annals of Surgery*, vol. 229, no. 6, pp. 880–888, 1999.

[27] D. J. Marsh, D. L. Learoyd, S. D. Andrew et al., "Somatic mutations in the RET proto-oncogene in sporadic medullary thyroid carcinoma," *Clinical Endocrinology*, vol. 44, no. 3, pp. 249–257, 1996.

[28] H. J. Wolfe, K. E. Melvin, S. J. Cervi-Skinner et al., "C-cell hyperplasia preceding medullary thyroid carcinoma," *New England Journal of Medicine*, vol. 289, no. 9, pp. 437–441, 1973.

[29] M. Drosten and B. M. Pützer, "Mechanisms of disease: cancer targeting and the impact of oncogenic RET for medullary thyroid carcinoma therapy," *Nature Clinical Practice Oncology*, vol. 3, no. 10, pp. 564–574, 2006.

[30] A. M. Hennige, R. Lammers, D. Arlt et al., "Ret oncogene signal transduction via a IRS-2/PI 3-kinase/PKB and a SHC/Grb-2 dependent pathway: possible implication for transforming activity in NIH3T3 cells," *Molecular and Cellular Endocrinology*, vol. 167, no. 1-2, pp. 69–76, 2000.

[31] H. Murakami, T. Iwashita, N. Asai et al., "Enhanced phosphatidylinositol 3-kinase activity and high phosphorylation state of its downstream signalling molecules mediated by Ret with the MEN 2B mutation," *Biochemical and Biophysical Research Communications*, vol. 262, no. 1, pp. 68–75, 1999.

[32] R. N. Jorissen, F. Walker, N. Pouliot, T. P.J. Garrett, C. W. Ward, and A. W. Burgess, "Epidermal growth factor receptor: mechanisms of activation and signalling," *Experimental Cell Research*, vol. 284, no. 1, pp. 31–53, 2003.

[33] T. Holbro, G. Civenni, and N. E. Hynes, "The ErbB receptors and their role in cancer progression," *Experimental Cell Research*, vol. 284, no. 1, pp. 99–110, 2003.

[34] G. Vlahovic and J. Crawford, "Activation of tyrosine kinases in cancer," *Oncologist*, vol. 8, no. 6, pp. 531–538, 2003.

[35] C. L. Arteaga, "ErbB-targeted therapeutic approaches in human cancer," *Experimental Cell Research*, vol. 284, no. 1, pp. 122–130, 2003.

[36] I. Vivanco and I. K. Mellinghoff, "Epidermal growth factor receptor inhibitors in oncology," *Current Opinion in Oncology*, vol. 22, no. 6, pp. 573–578, 2010.

[37] P. Traxler, "Tyrosine kinases as targets in cancer therapy—successes and failures," *Expert Opinion on Therapeutic Targets*, vol. 7, no. 2, pp. 215–234, 2003.

[38] M. Croyle, N. Akeno, J. A. Knauf et al., "RET/PTC-induced cell growth is mediated in part by epidermal growth factor receptor (EGFR) activation: evidence for molecular and functional interactions between RET and EGFR," *Cancer Research*, vol. 68, no. 11, pp. 4183–4191, 2008.

[39] C. Rodríguez-Antona, J. Pallares, C. Montero-Conde et al., "Overexpression and activation of EGFR and VEGFR2 in medullary thyroid carcinomas is related to metastasis," *Endocrine-Related Cancer*, vol. 17, no. 1, pp. 7–16, 2010.

[40] B. I. Terman, M. Dougher-Vermazen, M. E. Carrion et al., "Identification of the KDR tyrosine kinase as a receptor for vascular endothelial cell growth factor," *Biochemical and Biophysical Research Communications*, vol. 187, no. 3, pp. 1579–1586, 1992.

[41] M. Shibuya and L. Claesson-Welsh, "Signal transduction by VEGF receptors in regulation of angiogenesis and lymphangiogenesis," *Experimental Cell Research*, vol. 312, no. 5, pp. 549–560, 2006.

[42] R. S. Kerbel, "Tumor angiogenesis," *New England Journal of Medicine*, vol. 358, no. 19, pp. 2039–2049, 2008.

[43] K. Alitalo and P. Carmeliet, "Molecular mechanisms of lymphangiogenesis in health and disease," *Cancer Cell*, vol. 1, no. 3, pp. 219–227, 2002.

[44] C. Capp, S. M. Wajner, D. R. Siqueira, B. A. Brasil, L. Meurer, and A. L. Maia, "Increased expression of vascular endothelial growth factor and its receptors, VEGFR-1 and VEGFR-2, in medullary thyroid carcinoma," *Thyroid*, vol. 20, no. 8, pp. 863–871, 2010.

[45] G. Bunone, P. Vigneri, L. Mariani et al., "Expression of angiogenesis stimulators and inhibitors in human thyroid tumors and correlation with clinical pathological features," *American Journal of Pathology*, vol. 155, no. 6, pp. 1967–1976, 1999.

[46] D. P. Bottaro, J. S. Rubin, D. L. Faletto et al., "Identification of the hepatocyte growth factor receptor as the c-met proto-oncogene product," *Science*, vol. 251, no. 4995, pp. 802–804, 1991.

[47] M. Sattler and R. Salgia, "The MET axis as a therapeutic target," *Update on Cancer Therapeutics*, vol. 3, no. 3, pp. 109–118, 2009.

[48] S. Corso, C. Migliore, E. Ghiso, G. De Rosa, P. M. Comoglio, and S. Giordano, "Silencing the MET oncogene leads to regression of experimental tumors and metastases," *Oncogene*, vol. 27, no. 5, pp. 684–693, 2008.

[49] M. Papotti, M. Olivero, M. Volante et al., "Expression of hepatocyte growth factor (HGF) and its receptor (MET) in medullary carcinoma of the thyroid," *Endocrine Pathology*, vol. 11, no. 1, pp. 19–30, 2000.

[50] D. Vitagliano, V. De Falco, A. Tamburrino et al., "The tyrosine kinase inhibitor ZD6474 blocks proliferation of RET mutant medullary thyroid carcinoma cells," *Endocrine-Related Cancer*, vol. 18, no. 1, pp. 1–11, 2011.

[51] A. Ocana, E. Amir, B. Seruga, and A. Pandiella, "Do we have to change the way targeted drugs are developed?" *Journal of Clinical Oncology*, vol. 28, no. 24, pp. e420–e421, 2010.

[52] R. S. Herbst, J. V. Heymach, M. S. O'Reilly, A. Onn, and A. J. Ryan, "Vandetanib (ZD6474): an orally available receptor tyrosine kinase inhibitor that selectively targets pathways critical for tumor growth and angiogenesis," *Expert Opinion on Investigational Drugs*, vol. 16, no. 2, pp. 239–249, 2007.

[53] P. P. Knowles, J. Murray-Rust, S. Kjær et al., "Structure and chemical inhibition of the RET tyrosine kinase domain," *Journal of Biological Chemistry*, vol. 281, no. 44, pp. 33577–33587, 2006.

[54] F. Carlomagno, D. Vitagliano, T. Guida et al., "ZD6474, an orally available inhibitor of KDR tyrosine kinase activity, efficiently blocks oncogenic RET kinases," *Cancer Research*, vol. 62, no. 24, pp. 7284–7290, 2002.

[55] F. Carlomagno, T. Guida, S. Anaganti et al., "Disease associated mutations at valine 804 in the RET receptor tyrosine kinase confer resistance to selective kinase inhibitors," *Oncogene*, vol. 23, no. 36, pp. 6056–6063, 2004.

[56] V. Johanson, H. Ahlman, P. Bernhardt et al., "A transplantable human medullary thyroid carcinoma as a model for RET tyrosine kinase-driven tumorigenesis," *Endocrine-Related Cancer*, vol. 14, no. 2, pp. 433–444, 2007.

[57] S. N. Holden, S. G. Eckhardt, R. Basser et al., "Clinical evaluation of ZD6474, an orally active inhibitor of VEGF and EGF receptor signaling, in patients with solid, malignant tumors," *Annals of Oncology*, vol. 16, no. 8, pp. 1391–1397, 2005.

[58] S. A. Wells Jr., J. E. Gosnell, R. F. Gagel et al., "Vandetanib for the treatment of patients with locally advanced or metastatic hereditary medullary thyroid cancer," *Journal of Clinical Oncology*, vol. 28, no. 5, pp. 767–772, 2010.

[59] P. Therasse, S. G. Arbuck, E. A. Eisenhauer et al., "New guidelines to evaluate the response to treatment in solid tumors," *Journal of the National Cancer Institute*, vol. 92, no. 3, pp. 205–216, 2000.

[60] B. G. Robinson, L. Paz-Ares, A. Krebs, J. Vasselli, and R. Haddad, "Vandetanib (100 mg) in patients with locally advanced or metastatic hereditary medullary thyroid cancer," *Journal of Clinical Endocrinology and Metabolism*, vol. 95, no. 6, pp. 2664–2671, 2010.

[61] N. Akeno-Stuart, M. Croyle, J. A. Knauf et al., "The RET kinase inhibitor NVP-AST487 blocks growth and calcitonin gene expression through distinct mechanisms in medullary thyroid cancer cells," *Cancer Research*, vol. 67, no. 14, pp. 6956–6964, 2007.

[62] L. Ludwig, H. Kessler, M. Wagner et al., "Nuclear factor-κB is constitutively active in C-cell carcinoma and required for RET-induced transformation," *Cancer Research*, vol. 61, no. 11, pp. 4526–4535, 2001.

[63] C. S. Mitsiades, D. McMillin, V. Kotoula et al., "Antitumor effects of the proteasome inhibitor bortezomib in medullary and anaplastic thyroid carcinoma cells in vitro," *Journal of Clinical Endocrinology and Metabolism*, vol. 91, no. 10, pp. 4013–4021, 2006.

[64] F. Carlomagno, S. Anaganti, T. Guida et al., "BAY 43-9006 inhibition of oncogenic RET mutants," *Journal of the National Cancer Institute*, vol. 98, no. 5, pp. 326–334, 2006.

[65] A. Degen, M. Alter, F. Schenck et al., "The hand-foot-syndrome associated with medical tumor therapy—classification and management," *Journal of the German Society of Dermatology*, vol. 8, no. 9, pp. 652–662, 2010.

[66] D. Strumberg, J. W. Clark, A. Awada et al., "Safety, pharmacokinetics, and preliminary antitumor activity of sorafenib: a review of four phase I trials in patients with advanced refractory solid tumors," *Oncologist*, vol. 12, no. 4, pp. 426–437, 2007.

[67] F. Kober, M. Hermann, A. Handler, and G. Krotla, "Effect of sorafenib in symptomatic metastatic medullary thyroid cancer," *Journal of Clinical Oncology*, vol. 25, abstract 14065, 2007.

[68] E. T. Lam, M. D. Ringel, R. T. Kloos et al., "Phase II clinical trial of sorafenib in metastatic medullary thyroid cancer," *Journal of Clinical Oncology*, vol. 28, no. 14, pp. 2323–2330, 2010.

[69] S. I. Sherman, "NCCN Practice guidelines for thyroid cancer," Version 1.2011. 2011.

[70] D. S. Hong, S. M. Sebti, R. A. Newman et al., "Phase I trial of a combination of the multikinase inhibitor sorafenib and the farnesyltransferase inhibitor tipifarnib in advanced malignancies," *Clinical Cancer Research*, vol. 15, no. 22, pp. 7061–7068, 2009.

[71] D. Hong, L. Ye, R. Gagel et al., "Medullary thyroid cancer: targeting the RET kinase pathway with sorafenib/tipifarnib," *Molecular Cancer Therapeutics*, vol. 7, no. 5, pp. 1001–1006, 2008.

[72] A. M. Tsimberidou, C. Chandhasin, and R. Kurzrock, "Farnesyltransferase inhibitors: where are we now?" *Expert Opinion on Investigational Drugs*, vol. 19, no. 12, pp. 1569–1580, 2010.

[73] C. Lanzi, G. Cassinelli, V. Nicolini, and F. Zunino, "Targeting RET for thyroid cancer therapy," *Biochemical Pharmacology*, vol. 77, no. 3, pp. 297–309, 2009.

[74] C. Romei, S. Mariotti, L. Fugazzola et al., "Multiple endocrine neoplasia type 2 syndromes (MEN 2): results from the ItaMEN network analysis on the prevalence of different genotypes and phenotypes," *European Journal of Endocrinology*, vol. 163, no. 2, pp. 301–308, 2010.

[75] D. B. Mendel, A. D. Laird, X. Xin et al., "In vivo antitumor activity of SU11248, a novel tyrosine kinase inhibitor targeting vascular endothelial growth factor and platelet-derived growth factor receptors: determination of a pharmacokinetic/pharmacodynamic relationship," *Clinical Cancer Research*, vol. 9, no. 1, pp. 327–337, 2003.

[76] E. E. Cohen, B. M. Needles, K. J. Cullen et al., "Phase 2 study of sunitinib in refractory thyroid cancer," *Journal of Clinical Oncology*, vol. 26, abstract 6025, 2008.

[77] J. A. De Souza, N. Busaidy, A. Zimrin et al., "Phase II trial of sunitinib in medullary thyroid cancer (MTC)," *Journal of Clinical Oncology*, vol. 28, abstract 5504, 2010.

[78] L. L. Carr, D. A. Mankoff, B. H. Goulart et al., "Phase II study of daily sunitinib in FDG-PET-positive, iodine-refractory differentiated thyroid cancer and metastatic medullary carcinoma of the thyroid with functional imaging correlation," *Clinical Cancer Research*, vol. 16, no. 21, pp. 5260–5268, 2010.

[79] J. P. Eder, G. F. Vande Woude, S. A. Boerner, and P. M. Lorusso, "Novel therapeutic inhibitors of the c-Met signaling pathway in cancer," *Clinical Cancer Research*, vol. 15, no. 7, pp. 2207–2214, 2009.

[80] S. I. Sherman, "Targeted therapy of thyroid cancer," *Biochemical Pharmacology*, vol. 80, no. 5, pp. 592–601, 2010.

[81] J. Matsui, Y. Yamamoto, Y. Funahashi et al., "E7080, a novel inhibitor that targets multiple kinases, has potent antitumor activities against stem cell factor producing human small cell lung cancer H146, based on angiogenesis inhibition," *International Journal of Cancer*, vol. 122, no. 3, pp. 664–671, 2008.

[82] R. J. Keizer, A. Gupta, M. R. Mac Gillavry et al., "A model of hypertension and proteinuria in cancer patients treated with the anti-angiogenic drug E7080," *Journal of Pharmacokinetics and Pharmacodynamics*, vol. 37, no. 4, pp. 347–363, 2010.

[83] G. Sonpavde, T. E. Hutson, and C. N. Sternberg, "Pazopanib, a potent orally administered small-molecule multitargeted tyrosine kinase inhibitor for renal cell carcinoma," *Expert Opinion on Investigational Drugs*, vol. 17, no. 2, pp. 253–261, 2008.

[84] K. C. Bible, V. J. Suman, J. R. Molina et al., "Efficacy of pazopanib in progressive, radioiodine-refractory, metastatic differentiated thyroid cancers: results of a phase 2 consortium study," *The Lancet Oncology*, vol. 11, no. 10, pp. 962–972, 2010.

25

Thyroid Antibodies and Miscarriage: Where Are We at a Generation Later?

Alex Stagnaro-Green

George Washington University School of Medicine and Health Sciences, 2300 Eye Street, Ross Hall, Suite 712, Washington, DC 20037, USA

Correspondence should be addressed to Alex Stagnaro-Green, msdasg@gwumc.edu

Academic Editor: Bijay Vaidya

In 1990, an association between thyroid antibody positivity and spontaneous miscarriage was first reported. A generation has passed since the initial observation. Over that time a robust literature has developed which has confirmed the initial finding and expanded upon it. The present paper reviews the literature that has been generated over the last twenty years on the following topics: (1) thyroid antibodies and spontaneous miscarriage, (2) thyroid antibodies and recurrent abortion, (3) etiology of pregnancy loss in thyroid antibody positive women, and (4) discussion of future research directions.

1. Introduction

It has been twenty years since the first paper reporting an association between thyroid antibodies and spontaneous miscarriage in euthyroid women was published [1]. The finding was serendipitous as the study was designed to evaluate the prevalence and etiology of postpartum thyroiditis. Five hundred and fifty-two women in the New York metropolitan area were screened in the first trimester of pregnancy for thyroid function and thyroid antibody status. A cohort of antibody positive and antibody negative women were selected and followed prospectively throughout pregnancy and into the postpartum period. As the study progressed, a high incidence of spontaneous miscarriage was observed in the cohort. In particular, it appeared that the miscarriage rate was disproportionately higher in women who were thyroid antibody positive. Following much discussion within the research team, as there was no known association between thyroid autoimmunity and miscarriage, nor was there a plausible mechanism, it was decided to examine the pregnancy outcome in the 552 women who were initially screened. A doubling of the miscarriage rate was found (17% versus 8.4%, $P = .011$) and reported in the Journal of the American Medical Association. It was unclear at the time if the finding was a statistical fluke or in fact represented an important association.

A generation has passed since the initial observation. Over that time a robust literature has developed which has not only confirmed the initial observation but expanded upon it. The present paper will summarize the data that has been published over the ensuing 20 years and speculate upon future directions. In particular, the areas of focus will be (1) thyroid antibodies and spontaneous miscarriage, (2) thyroid antibodies and recurrent abortion, (3) etiology of pregnancy loss, and (4) future directions. A comprehensive meta-analysis was published last year on the relationship between thyroid antibodies and in vitro fertilization (IVF) demonstrating that thyroid autoimmunity in women undergoing IVF is associated with an increased rate of pregnancy loss [2]. Consequently, the present discussion will not include a review of the IVF and thyroid antibody literature on spontaneous miscarriage.

2. Thyroid Antibodies and Pregnancy Loss

As noted above, Stagnaro-Green et al. reported a statistically significant doubling in the miscarriage rate in American euthyroid women in the first trimester of pregnancy who were thyroid antibody positive. Of the 552 women initially screened, 57 were unavailable for followup. One hundred women were thyroid antibody positive (with a miscarriage rate of 17/100 or 17%), and 392 women were antibody negative (with a miscarriage rate of 33/392 or 8.4%). Prior to the 1990 paper the only antibody shown to be associated with spontaneous miscarriage was anticardiolipin antibody. Analysis of the sera of the 50 women who miscarried revealed no difference in percentage of women who were cardiolipin antibody positive between women who were thyroid antibody positive and miscarried versus women who were thyroid antibody negative and miscarried. There were also no demographic differences between the groups. The TSH level was slightly, but not significantly, higher in the thyroid antibody positive women as compared to thyroid antibody negative controls (TSH-2.35 mIU/L versus 1.60 mIU/L, resp., $P = .12$). Finally, no difference in thyroid antibody titers were noted in antibody positive women who miscarried as compared to antibody women who carried to term.

Glinoer and colleagues in 1991 [3] reported findings of a prospective study of 120 Belgian euthyroid women with mild thyroid abnormalities (nodules, goiter or thyroid antibody positivity) and 630 euthyroid controls. The goal of the study was to evaluate the progression of thyroid function tests throughout pregnancy and assess for adverse obstetrical and/or neonatal outcomes. Women with thyroid autoimmunity ($n = 45$) were found to have a dramatic increase in spontaneous miscarriage when contrasted to controls (13.3% versus 3.3%, $P < .001$). As found in the study by Stagnaro-Green et al. there was no association with anticardiolipin antibody or thyroid antibody titer. Further analysis of the study was published by Lejeune et al. in 1993 [4]. Specifically, analysis of first trimester pregnancy loss revealed a spontaneous miscarriage rate of 24% in thyroid antibody positive women when compared to 5% in controls ($P < .005$).

In 1997, Iijima and colleagues evaluated 1179 healthy pregnant Japanese women between 6-14 weeks gestation for the presence of seven autoantibodies [5]. A doubling of the miscarriage rate was reported in antithyroid microsomal antibody positive women as contrasted to women who were negative for all seven autoantibodies (10.4% versus 5.5%, resp., $P < .05$). Furthermore, the rate of small for gestational age births (SGA) was increased in microsomal antibody women when compared to controls (7.1% versus 3.4%). The thyroid antibody titer was related to neither the rate of spontaneous miscarriage nor the rate of SGA.

Bagis and colleagues published a study of 876 Turkish women initially screened at 12 weeks gestation [6]. All women had thyroid function tests and thyroid autoantibodies performed at 12 weeks gestation, revealing an antibody positive rate in the entire cohort of 12.3% ($P < .0001$). Fifty percent of the antibody-positive group had a history of a prior miscarriage as contrasted to only 14.1% in the antibody negative group ($P < .0001$). TSH levels were significantly higher in antibody-positive women with a history of miscarriage as compared to antibody women who had carried to term (1.90 μU/mL versus 1.2 μU/mL,

$P < .006$). Free T4 values were also lower in the antibody positive women with a history of miscarriage (11.0 pmol/L versus 12.7 pmol/L, $P < .05$).

In 2006, Ghafoor et al. evaluated 1500 Pakistani women for thyroid peroxidase antibodies and thyroid function tests during pregnancy. Women were followed throughout gestation to determine pregnancy outcome [7]. Thyroid antibody positive women, which comprised 11.2% of the cohort, had a spontaneous miscarriage rate of 36.3% as compared to 1.8% in antibody negative women ($P < .01$). A significantly higher rate of prematurity was also reported (26.8% versus 8.0, $P < .01$) in antibody positive women. All 1500 women in the study were euthyroid.

In 2006, Negro et al. reported the findings of a prospective intervention trial. Nine hundred and eighty-four women from southern Italy in the first trimester of pregnancy were evaluated for thyroid function and thyroid peroxidase [8]. Women who were antibody positive ($n = 115$) were divided into two groups. Half of the antibody positive women were given levothyroxine during pregnancy ($n = 57$), the dose of which was determined by their initial TSH level and thyroid antibody titer. The remaining antibody positive women ($n = 58$), along with 869 antibody negative controls, did not receive levothyroxine intervention. The rate of spontaneous miscarriage was 13.8% in untreated thyroid antibody positive women and 2.4% in the 890 controls ($P < .05$). Thyroid antibody positive women who received levothyroxine had a spontaneous miscarriage rate of 3.5% which was similar to controls (2.4%), and statistically lower then the miscarriage rate in the untreated thyroid antibody positive group (13.8%) ($P < .05$). Thyroid antibody positive women who were not treated with levothyroxine had higher TSH levels at 20 weeks, 30 weeks, and three days postdelivery when compared to controls or thyroid antibody-positive women who were given levothyroxine. The largest difference was seen postdelivery (TSH-1.9 mIU/L in levothyroxine treated antibody positive women, TSH-3.5 mIU/L in untreated antibody positive women, TSH-2.1 mIU/L in controls, $P < .01$). Free T4 values were also lower in the untreated group at 30 weeks and postdelivery when compared to treated antibody positive women or controls (postdelivery values were 10.2 ng/liter, 14.3 ng/liter, and 14.6 ng/liter, resp., $P < .01$)

In summary, a total of seven studies (see Table 1) in six different countries have reported an association between thyroid antibody positivity in unselected women in the first trimester of pregnancy and spontaneous miscarriage (see Figure 1). It can therefore be concluded that there is a clear and consistent association between thyroid antibody positivity and pregnancy loss. Studies have excluded cardiolipin antibody as a potential explanation for the pregnancy loss.

3. Recurrent Abortion

Shortly after the initial publication demonstrating an association between thyroid antibody positivity and spontaneous miscarriage, researchers began evaluating women with recurrent abortion. Recurrent abortion occurs in 0.5–1%

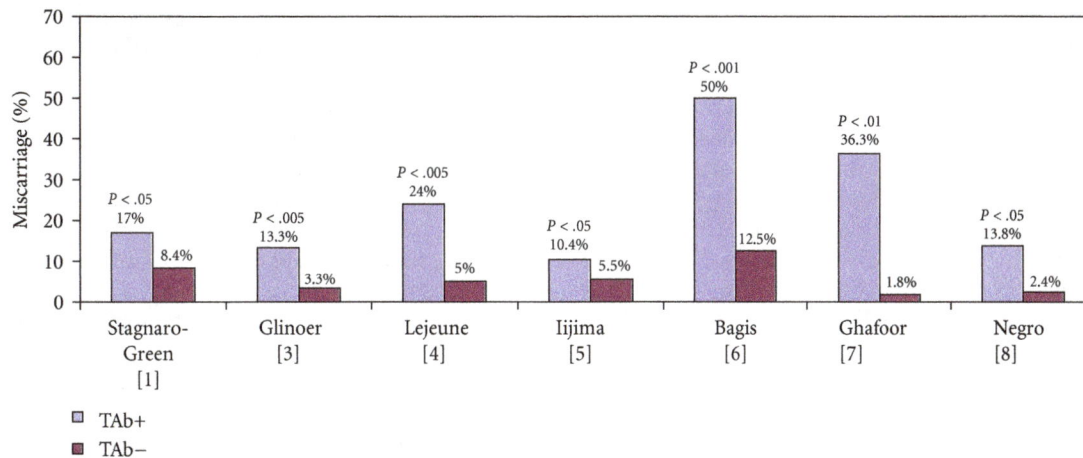

FIGURE 1: Percentage of spontaneous miscarriage in unselected pregnancies in women who were thyroid antibody positive (TAb+) and thyroid antibody negative (TAB−).

TABLE 1: Country of origin and number of women in each study of Figure 1.

Author	Country	TAb+	TAb−
Stagnaro-Green et al. [1]	USA	100	392
Glinoer et al. [3]	Belgium	45	360
Lejeune et al. [4]	Belgium	23	340
Iijima et al. [5]	Japan	24	52
Bagis et al. [6]	Turkey	108	768
Ghafoor et al. [7]	Pakistan	212	1288
Negro et al. [8]	Italy	115	869

of all women and is defined as three or more spontaneous miscarriages. The etiology is multifactorial, and includes uterine anomalies, endocrine disorders, genetic defects, and the anticardiolipin antibody. Nevertheless, despite comprehensive workups, approximately 50% of women with recurrent abortion will have no identified etiology. It is therefore not surprising that multiple research groups have studied the relationship between thyroid antibody positivity in women with recurrent abortion.

The first two studies investigating women with recurrent abortion were published in 1993 and performed by Pratt and colleagues in Chicago. The first study examined 45 women with recurrent abortion for four polynucleotides, five histones, six phospholipids, and thyroid antibodies [20]. Thirty-one percent of the recurrent aborters were thyroid antibody positive as compared to 19% in a control group of 100 normal blood donors (P = ns). The study was limited by the composition of the controls which included 46 men, and the small size of the group of women with recurrent abortion. Pratt and colleagues then performed a prospective study evaluating the outcome of a subsequent pregnancy in 42 women with recurrent abortion [9]. Thirty-one percent of the 42 women were thyroid antibody positive (n = 13) with 12 of the 42 women experienced a recurrent abortion in the subsequent pregnancy. Of the twelve women who miscarried,

eight were thyroid antibody positive (8/12 = 67%). In comparison, only five of the thirty who went to term were thyroid antibody positive (17%) (P = .003). The authors concluded that in women with recurrent abortion the presence of thyroid antibody positivity was associated with an increased rate of pregnancy loss in a subsequent pregnancy.

Bussen and Steck also published two papers on the topic of thyroid antibodies and recurrent abortion. The first study was published in 1995 and evaluated 66 German women for thyroid antibody positivity. Three groups were studied, including 22 euthyroid nonpregnant women with recurrent abortion, 22 multigravida women without endocrine disorders, and 22 nulligravida women [10]. The recurrent abortion group had a significantly higher rate of antibody positivity (36%) then either the euthyroid nonpregnant controls (5%) (36% versus 5%, P < .01), or the nulligravida controls (9%) (36% versus 9%, P < .01). In their 1997 paper, Bussen and Steck evaluated 28 euthyroid nonpregnant women with recurrent abortion for thyroid antibodies and nonorgan specific antibodies [12]. Secondary causes of recurrent abortion were excluded in all 28 women. Thirty-nine percent (n = 11/28) of the women with recurrent abortion were positive for thyroid antibodies versus 7% (n = 2/28) of multigravida controls (P < .01). No correlation was found between the presence of phospholipid antibodies and thyroid antibody positivity.

In a small study performed by Roberts et al. in Scotland in 1996, thyroid antibody positivity rate was evaluated in 11 women with recurrent abortion, 11 healthy pregnant women, 10 nonpregnant women, 11 women with a spontaneous miscarriage, and 10 women who had an elective termination of pregnancy [11]. Thirty-six percent (4/11) of the women with a history of recurrent abortion were thyroid antibody positive as opposed to five percent (2/41) of the women in the other four groups (P < .01). Roussev et al. also performed a small study consisting of 45 women with recurrent abortion and 15 healthy controls [21]. No difference was found in the thyroid antibody positivity rate between the two groups (9% versus 0%, P = ns).

Interpretation of the results of both studies are limited by their small sample size.

In 1998, Esplin et al. published a study performed in Salt Lake City, Utah comparing the incidence of thyroid antibody positivity in 74 nonpregnant women with recurrent abortion with 75 healthy nonpregnant controls of similar gravidity [13]. Women included in the recurrent abortion group had all tested negative for secondary causes of pregnancy loss. Although the thyroid antibody positivity rate in the recurrent abortion group was elevated at 29% the control group had an unusually high rate of thyroid antibody positivity of 37% (P = ns). It is unclear if geographic differences in rates of thyroid antibody positivity was a confound in this study.

In the largest study performed to date, Kutteh and colleagues in 1999 compared the rate of thyroid antibody positivity in 700 women with a minimum of two spontaneous miscarriages and in whom secondary causes of pregnancy loss were excluded, to 200 healthy controls [14]. All sera were obtained at least three months following a spontaneous miscarriage or birth. Thyroid antibody positive rate was significantly higher in the recurrent abortion group when compared to the controls (22.5% versus 14.5%, P = .01). There was no difference between the groups in regards to percentage of women with abnormally elevated TSH values; however women with a history of recurrent abortion were older then controls (33.3 years versus 30.8 years, P < .01).

Four more studies with either limited numbers of participants, or lack of a control group, were published in 1999 and 2000. Rushworth et al. evaluated the pregnancy outcome of 24 antibody-positive euthyroid British women with a history of recurrent abortion through a subsequent pregnancy. Eighty-one thyroid antibody negative women with recurrent abortion served as controls [22]. The live birth rate of the two groups was identical at 58%. Although the authors concluded that thyroid antibody positivity in women with recurrent abortion does not portend a worse outcome when compared to women who are thyroid antibody negative, interpretation of the results are limited by the small number of thyroid antibody positive women evaluated (n = 24). Reznikoff-Etievant et al. evaluated 678 French women with recurrent abortion and found a prevalence rate of thyroid antibody positivity of 2.9%. The study did not include a control group and did not address the unusually low rate of thyroid anitbody positivity [23]. Dendrinos et al. reported a thyroid antibody positivity rate of 37% in 30 Greek women with recurrent abortion as compared to 13% of 15 age-matched controls (P < .05) [15]. Finally, Mecacci reported that 37.9% (11/29) of women with recurrent abortion were antithyroid antibody positive as compared to 14.5% (10/69) of controls (P < .02) [16].

In 2002, Abdel Aziz et al. [24] performed a prospective study that was similar in design to the second investigation performed by Pratt et al. in 1993 [9]. Fifty Egyptian women with a history of recurrent abortion were tested for thyroid antibodies and followed until the 20th week of pregnancy. Eighteen (36%) of the women had the presence of thyroid antibodies. Twelve of the eighteen women (67%) went on to have another spontaneous miscarriage as compared to 15.6%

(5/32) of the thyroid antibody negative women (P < .001). These results are almost identical to the findings reported by Pratt and colleagues [9]. Antibody-positive women were older (33.1 years versus 29.0 years, P < .01), had a larger thyroid volume (23.9 mL versus 19.3 mL, P < .001) and reported a higher number of prior abortions (5.1 versus 3.9, P < .05) as compared to antibody-negative women.

A large scale study prospective trial comparing successful pregnancy in three groups of women with recurrent abortion was performed by De Carolis et al. in 2004 [25]. Group 1 consisted of women who were thyroid antibody positive but antiphospholipid syndrome (APS) negative (n = 162), group 2 women were APS positive but antithyroid antibody negative (n = 149), and group 3 women were both APS and thyroid antibody positive (n = 54). The group with the highest percentage of successful pregnancy outcome was Group 2 (92%), whereas the two groups of women who were thyroid antibody positive had significantly lower rates of successful pregnancies (Group 1–57%, Group 3–60%, P = .0003).

Another study published in 2004 was conducted by Marai et al. who evaluated 58 Israeli women [17]. Thirty-eight of the women had a history of recurrent abortion and 20 women had a history of infertility but no pregnancy losses. Thyroid antibody positivity rate was significantly higher in the women with recurrent abortion (21%) when compared to the thyroid antibody positive rate in women with a history of infertility (0%) (P = .001).

Shoenfeld and colleagues evaluated 109 women with recurrent pregnancy loss and compared the rate of thyroid antibody positivity to 120 healthy controls. Results on the presence of thyroid peroxidase or antithyroglobulin antibodies were only presented for 24 of the women with recurrent abortion. Thirty-three percent of the 24 women (8/24) were positive for thyroid antibodies as compared to only 11.2% (14/120) of the healthy controls (OR-3.79 {CI-1.2–11.7}) [18].

The most recent papers on thyroid antibodies and recurrent abortion were published in 2008. The first was a case control study performed by Iravani et al. [19] in Iran which included 641 women with three or more consecutive pregnancy losses and 269 age-matched controls. Women in the recurrent abortion group had a rate of thyroid antibody positivity almost twice that of the control group (24.5% versus 12.6%, P < .001). Mean TSH levels were higher in the recurrent abortion group when compared to controls (TSH-1.93 mIU/L versus 1.3 mIU/L, P < .001) and was independently associated with both pregnancy loss and autoimmunity. In a much smaller study, Bellver et al. found no difference in thyroid antibody positivity between 30 Spanish women with recurrent abortion and 32 controls (3.6% versus 15.6%) [26].

In conclusion, there have been 17 studies performed to date comparing thyroid antibody positivity rate in women with recurrent abortion as compared to control groups. The studies vary markedly in regards to the size of the population studied and have taken place in five different countries. Thirteen of the seventeen studies performed demonstrated a significant increase in the thyroid antibody positivity rate in women with recurrent abortion (Table 2, Figure 2). Of

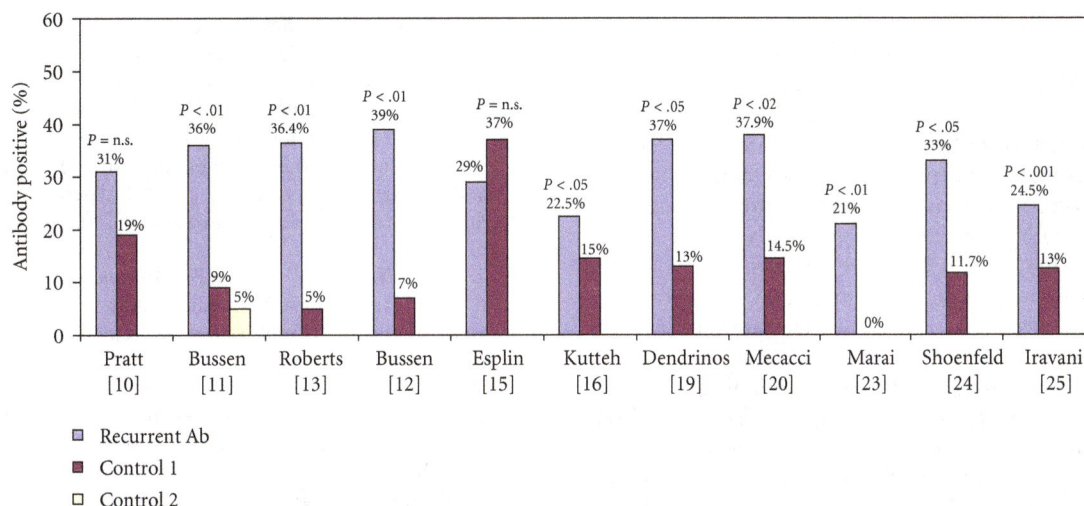

FIGURE 2: Percentage of thyroid antibody positivity in women with recurrent abortion (Recurrent Ab) and controls.

interest, the three negative studies were all performed in the United States.

4. Etiology of Pregnancy Loss

The etiology of pregnancy loss in thyroid antibody-positive women remains to be elucidated. Two meta-analyses have reported a difference in the mean age and mean TSH level between thyroid antibody-positive and thyroid antibody-negative women who miscarry [27, 28]. In the most recent meta-analysis, the mean TSH difference between groups was 0.61 mIU/L (1.7 mIU/L versus 1.1 mIU/L, $P < .00001$) [28]. Although the TSH levels are well within the normal range, a 2009 study by Benhadi et al. reported a statistically significant increase in child loss (defined as miscarriage, fetal, or neonatal death) with increasing levels of TSH between 0.34–5.60 mIU/L [29]. Similarly, Negro et al. found a 69% increase in the rate of miscarriage in thyroid antibody negative women with TSH values between 2.5–5.0 mIU/L as compared to thyroid antibody negative women with TSH values below 2.5 mIU/L (6.1% versus 3.6%, $P = .006$) [30]. Consequently, it is feasible that a component of the increased risk of pregnancy loss in thyroid antibody positive women could be attributable to increased TSH levels. On the other hand, the age difference reported in the meta-analysis of 1.3 years ($P < .003$) [28] appears to be limited to explain the marked difference in pregnancy loss between thyroid antibody positive and negative women. In support of this contention, Nybo Anderson et al. evaluated pregnancy outcome in 634,272 women and found only a minimal increase in the miscarriage rate between maternal ages 20 to 30 and approximately a 1.5%–2.0% increase in the miscarriage rate for each year between the maternal age of 30 to 40 [31].

Three research groups have evaluated the role of thyroid antibodies in pregnancy loss in an animal model. In 2001,

TABLE 2: Country of origin and number of women in each study of Figure 2.

Author	Country	TAb+	TAb−
Pratt et al. [9]	USA	45	100
Bussen et al. [10]	Germany	22	22
Roberts et al. [11]	Scotland	11	41
Bussen et al. [12]	Germany	28	28
Esplin et al. [13]	USA	74	75
Kutteh et al. [14]	USA	700	200
Dendrinos et al. [15]	Greece	30	15
Mecacci et al. [16]	Italy	29	69
Marai et al. [17]	Israel	38	20
Shoenfeld et al. [18]	Italy	33	120
Iravani et al. [19]	Iran	64	269

Imaizumi and colleagues evaluated the effect of experimental autoimmune thyroiditis on pregnancy outcome in a murine model of thyroglobulin immunized female mice [32]. Autoimmune thyroiditis and pregnancy loss were enhanced, but only when specific strains of mice were mated. Class II MHC antigens were found on placental cells from thyroglobulin induced mice but not on controls. The authors concluded that the pregnancy loss detected in the murine model of autoimmune thyroiditis was related to paternal antigens.

Matalon et al. in 2003 immunized and mated BALB/c mice with either human thyroglobulin or complete Freund's adjuvant (the control group) [33]. No difference in thyroid function tests were found between the two groups of mice. Animals immunized with human thyroglobulin developed high titers of antithyroglobulin antibodies and antibodies to thyroglobulin on the placenta. The rate of resorbed fetuses was higher in the immunized animals. Immunized animals also had lower placental and fetal weights. Interestingly, Mannisto et al. reported higher placental weights in thyroid peroxidase antibody mothers, but not in thyroglobulin antibody women [34]. In 2009, Lee et al. reported similar findings to Matalon et al. in a study that immunized female C57bl/6 mice with recombinant mouse thyroid peroxidase [35]. Compared to controls, immunized mice had a significantly higher rate of resorped fetuses and a reduced liter size. The authors concluded that antithyroid peroxidase antibody may impact embryo development postimplantation.

To date, the only prospective randomized controlled treatment in thyroid antibody-positive euthyroid women was performed by Negro et al. in 2006 [8]. The rate of miscarriage was compared between 57 thyroid peroxidase antibody women who were given levothyroxine beginning in the first trimester of pregnancy with 58 euthyroid thyroid antibody positive women who were not given levothyroxine (the control group). As noted earlier, the dose of levothyroxine administered was based on a combination of initial TSH level and titer of thyroid antibody. A statistically significant decrease in spontaneous miscarriage was seen in the group of treated women as compared to the controls (3.5% versus 13.8%, $P < .05$).

5. Future Directions

Summarizing the studies which have been published over the last generation, the following can be concluded: (1) thyroid antibody positivity is associated with pregnancy loss in unselected pregnancies, (2) thyroid antibody positivity is associated with pregnancy loss in women with recurrent miscarriage, (3) murine data have demonstrated a direct impact of immunization of female mice, with either thyroglobulin or thyroid peroxidase, and the development of thyroid antibodies along with decreased litter size, fetal resorption, and diminished placental weight, and (4) the results of the study by Negro et al. demonstrating a decreased rate of pregnancy loss in euthyroid thyroid antibody-positive women are exciting initial data but need to be replicated. Future directions should include the following: (1) an expansion of the murine model in order to further elucidate potential pathophysiological etiologies, (2) studies of immune markers in thyroid antibody-positive pregnant women, (3) studies of placentas of thyroid antibody positive pregnant women who miscarry, (4) studies further separating the impact of thyroid antibodies and TSH differences (within the reported normal range for pregnancy) on miscarriage, and (5) replication of the study by Negro et al. Many answers should be forthcoming in the generation ahead.

References

[1] A. Stagnaro-Green, S. H. Roman, R. H. Cobin, E. El-Harazy, A. Alvarez-Marfany, and T. F. Davies, "Detection of at-risk pregnancy by means of highly sensitive assays for thyroid autoantibodies," *Journal of the American Medical Association*, vol. 264, no. 11, pp. 1422–1425, 1990.

[2] K. A. Toulis, D. G. Goulis, C. A. Venetis et al., "Risk of spontaneous miscarriage in euthyroid women with thyroid autoimmunity undergoing IVF: a meta-analysis," *European Journal of Endocrinology*, vol. 162, no. 4, pp. 643–652, 2010.

[3] D. Glinoer, M. F. Soto, P. Bourdoux et al., "Pregnancy in patients with mild thyroid abnormalities: maternal and neonatal repercussions," *Journal of Clinical Endocrinology and Metabolism*, vol. 73, no. 2, pp. 421–427, 1991.

[4] B. Lejeune, J. P. Grun, P. De Nayer, G. Servais, and D. Glinoer, "Antithyroid antibodies underlying thyroid abnormalities and miscarriage or pregnancy induced hypertension," *British Journal of Obstetrics and Gynaecology*, vol. 100, no. 7, pp. 669–672, 1993.

[5] T. Iijima, H. Tada, Y. Hidaka, N. Mitsuda, Y. Murata, and N. Amino, "Effects of autoantibodies on the course of pregnancy and fetal growth," *Obstetrics and Gynecology*, vol. 90, no. 3, pp. 364–369, 1997.

[6] T. Bagis, A. Gokcel, and E. S. Saygili, "Autoimmune thyroid disease in pregnancy and the postpartum period: relationship to spontaneous abortion," *Thyroid*, vol. 11, no. 11, pp. 1049–1053, 2001.

[7] F. Ghafoor, M. Mansoor, T. Malik et al., "Role of thyroid peroxidase antibodies in the outcome of pregnancy," *Journal of the College of Physicians and Surgeons Pakistan*, vol. 16, no. 7, pp. 468–471, 2006.

[8] R. Negro, G. Formoso, T. Mangieri, A. Pezzarossa, D. Dazzi, and H. Hassan, "Levothyroxine treatment in euthyroid pregnant women with autoimmune thyroid disease: effects on obstetrical complications," *Journal of Clinical Endocrinology and Metabolism*, vol. 91, no. 7, pp. 2587–2591, 2006.

[9] D. E. Pratt, G. Kaberlein, A. Dudkiewicz, V. Karande, and N. Gleicher, "The association of antithyroid antibodies in euthyroid nonpregnant women with recurrent first trimester abortions in the next pregnancy," *Fertility and Sterility*, vol. 60, no. 6, pp. 1001–1005, 1993.

[10] S. Bussen and T. Steck, "Thyroid autoantibodies in euthyroid non-pregnant women with recurrent spontaneous abortions," *Human Reproduction*, vol. 10, no. 11, pp. 2938–2940, 1995.

[11] J. Roberts, C. Jenkins, R. Wilson et al., "Recurrent miscarriage is associated with increased numbers of CD5/20 positive lymphocytes and an increased incidence of thyroid antibodies," *European Journal of Endocrinology*, vol. 134, no. 1, pp. 84–86, 1996.

[12] S. S. Bussen and T. Steck, "Thyroid antibodies and their relation to antithrombin antibodies, anticardiolipin antibodies and lupus anticoagulant in women with recurrent spontaneous abortions (antithyroid, anticardiolipin and antithrombin autoantibodies and Lupus anticoagulant in habitual aborters)," *European Journal of Obstetrics Gynecology and Reproductive Biology*, vol. 74, no. 2, pp. 139–143, 1997.

[13] M. S. Esplin, D. W. Branch, R. Silver, and A. Stagnaro-Green, "Thyroid autoantibodies are not associated with recurrent pregnancy loss," *American Journal of Obstetrics and Gynecology*, vol. 179, no. 6, pp. 1583–1586, 1998.

[14] W. H. Kutteh, D. L. Yetman, A. C. Carr, L. A. Beck, and R. T. Scott Jr., "Increased prevalence of antithyroid antibodies identified in women with recurrent pregnancy loss but not in women undergoing assisted reproduction," *Fertility and Sterility*, vol. 71, no. 5, pp. 843–848, 1999.

[15] S. Dendrinos, C. Papasteriades, K. Tarassi, G. Christodoulakos, G. Prasinos, and G. Creatsas, "Thyroid autoimmunity in patients with recurrent spontaneous miscarriages," *Gynecological Endocrinology*, vol. 14, no. 4, pp. 270–274, 2000.

[16] F. Mecacci, E. Parretti, R. Cioni et al., "Thyroid autoimmunity and its association with non-organ-specific antibodies and subclinical alterations of thyroid function in women with a history of pregnancy loss or preeclampsia," *Journal of Reproductive Immunology*, vol. 46, no. 1, pp. 39–50, 2000.

[17] I. Marai, H. Carp, S. Shai, R. Shabo, G. Fishman, and Y. Shoenfeld, "Autoantibody panel screening in recurrent miscarriages," *American Journal of Reproductive Immunology*, vol. 51, no. 3, pp. 235–240, 2004.

[18] Y. Shoenfeld, H. J. A. Carp, V. Molina et al., "Autoantibodies and prediction of reproductive failure," *American Journal of Reproductive Immunology*, vol. 56, no. 5-6, pp. 337–344, 2006.

[19] A. T. Iravani, M. M. Saeedi, J. Pakravesh, S. Hamidi, and M. Abbasi, "Thyroid autoimmunity and recurrent spontaneous abortion in Iran: a case-control study," *Endocrine Practice*, vol. 14, no. 4, pp. 458–464, 2008.

[20] D. Pratt, M. Novotny, G. Kaberlein, A. Dudkiewicz, and N. Gleicher, "Antithyroid antibodies and the association with non-organ-specific antibodies in recurrent pregnancy loss," *American Journal of Obstetrics and Gynecology*, vol. 168, no. 3, pp. 837–841, 1993.

[21] R. G. Roussev, B. D. Kaider, D. E. Price, and C. B. Coulam, "Laboratory evaluation of women experiencing reproductive failure," *American Journal of Reproductive Immunology*, vol. 35, no. 4, pp. 415–420, 1996.

[22] F. H. Rushworth, M. Backos, R. Rai, I. T. Chilcott, N. Baxter, and L. Regan, "Prospective pregnancy outcome in untreated recurrent miscarriers with thyroid autoantibodies," *Human Reproduction*, vol. 15, no. 7, pp. 1637–1639, 2000.

[23] M. F. Reznikoff-Etievant, V. Cayol, G. M. Zou et al., "Habitual abortions in 678 healthy patients: investigation and prevention," *Human Reproduction*, vol. 14, no. 8, pp. 2106–2109, 1999.

[24] S. F. Abdel Aziz, A. A. Moussa, H. O. Kandil, M. Y. Shaheen, and M. M. Abou Zeid, "Antithyroid Autoantibodies in Unexplained Recurrent Abortion," 2002, http://www.obgyn.net/women/women.asp?page=/pb/cotm/9905/Antithyrod1.

[25] C. De Carolis, E. Greco, M. D. Guarino et al., "Antithyroid antibodies and antiphospholipid syndrome: evidence of reduced fecundity and of poor pregnancy outcome in recurrent spontaneous aborters," *American Journal of Reproductive Immunology*, vol. 52, no. 4, pp. 263–266, 2004.

[26] J. Bellver, S. R. Soares, C. Álvarez et al., "The role of thrombophilia and thyroid autoimmunity in unexplained infertility, implantation failure and recurrent spontaneous abortion," *Human Reproduction*, vol. 23, no. 2, pp. 278–284, 2008.

[27] M. F. Prummel and W. M. Wiersinga, "Thyroid autoimmunity and miscarriage," *European Journal of Endocrinology*, vol. 150, no. 6, pp. 751–755, 2004.

[28] L. Chen and R. Hu, "Thyroid autoimmunity and miscarriage: a meta-analysis," *Clinical Endocrinology*, vol. 74, no. 4, pp. 513–519, 2011.

[29] N. Benhadi, W. M. Wiersinga, J. B. Reitsma, T. G. M. Vrijkotte, and G. J. Bonsel, "Higher maternal TSH levels in pregnancy are associated with increased risk for miscarriage, fetal or neonatal death," *European Journal of Endocrinology*, vol. 160, no. 6, pp. 985–991, 2009.

[30] R. Negro, A. Schwartz, R. Gismondi, A. Tinelli, T. Mangieri, and A. Stagnaro-Green, "Increased pregnancy loss rate in thyroid antibody negative women with TSH levels between 2.5 and 5.0 in the first trimester of pregnancy," *Journal of Clinical Endocrinology and Metabolism*, vol. 95, no. 9, pp. E44–E48, 2010.

[31] A.-M. Nybo Andersen, J. Wohlfahrt, P. Christens, J. Olsen, and M. Melbye, "Maternal age and fetal loss: population based register linkage study," *British Medical Journal*, vol. 320, no. 7251, pp. 1708–1712, 2000.

[32] M. Imaizumi, A. Pritsker, M. Kita, L. Ahmad, P. Unger, and T. F. Davies, "Pregnancy and murine thyroiditis: thyroglobulin immunization leads to fetal loss in specific allogeneic pregnancies," *Endocrinology*, vol. 142, no. 2, pp. 823–829, 2001.

[33] S. T. Matalon, M. Blank, Y. Levy et al., "The pathogenic role of anti-thyroglobulin antibody on pregnancy: evidence from an active immunization model in mice," *Human Reproduction*, vol. 18, no. 5, pp. 1094–1099, 2003.

[34] T. Mannisto, M. Vaarasmaki, A. Pouta et al., "Perinatal outcome of children born to mothers with thyroid dysfunction or antibodies: a prospective population-based cohort study," *Journal of Clinical Endocrinology and Metabolism*, vol. 94, no. 3, pp. 772–779, 2009.

[35] Y. L. Lee, H. P. Ng, K. S. Lau et al., "Increased fetal abortion rate in autoimmune thyroid disease is related to circulating TPO autoantibodies in an autoimmune thyroiditis animal model," *Fertility and Sterility*, vol. 91, no. 5, pp. 2104–2109, 2009.

26

Thyroid Cancer: Molecular Aspects and New Therapeutic Strategies

Enrique Grande,[1] Juan José Díez,[2] Carles Zafon,[3] and Jaume Capdevila[4]

[1] *Department of Medical Oncology, Ramón y Cajal University Hospital, 28034 Madrid, Spain*
[2] *Department of Endocrinology, Ramón y Cajal University Hospital, 28034 Madrid, Spain*
[3] *Department of Endocrinology, Vall d'Hebron University Hospital, 08035 Barcelona, Spain*
[4] *Department of Medical Oncology, Vall d'Hebron University Hospital, 08035 Barcelona, Spain*

Correspondence should be addressed to Enrique Grande, egrande@oncologiahrc.com

Academic Editor: Fausto Bogazzi

Despite that thyroid cancer accounts for over 90% of tumors that arise from the endocrine system, these tumors barely represent 2% of solid tumors in adults. Many entities are grouped under the general term of thyroid cancer, and they differ in histological features as well as molecular and clinical behavior. Thus, the prognosis for patients with thyroid cancer ranges from a survival rate of >97% at 5 years, in the case of differentiated thyroid tumors sensitive to radioactive iodine, to a 4-month median survival for anaplastic tumors. The high vascularity in these tumors and the important role that oncogenic mutations may have in the RAS/RAF/MEK pathway and oncogenicity (as suggested by activating mutations and rearrangements of the *RET* gene) have led to the development of multitarget inhibitors in different histological subgroups of patients. The correct molecular characterization of patients with thyroid cancer is thought to be a key aspect for the future clinical management of these patients.

1. Introduction

Three different types of thyroid cancer have been defined according to their histological features: differentiated thyroid cancer (DTC) deriving from epithelial cells from the thyroid follicles; medullary thyroid cancer (MTC); anaplastic thyroid cancer (ATC). Approximately 90% of diagnosed thyroid cancers correspond to DTC, with papillary (PTC) histology being the most frequent (75%), followed by follicular (FTC) (10%), Hürthle cells (5%), and poorly differentiated carcinomas (1–6%) [1, 2]. Overall, MTC accounts for approximately 10% of all thyroid tumors and ATC barely 1% [2].

Thyroid cancer is considered a nonfrequent entity because it represents only 1% of all solid tumors in adults. Women are three-times more likely to suffer this disease, and the incidence of DTC has increased 2.4-fold over the past 30 years [3]. Most DTC patients have a very good prognosis if diagnosed at early stages, and 91% of patients are alive at 20 years when the classical treatment with surgery followed by radioiodine ablation and suppression of thyroid

stimulating hormone (TSH) is employed. However, patients with DTC resistant to radioactive iodine, or those with MTC or ATC, have limited options for treatment. Up to now, the chemotherapy drugs most often used worldwide to treat thyroid cancer are doxorubicin and cisplatin. However, the most referenced guidelines in the field do not always recommend the routine use of these agents in the clinic. Doxorubicin and cisplatin showed some activity in a study conducted in the 1970s in a total of 92 patients with all types of thyroid cancer; a progression-free survival of 3 months; an overall survival of 7 months being achieved following treatment [4]. Currently, the use of chemotherapy in patients with thyroid cancer is limited to patients with ATC, those with poorly differentiated histology with a high rate of proliferation, or in highly symptomatic patients who are not candidates for other local or systemic therapies.

The last decade has seen advances in the molecular biology that may underlie the development and progression of these tumors. For example, DTC is mainly associated with mutations in the RAS/RAF/MAPK intracellular signaling

TABLE 1: Inhibitory concentration 50 (IC_{50}) of the major pharmaceutical compounds in clinical development for the treatment of thyroid cancer segregated with respect to the kinase activity required to inhibit different molecular targets (nmol/L).

Pharmaceutical compound	VEGFR1	VEGFR2	VEGFR3	RET	RET/PTC	PDGFRβ	BRAF	KIT	Others (IC_{50})
Sorafenib	26	90	20	47	50	57	25	68	—
Motesanib	2	3	6	59	—	84	—	8	—
Axitinib	0.1	0.2	0.29	1.2	—	2	—	1.7	—
Sunitinib	10	10	10	100	224	39	—	1–10	—
Vandetanib	—	40	110	130	100	—	—	—	EGFR (500)
Pazopanib	10	30	47	—	—	84	—	74	—
Lenvatinib (E7080)	22	4	5.2	35	—	39	—	—	FGFR1 (46)
Cabozantinib (XL-184)	—	0.035	—	4	—	—	—	—	C-MET (1.8)

pathway or with gene rearrangements such as RET/PTC. Virtually all MTC tumors associated with hereditary syndromes and about 45% of sporadic MTC are associated with mutations activating the RET gene [5].

Classically, thyroid tumors are associated with high vascularization and high levels of vascular endothelial growth factor, fibroblast growth factor, and platelet-derived growth factor (VEGF, FGF, and PDGF, resp.) [6]. The importance of angiogenesis in these neoplasms became clear when several studies showed that tumors with high levels of VEGF in the stroma correlated with a greater propensity towards metastases at distance, as well as with other markers of tumor aggressiveness. Of considerable note is that thyroid cell cultures have a reduced proliferation when the VEGF pathway is blocked, thus demonstrating a direct antitumor activity of antiangiogenic drugs on thyroid tumor cells [7]. Additionally, VEGFR3 is involved in the lymphangiogenesis process, that is, of special interest in papillary thyroid carcinomas that commonly metastasizes in regional lymph nodes [8].

Tyrosine kinases are enzymes that transfer phosphate groups from adenosine triphosphate (ATP) to tyrosine residues of another protein. Many tyrosine kinases are documented in humans as being involved in key processes of cellular control such as survival, proliferation, differentiation, function, and cell motility. In recent years, a large group of low molecular weight agents capable of inhibiting the function of tyrosine kinases have changed the natural history and management of various solid tumors such as kidney cancer, liver cancer, gastrointestinal stromal tumor (GIST), and, more recently, pancreatic neuroendocrine tumor. These drugs are called multitarget tyrosine kinase inhibitors and, due to their biochemical structure being similar to that of ATP, they are able to block the intracellular activation of several membrane receptors or proteins in the intracellular signaling cascade with tyrosine kinase activity. The degree of affinity and selectivity of this inhibitory activity is very variable (Table 1) [6].

Advances in understanding the molecular pathogenesis of different subtypes of thyroid cancer have, currently, made this field of research one of the busiest in the world of endocrine oncology. The application of discoveries in the laboratory to the patient (the "bench-to-bed" transfer) is one of the biggest challenges in translational research area, since

these tumors can become a paradigm of therapy based on molecular features that govern the development and growth of tumors in each individual patient. This paper aims to summarize the key molecular determinants of each histological subtype of thyroid cancer and the data derived in recent years from clinical studies conducted with multitarget agents.

2. Differentiated Thyroid Cancer (DTC)

2.1. Clinical Management of DTC Patients Sensitive to Radioactive Iodine. DTC represents the vast majority of thyroid tumors. Treatment is based on thyroidectomy with or without lymphadenectomy regarding papillary or follicular histology, followed by radioiodine ablation in those patients at high risk of lymph node metastases and levothyroxine in doses that suppress TSH levels. The semiannual or annual monitoring using cervical ultrasound, measurement of thyroglobulin levels as a tumor marker, and whole-body iodine scan is appropriate for these patients.

It is estimated that between 10 and 15% of patients undergoing DTC will have disease relapse. In 3 out of 4 cases, recurrence occurs at the cervical level in the thyroid bed or lymph node level. In these patients salvage surgery, radioiodine therapy and external radiotherapy is recommended in highly selected patients.

Distant metastases occur in <10% of DTC patients, and only half of them are apparent at the time of diagnosis. The lungs are the main receptor organs of these tumor metastases (50%), followed by bone (25%). Initial treatment of patients with disseminated disease includes TSH-suppressive doses of levothyroxine plus radioiodine administered in conditions of high serum TSH levels in those patients with positive total body scan uptake, albeit complete remission is achieved in only 30% of subjects [9].

2.2. Clinical Management of Patients with Radioactive Iodine-Refractory DTC. A patient is considered resistant to the use of radioactive iodine when at least one tumor lesion is observed that does not show uptake of radioiodine, or when the lesion radiologically progresses in the first 12 months post-radioiodine administration, or when the patient has persistent disease following the administration of an accumulated dose of radioactive iodine of >600 mCi

[10]. The median survival of patients with radioiodine-resistant DTC and distant metastases ranges between 3 and 6 years. It is in these patients that the application of new multitarget inhibitors has its main testing ground [8]. The use of classical chemotherapy, both as monotherapy and in combination with other treatments, in patients with radioiodine-refractory DTC has not shown any significant benefit in these patients and, conversely, has shown high toxicity. The most recent study conducted with doxorubicin was published in 2008 by Matuszczyk et al. [11]. Among the 22 recruited patients with radioiodine-refractory DTC, only one (5%) achieved a partial positive response that lasted for 6 months. Adverse effects included alopecia (42%), nausea (23%), pneumonia (20%), and neutropenia (10%). Of the 22 patients, 12 showed disease progression during the first measurement of treatment response, and only 42% of the patients recruited for the trial had stable disease for a median of 7 months. Other authors have also tested several combination regimes with specific chemotherapy agents such as taxanes, platinum, or gemcitabine, with little added clinical benefit; response rates ranging between 0 and 22% and without an amelioration of progression-free survival (PFS) of the disease [12].

2.3. Molecular Biology of DTC (Figure 1). In recent years, several different genetic events have been identified as being related to the genesis of the DTC. Further, a correlation has been reported between the manifestation of histological alterations of the disease and the presence of changes in the regulation of intracellular molecular pathways that confer a distinct clinical behavior. Two major molecular determinants that involve the same molecular pathway are responsible for the appearance of a PTC: the alteration of gene regulation of the *RET* gene expression and the abnormal activation of signaling pathways, RAS/RAF/MAPK. There is an increasing body of evidence showing that the role of PI3K/Akt/mTOR pathway may be crucial for tumor development and may become an attractive target in the future [13].

The abnormal chromosome rearrangement of proto-oncogene *RET* (rearranged during transfection) with the tyrosine kinase domain of other genes located in the same or other chromosomes results in the fusion oncogene *RET/PTC* that plays a key role in the pathogenesis of up to 30% of patients with PTC [14]. Their involvement is even greater in childhood PTC and in patients whose tumor results from exposure to ionizing radiation (approximately 50–80% of cases). The *RET* proto-oncogene is activated by fusion of the RET TK domain with the 5′-terminal sequence of one of different heterologous genes via rearrangements that generate a series of chimeric-transforming oncogenes collectively described as *RET/PTCs*. The results of *RET/PTC* reorganization are abnormal proteins constitutively activated from RET kinase, independently of the binding to extracellular ligands, that activate multiple intracellular signaling pathways leading to clonal expansion and neoplastic transformation of the thyroid follicle cells. It is widely known that *RET* oncogene rearrangements plays a crucial role in radiation-associated papillary thyroid carcinogenesis.

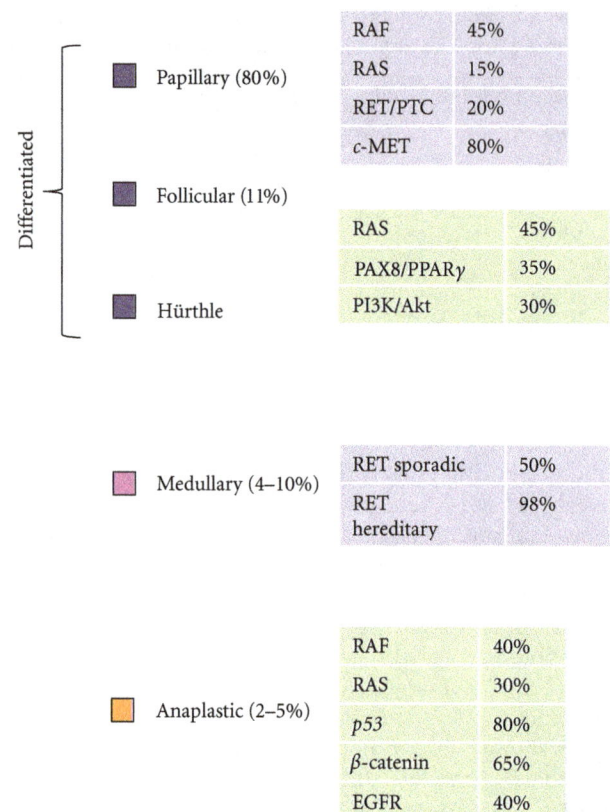

Differentiated

Papillary (80%)		
RAF	45%	
RAS	15%	
RET/PTC	20%	
c-MET	80%	

Follicular (11%)

RAS	45%	
PAX8/PPARγ	35%	
PI3K/Akt	30%	

Hürthle

Medullary (4–10%)	
RET sporadic	50%
RET hereditary	98%

Anaplastic (2–5%)	
RAF	40%
RAS	30%
p53	80%
β-catenin	65%
EGFR	40%

Figure 1: Molecular alterations present in different histological types of thyroid cancer.

Other proto-oncogene rearrangements have been identified affecting to the *NTRK1* gene in PTCs. The frequency of these rearrangements could be seen in up to 25% of patients with PTC. *NTRK1* proto-oncogene rearrangements result in the formation of chimeric genes composed of the tyrosine kinase domain of NTRK1 fused to 5′ sequences of different genes (*TPM3, MET,* and *TRK-T2*). It is estimated that *NTRK1* proto-oncogene is activated by rearrangement with a similar frequency in "spontaneous" and radiation-associated thyroid tumours. Moreover, *NTRK1* proto-oncogene activating rearrangements play a role in the development of a minority of radiation-associated PTC but not in adenomas [15].

Molecular aberrations observed in FTC are significantly different from those described in PTC, including RAS mutations in up to 45% of patients and rearrangements involving the transcription factor gene of the paired-box 8 *(PAX8)* and peroxisome proliferator-activated receptor-*γ* *(PPARγ)* resulting in a *PAX8/PPARγ* rearrangement observed in up to 35% of FTC [12].

Genetic alterations in the signaling pathway of RAS/RAF/MAPK constitute the most frequent genetic/molecular anomaly in patients with DTC. BRAF is a serine-threonine kinase that is key in the intracellular regulation of this cellular pathway. Activating mutations have been observed in the V600E codon of the *BRAF* gene in up to 70% of patients with PTC. Similarly, patients with mutations in *BRAF* have more chances of developing resistance to radioactive

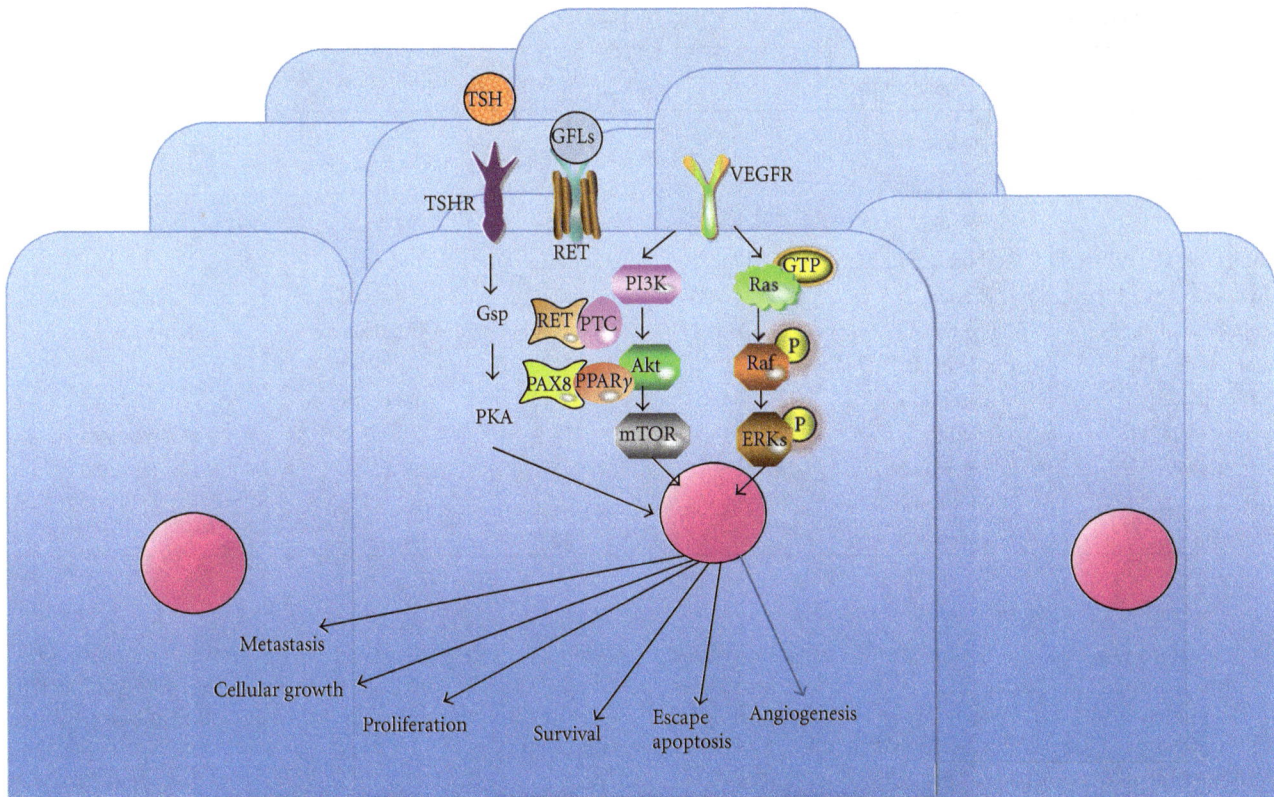

FIGURE 2: Schematic representation of the follicular tumor cell.

iodine resulting from alterations in the normal patterns of mobilization and metabolism of iodine in the thyroid follicle cell. These features confer poorer clinical prognosis to patients carrying the mutation. The *V600E BRAF* activating mutation is associated with a loss of expression of the unidirectional cotransporter (symport) sodium iodine and, consequently, a lower uptake of radioiodine by the metastatic lesions of tumors that harbor the mutation. This decreased expression of symport is mediated via the TGFβ autocrine pathway.

Point mutations in the gene encoding the *RAS* oncoprotein occur to a lesser extent (15%) in PTC, but their frequencies are increased in patients with FTC and less differentiated histologies. Mutations in any gene encoding for *RAS* (*HRAS*, *KRAS* and *NRAS*) involve abnormal activation of mitogen-activated protein kinase (MAPK) and the PI3K/Akt/mTOR alternative parallel route [12, 33].

Mutations in *BRAF*, *RAS* and *RET* rearrangements are involved in >70% of PTC. However, these molecular alterations are mutually exclusive in most cases and are rarely expressed simultaneously within the same tumor. As such, they are independently able to promote PTC.

Activation and dysregulation of the intracellular signaling cascade PI3K/Akt/mTOR through loss of expression of tumor suppressor phosphatase PTEN has been implicated in the development of DTC and undifferentiated tumors of the thyroid. Likewise, mutations in the gene *PI3CA*, encoding for the phosphatidyl-inositol-tri-phosphate kinase (PI3K), play

a role as initial triggers that activate the intracellular signaling pathway (Figure 2).

Another molecular alteration frequently found in DTC is amplification of the gene encoding for the hepatocyte growth factor (*c*-MET) receptor. The MET membrane receptor cooperates with VEGF receptor to promote angiogenesis, cell mobility, and survival of thyroid cells. Amplification occurs in 80% of papillary thyroid tumors, while its silencing in animal models induces tumor regression, reduction in tumor size, and the appearance of new distant metastases [12].

Angiogenesis is another potential area for the design of new molecular targets. Known receptors for VEGF (VEGFR-1, -2, and -3) and the FGF (FGFR) and PDGF (PDGFR-α and -β) have been shown to be associated with an increased risk of distant metastases, an increased risk of disease recurrence, less protracted PFS, and increased presence of mutations in BRAF. In *in vitro* experimental models, blockade of the VEGF pathway has succeeded in delaying DTC growth [10].

2.4. Multitarget Agents in Current Clinical Development for the Treatment of DTC (Table 2)

2.4.1. Sorafenib. Sorafenib is a multitarget agent for several major molecular pathways involved in the development and progression of PTC, including the serine-threonine kinase BRAF and the tyrosine kinases from the membrane receptors VEGFR-2 and PDGFR-β (Table 1). From

TABLE 2: Clinical data from studies with the main agents in clinical development in differentiated thyroid cancer.

Author (ref)	Pharmaceutical compound	N	Response rate (%)	Stabilizations (%)	Progression-free survival (months)
Gupta-Abramson et al. [16]	Sorafenib	30	23	53	20
Kloss et al. [17]	Sorafenib	41	15	56	15
Ahmed et al. [18]	Sorafenib	34	20 (DTC)	48	12
Hoftijzer et al. [19]	Sorafenib	31	24	34	14
Capdevila et al. [20]	Sorafenib	34 (16 DTC)	19 (DTC)	50 (DTC)	13.5
Leboulleux et al. [21]	Vandetanib	145	8.3 versus 5.5	48 versus 37	11 versus 5.8
Cohen et al. [22]	Axitinib	60	30	38	18
Carr et al. [23]	Sunitinib	33	13 (DTC)	68 (DTC)	12.8
Cohen et al. [24]	Sunitinib	31	13	63	Not reported
Sherman et al. [25]	Lenvatinib	56	47 (DTC)	36 (DTC)	Not reported
Sherman et al. [26]	Motesanib	93	24	67	10
Bible et al. [27]	Pazopanib	37	49	46	11.8

a biological standpoint, the action profile of sorafenib is the most complete in terms of activity on key molecular targets involved in PTC. Data are available from at least 4 nonrandomized phase II studies which used a dose of sorafenib 800 mg/day as a single agent in patients with DTC refractory to radioactive iodine. In the 30 patients treated by the group of Gupta-Abramson et al. in Philadelphia, a median PFS of 18.4 months was achieved; 7 (23%) patients achieving an objective radiological partial response and 16 patients (53%) achieving disease stabilization of >6 months. Those patients with BRAF mutation (n = 16) achieved a median PFS of 84 weeks versus 54 weeks for those who did not have this mutation [16]. In a more recent study, also conducted in the USA, similar results were observed in 41 patients with PTC. In these patients, the objective radiological response rate was 15%, and disease stabilization was observed in 56% of patients. The median PFS was 15 months; the presence of BRAF mutation was observed in 17 (77%) of the 22 patients analyzed [17]. In the UK Matisse study (Safety and Efficacy of Sorafenib in Advanced Metastatic Thyroid Cancer), a total of 30 patients with thyroid cancer were treated, up to 14 with DTC. The objective response rate was 18% [18]. In a more recent study conducted in 31 patients, the response rate achieved was 24%, with a median PFS of 14 months [19]. Most adverse effects occurring in these 4 studies were consistent with the already-known safety profile of the drug; the majority of toxicities found were grade I and II and easily manageable with a delay or dose reduction of sorafenib administration. The data from a retrospective analysis of 34 patients with refractory thyroid cancer treated with sorafenib in Spain have recently been published. Clinical benefit of sorafenib was 73% with a response rate in DTC of 19% and 47% in MTC [20]. Taken together, these results formed the scientific basis for the launch of a phase III registration. Termed DECISION (Study of Sorafenib in Metastatic or Locally Advanced, Refractory Patients with Thyroid Cancer RAI), the study compared the administration of sorafenib versus placebo in 380 patients with radioiodine-refractory DTC with PFS as the primary endpoint (NCT00984282). This study has just completed recruitment, and results are awaited with interest.

2.4.2. Vandetanib. Vandetanib (ZD6474) is a low molecular weight inhibitor of tyrosine kinases, which acts mainly against VEGFR-2, VEGFR-3, and RET and, in higher concentrations, on the epidermal growth factor receptor (EGFR) (Table 1). Vandetanib was one of the first drugs to demonstrate activity in thyroid cancer cell lines, mainly through its action on the rearrangements *RET/PTC* and on RET mutations. Vandetanib has been the subject of report of the largest randomized clinical trial conducted to date in patients with DTC refractory to radioiodine. A total of 145 patients received vandetanib at doses of 300 mg/day or placebo. PFS, which was the primary endpoint, was significantly higher from the clinical as well as statistical point of view, in patients receiving the study drug (11 months) as compared to those receiving placebo (5.8 months) with a relative risk (hazard ratio) of 0.63 (95% CI: 0.43–0.92). However, the objective response rate was less than 5% in the vandetanib arm, and is difficult to explain. The most frequent adverse events found in the vandetanib arm were diarrhea (74%), asthenia (26%), fatigue (23%), nausea (25%), hypertension (34%), hyporexia (26%), and skin rash (25%). Updates from this study are expected in the near future [21].

2.4.3. Axitinib. Axitinib is one of the most selective and potent tyrosine kinase inhibitors currently under clinical development. The main targets blocked by axitinib are VEGFR-2, PDGFR-β, and c-KIT, in the subnanomolar range (Table 1). In a prospective noncontrolled phase II trial, axitinib was the first drug that demonstrated clinical activity by inducing objective radiological response in all histological subtypes of thyroid cancer (DTC, MTC, and ATC). Of a total of 60 patients who entered the study, 37 patients had

DTC refractory to radioactive iodine; 15 of 47 (31%) patients achieved an objective response rate (by RECIST criteria); 20 (42%) had disease stabilization beyond 6 months when treated with 5 mg of axitinib every 12 hours as a single agent. The median PFS was 18 months, if all histologies were included. Of note is the finding that the median time on treatment with the drug was only 4.8 months, especially considering the high median PFS achieved. The most common adverse events found were asthenia, diarrhea, nausea, anorexia, hypertension, and mucositis [22].

2.4.4. Sunitinib. Sunitinib is a multitarget inhibitor of 3 known receptors of VEGF, as well as of RET and PDGFR-α and -β, and of the protein derived from the *RET/PTC* realignment (Table 1). In a phase II study [23], sunitinib, administered at a dose of 37.5 mg/day in continuous schedule, induced metabolic complete response in 28 DTC patients, with uptake of distant disease on PET/CT scan a partial response in 7 cases (25%), and disease stabilization in 14 (50%). The median time to progression (TTP) was 12.8 months, and the decline in the uptake of fluorodeoxyglucose (FDG) at 7 days of treatment with sunitinib was superior in those patients who subsequently achieved positive radiological response (by RECIST criteria). In another phase II study conducted in 31 evaluable patients with DTC with metastatic disease progression, sunitinib administered at a dose of 50 mg/day for 4 weeks followed by 2 weeks off treatment, achieved a partial response rate of 13%, with 63% stabilizations [24]. In a retrospective analysis that we conducted in 17 patients with thyroid cancer of different histologies treated with sunitinib for advanced disease, we found an objective reduction of the size of metastases in 4 (33%) of the evaluable patient, and a median PFS of 13.3 months in the overall patient groups, 8.6 months being the PFS in those patients who had failed to one prior systemic treatment with sorafenib. The main grade 3-4 toxicities found in the study were asthenia (7.1%), thrombocytopenia (7.1%), and mucositis (5.9%) [34].

2.4.5. Lenvatinib (E7080). Lenvatinib (E7080) is a potent inhibitor in the nanomolar range of VEGFR-1 and -2 as well as PDGFR-β and the fibroblast growth factor receptor-1 (FGFR-1) (Table 1). In an international, open, phase II study which treated a total of 99 patients who had advanced thyroid cancer, lenvatinib showed an objective reduction in the size of metastases (according to RECIST criteria 1.1) in 29 (50%) of the 58 patients with histology of DTC. Also, 21 (36%) patients achieved disease stabilization, and the median PFS in all DTC patients was 12.6 months [25]. Among the 41 (70%) patients who had not received prior antiangiogenic therapy for advanced disease, the radiological objective response rate was 54% while, in the 17 patients who had previously received anti-VEGF, the observed partial response rate was 41%. However, dose reduction was required in 35% of patients, and 23% of them discontinued treatment due to toxicity. The most frequent grade 3 or 4 toxicities that led to dose reductions were hypertension (10%), proteinuria (10%), decreased weight (7%), diarrhea (10%), and fatigue

(7%). Based on these promising data, we began a phase III registration study in which 360 patients with DTC refractory to radioactive iodine, which had been previously treated with other anti-VEGF agents, were randomized to receive lenvatinib or placebo. PFS was the primary aim of the study (NCT01321554).

2.4.6. Motesanib. Motesanib (AMG706) is an oral inhibitor of multiple kinases, including VEGFR-1, -2, and -3 as well as the wild and mutant forms of the membrane receptor RET. In one of the initial phase I studies, focusing on recommended doses and major toxicities, motesanib was shown to achieve objective radiographic partial response in 3 of the 5 patients with thyroid cancer. This activity was not expected in these patients and led on to a prospective phase II study in 93 patients with DTC being carried out. One in every 3 patients remained on treatment for 48 weeks after commencement. The most common adverse events found at any grade were diarrhea (59%), hypertension (56%), fatigue (46%), and weight loss (40%). The radiological response rate assessed by independent reviewers was 14%, and up to 35% of patients benefited from a stabilization of their disease beyond 6 months. The median PFS was 9.3 months and, although the drug does not inhibit BRAF, the investigators observed that patients carrying a mutation in this pathway were less likely to progress if they received motesanib than patients without the mutation This finding suggested a greater involvement of angiogenesis in patients with the BRAF mutation [26].

2.4.7. Pazopanib. Pazopanib shares the main targets with the other agents discussed above. However, it appears to have a marginal activity on *RET/PTC* and BRAF that is, its activity in these tumors is due mainly to its antiangiogenic effect rather than any intrinsic antitumor effect (Table 1). In a phase II study, pazopanib administered at a dose of 800 mg/day, induced a radiographic response rate of 49% in 37 patients with DTC who had disease progression over the previous 12 months. This response rate is among the highest achieved by any multitarget agent reported in this context. Up to 66% of patients who achieved a positive objective radiological response rate were able to maintain the response one year from the commencement of treatment. The median PFS in the total patient sample was 11.8 months. The most frequent toxicities found were fatigue (78%), skin rash (75%), diarrhea (73%), and nausea (73%). Contrary to that observed with axitinib, patients treated with pazopanib received the drug for a median of 12 months [27].

3. Medullary Thyroid Cancer (MTC)

3.1. Clinical Management of Patients with MTC. Currently, there were no officially approved therapy for the treatment of metastatic MTC until the recent approval of vandetanib by the American Food and Drugs Administration (FDA) and the European Medicine Agency (EMA). Following the failure of initial treatment by thyroidectomy and cervical lymphadenectomy, patients have received only symptomatic

TABLE 3: Clinical data from studies with the main multi-target agents in clinical development for the treatment of medullary thyroid cancer.

Author (ref)	Pharmaceutical compound	N	Response rate (%)	Stabilizations (%)	Progression-free survival (months)
Wells Jr. et al. [28]	Vandetanib	231	45	—	Not achieved at 24 months. HR versus placebo = 0.46 $P < 0.001$
Kurzrock et al. [29]	Cabozantinib	37	49	41	Not reported
Lam et al. [30]	Sorafenib	16	6	62	17.9
Capdevila et al. [20]	Sorafenib	34 (15 MTC)	47	40	10.5
Schlumberger et al. [31]	Motesanib	91	2	48	11.2
Carr et al. [23]	Sunitinib	7	37.5	—	Not reported
De Souza et al. [32]	Sunitinib	25	35	57	Not reported

care measures. Therefore, this tumor has represented, and currently represents, a niche for the development of new active drugs, especially considering that between 35 and 50% of patients diagnosed with metastatic disease are likely to be diagnosed as having lympho-ganglionar metastases, and up to 15% of patients will develop distant metastases after diagnosis. Half of the patients diagnosed with MTC will ultimately present distant metastases during the clinical evolution of the disease.

MTC is considered a neuroendocrine tumor caused by the uncontrolled proliferation of para-follicular C cells producing calcitonin derived from the neural crest. It accounts for between 4 and 10% of thyroid cancers. In up to 30% of cases, the CMT is associated with an inherited syndrome and multiple endocrine neoplasia type 2 (MEN 2A or 2B) or with familial MTC (FMTC). Most hereditary MTC occur within MEN 2A that is often associated with pheochromocytoma or hyperparathyroidism [35].

Sporadic MTC is diagnosed in the 5th or 6th decade of life, while the hereditary versions of the disease can be diagnosed in 5-year-old children. Conventional therapy with chemotherapy has not proven to be particularly useful in patients with metastatic MTC. The most commonly used chemotherapy regimen has traditionally been that of doxorubicin monotherapy. This treatment achieves a clinical benefit, including the partial responses plus stable disease of 6 months, in about 21% of patients, with 79% of patients progressing within 5 months of treatment [27]. Regimens for neuroendocrine tumors have also been used for MTC, including a combination of streptozocin, dacarbazine, and 5-fluorouracil. Up to 30% of patients achieved objective response rates in small nonrandomized studies [36].

3.2. Molecular Biology of MTC (Figure 1).

Approximately 50% of patients with sporadic MTC have a somatic mutation at codon 918 of the RET gene. These mutations are considered "gain of function" type. The presence of this mutation is also associated with a high probability of lympho-ganglionary metastases, recurrent/persistent disease, and decreased survival. By contrast, germinal mutations at different loci of the RET gene are present in virtually all hereditary syndromes associated with MTC. There is a strong genotype-phenotype correlation between the location of the mutation in RET and the associated MEN2 type. This enables the patients to be classified into different risk groups according to the mutation they carry and as such, to be referred (or not) for prophylactic thyroidectomy [35, 37].

The abnormal activation of RET by any of the several mutations affecting the coding part of the gene can trigger activation of multiple intracellular signaling pathways such as RAS/RAF/MAPK, PI3K/Akt/mTOR, or Rac/JNK.

3.3. Multitarget Agents in Clinical Development of MTC (Table 3)

3.3.1. Vandetanib. Vandetanib is the first drug approved in the US by the FDA and in Europe by the EMA for treatment of MTC in the last 30 years. The approval was as a consequence of the data reported in the ZETA study which was a phase III, double-blind trial with 2 : 1 randomization of patients to receive vandetanib at doses of 300 mg/day versus placebo. Between December 2006 and November 2007, a total of 331 patients with sporadic or inherited MTC were enrolled. The median PFS in the placebo arm was 19.3 months while the vandetanib treatment arm has not yet been concluded (HR: 0.46; 95% CI: 0.31–0.69; $P < 0.0001$) after 24 months of followup. The objective radiological response rate was also higher in the vandetanib treatment arm (45% versus 13%; $P < 0.0001$). Patients receiving vandetanib showed a statistically significant delay in time-to-pain worsening compared with patients receiving placebo (7.85 versus 3.25 months, HR: 0.61; 95% CI: 0.43–0.87; $P = 0.006$). Patients receiving this agent also showed significant decreases in serum concentrations of calcitonin and carcinoembryonic antigen (CEA). Adverse effects found were asthenia, weight loss, diarrhea, mucositis, hand-foot syndrome, and hypertension, most of them of grades 1 and 2 severity. Very rarely, some grade 3/4 events were observed. Interestingly, those patients harboring M918T mutation in RET had higher objective response rate (54.5%) than those with RET mutation unknown (34.1%) or negative (0%) [28].

3.3.2. Cabozantinib (XL184). Cabozantinib is an oral inhibitor that, in addition to acting against VEGFR-1 and -2, and c-KIT as are most of the drugs discussed above, is able to inhibit c-MET which, as also discussed above, is amplified in a large proportion of patients with DTC and MTC. It also acts against RET and against *RET/PTC* rearrangements (Table 1). In the extension phase of a phase I study containing 37 patients with MTC, we observed that 17 (49%) of 35 evaluable patients achieved an objective radiological response that, together with the 15 (41%) patients achieving stable disease over 6 months, totaled an overall clinical benefit of 90% of patients [29]. However, no significant correlation was observed between the presence of mutations in *RET* (in both sporadic and hereditary cases) and tumor response to cabozantinib. A phase III study comparing cabozantinib and placebo in patients with metastatic MTC is currently recruiting patients (NCT00215605).

3.3.3. Sorafenib.
The observed *in vitro* activity of sorafenib in MTC cell lines has stimulated investigators to design a phase II study in patients with hereditary ($n = 5$) and sporadic ($n = 16$) MTC. Analysis of the M918T mutation of the *RET* gene was performed in 12 of these patients, with 8 showing positive for the mutation. Preliminary results of the activity of sorafenib as a single agent in patients with MTC show that one (6%) patient achieved a partial positive response and 10 (62%) of 16 patients with sporadic MTC obtained a stabilization of their disease for >6 months. Serum levels of calcitonin and CEA decreased by over 62% and 44%, respectively [30].

3.3.4. Motesanib.
In a multicentered, international, open-label phase II trial, motesanib demonstrated that it was able to induce a clinical benefit in 50% of 91 patients with locally advanced or metastatic MTC. The PFS was 12 months. Most study patients (84%) corresponded to sporadic MTC in 72% of whom the *RET* mutation was present. There were no significant differences between the effectiveness of motesanib in patients in relation to the presence or absence of the *RET* mutation [31].

3.3.5. Sunitinib.
In the study by Carr et al. [23] that measured metabolic activity level in MTC patients, sunitinib showed a metabolic response (as measured by FDG uptake analyzed by PET) in the 3 of 8 patients in whom this measurement was performed. Subsequently, a phase II study specific for patients with MTC with disease progression over the previous 6 months was undertaken. Patients were treated with sunitinib at doses of 50 mg/day for 4 weeks followed by 2 weeks off drug. A total of 25 patients with MTC were recruited into the study. A partial response rate of 35% was achieved, with median response duration of 37 weeks; 57% of patients had stable disease as best response to treatment [32]. In patients with *RET* mutation and treated with sunitinib, the probability of remaining progression-free at one year was 88% (95% CI: 43%–98%).

4. Anaplastic Thyroid Cancer (ATC)

4.1. Clinical Management of Patients with ATC.
ATC contributes less than 2% of all thyroid-derived tumors but is responsible for 14 to 39% of deaths from thyroid cancer. With a frequency 5-fold higher in men than in women, the median survival range depends on status between 3 and 9 months after diagnosis. Approximately 50% of patients diagnosed with ATC already have metastases at the time of diagnosis, and another 25% will eventually develop metastases. Treatment options are surgery, palliative radiotherapy, and chemotherapy. ATC tumors are considered chemo resistant. Doxorubicin in monotherapy achieves positive radiological response rates in <20% of patients, and this response is rarely protracted. Other platinum-based combinations such as taxanes, gemcitabine or vinorelbine can achieve up to 53% radiological response but does not have much impact on the overall survival of patients [38].

4.2. Molecular Biology of ATC (Figure 1).
Most frequent mutations observed in ATC affect *p53* gene in up to 70% of patients. Genomic aberrations of ATC also include RAS and β-catenin mutations in more than 50% of cases, and mutations in the oncogene *BRAF* have only been observed in around 20% of patients. Different genomic profiles between DTC or MTC and ATC probably are related with the higher aggressiveness of these tumors. Similarly, histological findings indicate high vascularity with overexpression of VEGF, the levels of which appear to correlate with stage and tumor size, lymph node, and distant metastases. Finally, EGFR is overexpressed in most of the patients with ATC. The implication of overexpression of EGFR on the clinical and biological behavior of these tumors is not known [38].

4.3. Multitarget Agents in Clinical Development in ATC

4.3.1. Axitinib.
In a phase II study conducted with single-agent axitinib in patients with thyroid cancer of all histology subtypes, there was an objective radiological response in approximately 50% patients with ATC who entered the study [22].

4.3.2. Sorafenib.
In the only study performed specifically in patients with ATC, 16 patients were treated with sorafenib alone. The rate of control of the disease was 40%, although time-to-progression barely reached 1.5 months. Of the 15 evaluable patients, 2 (13%) showed an objective radiological response that was maintained for a median of 5.3 months. The most frequently observed grade 3 and 4 adverse events were lymphopenia (31%), skin rash (12%), weight loss (12%), and chest pain (12%) [39].

4.3.3. Combretastatin A4 Phosphate (CA4P).
CA4P is a vascular-disrupting agent, also called fosbretabulin tromethamine or combretastatin A4 phosphate. Unlike other antiangiogenesis agents that block tumor blood vessel formation, CA4P prevents blood flow in existing vessels. This drug has shown some activity as a single agent in patients with metastatic ATC who have not responded to at least one prior systemic therapy but in whom, on rare occasions, positive responses were observed and objective radiological PFS of 3 months was achieved. The final results in overall survival of the largest randomized trial conducted in patients

with metastatic ATC were presented at American Society of Clinical Oncology (ASCO) annual meeting in 2011. A total of 80 of the planned 180 patients with ATC were recruited and randomized to receive carboplatin + paclitaxel with or without associated CA4P in a 2 : 1 randomization. The median overall survival was higher in the CA4P arm but did not reach statistical significance (5.2 versus 4.0 months; HR 0.65; 95% CI: 0.38–1.10); 27% of patients were alive at 1 year in the arm that received the experimental therapy compared to 9% in the standard treatment arm. The planned total patient sample could not be reached due to low recruitment [40].

5. Conclusion

Thyroid cancers are one of the greatest challenges for those treating advanced tumors. Thyroid cancer offers extensive opportunities to work in interdisciplinary teams that include not only oncologists and endocrinologists but also specialists in pathology, nuclear medicine, surgery, otolaryngology, radiology, clinical laboratory, and radiotherapy. Coordinated administration (whether concomitant or sequential) of the different therapeutic options for these patients make collaborative and efficient functioning of surgical and medical professionals more important than ever. The opportunity that presents itself is to apply the various treatments becoming available based on the genotypic characteristics of patients. Moreover, we have to consider the possibility of administering tyrosine kinase inhibitors for a long time with caution. We assume that these drugs are quite specific cytostatic and not cytotoxic agents, therefore, there is a need to give these agents until progression of the disease or toxicity. The concept of long-term treatment management of these new agents to patients in a childbearing age, with known cardiovascular toxicity, and perhaps many different side effects that could arise in the long-time followup, makes the monitoring of patients receiving inhibitors tyrosine kinase a must to be done very closely.

Maximizing clinical outcomes of tyrosine kinase therapy requires clear, effective communication, anticipation of side effects, and early intervention to avoid treatment delays and dose-limiting toxicities. There is a direct correlation between the plasmatic levels of the tyrosine kinase inhibitors with the activity of the drug, therefore, we would need to maintain as far as we can the highest dose of the targeted agent we consider is the most appropriate to our patients. In this sense, the experience in the management of tyrosine kinase inhibitors is crucial and probably the development of therapy management guidelines would be necessary in the next years.

To summarize, there is a need for a greater understanding of the molecular basis of the disease by the various health professionals charged with the care of these patient that could lead to a better optimization of treatment options in the advanced setting.

Acknowledgments

The authors declare that have no relevant conflict of interests in this paper. Pfizer funded the submission of the manuscript.

References

[1] S. Asioli, L. A. Erickson, A. Righi et al., "Poorly differentiated carcinoma of the thyroid: validation of the Turin proposal and analysis of IMP3 expression," *Modern Pathology*, vol. 23, no. 9, pp. 1269–1278, 2010.

[2] A. Y. Chen, A. Jemal, and E. M. Ward, "Increasing incidence of differentiated thyroid cancer in the United States, 1988–2005," *Cancer*, vol. 115, no. 16, pp. 3801–3807, 2009.

[3] L. Enewold, K. Zhu, E. Ron et al., "Rising thyroid cancer incidence in the United States by demographic and tumor characteristics, 1980–2005," *Cancer Epidemiology Biomarkers and Prevention*, vol. 18, no. 3, pp. 784–791, 2009.

[4] K. Shimaoka, D. A. Schoenfeld, and W. D. DeWys, "A randomized trial of doxorubicin versus doxorubicin plus cisplatin in patients with advanced thyroid carcinoma," *Cancer*, vol. 56, no. 9, pp. 2155–2160, 1985.

[5] T. Kondo, S. Ezzat, and S. L. Asa, "Pathogenetic mechanisms in thyroid follicular-cell neoplasia," *Nature Reviews Cancer*, vol. 6, no. 4, pp. 292–306, 2006.

[6] J. A. Sipos and M. H. Shah, "Thyroid cancer: emerging role for targeted therapies," *Therapeutic Advances in Medical Oncology*, vol. 2, no. 1, pp. 3–16, 2010.

[7] E. Y. Soh, M. S. Eigelberger, K. J. Kim et al., "Neutralizing vascular endothelial growth factor activity inhibits thyroid cancer growth in vivo," *Surgery*, vol. 128, no. 6, pp. 1059–1066, 2000.

[8] X. M. Yu, C. Y. Lo, W. F. Chan, K. Y. Lam, P. Leung, and J. M. Luk, "Increased expression of vascular endothelial growth factor C in papillary thyroid carcinoma correlates with cervical lymph node metastases," *Clinical Cancer Research*, vol. 11, no. 22, pp. 8063–8069, 2005.

[9] M. S. Haq, R. V. McCready, and C. L. Harmer, "Treatment of advanced differentiated thyroid carcinoma with high activity radioiodine therapy," *Nuclear Medicine Communications*, vol. 25, no. 8, pp. 799–805, 2004.

[10] M. Schlumberge and S. Sherman, "Approach to the patient with advanced differentiated thyroid cancer," *European Journal of Endocrinology*, vol. 166, no. 1, pp. 5–11, 2011.

[11] A. Matuszczyk, S. Petersenn, A. Bockisch et al., "Chemotherapy with doxorubicin in progressive medullary and thyroid carcinoma of the follicular epithelium," *Hormone and Metabolic Research*, vol. 40, no. 3, pp. 210–213, 2008.

[12] L. Licitra, L. D. Locati, A. Greco, R. Granata, and P. Bossi, "Multikinase inhibitors in thyroid cancer," *European Journal of Cancer*, vol. 46, no. 6, pp. 1012–1018, 2010.

[13] E. C. L. De Souza, A. C. Ferreira, and D. P. De Carvalho, "The mTOR protein as a target in thyroid cancer," *Expert Opinion on Therapeutic Targets*, vol. 15, no. 9, pp. 1099–1112, 2011.

[14] V. Marotta, A. Guerra, M. R. Sapio, and M. Vitale, "RET/PTC rearrangement in benign and malignant thyroid diseases: a clinical standpoint," *European Journal of Endocrinology*, vol. 165, no. 4, pp. 499–507, 2011.

[15] A. Bounacer, M. Schlumberger, R. Wicker et al., "Search for NTRK1 proto-oncogene rearrangements in human thyroid tumours originated after therapeutic radiation," *British Journal of Cancer*, vol. 82, no. 2, pp. 308–314, 2000.

[16] V. Gupta-Abramson, A. B. Troxel, A. Nellore et al., "Phase II trial of sorafenib in advanced thyroid cancer," *Journal of Clinical Oncology*, vol. 26, no. 29, pp. 4714–4719, 2008.

[17] R. T. Kloos, M. D. Ringel, M. V. Knopp et al., "Phase II trial of sorafenib in metastatic thyroid cancer," *Journal of Clinical Oncology*, vol. 27, no. 10, pp. 1675–1684, 2009.

[18] M. Ahmed, Y. Barbachano, A. Riddell et al., "Analysis of the efficacy and toxicity of sorafenib in thyroid cancer: a phase II study in a UK based population," *European Journal of Endocrinology*, vol. 165, no. 2, pp. 315–322, 2011.

[19] H. Hoftijzer, K. A. Heemstra, H. Morreau et al., "Beneficial effects of sorafenib on tumor progression, but not on radioiodine uptake, in patients with differentiated thyroid carcinoma," *European Journal of Endocrinology*, vol. 161, no. 6, pp. 923–931, 2009.

[20] J. Capdevila, L. Iglesias, I. Halperin et al., "Sorafenib in metastatic thyroid cancer," *Endocrine-Related Cancer*, vol. 19, no. 2, pp. 209–216, 2012.

[21] S. Leboulleux, L. Bastholt, T. M. Krause et al., "Vandetanib in locally advanced or metastatic differentiated thyroid cancer (papillary or follicular; DTC): a randomized, double-blind phase II trial," in *Proceedings of the 4th International Thyroid Congress*, Abstract OC-023, Paris, France, 2010.

[22] E. E. W. Cohen, L. S. Rosen, E. E. Vokes et al., "Axitinib is an active treatment for all histologic subtypes of advanced thyroid cancer: results from a phase II study," *Journal of Clinical Oncology*, vol. 26, no. 29, pp. 4708–4713, 2008.

[23] L. L. Carr, D. A. Mankoff, B. H. Goulart et al., "Phase II study of daily sunitinib in FDG-PET-positive, iodine-refractory differentiated thyroid cancer and metastatic medullary carcinoma of the thyroid with functional imaging correlation," *Clinical Cancer Research*, vol. 16, no. 21, pp. 5260–5268, 2010.

[24] E. E. Cohen, B. M. Needles, K. J. Cullen et al., "Phase 2 study of sunitinib in refractory thyroid cancer," *Journal of Clinical Oncology*, vol. 26, supplement, abstract 6025, 2008.

[25] S. I. Sherman, B. Jarzab, M. E. Cabanillas et al., "A phase II trial of the multitargeted kinase inhibitor E7080 in advanced radioiodine (RAI)-refractory differentiated thyroid cancer (DTC)," *Journal of Clinical Oncology*, vol. 29, supplement, abstract 5503, 2011.

[26] S. I. Sherman, L. J. Wirth, J. P. Droz et al., "Motesanib diphosphate in progressive differentiated thyroid cancer," *New England Journal of Medicine*, vol. 359, no. 1, pp. 31–42, 2008.

[27] K. C. Bible, V. J. Suman, J. R. Molina et al., "Efficacy of pazopanib in progressive, radioiodine-refractory, metastatic differentiated thyroid cancers: results of a phase 2 consortium study," *The Lancet Oncology*, vol. 11, no. 10, pp. 962–972, 2010.

[28] S. A. Wells Jr., B. G. Robinson, R. F. Gagel et al., "Vandetanib in patients with locally advanced or metastatic medullary thyroid cancer: a randomized, double-blind phase III trial," *Journal of Clinical Oncology*, vol. 30, no. 2, pp. 134–141, 2012.

[29] R. Kurzrock, S. I. Sherman, D. W. Ball et al., "Activity of XL184 (cabozantinib), an oral tyrosine kinase inhibitor, in patients with medullary thyroid cancer," *Journal of Clinical Oncology*, vol. 29, no. 19, pp. 2660–2666, 2011.

[30] E. T. Lam, M. D. Ringel, R. T. Kloos et al., "Phase II clinical trial of sorafenib in metastatic medullary thyroid cancer," *Journal of Clinical Oncology*, vol. 28, no. 14, pp. 2323–2330, 2010.

[31] M. J. Schlumberger, R. Elisei, L. Bastholt et al., "Phase II study of safety and efficacy of motesanib in patients with progressive or symptomatic, advanced or metastatic medullary thyroid cancer," *Journal of Clinical Oncology*, vol. 27, no. 23, pp. 3794–3801, 2009.

[32] J. A. De Souza, N. Busaidy, A. Zimrin et al., "Phase II trial of sunitinib in medullary thyroid cancer (MTC)," *Journal of Clinical Oncology*, vol. 28, supplement, abstract 5504, no. 15s, 2010.

[33] L. Santarpia, J. N. Myers, S. I. Sherman, F. Trimarchi, G. L. Clayman, and A. K. El-Naggar, "Genetic alterations in the Ras/Raf/mitogen-activated protein kinase and phosphatidylinositol 3-kinase/Akt signaling pathways in the follicular variant of papillary thyroid carcinoma," *Cancer*, vol. 116, no. 12, pp. 2974–2983, 2010.

[34] E. Grande-Pulido, B. Castelo, and P. J. Fonseca, "Efficacy and tolerability of sunitinib in patients with advanced thyroid cancer out of a trial: a Spanish multicenter cohort," *Journal of Clinical Oncology*, vol. 29, supplement, abstract e16024, 2011.

[35] M. Cakir and A. B. Grossman, "Medullary thyroid cancer: molecular biology and novel molecular therapies," *Neuroendocrinology*, vol. 90, no. 4, pp. 323–348, 2009.

[36] F. Pacini, M. G. Castagna, C. Cipri, and M. Schlumberger, "Medullary thyroid carcinoma," *Clinical Oncology*, vol. 22, no. 6, pp. 475–485, 2010.

[37] J. E. Phay and M. H. Shah, "Targeting RET receptor tyrosine kinase activation in cancer," *Clinical Cancer Research*, vol. 16, no. 24, pp. 5936–5941, 2010.

[38] F. Perri, G. D. Lorenzo, G. D. Scarpati, and C. Buonerba C, "Anaplastic thyroid carcinoma: a comprehensive review of current and future therapeutic options," *World Journal of Clinical Oncology*, vol. 2, no. 3, pp. 150–157, 2011.

[39] G. Nagaiah, P. Fu, J. K. Wasman et al., "CTRU Research Nurses. Phase II trial of sorafenib (bay 43-9006) in patients with advanced anaplastic carcinoma of the thyroid," *Journal of Clinical Oncology*, vol. 27, supplement, abstract 6058, no. 15s, 2009.

[40] J. A. Sosa, R. Elisei, B. Jarzab et al., "A randomized phase II/III trial of a tumor vascular disrupting agent fosbretabulin tromethamine (CA4P) with carboplatin (C) and paclitaxel (P) in anaplastic thyroid cancer (ATC): final survival analysis for the FACT trial," *Journal of Clinical Oncology*, vol. 29, supplement, abstract 5502, 2011.

27

Cell-Type-Dependent Thyroid Hormone Effects on Glioma Tumor Cell Lines

Liappas Alexandros,[1,2] Mourouzis Iordanis,[1] Zisakis Athanasios,[1] Economou Konstantinos,[1] Lea Robert-William,[2] and Pantos Constantinos[1]

[1] *Department of Pharmacology, University of Athens, 75 Mikras Asias Avenue, 11527 Goudi, Athens, Greece*

[2] *School of Pharmacy and Biomedical Sciences, University of Central Lancashire, Preston PR1 2HE, Lancashire, UK*

Correspondence should be addressed to Pantos Constantinos, cpantos@med.uoa.gr

Academic Editor: Fausto Bogazzi

Purpose. The present study investigated the potential effects of long-term T3 treatment on glioma tumor cell lines. Thyroid hormone action on cell growth, differentiation and survival during development may be of therapeutic relevance *Methods and Results* 1321N1 cell line, an astrocytoma grade II, and U87MG, a glioblastoma grade IV, were exposed for 2 and 4 days in medium deprived of T3 and in medium containing 1 nM T3. T3 promoted re-differentiation in both cell lines. However, T3 increased cell proliferation in 1321N1 (2 days) which declined thereafter (4 days) while in U87MG resulted in suppression of cell proliferation. At the molecular level, a 2.9 fold increase in the expression of TRα1 receptor was observed in U87MG versus 1321N1, $P<0.05$. TRβ1 receptor was undetectable. These changes corresponded to a distinct pattern of T3-induced kinase signaling activation; T3 had no effect on ERK activation in both cell lines but significantly increased phospho-Akt levels in 1321N1. *Conclusion.* In conclusion, T3 can re-differentiate glioma tumor cells, whereas its effect on cell proliferation appears to be dependent on the type of tumor cell line with aggressive tumors being more sensitive to T3. TRα1 receptor may, at least in part, be implicated in this response.

1. Introduction

It is now recognized that thyroid hormone (TH) may have a critical role in the pathogenesis and the progression of the diseases due to its regulatory action on cell differentiation, proliferation, and survival [1]. Experimental and clinical studies provide a growing body of evidence that TH signaling may be altered in heart failure with important physiological and therapeutic consequences [2]. Similarly, alterations in TH signaling have been observed in malignancies [3, 4], and hypothyroidism is shown to enhance tumor invasiveness and metastasis development [5, 6]. Furthermore, in 1896, thyroxine (horse thyroid extract) was the first successful hormonal product to be used against a fulminating breast cancer [7]. Similar results were thereafter reported for a series of patients with breast cancer in 1954 [8]. However, until now, the potential of TH as cancer therapy has not been adequately explored.

Gliomas represent the most common primary brain tumor and are among the most aggressive of cancers. Patients with glioma typically relapse within a year of initial diagnosis [9]. Although neurosurgical resection, radiation, and chemotherapy provide clear benefit, prognosis remains disappointing. TH levels are shown to be low in patients with gliomas but the relevance of this response to the pathophysiology of the disease remains largely unknown [10]. However, recent experimental studies provide evidence showing that acute, short-term TH treatment may increase cell proliferation and survival via its nongenomic action [11–13]. In contrast, long-term TH treatment appears to suppress cell proliferation in neuroblastoma cells [5]. Based on this evidence, in the present study, we further explored the long-term T3 effects on glioma tumors in relation to the degree of tumor aggressiveness and potential alterations in thyroid hormone nuclear receptor (TR) expression which may characterize different types of glioma cell lines. This issue although of clinical and therapeutic relevance has not been previously addressed.

2. Materials and Methods

2.1. Cell Culture. 1321N1 cell line, an astrocytoma grade II, and U87MG, a glioblastoma grade IV, were used in this study. Glioma cell line U87MG was obtained from the American Type Culture Collection (ATCC) (Manassas, VA), and glioma cell line 1321N1 was obtained from the European Collection of Cell Culture (ECACC) (Salisbury, Wiltshire, UK). All cell lines were maintained in 150 cm^2 cell culture flasks (CORNING). U87MG was maintained in Eagle's Essential Minimum Medium (MEM) with Earle's salts supplemented with 10% fetal bovine serum (GIBCO), 1 mM sodium pyruvate, streptomycin and penicillin (5% v/v), 0.1 mM nonessential amino acids, 2 mM L-glutamine, and amphotericin B (5% v/v).

1321N1 was maintained in Dulbecco's Modified Eagle's Medium (DMEM) with glucose and sodium bicarbonate supplemented with 10% FBS, 2 mM L-glutamine, 5% penicillin and streptomycin, and 5% amphotericin B.

All cell lines were maintained in a 37°C humidified incubator with 5% CO$_2$. For all experiments, each of the glioma cell lines was used between passages 20–30. Once cells were 70–80% confluent, they were trypsinized using 1X Trypsin. Cells were settled for 24 h in stripped medium (using charcoal FBS, GIBCO) before the initiation of treatment. Cells were cultured for 48 h and 96 h either in stripped medium only (nontreated) or in stripped medium in which 1 nM of T3 was added.

2.2. Cell Morphology. Cell morphology was used to assess cell differentiation. Cells were fixed in, before being viewed with an inverted light microscope fitted with phase contrast optics. Five random fields, each containing no more than 50 cells, were examined in each well, and the total number of cells as well as the total number of extensions that were greater than two cell body diameters in length were recorded. Data were derived from approximately 100 cells in each group. Cell morphology could not be reliably assessed at 96 h due to more than 80% confluency in non-treated cells.

2.3. Cell Proliferation. In order to measure cell proliferation, BrdU labeling reagent (RPN20 kit, GE Healthcare, Piscataway, NJ) was added to the medium. Cells were incubated for 30 min and then fixed using 4% paraformaldehyde for 15 min. Primary antibody (anti-BrdU monoclonal antibody, dilution 1 : 100) was applied for 1 h at room temperature. Samples were washed 3 × 5 min with PBS. Secondary antibody (peroxidase anti-mouse IgG2a) was then applied for 30 min at room temperature, followed by washing 3 × 5 min. Finally, BrdU-immunostained cultures were visualized using DAB and photographs taken with a digital camera (Zeiss Axiovert) attached to an inverted microscope fitted with phase contrast optics. BrdU-positive nuclei were counted as a percentage of total nuclei. Proliferation data are derived from between 450 to 600 cells measured in each group.

2.4. Measurement of Total Cell Number. At 2 and 4 days after treatment, cells were washed twice with PBS, and 100 μL

trypsin 0.25% were added to each plate and incubated for 37°C until the cells were detached. A solution of 10% FBS in PBS was added to each plate to inhibit the trypsin action. Then, cells were harvested, and the cell number was determined after several counts of a certain volume in Neubauer hematocytometer.

2.5. Cell Apoptosis. Apoptotic cell nuclei were assessed by Tunnel staining using the In Situ Cell Death Detection Kit, according to standard protocol based on manufacturer's instructions (ROCHE, Cat. No. 11 684 795 910). Cell cultures were counterstained with Hoechst 33358 (5 μg/mL) which stained the nuclei of all cells. Administration of doxorubicin is known to induce apoptosis and was used as a positive control in order to certify the selected method.

2.6. Cell Injury. Cellular injury was assessed by LDH enzyme release in cultured medium. Culture medium was collected at the end of the experiment for the measurement of lactate dehydrogenase (LDH) activity (IU/L) using an ELISA kit (Quantichrom LDH Kit, DLDH-100, BioAssay Systems, USA). Measurements were performed with Tecan Genios system. LDH release was expressed in each group as percentage of the non-treated group.

2.7. Protein Isolation and Measurement of Thyroid Hormone Receptors. After washing twice with PBS, the cells were scraped into 400 μL lysis buffer containing 20 mM HEPES, pH 7.9, 10 mM KCl, 1 mM EDTA, 10% glycerol, 0.2% NP-40, 0.5 mM DTT, 0.5 mM PMSF, 5 μg/mL aprotinin, and 5 μg/mL leupeptin. A small quantity of total lysate was kept and the remainder centrifuged at 12000 g for 1 min at 4°C. The nuclear fraction was prepared by resuspension of the pellet in buffer containing 20 mM HEPES, pH 7.9, 0.42 M NaCl, 0.2 mM EDTA, 1.5 mM MgCl$_2$, 25% glycerol, 0.5 mM DTT, 0.5 mM PMSF, 5 μg/mL aprotinin, and 5 μg/mL leupeptin and incubated with agitation for 1 hour at 4°C before centrifugation for 10 min at 12,000 g. The resulting supernatants were collected and used for protein analysis of the nuclear fraction. Protein concentrations were determined by the BCA assay method. After boiling for 5 min (with 4% SDS, 2% mercaptoethanol, and 0.004% bromophenol blue), a quantity of 15 μg protein from nuclear or total fraction was separated on 7.5% SDS-PAGE using a Bio-Rad Mini-Protean gel apparatus. For Western blotting, proteins were transferred electrophoretically to a nitrocellulose membrane (Hybond ECL) at 100 V and 4°C, for 1.5 h using Towbin buffer. After Western blotting, filters were probed with specific antibodies against TRα1 (Abcam Rabbit polyclonal to TRα1, ab53729, dilution 1 : 1000, o/n at 4°C) and TRβ1 (Affinity Bioreagents, MA1-216, dilution 1 : 1000, o/n at 4°C). Filters were incubated with appropriate anti-mouse (Amersham) or anti-rabbit (Cell Signaling) HRP secondary antibodies. Immunoreactivity was detected by enhanced chemiluminescence using Lumiglo reagents (New England Biolabs). Chemiluminescence was detected by the image analysis system FluorChem HD2 (Alpha Innotech Corporation, 14743, Catalina Street, San Leandro, CA) equipped with a CCD camera and analysis software. Five samples from each group were loaded on the same gel. Ponceau staining was used in order to normalize slight variations in protein loading.

2.8. Determination of Kinase Signaling Activation. Filters were probed with specific antibodies. Membranes with total protein extracts were blocked with 5% nonfat milk in TBS-Tween for 60 min and then probed with specific antibodies against total and phospho-ERK (Cell Signalling Technology, dilution 1 : 1000) and total and phospho-Akt (Cell Signalling Technology, dilution 1 : 1000), overnight at 4°C. Filters were incubated with appropriate anti-rabbit HRP secondary antibody (Cell Signaling, 1 : 4000, 1 h R.T.), and immunoreactivity was detected by enhanced chemiluminescence using Lumiglo reagents (New England Biolabs). Immunoblots were quantified using the FluorChem HD2 system (Alpha Innotech Corporation, 14743, Catalina Street, San Leandro, CA). Data were obtained from $n = 5$ samples for each group.

2.9. Statistics. Values are presented as mean (S.E.M.). Data were analyzed with single factor analysis of variance ANOVA across groups. An unpaired independent sample *t*-test or nonparametric Mann-Whitney test was performed, as appropriate. A two-tailed test with a P value less than 0.05 was considered significant.

3. Results

3.1. Cell Morphology. T3 induced cell redifferentiation in both cell lines studied as indicated by the significant increase in the number of perisomatal filopodia like neurites. Thus, in 1321N1 cells, the ratio of total number of projections to total number of cells was 1.04 (0.14) for non-treated versus 1.9 (0.11) in T3 treated, $P < 0.05$. In U87-MG cells, the ratio of total number of projections to total number of cells was 1.16 (0.14) for nontreated versus 1.83 (0.19) in T3 treated, $P < 0.05$ (Figure 1).

3.2. Cell Proliferation. In 1321N1 cell cultures, at two days, BrdU-immunostained cell nuclei were found to be 23.6% (3) in non-treated versus 30.5% (3) in T3 treated, $P < 0.05$. At 4 days, cell proliferation was shown to be 45.2% (5) in nontreated versus 40% (6) in T3 treated, $P > 0.05$ (Figure 2).

In U87MG cell cultures, at 2 days, BrdU-immunostained cell nuclei were 48% (5) in nontreated versus 23.6% (4) in T3 treated, $P < 0.05$. In addition, after 4 days, cell proliferation was shown to be 36.5% (6) in non-treated versus 16.3% (4) in T3 treated, $P < 0.05$. (Figure 2).

3.3. LDH Release and Apoptosis. No change in LDH release was observed either in 1321N1 or U87MG cell cultures (Figure 2). Apoptosis was not detected either in 1321N1 or U87MG cells (data not shown).

3.4. Total Cell Number. In 1321N1 cell cultures, at two days, total cell number was found to be 207183 (2145) in non-treated versus 232366 (2390) in T3 treated, $P < 0.05$. At 4 days, total cell number was 381105 (4100) in non-treated versus 372433 (2595) in T3 treated, $P > 0.05$ (Figure 2).

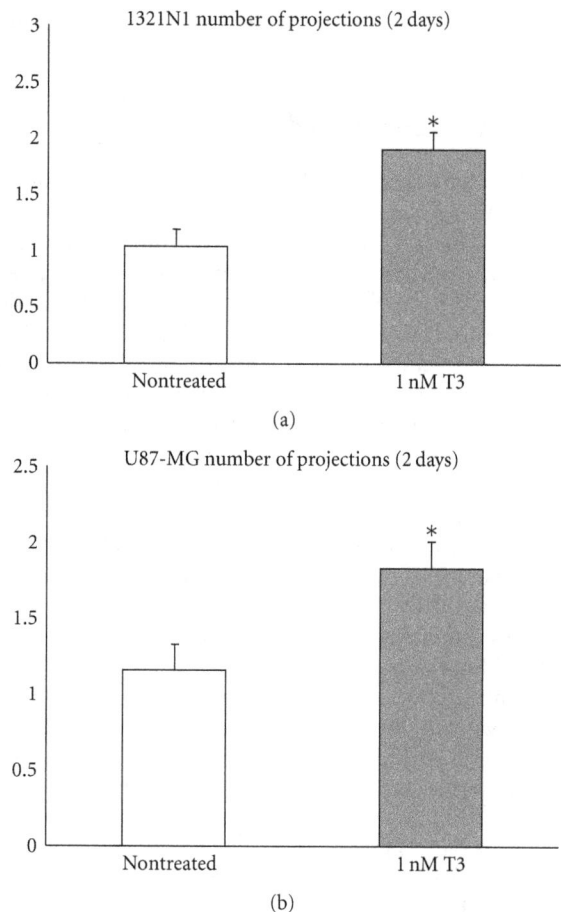

(a)

(b)

FIGURE 1: T3 induced cell re-differentiation as indicated by the significant increase in the ratio of number of projections to total cell number both in 1321N1 cells (a) and U87-MG cells (b) at 2 days. Data were derived from approximately 100 cells in each group. *$P < 0.05$ versus non-treated.

In U87MG cell cultures, at 2 days, total cell number was found to be 211300 (2078) in non treated versus 186166 (3122) in T3 treated, $P < 0.05$. In addition, after 4 days, total cell number was 396866 (5791) in non-treated versus 331133 (11652) in T3 treated, $P < 0.05$ (Figure 2).

3.5. Thyroid Hormone Receptors Expression. A 2.9-fold increase in the expression of TRα1 receptor was observed in U87MG cells as compared to 1321N1, $P < 0.05$. TRβ1 receptor was undetectable in both cell lines (Figure 3).

3.6. Levels of Phospho-Akt and Phospho-ERK after T3 Treatment. At two days, the ratio of p44 and p42 phospho-ERK to total ERK in 1321N1 cells was increased 2.0-fold in T3-treated cultures ($P > 0.05$) as compared to non-treated cells. Furthermore, the ratio of phospho-Akt to total Akt was found to be 1.4 higher in T3 treated cells as compared to non-treated cells, $P < 0.05$. At 4 days, no differences in the ratio of p44 and p42 phospho-ERK to total ERK and phospho-Akt to total Akt were observed between the two groups (Figure 4).

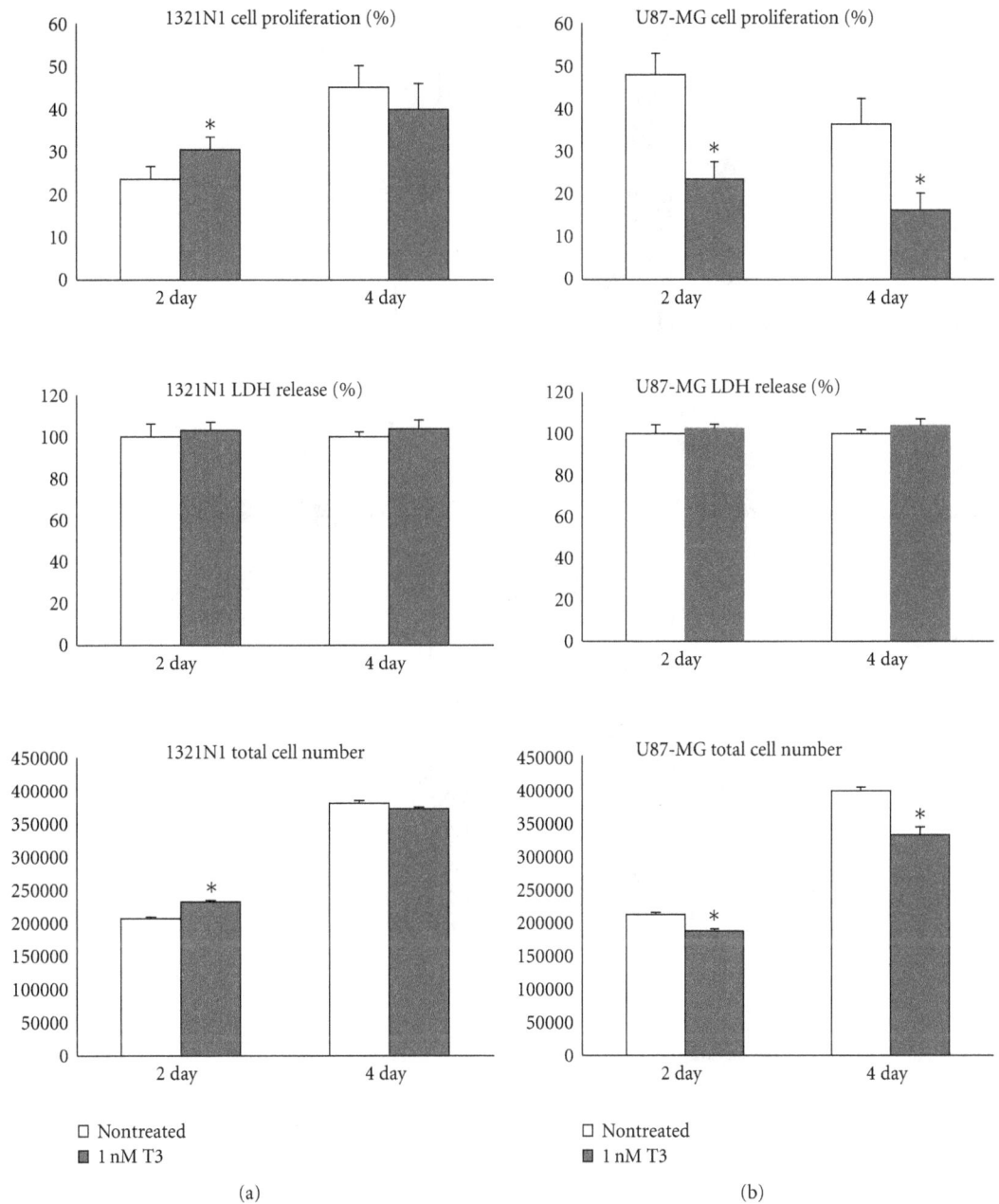

FIGURE 2: Cell proliferation index, LDH release, and total cell number in non-treated 1321N1 (a) and U87-MG (b) cells and after exposure to 1 nM T3 medium concentration for 48 h and 96 h. Cell proliferation index was assessed as the percentage of BrdU-positive nuclei to the total number of nuclei, while LDH release was expressed in each group as percentage of the untreated group. $^*P < 0.05$ versus non treated.

In U87MG cells, no differences in the ratio of p44 and p42 phospho-ERK to total ERK and phospho-Akt to total Akt were observed between the two groups either at 2 or 4 days (Figure 5).

4. Discussion

It is now recognized that TH has important regulatory actions beyond cell metabolism. TH is critical for cell differentiation, proliferation, and survival during development, and later in adult life may have regenerative/reparative action under pathological conditions [14–16]. This unique effect

could potentially be of therapeutic value in cancer therapy [17]. Thus, in the present study, we explored the effects of TH treatment on cell differentiation, proliferation, and survival using two different glioma cell lines, the 1321N1, an astrocytoma grade II, and U87MG, a glioblastoma grade IV cell line. T3 was used at medium concentration of 1 nM which is in the range of near physiological concentrations and has been previously shown to suppress cell proliferation in neuroblastoma cells [5]. This treatment resulted in cell redifferentiation in both cell lines studied as indicated by the morphological changes and the marked increase in the number of perisomatal filopodia like neurites. This finding is

(a)

(b)

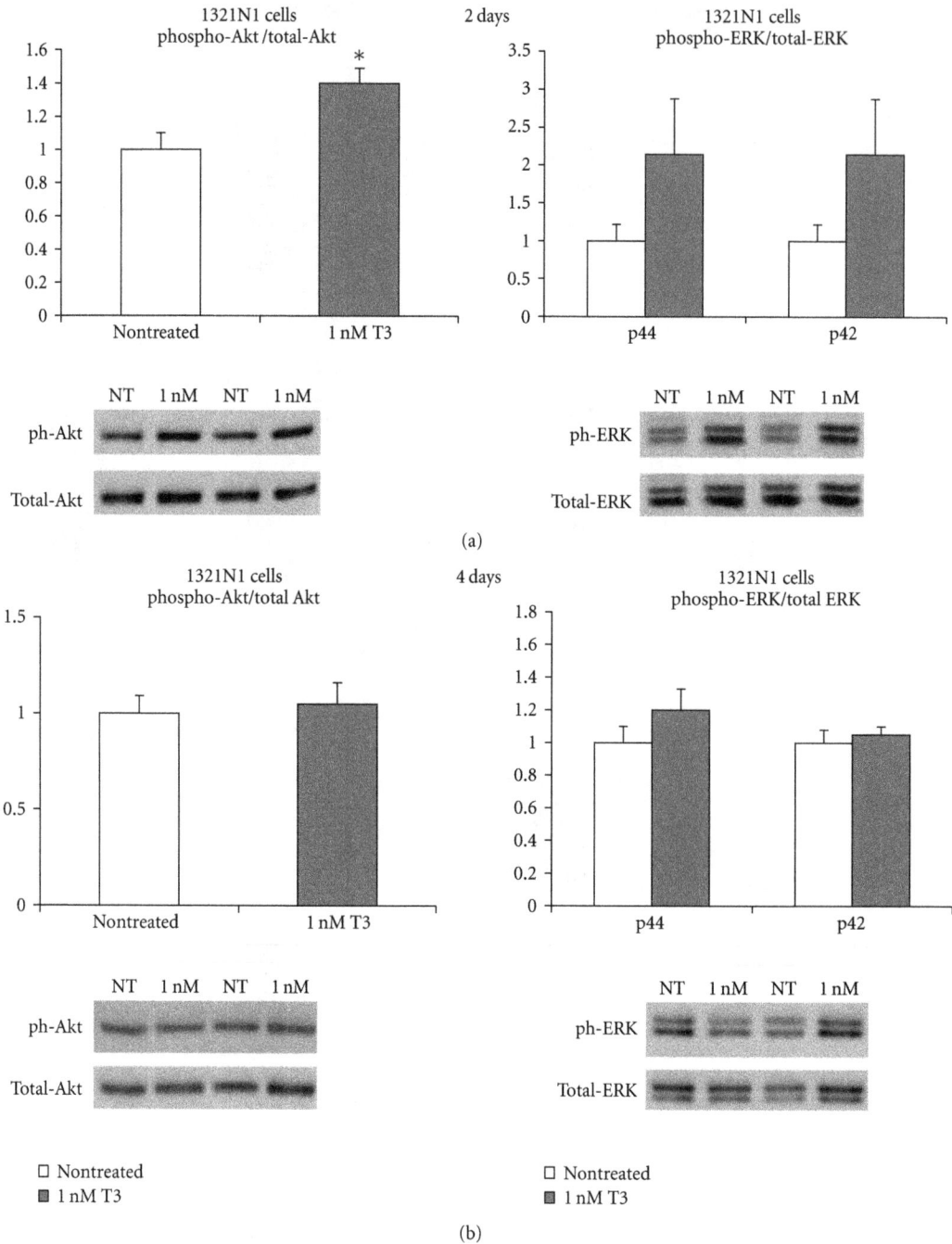

FIGURE 3: Thyroid hormone receptor $\alpha 1$ and $\beta 1$ expression in 1321N1 cells versus U87-MG cells. Representative western blotting images are shown. P.C. corresponds to positive control. *$P < 0.05$ versus 1321N1 cells.

in accordance with previous reports showing a transforming effect of T3 in neuroblastoma cells [5]. A series of genes related to neuroblastoma cell differentiation are shown to be responsive to TH [18]. It is of note that this unique effect of TH has also been shown in other cancer cells and may be of physiological and therapeutic relevance [19].

Our study further showed that the two cell lines responded differently to TH treatment as regards cell proliferation with the more aggressive tumor cells to be more sensitive. Thus, in 1321N1, T3 treatment resulted in increased cell

proliferation at two days which declined thereafter, while T3 had no effect on cell injury. In contrast, in the U87MG cell line, T3 markedly suppressed cell proliferation without increasing cell injury. The potential underlying mechanisms of this cell-type-dependent action of TH on cell proliferation are not fully understood. Long-term TH effects are mediated via thyroid hormone receptors (TRs). TRs are transcription factors which regulate important genes related to cell differentiation, proliferation, and survival [17]. It is now recognized that TRs are altered in pathological conditions with

(a)

(b)

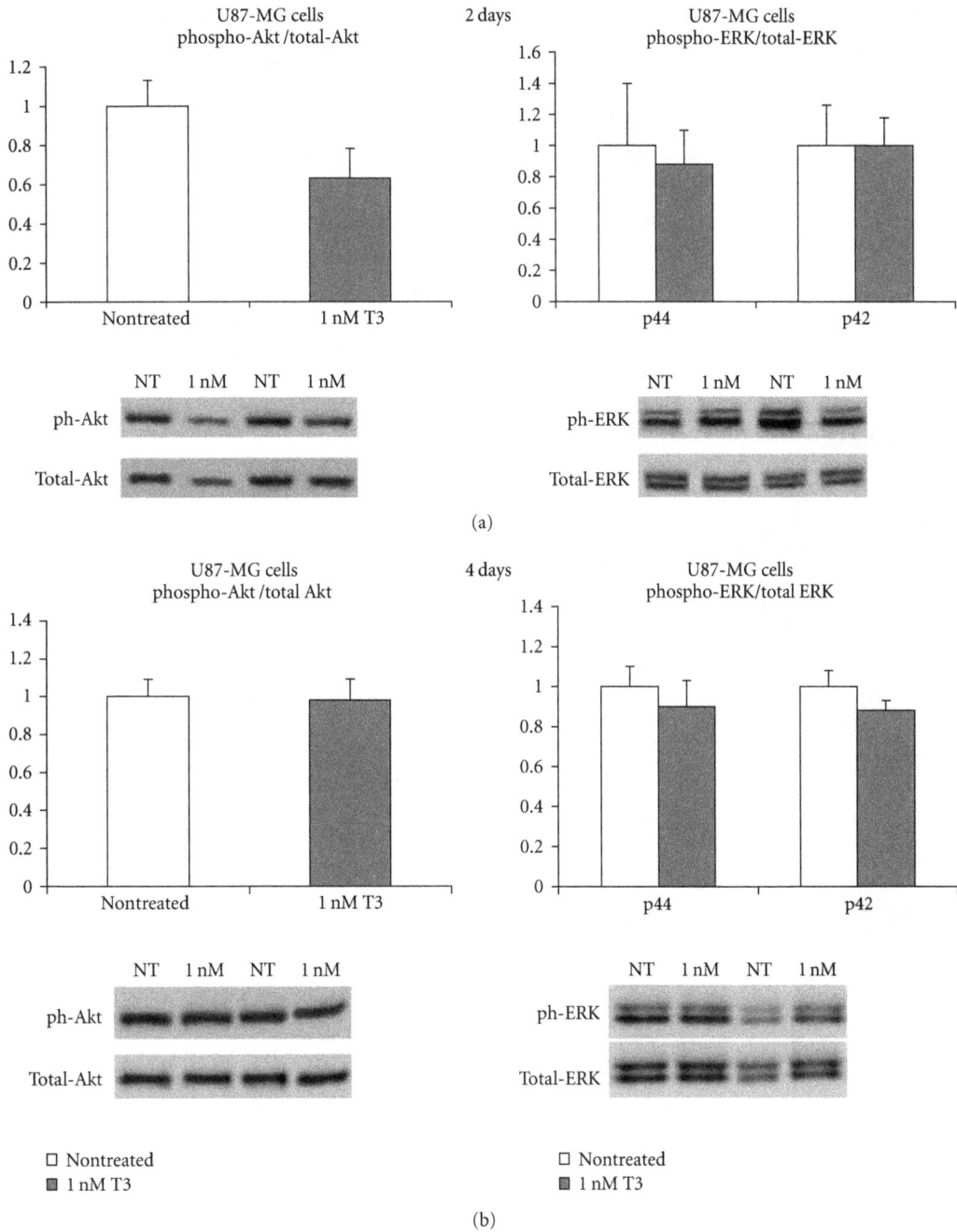

FIGURE 4: Phosphorylated levels of Akt and p44, p42 ERK after exposure of 1321N1 cells for 2 days (a) and 4 days (b) in 1 nM T3 as compared to non treated cells. Data were derived from $n = 5$ samples in each group. Representative Western blotting images are shown. $*P < 0.05$ versus non treated.

important physiological consequences. Thus, we have previously shown that TRs can change in the myocardium after ischaemic stress or in cardiac cells exposed to growth stimuli [20, 21]. Similarly, there is increasing evidence that alterations in TRs are common events in cancer [4]. On the basis of this evidence, we explored whether altered TR expression in these two cell lines could possibly underlie the differential T3 effect on cell proliferation. Interestingly, TRα1 was found to be overexpressed in U87MG cell line compared to 1321N1, while TRβ1 receptor was undetectable in both cell lines. This

finding may indicate a potential implication of TRα1 receptor in T3 action on glioma cell tumors. In fact, several lines of evidence support this notion. TRα1 receptor has a unique dual mode of function depending on thyroid hormone availability. Thus, TRα1 in its unliganded state (aporeceptor) instead of being inactive exerts repressive or inducible effect on the transcription of T3 inducible or repressive genes by recruiting corepressor complexes with histone deacetylase [22]. This is of important physiological relevance during development with TRα1 to be overexpressed at early

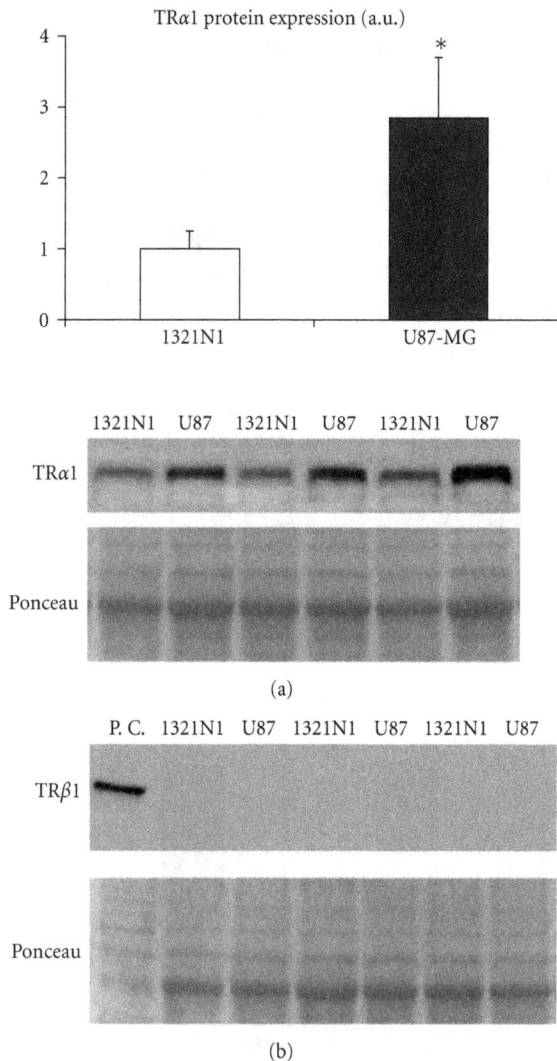

FIGURE 5: Phosphorylated levels of Akt and p44, p42 ERK after exposure of U87-MG cells for 2 days (a) and 4 days (b) in 1 nM T3 as compared to non treated cells. Data were derived from $n = 5$ samples in each group. Representative Western blotting images are shown. $*P < 0.05$ versus non treated, $**P < 0.05$ versus non treated and 1 nM T3 treated cells.

embryonic stages when TH is low, resulting in cell proliferation and declines thereafter with the rise of TH resulting in cell differentiation [1]. This fetal pattern of TRα1 expression reemerges under pathological conditions and may lead to pathological hypertrophy [20, 21] or promote cell cancer proliferation [5]. The addition of TH prevents the development of pathological cardiac hypertrophy [14] and suppresses cancer cell proliferation [5]. Taken together, these data reveal an important role of TRα1 in glioma cell aggressiveness and response to TH. However, this issue merits further investigation.

Our study further explored whether this differential expression of TRα1 had an impact on the activation of growth kinase (ERK and Akt) signaling activation induced by T3 treatment. These cascades are important regulators of cancer

growth and cancer cell survival [23–25]. Both Akt and ERK are active in gliomas and have been associated with tumor aggressiveness [26–29]. Interestingly, the present study showed that T3 could significantly increase p-Akt levels in 1321N1 and not in U87MG cell line while having no effect on ERK activation in either cell line. This is in contrast with the acute nongenomic effect of T3 on U87MG cell line which was shown to involve the activation of ERK cascade [12].

In conclusion, T3 can redifferentiate glioma tumor cells. However, the T3 effect on cell proliferation appears to be dependent on the type of tumor cell line with aggressive tumors to be more sensitive to thyroid hormone treatment. TRα1 receptor may, at least in part, be implicated in this response.

References

[1] I. Mourouzis, F. Forini, C. Pantos et al., "Thyroid hormone and cardiac disease: from basic concepts to clinical application," *Journal of Thyroid Research.* In press.

[2] C. Pantos, I. Mourouzis, C. Xinaris, Z. Papadopoulou-Daifoti, and D. Cokkinos, "Thyroid hormone and "cardiac metamorphosis": potential therapeutic implications," *Pharmacology and Therapeutics*, vol. 118, no. 2, pp. 277–294, 2008.

[3] A. Aranda, O. Martínez-Iglesias, L. Ruiz-Llorente, V. García-Carpizo, and A. Zambrano, "Thyroid receptor: roles in cancer," *Trends in Endocrinology and Metabolism*, vol. 20, no. 7, pp. 318–324, 2009.

[4] J. M. Gonzalez-Sancho, V. Garcia, F. Bonilla et al., "Thyroid hormone receptors/THR genes in human cancer," *Cancer Letters*, vol. 192, no. 2, pp. 121–132, 2003.

[5] S. Garcia-Silva and A. Aranda, "The thyroid hormone receptor is a suppressor of ras-mediated transcription, proliferation, and transformation," *Molecular and Cellular Biology*, vol. 24, no. 17, pp. 7514–7523, 2004.

[6] O. Martínez-Iglesias, S. García-Silva, J. Regadera, and A. Aranda, "Hypothyroidism enhances tumor invasiveness and metastasis development," *PLoS ONE*, vol. 4, no. 7, article e6428, 2009.

[7] G. Beatson, "On the treatment of inoperable cases of carcinoma of the mamma: suggestions for a new method of treatment with illustrative cases," *The Lancet*, vol. 148, no. 3802, pp. 101–107, 1896.

[8] A. A. Loeser, "A new therapy for prevention of post-operative recurrences in genital and breast cancer; a six-years study of prophylactic thyroid treatment," *British Medical Journal*, vol. 2, no. 4901, pp. 1380–1383, 1954.

[9] H. Ohgaki, "Epidemiology of brain tumors," *Methods in Molecular Biology*, vol. 472, pp. 323–342, 2009.

[10] P. Nauman, W. Bonicki, R. Michalik, A. Warzecha, and Z. Czernicki, "The concentration of thyroid hormones and activities of iodothyronine deiodinases are altered in human brain gliomas," *Folia Neuropathologica*, vol. 42, no. 2, pp. 67–73, 2004.

[11] F. B. Davis, H. Y. Tang, A. Shih et al., "Acting via a cell surface receptor, thyroid hormone is a growth factor for glioma cells," *Cancer Research*, vol. 66, no. 14, pp. 7270–7275, 2006.

[12] H. Y. Lin, M. Sun, H. Y. Tang et al., "L-thyroxine vs. 3,5,3′-triiodo-L-thyronine and cell proliferation: activation of mitogen-activated protein kinase and phosphatidylinositol 3-kinase," *American Journal of Physiology*, vol. 296, no. 5, pp. C980–C991, 2009.

[13] H. Y. Lin, H. Y. Tang, T. Keating et al., "Resveratrol is pro-apoptotic and thyroid hormone is anti-apoptotic in glioma cells: both actions are integrin and ERK mediated," *Carcinogenesis*, vol. 29, no. 1, pp. 62–69, 2008.

[14] C. Pantos, I. Mourouzis, and D. V. Cokkinos, "Rebuilding the post-infarcted myocardium by activating "physiologic" hypertrophic signaling pathways: the thyroid hormone paradigm," *Heart Failure Reviews*, vol. 15, no. 2, pp. 143–154, 2010.

[15] C. Pantos, I. Mourouzis, T. Saranteas et al., "Acute T3 treatment protects the heart against ischemia-reperfusion injury via TRα1 receptor," *Molecular and Cellular Biochemistry*, vol. 353, no. 1-2, pp. 235–241, 2011.

[16] A. Shulga, A. Blaesse, K. Kysenius et al., "Thyroxin regulates BDNF expression to promote survival of injured neurons," *Molecular and Cellular Neuroscience*, vol. 42, no. 4, pp. 408–418, 2009.

[17] E. Kress, J. Samarut, and M. Plateroti, "Thyroid hormones and the control of cell proliferation or cell differentiation: paradox or duality?" *Molecular and Cellular Endocrinology*, vol. 313, no. 1-2, pp. 36–49, 2009.

[18] G. Bedo, A. Pascual, and A. Aranda, "Early thyroid hormone-induced gene expression changes in N2a-beta neuroblastoma cells," *Journal of Molecular Neuroscience*, vol. 45, no. 2, pp. 76–86, 2011.

[19] A. Perra, M. A. Kowalik, M. Pibiri, G. M. Ledda-Columbano, and A. Columbano, "Thyroid hormone receptor ligands induce regression of rat preneoplastic liver lesions causing their reversion to a differentiated phenotype," *Hepatology*, vol. 49, no. 4, pp. 1287–1296, 2009.

[20] C. Pantos, I. Mourouzis, G. Galanopoulos et al., "Thyroid hormone receptor 1 downregulation in postischemic heart failure progression: the potential role of tissue hypothyroidism," *Hormone and Metabolic Research*, vol. 42, no. 10, pp. 718–724, 2010.

[21] C. Pantos, C. Xinaris, I. Mourouzis et al., "Thyroid hormone receptor α1: a switch to cardiac cell "metamorphosis"?" *Journal of Physiology and Pharmacology*, vol. 59, no. 2, pp. 253–269, 2008.

[22] J. Zhang and M. A. Lazar, "The mechanism of action of thyroid hormones," *Annual Review of Physiology*, vol. 62, pp. 439–466, 2000.

[23] W. H. Chappell, L. S. Steelman, J. M. Long et al., "Ras/Raf/MEK/ERK and PI3K/PTEN/Akt/mTOR inhibitors: rationale and importance to inhibiting these pathways in human health," *Oncotarget*, vol. 2, no. 3, pp. 135–164, 2011.

[24] I. Hers, E. E. Vincent, and J. M. Tavaré, "Akt signalling in health and disease," *Cellular Signalling*, vol. 23, no. 10, pp. 1515–1527, 2011.

[25] H. W. Lo, "Targeting Ras-RAF-ERK and its interactive pathways as a novel therapy for malignant gliomas," *Current Cancer Drug Targets*, vol. 10, no. 8, pp. 840–848, 2011.

[26] I. F. Pollack, R. L. Hamilton, P. C. Burger et al., "Akt activation is a common event in pediatric malignant gliomas and a potential adverse prognostic marker: a report from the Children's Oncology Group," *Journal of Neuro-Oncology*, vol. 99, no. 2, pp. 155–163, 2010.

[27] Q. W. Fan, C. Cheng, C. Hackett et al., "Akt and autophagy cooperate to promote survival of drug-resistant glioma," *Science Signaling*, vol. 3, no. 147, article ra81, 2010.

[28] E. A. El-Habr, P. Tsiorva, M. Theodorou et al., "Analysis of PIK3CA and B-RAF gene mutations in human astrocytomas: association with activation of ERK and AKT," *Clinical Neuropathology*, vol. 29, no. 4, pp. 239–245, 2010.

[29] J. P. Robinson, M. W. VanBrocklin, K. J. Lastwika, A. J. McKinney, S. Brandner, and S. L. Holmen, "Activated MEK cooperates with Ink4a/Arf loss or Akt activation to induce gliomas in vivo," *Oncogene*, vol. 30, no. 11, pp. 1341–1350, 2011.

28

Elevated Serum Thyroglobulin and Low Iodine Intake Are Associated with Nontoxic Nodular Goiter among Adults Living near the Eastern Mediterranean Coast

Yaniv S. Ovadia,[1,2] **Dov Gefel,**[1,2] **Svetlana Turkot,**[3] **Dorit Aharoni,**[4] **Shlomo Fytlovich,**[4] **and Aron M. Troen**[2]

[1]*Department of Internal Medicine "C", Barzilai Medical Center Ashkelon, Hahistadrout Street 2, 7830604 Ashkelon, Israel*
[2]*Nutrition and Brain Health Laboratory, School of Nutritional Sciences, Institute of Biochemistry,*
 Food Science and Nutrition, Robert H. Smith Faculty of Agriculture, Food and Environment, The Hebrew University of Jerusalem,
 P.O. Box 12, 76100 Rehovot, Israel
[3]*Endocrinology Clinic, Barzilai Medical Center Ashkelon, Hahistadrout Street 2, 7830604 Ashkelon, Israel*
[4]*Laboratory of Clinical Biochemistry, Barzilai Medical Center Ashkelon, Hahistadrout Street 2, 7830604 Ashkelon, Israel*

Correspondence should be addressed to Yaniv S. Ovadia; yaniv.ovadia@mail.huji.ac.il

Academic Editor: Noriyuki Koibuchi

Background. Information about iodine intake is crucial for preventing thyroid diseases. Inadequate iodine intake can lead to thyroid diseases, including nontoxic nodular goiter (NNG). *Objective.* To estimate iodine intake and explore its correlation with thyroid diseases among Israeli adults living near the Mediterranean coast, where iodine-depleted desalinated water has become a major source of drinking water. *Methods.* Cross-sectional study of patients attending Barzilai Medical Center Ashkelon. Participants, who were classified as either NNG ($n = 17$), hypothyroidism ($n = 14$), or control ($n = 31$), provided serum thyroglobulin (Tg) and completed a semiquantitative iodine food frequency questionnaire. *Results.* Elevated serum Tg values (Tg > 60 ng/mL) were significantly more prevalent in the NNG group than in the other groups (29% versus 7% and 0% for hypothyroidism and controls, resp., $P < 0.05$). Mean estimated iodine intake was significantly lower in the NNG group ($65 \pm 30\,\mu$g/d) than in controls ($115 \pm 60\,\mu$g/d) ($P < 0.05$) with intermediate intake in the hypothyroid group ($73 \pm 38\,\mu$g/d). *Conclusions.* Elevated serum Tg values and low dietary iodine intake are associated with NNG among adult patients in Ashkelon District, Israel. Larger studies are needed in order to expand on these important initial findings.

1. Introduction

Either high or low iodine intake can lead to thyroid disease (TD) [1]. Thus, assessment of iodine intake is crucial for TD prevention. One form of TD is nontoxic nodular goiter (NNG). Nontoxic nodular goiter is a benign thyroid enlargement [2] that may cause neck discomfort, respiratory symptoms, or dysphagia and can lead to thyroid dysfunction [2, 3]. Nontoxic nodular goiter is rarely reversible in adults [4, 5]. Hence, consuming the adequate amount of iodine should reduce NNG risk, perhaps decreasing TD incidence [4, 6]. Worldwide, long-term inadequate iodine intake (over months or years) is associated with high NNG rates [4], but

whether low or high intake is the major factor seems to depend on geographic region and timing. For example, NNG was attributed to iodine deficiency (ID) in Greece during the 1960s [6], whereas it was associated with excess iodine intake in Algeria during the previous decade [7]. The possibility that ID contributes to NNG in a developed state as Israel has global significance, given the drop in iodine intake in other industrialized countries in the recent decade [4].

The aim of this study was therefore to investigate the relationship between iodine intake and the presence of TD among Israeli adults, both inpatients and outpatients, within a single region (Ashkelon District). There is limited information about the extent of Israelis harboring TD and there are no national data on iodine intake; however, data from the first and second Israeli National Health Interview Surveys (INHIS-1) [8] (INHIS-2) [9] by Israel Center for Disease Control (ICDC) show that, in 2003–2010, the self-reported use of TD medication among Israeli adults increased from 2.9% to 4.7% (personal communication, ICDC 2013). Our literature review yielded only one study that found no correlation between iodine intake and NNG among Israeli adults (Benbassat et al. 2004) [10]. However, since then iodine-depleted desalinated water has become a major source of drinking water nationwide, particularly throughout the Ashkelon District (personal communication with Mr. Farkash, Israel's South Region Water Quality Engineer, 2011) [11].

Serum thyroglobulin (Tg) has been used as a sensitive marker for ID in many populations studies, and it positively correlates with ID severity as well as with some types of TD, including NNG [12, 13]. Furthermore, because serum Tg falls rapidly with iodine repletion, it is considered a more sensitive indicator of iodine repletion than serum thyrotropin (TSH) or free thyroxine (FT4) [13]. Therefore, we evaluated iodine intake by measuring serum Tg.

In addition to serum Tg values, we estimated habitual dietary iodine intake over the past year using a validated, semiquantitative, Iodine Food Frequency Questionnaire (sIFFQ) that we adapted to Israel. Although this sIFFQ does not include all foods consumed daily, it covers selected iodine-rich foods that provide the majority of dietary iodine, while the remaining food groups probably contain only about 3–6% of the total iodine amount consumed per day [14]. The approach presented here is sound in that it combines Tg and sIFFQ, two complementary indicators: Tg indicates intermediate (weeks to months) iodine intake [6], and the sIFFQ can classify longer-term (up to a year) intake to high and low intake [14]. Although urinary iodine concentration (UIC) is a common measure in many population studies [6, 7, 10], it was not suitable for this study, because of the high within-individual variability in UIC and because UIC indicates recent iodine intake (days), whereas NNG develops after long-term iodine inadequacy in the order of years [15].

2. Material and Methods

2.1. Settings. In this cross-sectional study, iodine status was assessed in a convenience sample of volunteers living in the Ashkelon District, Israel, who were prospectively recruited at Barzilai Medical Center in Ashkelon (BMCA). The Ashkelon District and city, where the BMCA is located, are shown in the accompanying map (Figure 1). Volunteers were enrolled over a period of 22 months (from March 2012 to January 2014).

2.2. Participants. The research was approved by the BMCA Medical Ethics Committee. All participants provided written informed consent after the protocol was carefully explained to them.

Participants included 62 euthyroid Jewish Caucasian adults (50 women, 12 men), aged 21–80. These participants were outpatients attending the endocrine clinic, inpatients,

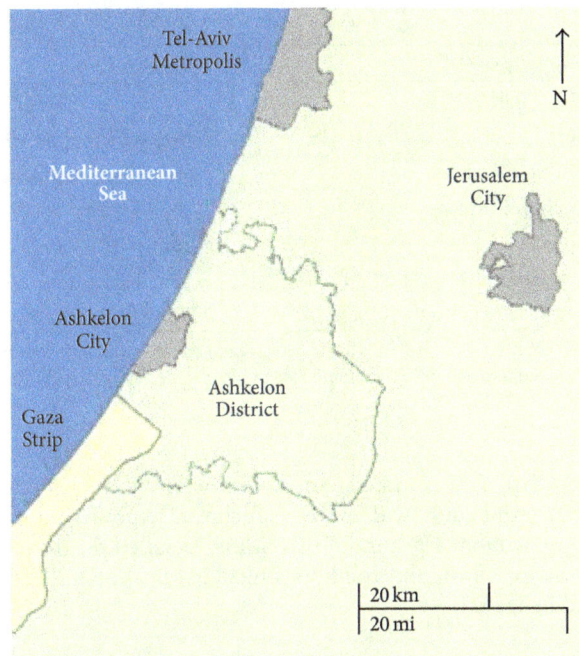

FIGURE 1: Map of Israel southern coastal area, showing Ashkelon District territory and location (reproduced with permission from The Israel Central Bureau of Statistics: http://gis.cbs.gov.il/benyam/).

and five hospital workers at BMCA. Every participant's medical file was carefully screened and all volunteers were interviewed with the aid of structured sociodemographic, health, and habits questionnaires. These questionnaires were based on previously validated governmental materials from the Israeli National Nutrition and Health Survey (MABAT) [16]. A series of multiple-choice and open-ended questions were used to collect information on demographic characteristics that could influence dietary and lifestyle practices. Self-reported health status and knowledge, attitudes, and behaviors regarding nutrition and health were also included in these questionnaires. Only volunteers who did not change their address or iodine intake habits (during the two years prior to initiating this study) were included in this study, as were those with BMI of 18.5–35 (kg/h^2), non-iodine-containing or steroidal drugs consumption, and without any past or current cancer diagnosis nor pregnancy. We also limited the study to those whose first diagnosis of any TD, by both medical file screen and self-reported TD status, took place less than five years prior to the study.

All participants were asked about TD risk factors. These included (a) daily dietary goitrogen exposure and a series of relevant items derived from MABAT [16] and INHIS-2 [9], including (b) previous X-ray examinations involving the jaw or neck area, (c) family history of TD, (d) current smoking habits, and (e) menopause (for women).

The diagnostic criterion for NNG was untreated euthyroid goiter consisting of a single benign nodule or multiple benign nodules. Each nodule was diagnosed as benign according to a fine needle aspiration (FNA) biopsy report. Hypothyroidism was diagnosed when past serum TSH higher

TABLE 1: Diagnostic criteria for thyroid diseases.

Thyroid disease	Diagnostic criteria
Nodular goiter	
Single nodule	Goiter with nodule >5 mm in diameter
Multiple nodules	≥2 nodules >5 mm in diameter
Hypothyroidism	
Overt	Serum TSH > 4 mIU/L, FT4 < 0.8 ng/dL
Subclinical	Serum TSH > 4 mIU/L, FT4 within the normal range*
With Hashimoto thyroiditis	TPOAb > 35 IU/mL with or without nodular goiter (with overt or subclinical hypothyroidism)

*The reference range for FT4 is 0.8 to 1.8 ng/dL; to convert values for FT4 from ng/dL to pmol/L, multiply by 12.87.
ng/dL: nanogram per deciliter; pmol/L: picomoles per liter; mIU/L: milli-international units per liter; FT4: free thyroxine; TPOAb: thyroid peroxidase antibody; TSH: thyrotropin.

than 4 mIU/L was first reported, within five years prior to initiating this study, with overt or subclinical hypothyroidism with or without Hashimoto thyroiditis. Detailed diagnostic criteria for all thyroid conditions included in this study are listed in Table 1.

2.3. Assays. Blood samples were taken from all participants without prior fasting and within 24 hours of the participant's signing the informed consent form. Samples were centrifuged immediately and serum was separated and stored at −20°C; serum values of TSH, FT4, thyroid peroxidase antibody (TPOAb), thyroglobulin antibody (TgAb), and Tg were measured for all participants, using the IMMULITE 2000 analyzer (Immunometric Chemiluminescent Assay (ICLA), Siemens Healthcare Diagnostics, Llanberis, UK; the Tg intra-assay CV 4.8%–6.8%, interassay CV 5.6%–10.0%).

Ranges for normal thyroid tests were TSH: 0.4 to 4 mIU/L; FT4: 0.8 to 1.8 ng/dL, according to the National Academy of Clinical Biochemistry [17]. Values of TPOAb above 35 IU/mL were considered positive [18]. Each volunteer with positive TgAb (>40 IU/mL) [18] was excluded. Serum Tg was detectable and available among all participants. Values of serum Tg above 60 ng/mL were considered abnormally elevated by the Laboratory of Clinical Biochemistry at BMCA.

2.4. Estimated Iodine Intake. The sIFFQ was designed to estimate participants' daily iodine intake during the one-year period prior to the administration of the questionnaire. This sIFFQ outline was adapted and translated from similar validated questionnaires [14, 19] with local modifications by one of the authors (YSO), a trained Registered Dietitian. A group of experts reviewed the sIFFQ instrument. The group included professional dietitians with experience working with in- and outpatients who were knowledgeable concerning the construction of validated questionnaires. The sIFFQ was pilot tested in a representative sample of both in- and outpatients for readability, clarity of instruction, ease of administration, and time needed for completion. It contained questions regarding the average frequency and amounts of 25 selected foods with relatively high iodine content which Israelis generally consume. The interview was conducted by a single RD (YSO) to minimize variability. Food models, measuring tools, and photographs were provided, when necessary, in

order to reduce variation among interviewees. Participants were not informed that the purpose of the interview was to estimate iodine intake. Follow-up phone calls to interviewees were made to clarify information, as, for example, when an interviewee had to check the manufacturer's label for iodine amounts in a dietary supplement. The mean estimated daily dietary intake level was calculated as follows:

$$I = \sum F_i \times Q_i \times C_i, \tag{1}$$

where I is iodine intake, $\sum$ is the amount or number of food items, F is the frequency per day, i represents food items, Q is the quantity or serving size, and C is the iodine content in the food.

The content of iodine in the participants' food was derived from multiple sources: specific food items from the Department of Nutrition at the Ministry of Health (iodine composition investigation in food by Dr. Eli Havivi 1989); fresh water fish from the Agricultural Service of Israel and the Israeli Fish Breeders Association (fresh water fish nutritional composition, 2012); tap drinking water from the Department of Environmental Health, Public Health Service at the Ministry of Health (survey of iodide levels of drinking water in the Ashkelon District by Israeli Drinking Water National Engineer, Mrs. Irit Hen, 2008); and other sources [10, 20–22].

2.5. Statistical Analysis. All statistical analyses were performed with JMP software (Version 7), except for prevalence of elevated serum Tg values for which a Fisher exact test was performed with SAS software (Version 9). A chi-square test was used to compare the prevalence of TD risk factors in the three groups. Age and estimated dietary iodine intake results are expressed as mean ± standard deviation (SD). Comparison of age, mean serum Tg values, and estimated mean dietary iodine intake for the three groups was performed by ANOVA, followed by pairwise comparisons using the Tukey-Kramer HSD method ($\alpha = 0.05$). Data of serum Tg values were log-transformed before analysis in order to stabilize variances. Mean and median of serum Tg were calculated on transformed data.

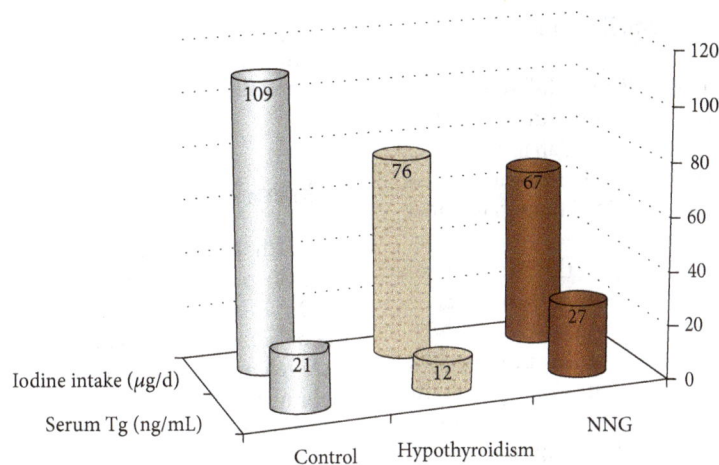

FIGURE 2: Medians of estimated dietary iodine intake and serum Tg by group. Numbers at the top of each column are median values. Tg: thyroglobulin; NNG: nontoxic nodular goiter; ng/mL: nanogram per milliliter; μg/d: microgram per day.

3. Results

The three study groups were similar in age and gender distribution, as well as in socioeconomic status. In addition, the prevalence of known risk factors for TD did not differ significantly between groups.

3.1. Serum Tg Values. A comparison of serum Tg concentrations between groups found a significant difference between the NNG and hypothyroidism groups ($P < 0.05$). The prevalence of elevated serum Tg values (Tg > 60 ng/mL) was significantly higher among the NNG group than in the other groups (29% versus 7% and 0% for hypothyroidism and controls, resp., $P < 0.05$) and the mean Tg concentration among NNG group (35 ng/mL) was significantly higher than in the hypothyroidism group (11 ng/mL).

3.2. Iodine Intake Estimation by the sIFFQ. At $65 \pm 30\,\mu$g/d, the mean estimated iodine intake of the NNG group was 42% lower than that of controls ($115 \pm 60\,\mu$g/d) with intermediate intake among hypothyroid patients (73 ± 38). Comparisons for all pair groups showed that these intakes differed significantly between the NNG group and the control group ($P < 0.05$).

A comparison by group of detailed mean, median, range, and prevalence of elevated serum Tg, as well as estimated iodine intake by sIFFQ, is given in Table 2. Median estimated dietary iodine intake and serum Tg are shown by group in Figure 2.

4. Discussion

In this study, we found a higher prevalence of elevated serum Tg values, as well as lower mean dietary iodine intake among NNG patients as compared with euthyroid controls and hypothyroid patients. Significantly increased serum Tg values among NNG patients compared with the controls have been

TABLE 2: Demographic characteristics, serum Tg values, and estimated dietary iodine intake of the study groups.

Characteristics	Control	Hypothyroidism	NNG
N	31	14	17
Gender (women, men)	25, 6	12, 2	13, 4
Age (years)			
Mean$^\pm$	58 ± 13	54 ± 17	60 ± 10
Range (years)	23–77	21–71	49–80
Serum Tg (ng/mL)			
Mean	17[AB]	11[B]	35[A]
Median	21	12	27
Range	2–59	1–101	2–792
25th–75th percentiles range	12–32	3–43	10–182
n (abnormally elevated values)^{P*}	0 (0%)	1 (7%)	5 (29%)
Estimated dietary iodine intake (μg/d)			
Mean$^\pm$	115 ± 60[B]	73 ± 38[AB]	65 ± 30[A]
Median	109	76	67
Range (μg/d)	27–263	29–165	10–113

$^\pm$Plus-minus values are mean $\pm$ SD.
[AB]Means without a common letter are significantly different (Tukey-Kramer, $\alpha = 0.05$).
n (abnormally elevated values) = number of participants with Tg values above 60 ng/mL.
[P]Prevalence displayed as number of positive cases (percentage in brackets).
*Groups are significantly different (Fisher exact test, $P < 0.05$).
Tg: thyroglobulin; NNG: nontoxic nodular goiter; ng/mL: nanogram per milliliter; μg/d: microgram per day.

reported in a comparable epidemiologic study in a Mediterranean population from Sicily, Italy [23]. As in that study, our present findings show the same general trend of elevated Tg among NNG patients compared to controls; however, our sample size is probably too small to reach statistical significance.

Our present results of a nonsignificant difference in Tg values between the hypothyroidism group and the controls resembled a similar Saudi study, among Jeddah area dwellers [19]. This apparent pattern may indicate that elevated serum Tg values are more closely linked with NNG than to hypothyroidism.

Serum Tg values of the NNG group in the current study (mean, median, and 25th–75th percentiles range: 35, 27, and 10–182 ng/mL) were higher than those of both NNG patients' groups in similar small-scale studies: in the greater area of Thessaloniki, Greece (median, 25th–75th percentiles range: 31, 13–70 ng/mL) [24], and in Sicily (mean, range: 34, 0–111 ng/mL) [23]. Destruction of the thyroid follicles and release of Tg in the circulation within 10–15 days after FNA have been suggested to cause serum Tg elevation [24, 25]. Nevertheless, none of the present studied blood samples was taken during 15 days after FNA. Therefore, the contrast between the low iodine intake in the present study and the habitual consumption of iodized salt and bread in Thessaloniki (personal communication, Athanasios D. Anastasilakis, Department of Endocrinology, 424 Military Hospital, Thessaloniki, 2014) and the iodine sufficiency known for Catania city area, Sicily [23], can explain our relatively higher serum Tg values.

The mean dietary iodine intake among NNG participants ($65 \pm 30 \, \mu g/d$) was estimated as significantly lower than among controls ($115 \pm 60 \, \mu g/d$) and both are much lower than the RDA, which is $150 \, \mu g/d$ [26]. These findings contradict the postulate that because Israel is on the Mediterranean it is an iodine-sufficient country [27]. Moreover, our present findings of low iodine intake among the overall sample and in the NNG group in particular differ from those previously reported about a decade ago by Benbassat et al. [10]. One explanation for this finding can be the increased use of iodine-depleted desalinated water in recent years as the dominant source of drinking water in the Ashkelon District [11]. Another explanation may be related to the fact that, in our study, unlike that of Benbassat et al. [10], we excluded patients who had received a diagnosis of NNG more than five years before study. Such exclusion decreases the likelihood of changes in dietary habits between the diagnosis of incident thyroid disease and the subsequent estimation of habitual dietary iodine intake. The time frame we used is appropriate for the natural history of acquired iodine deficiency disorders such as NNG.

5. Conclusions

The data presented in this study suggest that elevated serum Tg values are more prevalent among NNG adult patients in Ashkelon District, Israel. In addition, long-term low dietary iodine intake, rather than high intake, is associated with NNG among this population. It appears that proximity to a saltwater sea in and of itself cannot protect against ID and NNG. As this study comprises a relatively small sample, it cannot be extrapolated to the entire Israeli population. However, if, as it suggests, iodine intake is deficient in the population, then this must be urgently investigated in larger-scale studies. Such reinforcement may help to prevent TD in the future.

Acknowledgments

The authors are indebted to those who were attending or were hospitalized at BMCA who participated in this study; to Dr. Inbar Zucker from ICDC for her assistance with the background data regarding TD for Israel; to Dr. Hillary Voet from the Department of Agricultural Economics at the Hebrew University for assistance with the initial study design selection and the statistical analysis; and to Mrs. Nirit Nagar from the Department of Internal Medicine "C" at BMCA for assistance with the administration at BMCA.

References

[1] W. Teng, Z. Shan, X. Teng et al., "Effect of iodine intake on thyroid diseases in China," *The New England Journal of Medicine*, vol. 354, no. 26, pp. 2783–2793, 2006.

[2] R. S. Bahn and M. R. Castro, "Approach to the patient with non-toxic multinodular goiter," *The Journal of Clinical Endocrinology & Metabolism*, vol. 96, no. 5, pp. 1202–1212, 2011.

[3] A. Belfiore, G. L. La Rosa, G. Padova, L. Sava, O. Ippolito, and R. Vigneri, "The frequency of cold thyroid nodules and thyroid malignancies in patients from an iodine-deficient area," *Cancer*, vol. 60, no. 12, pp. 3096–3102, 1987.

[4] M. B. Zimmermann, "Iodine deficiency," *Endocrine Reviews*, vol. 30, no. 4, 2009.

[5] M. B. Zimmermann, S. Y. Hess, P. Adou, T. Toresanni, R. Wegmüller, and R. F. Hurrell, "Thyroid size and goiter prevalence after introduction of iodized salt: a 5-y prospective study in schoolchildren in Côte d'Ivoire," *The American Journal of Clinical Nutrition*, vol. 77, no. 3, pp. 663–667, 2003.

[6] M. Michalaki, V. Kyriazopoulou, P. Paraskevopoulou, A. G. Vagenakis, and K. B. Markou, "The odyssey of nontoxic nodular goiter (NTNG) in Greece under suppression therapy, and after improvement of iodine deficiency," *Thyroid*, vol. 18, no. 6, pp. 641–645, 2008.

[7] S. Henjum, I. Barikmo, T. A. Strand, A. Oshaug, and L. E. Torheim, "Iodine-induced goitre and high prevalence of anaemia among Saharawi refugee women," *Public Health Nutrition*, vol. 15, no. 8, pp. 1512–1518, 2012.

[8] "Israel National Health Interview Survey INHIS-1, 2003-2004—Selected Findings," Israel Center for Disease Control, Ministry of Health; 2013.

[9] *Israel National Health Interview Survey INHIS-2, 2007–2010—Selected Findings*, Israel Center for Disease Control, Ministry of Health, 2013.

[10] C. Benbassat, G. Tsvetov, B. Schindel, M. Hod, Y. Blonder, and B. Ami Sela, "Assessment of Iodine intake in the Israel coastal area," *Israel Medical Association Journal*, vol. 6, no. 2, pp. 75–77, 2004.

[11] E. Farkash and N. Eliyahu, "Drain project in eastern South Beach Aquifer restoration—Lahat desalination plant," *Mekorot Ba'Shetach—Southern Region*, vol. 5, no. 1, p. 1, 2010 (Hebrew), http://www.magazine-pro.com/13/45/A/390/Mekorot.

[12] N. Knudsen, I. Bülow, T. Jørgensen, H. Perrild, L. Ovesen, and P. Laurberg, "Serum Tg—a sensitive marker of thyroid abnormalities and iodine deficiency in epidemiological studies," *The Journal of Clinical Endocrinology and Metabolism*, vol. 86, no. 8, pp. 3599–3603, 2001.

[13] M. B. Zimmermann and M. Andersson, "Assessment of iodine nutrition in populations: past, present, and future," *Nutrition Reviews*, vol. 70, no. 10, pp. 553–570, 2012.

[14] L. B. Rasmussen, L. Ovesen, I. Bülow et al., "Evaluation of a semi-quantitative food frequency questionnaire to estimate iodine intake," *European Journal of Clinical Nutrition*, vol. 55, no. 4, pp. 287–292, 2001.

[15] World Health Organization (WHO), United Nations Children's Fund (UNICEF), and International Council for Control of iodine Deficiency Disorders (ICCIDD), *Assessment of the Iodine Deficiency Disorders and Monitoring Their Elimination. A Guide for Program Managers*, Report of Consultation, WHO/NHI/01.1, WHO, Geneva, Switzerland, 2nd edition, 1999.

[16] Israel Center for Disease Control, Ministry of Health, Israel, MABAT: First Israeli National Health and Nutrition Survey 1999–2001, Food & Nutrition Services 2003: Publication 225, http://www.health.gov.il/UnitsOffice/ICDC/mabat/Pages/Mabat1999_2001.aspx.

[17] L. M. Demers and C. A. Spencer, "National Academy of Clinical Biochemistry 2002 Laboratory support for the diagnosis and monitoring of thyroid disease," *Thyroid*, vol. 13, pp. 21–44, 2003.

[18] L. Giovanella, M. Imperiali, A. Ferrari et al., "Serum thyroglobulin reference values according to NACB criteria in healthy subjects with normal thyroid ultrasound," *Clinical Chemistry and Laboratory Medicine*, vol. 50, no. 5, pp. 891–893, 2012.

[19] E. M. Alissa, K. AlShali, and G. A. Ferns, "Iodine deficiency among hypothyroid patients living in Jeddah," *Biological Trace Element Research*, vol. 130, no. 3, pp. 193–203, 2009.

[20] N. Erkan, "Iodine content of cooked and processed fish in Turkey," *International Journal of Food Science & Technology*, vol. 46, no. 8, pp. 1734–1738, 2011.

[21] Centre for Food Safety—Food and Environmental Hygiene Department—The Government of the Hong Kong Special Administrative Region, "Dietary iodine intake in Hong Kong adults," Risk Assessment Studies Report 45, 2011.

[22] Norwegian Food Safety Authority, *The Norwegian Directorate for Health and the University of Oslo. The Iodine Table*, 2012, http://www.matvaretabellen.no/.

[23] V. Pezzino, R. Vigneri, S. Squatrito, S. Filetti, M. Camus, and P. Polosa, "Increased serum thyroglobulin levels in patients with nontoxic goiter," *The Journal of Clinical Endocrinology and Metabolism*, vol. 46, no. 4, pp. 653–657, 1978.

[24] A. D. Anastasilakis, S. A. Polyzos, S. Delaroudis et al., "Long-term effects of thyroid fine-needle biopsy on the thyroid-related biochemical parameters," *International Journal of Clinical Practice*, vol. 66, no. 6, pp. 602–609, 2012.

[25] R. Luboshitzky, I. Lavi, and A. Ishay, "Serum thyroglobulin levels after fine-needle aspiration of thyroid nodules," *Endocrine Practice*, vol. 12, no. 3, pp. 264–269, 2006.

[26] Standing Committee on the Scientific Evaluation of Dietary Reference Intakes and Institute of Health; The United States of America, *Iodine*, National Academy Press, 2001.

[27] Y. Zohar, "Endemic goiter in a non-goitrogenic country," *Harefuah*, vol. 127, no. 3-4, pp. 75–78, 1994 (Hebrew).

29

Challenges Associated with Tyrosine Kinase Inhibitor Therapy for Metastatic Thyroid Cancer

Maria E. Cabanillas,[1] Mimi I. Hu,[1] Jean-Bernard Durand,[2] and Naifa L. Busaidy[1]

[1] *Department of Endocrine Neoplasia and Hormonal Disorders, The University of Texas MD Anderson Cancer Center, Houston, TX 77030, USA*
[2] *Department of Cardiology, The University of Texas MD Anderson Cancer Center, Houston, TX 77030, USA*

Correspondence should be addressed to Maria E. Cabanillas, mcabani@mdanderson.org

Academic Editor: Maria João M. Bugalho

Tyrosine kinase inhibitors (TKIs) which target angiogenesis are promising treatments for patients with metastatic medullary and differentiated thyroid cancers. Sorafenib, sunitinib, and pazopanib are commercially available drugs which have been studied in these diseases. Vandetanib is the first drug approved in the United States for treatment of medullary thyroid cancer. These TKIs are used as chronic therapies, and therefore it is imperative to understand the adverse event profile in order to avoid excessive toxicity and maintain patients on therapy as long as it proves beneficial. Here we review common toxicities, management of these, and other challenging situations that arise when using TKIs in patients with thyroid cancer.

1. Introduction

Thyroid cancer is now the 5th most commonly diagnosed cancer in women and 9th in overall incidence in the United States; however, fewer than 2000 people die per year of their disease and mortality rates have remained fairly stable for the past several decades [1]. The most common form of thyroid cancer, differentiated thyroid cancer (DTC), is derived from the follicular cells of the thyroid, and it includes papillary and follicular thyroid cancers. While most patients are cured or have indolent disease, a small percentage develop metastases that no longer respond to treatment with radioactive iodine or TSH suppressive therapy. Medullary thyroid cancer (MTC) accounts for only about 2-3% of thyroid cancers and is derived from the neuroendocrine "C" cells of the thyroid gland. The only treatment with curative intent for medullary thyroid carcinoma is complete surgical resection.

Therapy with tyrosine kinase inhibitors (TKIs) has only recently been studied in thyroid cancer. The discovery that BRAF (in papillary and anaplastic thyroid cancers) and RET (in MTC) mutations, as well as angiogenesis, play a significant role in tumorigenesis in DTC and MTC led to

several clinical trials over the past decade with multikinase inhibitors. For purposes of this paper, TKIs refer to small molecule drugs, which target multiple pathways, including, but are not limited to, vascular endothelial growth factor receptor (VEGFR). Sorafenib, sunitinib, and pazopanib are three commercially available TKIs which have shown favorable results in phase II trials in DTC [2–4]. Although these small trials have reported favorable responses, at this time, there are no published results of large phase III trials in DTC. Favorable results of a phase III, randomization study of vandetanib versus placebo in MTC have been reported [5]; however, it is important to note that patients on this study were not required to have progressive disease prior to study entry. Vandetanib was recently approved by the Food and Drug Administration for symptomatic or progressive MTC, establishing it as the first drug to be approved for this disease. The drug is available only through the Vandetanib Risk Evaluation and Mitigation Strategy (REMS) Program due to the prolongation of the QT interval and reported cases of torsades de pointes and sudden death in clinical trials. Sorafenib has also been studied in MTC in a phase II trial [6], and encouraging results of sunitinib in MTC have been presented at a national meeting [7].

TABLE 1: Major adverse events associated with commercially available TKIs which have been studied in thyroid cancer.

Adverse event	Sorafenib (%)		Sunitinib (%)		Pazopanib (%)		Vandetanib (%)	
	All-grade	≥grade 3	All-grade	≥grade 3	All-grade	≥grade 3	All-grade	≥grade 3
Hypertension	17	4	30	12	40	4	33	9
CHF or LVEF decline	1.7	NR	13	3	<1%	NR	<1	NR
Proteinuria	NR	NR	NR	NR	9	<1	10	0
Hand-foot skin reaction	30	6	29	6	6	NR	NR	NR
Stomatitis	NR	NR	30	1	4	NR	NR	NR
Anorexia	16	<1	34	2	22	2	21	4
Weight loss	10	<1	12	<1	52	3.5	10	1
Diarrhea	43	2	61	9	52	3.5	57	11
AST elevation	NR	NR	56	2	53	7.5	NR	NR
ALT elevation	NR	NR	51	2.5	53	12	51	2
Fatigue	37	5	54	11	19	2	24	6
Hypothyroidism	NR	NR	14	2	7	NR	NR	NR
Arterial thromboembolism	2.9	NR	NR	NR	3	2	NR	NR
Hemorrhage/bleeding (all sites)	15	3	30	3	13	2	NR	NR

CHF: congestive heart failure; LVEF: left ventricular ejection fraction; AST: aspartate aminotransferase; ALT: alanine aminotransferase; NR: not reported.
Data extracted from the phase 3 trials or from the prescribing drug reference information [9, 28–30].
Table is adapted from [31].

There are many challenges posed by the use of TKIs, which we believe should be used with caution and reserved for patients with either advanced, progressive disease or bulky disease which may compromise organ function. This review focuses on highlighting the most common and problematic adverse events associated with TKIs with suggestions for management. Other dilemmas that often arise with use of these drugs will be described as well.

2. Adverse Event Management

Although TKIs are generally better tolerated than cytotoxic chemotherapy, many patients develop side effects from on-target and off-target effects which require aggressive management in order to maintain patient compliance, optimize therapy, and avoid potentially life-threatening consequences. Since many patients require long-term use of TKIs for continued control of disease, it is imperative for the treating clinician to be familiar with the potential side effects of these drugs. The most frequent side effects of TKIs are hypertension, dermatologic effects, fatigue, and diarrhea. In addition, the risk of bleeding and liver toxicity may be fatal. The clinician should conduct thorough physical and laboratory examinations prior to considering therapy with these drugs to identify the most appropriate choice of treatment and must monitor and treat adverse events during therapy. Treatment of all comorbid conditions should be optimized and drug-drug interaction, antifungals, antiemetics, and class III antiarrhythmic agents avoided to prevent interactions with TKIs. In this section we will discuss the most common and potentially fatal side effects of TKIs with management recommendations.

Table 1 lists adverse events of the commercially available TKIs relevant to thyroid cancer, their incidence, and grades (data extracted from phase III trials in renal cell carcinoma and package inserts) using Common Terminology Criteria for Adverse Events version 3.0 (CTCAE v3.0). The CTCAE is a list of descriptive terminology utilized for adverse event grading and reporting on clinical trials and is made available through the CTEP website at http://ctep.cancer.gov/proto-coldevelopment/electronic_applications/docs/ctcaev3.pdf.

2.1. Drug-Drug Interactions. Cytochrome P450 enzymes, expressed primarily in the liver, play a primary role in the metabolism of many drugs. Sunitinib, sorafenib, pazopanib, and vandetanib are all metabolized by cytochrome P450 3A4 (CYP3A4). Of the four drugs, sorafenib appears to be the least susceptible to CYP3A4 inducers or inhibitors, although the package labeling warns against concomitant use of CYP3A4 inducers [8]. Concomitant use of CYP3A4 inducers may decrease the plasma concentration of the TKI, resulting in decreased efficacy, while inhibitors may increase the plasma concentration, resulting in toxicity. Itraconazole, a potent inhibitor of CYP3A4, does not appear to affect the metabolism of vandetanib [9]. Table 2 lists the more common, clinically significant drugs metabolized via the CYP3A4 enzyme system.

The medical history should include a thorough review of medications which may affect the metabolism of the TKI. Concomitant drugs which are metabolized via CYP3A4 should be avoided or substituted for another drug. If a CYP3A4 inhibitor drug cannot be eliminated, a dose reduction in the TKI should be considered. Patients should also be monitored for increasing side effects if a CYP3A4 inhibitor is coadministered.

2.2. Cardiovascular. Hypertension is the most common cardiovascular side effect associated with antiangiogenic drugs.

TABLE 2: Clinically significant CYP3A4 inducers, inhibitors, and substrates.

CYP3A4 inducers	CYP3A4 inhibitors	CYP3A4 substrates
Dexamethasone	Calcium channel blockers: amiodarone, verapamil	Statins: atorvastatin, lovastatin, and simvastatin (not pravastatin) (not rosuvastatin)
Anticonvulsants: phenytoin, carbamazepine	Azole antifungals: itraconazole, voriconazole, and ketoconazole	Calcium channel blockers: amlodipine, diltiazem, felodipine, nifedipine, and verapamil
Phenobarbital		
Rifampin	Macrolide antibiotics: erythromycin, and clarithromycin (not azithromycin)	
St. John's wort		
HIV antivirals: nonnucleoside reverse transcriptase inhibitors: efavirenz, and nevirapine	HIV antivirals: protease inhibitors: indinavir, nelfinavir, and ritonavir	
Pioglitazone		

The mechanism of hypertension is not well understood, but it has been suggested that it is due to increased fluid retention, endothelial dysfunction, nitrous oxide inhibition, rarefaction [10], reduction of vascular surface area, and increase in peripheral vascular resistance caused by inhibition of angiogenesis [11–14]. A recent study by Rini et al. suggests that the rise in blood pressure above 140/90 may be a biomarker for anticancer therapy and was associated with significant survival benefit even with treatment of antihypertensives. The use of antihypertensives did not reduce the efficacy of sunitinib in metastatic renal cell carcinoma [15].

The onset of hypertension is variable. Blood pressure may begin to rise within days of therapy prior to steady state or the onset of the therapies' biological effects or may be more indolent. There are no clear guidelines for managing TKI-induced hypertension. It is our clinical practice to use ACE inhibitors, angiotensin receptor blockers (ARBs) or a beta blocker as first-line therapy for hypertension since these drugs are not metabolized via the CYP3A4 enzyme system. However, the choice of an antihypertensive should be individualized. The Angiogenesis Task Force of the National Cancer Institute Investigational Drug Steering Committee recently published guidelines for management of hypertension with TKIs [16]. Hypertension should be controlled based on compelling and noncompelling indications to a goal of <140/90 prior to starting TKIs. Once a TKI is initiated, patients should have the blood pressure monitored within 1 week. Blood pressure monitoring at home may be more effective at prediction of outcomes from cardiovascular disease than clinic blood pressure monitoring [17]. If the blood pressure is above goal, antihypertensive therapy should be initiated or adjusted. Patients should continue to check their blood pressure daily (with brachial blood pressure device) and report results on a weekly basis (until adequate blood pressure control is achieved), and antihypertensive drugs should be rapidly titrated or new drugs added to the regimen. Once control of blood pressure is obtained, the blood pressure should be monitored on a monthly basis. Interruption or dose reduction of the TKI

may be necessary in order to achieve adequate blood pressure control. Some calcium-channel blockers, such as felodipine, diltiazem, nifedipine, and verapamil, are CYP3A4 substrates or inhibitors and should be avoided.

Sunitinib and pazopanib can lead to QT interval prolongation; therefore, they should be used with caution in patients with a history of QT prolongation and patients taking antiarrhythmic drugs. Torsade de pointes was seen in <0.1% of patients exposed to sunitinib and <2% of patients treated with pazopanib. Vandetanib carries a black box warning due to QT interval prolongation, Torsade de pointes, and sudden death observed in clinical trials involving patients with a broad variety of solid malignancies. Serial monitoring of electrocardiograms and electrolytes is mandated and electrolyte abnormalities should be corrected [9, 18, 19]. In a phase III trial that examined the efficacy and safety of vandetanib 300 mg in the treatment of unresectable locally advanced or metastatic MTC, QT prolongation was reported in 14% of patients randomized to vandetanib and in 1% of patients randomized to placebo, with 8% (18/231) and 1% (1/99), respectively, being ≥grade 3 events. Vandetanib should not be given to patients who have a history of Torsades de pointes, congenital long QT syndrome, bradyarrhythmias, or uncompensated heart failure. Vandetanib should not be started in patients whose corrected QT interval (QTcF, Fridericia formula) is greater than 450 ms. Specific guidelines for monitoring of QT abnormalities and electrolytes in patients taking vandetanib are specified in the package insert [9]. In addition, use of concomitant drugs known to prolong the QT interval, such as amiodarone and erythromycin, should be avoided.

A less common but serious adverse event associated with TKIs is systolic and diastolic congestive heart failure. It appears to be more common with sunitinib but has been reported with sorafenib and pazopanib. Patients may present with very dramatic symptoms of heart failure, while others demonstrate mild symptoms which may be difficult to differentiate from fatigue due to the TKI or the tumor itself [20]. Cardiac toxicity, although not always completely reversible, is often a manageable condition if patients have careful monitoring and treatment with routine heart failure therapies with beta blockers and ACE inhibitors/ARB as recommended by the guidelines of heart failure management by the American College of Cardiology. The etiology of the heart failure is thought to be due to direct reversible cardiomyocyte toxicity, possibly exacerbated by hypertension which may progress to irreversible, progressive injury if not treated with standard heart failure therapy [21]. This toxicity is not completely understood, but platelet-derived growth factor receptor-β (PDGFR-β) inhibition has been implicated as playing a role in the response to pressure-overload-induced stress [22]. We recommend that all patients initiating TKIs have a baseline echocardiogram and periodic monitoring while they are on therapy. Furthermore, aggressive management of hypertension may help reduce cardiomyocyte damage.

Case Number 1. A 69-year-old woman with a history of hypertension and premature ventricular contractions was referred to our center. She had a history of T4a, N0, M0, stage IVA papillary thyroid cancer for 10 years prior. The patient's thyroid cancer was initially managed with total thyroidectomy and radioactive iodine ablation, but she developed local recurrence and pulmonary metastases several years later. She continued to have progressive disease in the lungs and neck and was referred to our center. The patient was enrolled into a phase II clinical trial with an investigational TKI targeting VEGFRs, PDGFR, and others. The patient's blood pressure was normal prior to initiation of the investigational TKI, but one week later she developed grade 2 hypertension which was difficult to control despite treatment with multiple antihypertensive agents. Her pretreatment echocardiogram demonstrated an ejection fraction of 55–60%. Nearly 4 months after starting on the investigational agent, she underwent adenosine stress test which identified a 30% ejection fraction with hypokinesia in the anterior septal segments which partially reversed with rest. Because of the presence of a left bundle branch block at baseline, definitive diagnosis of ischemia was not possible from the images. Carvedilol was initiated, and the investigational TKI was held. Echocardiogram confirmed the low ejection fraction. A cardiac catheterization with myocardial biopsy was performed. She was found to have mild ischemic heart disease (defined as less than 50% stenosis in any coronary) which was disproportionate to her degree of heart failure, and therefore the heart failure was attributed to the TKI. Direct cardiomyocyte toxicity was confirmed with the biopsy, demonstrating hypertrophy and interstitial edema, increased lipid droplets, and dilatation of sarcotubular elements (Figure 1). Since the biopsy showed no myocyte death (indicating reversibility) and the echocardiogram showed a return to baseline, after 3 weeks, the investigational agent was reintroduced at a reduced dose. Two months later she was found to have progression of disease, and the investigational agent was discontinued permanently.

2.3. Renal. Proteinuria associated with antiangiogenic therapies was first described with bevacizumab, a monoclonal

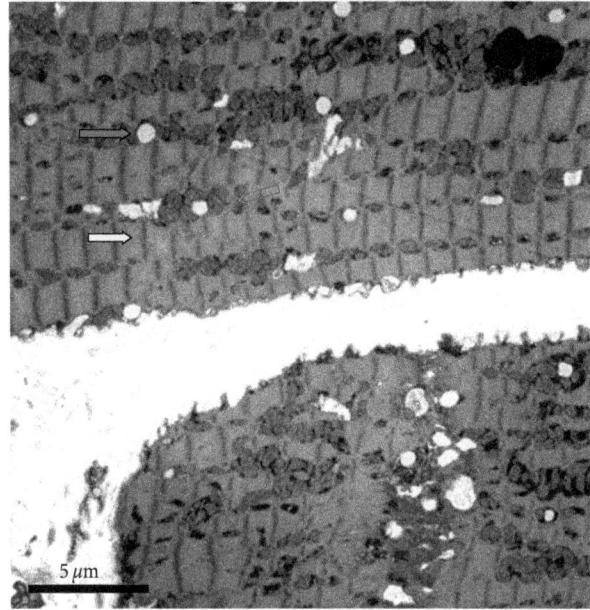

FIGURE 1: Transmission electron micrographs of endomyocardial biopsy from patient with systolic heart failure treated with a TKI. Section shows hypertrophy and interstitial edema with edematous mitochondria (open red arrow), with increased lipid droplets (solid red arrow) and dilatation of sarcotubular elements (yellow arrow). These findings are consistent with acute but reversible injury.

antibody against VEGF [23]. Small-molecule tyrosine kinase inhibitors, which inhibit VEGF-R, lead to proteinuria as well [24]. Thrombotic microangiopathy and acute interstitial nephritis have been reported with sorafenib and sunitinib [25, 26]. The glomerular podocytes express VEGF, and glomerular endothelial cells express VEGF receptors. Thus, a proposed mechanism of proteinuria is that deletion of VEGF allele in podocytes or inhibited VEGF signaling leads to proteinuria and capillary endotheliosis [27].

All patients who will receive antiangiogenic therapies should have a baseline urinalysis and protein to creatinine ratio, with routine monitoring for development of proteinuria while on treatment. A urine protein to creatinine ratio of ≥ 1 or 24-hour urine with ≥ 1 gram/dL/24 hours of protein should prompt intervention. The decision to hold drug should be considered on a case-by-case basis. Treatment with an ACE inhibitor or ARB should be initiated and consultation with nephrology may be warranted. As proteinuria is a class effect of antiangiogenic treatments, changing from one agent to another may not prevent this effect in a patient.

2.4. Dermatologic. Dermatologic reactions observed with TKIs include hand-foot syndrome (HFS), skin induration or callous formation, rash, alopecia, hair texture and color changes, and skin discoloration. HFS, the most common and potentially most debilitating dermatologic effect, presents as desquamating lesions in a palmoplantar distribution typically at pressure points or areas of friction or trauma. The lesions can significantly affect a patient's quality of life, thus

TABLE 3: Suggested dose modification for skin toxicity for sorafenib [8].

Skin toxicity grade	Occurrence	Suggested dose modification
Grade 1: numbness, dysesthesia, paresthesia, tingling, painless swelling, erythema or discomfort of the hands or feet which does not disrupt the patient's normal activities	Any occurrence	Continue sorafenib and consider topical therapy for symptomatic relief
Grade 2: Painful erythema and swelling of the hands or feet and/or discomfort affecting the patient's normal activities	1st occurrence	Continue sorafenib and consider topical therapy for symptomatic relief. If no improvement within 7 days, see below
	No improvement within 7 days or 2nd or 3rd occurrence	Interrupt sorafenib until toxicity resolves to grade 0-1. When resuming treatment, decrease sorafenib dose by one dose level (400 mg daily or 400 mg every other day)
	4th occurrence	Discontinue sorafenib treatment
Grade 3: Moist desquamation, ulceration, blistering or severe pain of the hands or feet, or severe discomfort that causes the patient to be unable to work or perform activities of daily living	1st or 2nd occurrence	Interrupt sorafenib until toxicity resolves to grade 0-1. When resuming treatment, decrease sorafenib dose by one dose level (400 mg daily or 400 mg every other day)
	3rd occurrence	Discontinue sorafenib treatment

necessitating drug discontinuation or dose reduction. The pathogenesis of HFS is not entirely clear. Preventive application of hand and foot lubricants should be implemented at time of drug initiation. The package insert for sorafenib gives clear recommendations on dose modifications and holds for skin toxicity (Table 3). It has been the authors' experience with sorafenib that when patients develop grade ≥3 HFS, drug interruption until skin toxicity declines to grade ≤1 with reinitiation at 200 mg daily, and titration by 200 mg every 3–5 days can prevent further escalation of skin toxicity (unpublished data). Stevens-Johnson syndrome, characterized by a prodrome of malaise and fever, followed by rapid development of erythematous or purpuric macules, which can progress to epidermal necrosis or sloughing, has been reported with vandetanib. A patient with these signs and/or symptoms should discontinue drug therapy immediately and seek medical attention, as this could be a life-threatening adverse effect.

Skin induration and callous formation can lead to pain at pressure points and limit mobility. Referral to podiatry can be considered to reduce callous size. Skin evaluation for development of actinic keratoses or keratoacanthoma-type squamous cell carcinomas (KA-SCC) should be performed regularly while being treated with sorafenib and BRAF inhibitors, as these lesions have been described primarily with targeted therapy against Raf kinase or mutant BRAF [32–35]. These lesions can develop as solitary or multiple lesions, weeks to months after starting drug therapy, and do not need to be confined to sun-exposed areas. Fortunately, KA-SCC has not been reported to metastasize, and spontaneous regression has been reported [32]. KA-SCCs should be completely excised. It has not been uniformly recommended that drug discontinuation occur when KA-SCCs develop due to the low metastatic potential; however, patients should be made aware of this effect and maintain routine skin evaluations.

2.5. Gastrointestinal System. Diarrhea, nausea, mucositis, stomatitis, dysgeusia, anorexia, abdominal discomfort, and weight loss may develop with the use of these drugs. Reduced side effects may occur if medication is taken with a large meal and water, if appropriate for administration per package insert. Appropriate use of supportive therapies with antidiarrheal or antiemetic medications may prevent the need for dose reduction or discontinuation. In the case of severe, unresponsive gastrointestinal effects, drug discontinuation should be implemented and reinitiated at a reduced dose once symptoms resolve to baseline or grade 1 level. Gastrointestinal perforation or fistula development is a rare, but potentially life-threatening, adverse event reported with TKIs. Risk factors include underlying tumor at perforation, diverticulitis, bowel obstruction, recent sigmoidoscopy or colonoscopy, and historical abdominal/pelvic irradiation [36]. Drug discontinuation is warranted if perforation event occurs. Consideration for a different TKI will need to be done with caution.

Hepatic toxicity or abnormalities, demonstrated by elevations in aspartate aminotransferase (AST) and alanine aminotransferase (ALT) and bilirubin, can occur. Elevations in AST or ALT were the most common metabolic abnormality requiring treatment seen in the phase III trial of pazopanib in renal cell carcinoma [28]. Although isolated elevations of total bilirubin were also seen at a similar frequency, concurrent elevations of ALT and total bilirubin were rare. The presence of a polymorphism in the uridine diphosphate glucuronosyltransferase 1A1 (UGT1A1) gene, which predisposes to Gilbert's syndrome, leads to reduced enzymatic activity necessary for the conjugation of bilirubin allowing it to be excreted in bile. Xu et al. reported that the presence of a polymorphism in UGT1A1 was significantly associated with pazopanib-induced hyperbilirubinemia, indicating that isolated unconjugated hyperbilirubinemia was a benign finding associated with Gilbert's syndrome, which did not require discontinuation of drug therapy [37]. Conjugated hyperbilirubinemia would require further investgation. None of the genetic markers evaluated in this study were associated with hepatic transaminase elevation, thus leaving the etiology still to be determined.

TKIs can lead to asymptomatic increases in pancreatic enzymes or rarely acute pancreatitis, most commonly reported with sorafenib and pazopanib. Standard treatment for pancreatitis and evaluation with endoscopic ultrasonography and other diagnostic testings for underlying causes of pancreatitis should be implemented. However, radiologic evidence of pancreatic damage or pancreatitis often is not found. Thus, dose-limiting toxicity for pancreatic enzyme elevation should be applied to grade 4 levels associated with clinical findings of pancreatitis, or if considered to be life threatening [38]. The cause of elevation in amylase and lipase is unclear, although some have attributed it to pancreatic ischemia from antiangiogenesis or to other drug-related effects.

2.6. Hematologic.
Mucosal bleeding (e.g., epistaxis) to hemorrhage (i.e., gastrointestinal, pulmonary, cerebral, vaginal) has been reported with TKIs. Although mild mucosal bleeding could be attributed to inhibition of VEGFR-2 causing microvascular leaks from endothelial cell damage, clinically more severe hemorrhage is attributed to tumoral invasion of large vessels or other concurrent pathological conditions [36]. Additionally, thrombosis has been identified with TKI use. Inhibition of VEGF signaling could lead to overproduction of erythropoietin in the liver, which increases hematocrit and blood viscosity [39, 40]. Additionally, as wound healing is dependent upon angiogenesis, VEGF-inhibitors can impair or delay wound healing after surgery or other invasive procedures. Thus, drug should be withheld before and after surgery to optimize wound healing [36].

Hematologic laboratory abnormalities with neutropenia, lymphopenia, and thrombocytopenia are associated with TKIs. In contrast, anemia occurs less frequently, which may be explained by the relative increased erythrocytosis seen with this class of drugs. As patients with differentiated thyroid carcinoma may have received large cumulative doses of radioactive iodine and thyroid cancer patients may have received external beam radiation therapy, myelosuppression may be present prior to TKI initiation. Thus, routine monitoring of complete blood count and differential is required while on therapy.

2.7. Miscellaneous.
Hypothyroidism or rising thyroid stimulating hormone (TSH), requiring increasing the thyroid hormone replacement doses, is seen as a class effect. Suggested etiologies have been poor absorption of levothyroxine from concomitant treatment-related diarrhea, or in patients with intact thyroid glands, regression of thyroid capillaries, or inhibition of thyroid peroxidase [36, 41]. Thyroid function should be monitored routinely while on TKI treatment to maintain a suppressed TSH in patients with DTC and a normal TSH in MTC patients.

Fatigue is a pervasive and often difficult-to-manage problem in cancer patients and may be related to many factors, in addition to direct toxicity of targeted drug therapy. Investigation for causes (e.g., anemia, hypothyroidism, cardiac dysfunction, renal dysfunction) should be performed. Supportive care with adequate nutrition, exercise, and stress reducing techniques is encouraged.

3. Recommendations for Dose Modifications or Discontinuation of TKIs due to Intolerance

Nonhematologic Adverse Events (AEs). Patients with tolerable grade 1-2 nonhematologic AEs may continue TKI therapy while treatment for the AE is being optimized. For example, grade 1–3 hypertension does not necessarily require a dose modification or drug hold if the patient can be managed with antihypertensive agents. On the other hand, adverse events such as grade 1-2 skin rash, which have minimally effective treatments and/or are distressful or embarrassing to patients, may require drug interruptions. Although the package insert for sorafenib describes dose modification recommendation for cutaneous toxicity [8] (Table 3), others do not have clearly defined dose modifications for this toxicity. Recurrent grade 2 AEs require drug hold and often dose reduction if they are possibly related to the TKI and not responding to optimal supportive therapy. However, since TKIs are often chronic treatments for patients with thyroid cancer, the decision to hold and reduce the dose is often dictated in part by the patient's quality of life and physician judgment. Most grade 3 toxicities will require a drug hold until the AE improves significantly with resumption of the TKI at a reduced dose. However, grade 3 toxicities which can be readily managed (such as correction of hypokalemia arising from diarrhea which can be controlled) do not require a drug hold. Second occurrence of grade 3 toxicity should be managed again with drug hold and reduction of the dose. Third occurrences which cannot be effectively managed often require discontinuation of the TKI. Grade 4 AEs are life-threatening events, and if related to the TKI, require discontinuation of drug. However, in some select cases, it may be appropriate to resume treatment after reduction of the dose by two dose levels and if other interventions are implemented to prevent recurrence of the event. Thus, the decision to resume drug in patients with manageable grade 4 AEs, even when drug related, must be individualized and the benefit/risk ratio should be considered. Careful review of concomitant medications and herbal remedies which may cause increases in the drug levels of the TKI should also be given consideration.

Hematologic Adverse Events. Grade 2 hematologic toxicities do not require dose reduction. Grade 3-4 neutropenia and thrombocytopenia and grade 4 anemia require dose reductions upon first and second occurrences. Grade 3 and 4 hematologic toxicities are rare in thyroid cancer patients receiving TKIs; thus, other causes such as myelodysplasia should be ruled out.

Intolerance to TKIs. The definition of intolerance, proposed by Jabbour et al. in the context of leukemia, is met if the patient has one or more criterion as delineated in the manuscript [19]. We propose the following modified criteria as a definition of TKI intolerance: presence of one or more of the following criteria: (i) any grade 3-4 non-hematologic toxicity related to TKI therapy that has recurred despite dose reduction and optimal symptomatic measures, (ii) any grade 2 non-hematologic, intolerable toxicity, related to TKI therapy, that persists for more than a month despite optimal supportive measures, or (iii) grade 3-4 hematologic toxicity, related to TKI therapy, that is unresponsive to supportive measures and would require dose reductions below the accepted minimal effective dose, (iv) any life-threatening grade 4 non-hematological toxicity related to TKI therapy.

4. Variable Responses in Different Tissues

Case Number 2. A 54-year-old man with a history of stage IV papillary thyroid carcinoma was seen at our institution. He developed progressive disease that was noted to be nonavid to radioactive iodine. He was initiated on a clinical trial investigating a TKI in metastatic progressive thyroid carcinoma. He developed an excellent response (48% decrease in target lesion by RECIST), but his spinal bone metastasis continued to progress and became symptomatic (Figures 2(a) and 2(b)). His TKI therapy was held, and his progressive bone lesion was treated with external beam radiation. Due to overall favorable response in soft tissues, the TKI was restarted. The patient is still on therapy 24 months later with stabilization of disease in his bone and soft tissue lesions.

This case illustrates two points. First, tumor regression in response to TKI therapy can occur in some organs but not in other areas in the same patient. Additionally, TKI therapy can be continued in a patient with differential responses in various organs provided that local therapy is initiated for the region of progressive disease. This case is not unique; this scenario of varying responses to therapy in different organs is often encountered in metastatic thyroid cancer patients treated with TKI therapy. For example, lung metastases respond more favorably to sorafenib and sunitinib than do bone or pleura [42]. It has been noted that TKIs may lead to varying responses in different tissue sites in other cancers as well [43] and that continuation of systemic therapy after appropriate local therapy could be beneficial [44]. This differential response may not be unique to TKIs [45]. The pathophysiologic mechanism behind this variable response is not well elucidated. Some theories include host, tumor, and stroma factors. Resistance to TKI therapy has proven mechanisms in tumor and stroma as well. Some postulated theories include varying hepatocyte growth factor (HGF), VEGF receptors or serum levels, decreased drug bioavailability in certain organs, and organ-specific tumor resistance.

Until mechanisms are better elucidated to direct therapy for organ-specific TKI selection, consideration should be given to local therapies for areas of progressive disease. Clinically, one should consider irradiating bone lesions

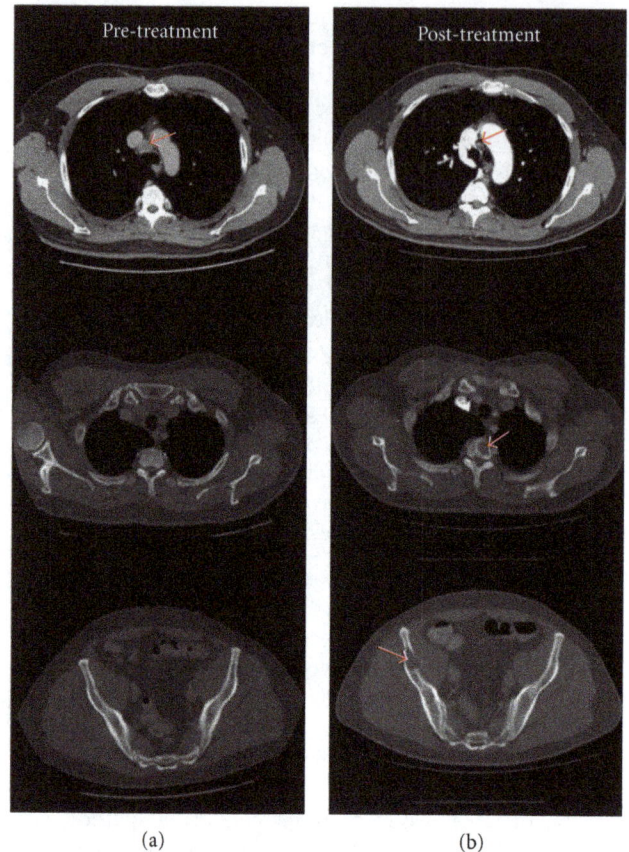

(a)   (b)

FIGURE 2: Patient with partial response in lymph nodes but progression in bone. CT scans before (a) and after (b) 6 months of therapy with a TKI. The patient had a partial response in mediastinal and hilar adenopathy but progression in bone with cortical destruction. The patient's bone lesions were irradiated, and he was restarted on the TKI. The patient continues on the TKI after 24 months and has no further evidence of progression.

(especially if symptomatic) if they progress on TKI therapy. If a bone lesion is threatening vital structures (i.e., the spinal cord), consideration should be given to treating the bone lesion prior to TKI therapy. This may avoid a drug hold later and further compromise of vital structures. In general, the TKI is held during radiation therapy, although there are upcoming trials that may inform us differently. Bony metastatic lesion may also be treated with bisphosphonates or denosumab. This may decrease pain in the bony lesions or may decrease rate of progression, although trials are needed to determine efficacy of these therapies and frequency of dosing.

5. Sequential Use of TKIs

The former belief that if a patient has progressed through one TKI, he/she will fail with another TKI is false and outdated. Due to the many overlapping targets it was assumed that there would be complete cross-resistance. There is increasing evidence that with sequential application of these drugs, a patient who had progressive disease with one TKI may still respond to the next one. In a cohort of metastatic renal cell carcinoma treated with sunitinib after progression through sorafenib, the response rate (or efficacy) seen with second-line sunitinib after sorafenib was similar to that of first line sunitinib [46]. Investigations are under way to determine the best order for sequential TKI and other targeted therapies.

6. Summary

Drug development in oncology has led to several new targeted agents which have demonstrated efficacy in progressive thyroid cancer. Although it was initially thought that these drugs would prove to be less toxic than cytotoxic chemotherapy, the fact that these drugs have many off-target effects and the likelihood that most patients will be treated chronically beg the need for further research to better understand the cause of these toxicities and their optimal management. It also underscores the importance of appropriate patient selection.

Patients and physicians must understand the possible adverse effects and weigh the advantages versus the risks of these drugs. Alternatives to systemic therapy for localized disease, such as external beam radiation or embolization should be considered when appropriate. Until prolongation of overall survival can be demonstrated with the use of the drugs, physicians should exercise caution in the selection of patients to undergo therapy with a TKI.

Finally, more optimal drug selection should be personalized for the individual patient and tumor. Further research is needed to determine the ideal targeted therapy for an individual based on the molecular characterization of the tumor, stroma, and host factors. Future targeted therapy development may require that the on-target and off-target effects may be reengineered to enhance antiangiogenesis pathways and avoid cardiovascular, renal, and dermatologic pathways [47].

Acknowledgments

The authors would like to acknowledge Dr. Steven I. Sherman for his assistance with this manuscript.

Disclosures

M. E. Cabanillas, M. I. Hu, and J. B. Durand have no conflicts to disclose. N. L. Busaidy has received research support from Bayer.

References

[1] American Cancer Society, *Cancer Facts and Figures*, American Cancer Society, 2010.

[2] K. C. Bible, V. J. Suman, J. R. Molina et al., "Efficacy of pazopanib in progressive, radioiodine-refractory, metastatic differentiated thyroid cancers: results of a phase 2 consortium study," *The Lancet Oncology*, vol. 11, no. 10, pp. 962–972, 2010.

[3] L. L. Carr, D. A. Mankoff, B. H. Goulart et al., "Phase II study of daily sunitinib in FDG-PET-positive, iodine-refractory differentiated thyroid cancer and metastatic medullary carcinoma of the thyroid with functional imaging correlation," *Clinical Cancer Research*, vol. 16, no. 21, pp. 5260–5268, 2010.

[4] R. T. Kloos, M. D. Ringel, M. V. Knopp et al., "Phase II trial of sorafenib in metastatic thyroid cancer," *Journal of Clinical Oncology*, vol. 27, no. 10, pp. 1675–1684, 2009.

[5] S. A. Wells, B. G. Robinson, R. F. Gagel et al., "Vandetanib (VAN) in locally advanced or metastatic medullary thyroid cancer (MTC): a randomized, double-blind phase III trial (ZETA)," *Journal of Clinical Oncology*, vol. 28, supplement, 2010.

[6] E. T. Lam, M. D. Ringel, R. T. Kloos et al., "Phase II clinical trial of sorafenib in metastatic medullary thyroid cancer," *Journal of Clinical Oncology*, vol. 28, no. 14, pp. 2323–2330, 2010.

[7] J. A. De Souza, N. Busaidy, A. Zimrin et al., "Phase II trial of sunitinib in medullary thyroid cancer (MTC)," *Journal of Clinical Oncology*, vol. 28, supplement, 2010.

[8] Package insert sorafenib (Nexavar). In: Bayer HealthCare and Onyx Pharmaceuticals.

[9] Package insert vandetanib (Vandetanib). In: AstraZeneca Pharmaceuticals.

[10] R. J. Johnson, S. D. Kivlighn, Y. G. Kim, S. Suga, and A. B. Fogo, "Reappraisal of the pathogenesis and consequences of hyperuricemia in hypertension, cardiovascular disease, and renal disease," *American Journal of Kidney Diseases*, vol. 33, no. 2, pp. 225–234, 1999.

[11] D. C. Sane, L. Anton, and K. B. Brosnihan, "Angiogenic growth factors and hypertension," *Angiogenesis*, vol. 7, no. 3, pp. 193–201, 2004.

[12] M. Schmidinger, D. Arnold, C. Szczylik, J. Wagstaff, and A. Ravaud, "Optimizing the use of sunitinib in metastatic renal cell carcinoma: an update from clinical practice," *Cancer Investigation*, vol. 28, no. 8, pp. 856–864, 2010.

[13] M. L. Veronese, A. Mosenkis, K. T. Flaherty et al., "Mechanisms of hypertension associated with BAY 43-9006," *Journal of Clinical Oncology*, vol. 24, no. 9, pp. 1363–1369, 2006.

[14] H. A. J. Struijker Boudier, J. L. M. L. Le Noble, M. W. J. Messing, M. S. P. Huijberts, F. A. C. Le Noble, and H. Van Essen, "The microcirculation and hypertension," *Journal of Hypertension*, vol. 10, no. 7, supplement, pp. S147–S156, 1992.

[15] B. I. Rini, D. P. Cohen, D. R. Lu et al., "Hypertension as a biomarker of efficacy in patients with metastatic renal cell carcinoma treated with sunitinib," *Journal of the National Cancer Institute*, vol. 103, no. 9, pp. 763–773, 2011.

[16] M. L. Maitland, G. L. Bakris, H. R. Black et al., "Initial assessment, surveillance, and management of blood pressure in patients receiving vascular endothelial growth factor signaling pathway inhibitors," *Journal of the National Cancer Institute*, vol. 102, no. 9, pp. 596–604, 2010.

[17] S. Mallick, R. Kanthety, and M. Rahman, "Home blood pressure monitoring in clinical practice: a review," *American Journal of Medicine*, vol. 122, no. 9, pp. 803–810, 2009.

[18] Package insert sunitinib (Sutent). In: Pfizer Labs.

[19] Package insert pazopanib (Votrient). In: GlaxoSmithKline.

[20] A. Y. Khakoo, C. M. Kassiotis, N. Tannir et al., "Heart failure associated with sunitinib malate: a multitargeted receptor tyrosine kinase inhibitor," *Cancer*, vol. 112, no. 11, pp. 2500–2508, 2008.

[21] T. F. Chu, M. A. Rupnick, R. Kerkela et al., "Cardiotoxicity associated with tyrosine kinase inhibitor sunitinib," *The Lancet*, vol. 370, no. 9604, pp. 2011–2019, 2007.

[22] V. Chintalgattu, D. Ai, R. R. Langley et al., "Cardiomyocyte PDGFR-β signaling is an essential component of the mouse

cardiac response to load-induced stress," *Journal of Clinical Investigation*, vol. 120, no. 2, pp. 472–484, 2010.

[23] X. Zhu, S. Wu, W. L. Dahut, and C. R. Parikh, "Risks of proteinuria and hypertension with bevacizumab, an antibody against vascular endothelial growth factor: systematic review and meta-analysis," *American Journal of Kidney Diseases*, vol. 49, no. 2, pp. 186–193, 2007.

[24] T. V. Patel, J. A. Morgan, G. D. Demetri et al., "A preeclampsia-like syndrome characterized by reversible hypertension and proteinuria induced by the multitargeted kinase inhibitors sunitinib and sorafenib," *Journal of the National Cancer Institute*, vol. 100, no. 4, pp. 282–284, 2008.

[25] C. Frangié, C. Lefaucheur, J. Medioni, C. Jacquot, G. S. Hill, and D. Nochy, "Renal thrombotic microangiopathy caused by anti-VEGF-antibody treatment for metastatic renal-cell carcinoma," *The Lancet Oncology*, vol. 8, no. 2, pp. 177–178, 2007.

[26] S. K. Winn, S. Ellis, P. Savage, S. Sampson, and J. E. Marsh, "Biopsy-proven acute interstitial nephritis associated with the tyrosine kinase inhibitor sunitinib: a class effect?" *Nephrology Dialysis Transplantation*, vol. 24, no. 2, pp. 673–675, 2009.

[27] V. Eremina, M. Sood, J. Haigh et al., "Glomerular-specific alterations of VEGF-A expression lead to distinct congenital and acquired renal diseases," *Journal of Clinical Investigation*, vol. 111, no. 5, pp. 707–716, 2003.

[28] C. N. Sternberg, I. D. Davis, J. Mardiak et al., "Pazopanib in locally advanced or metastatic renal cell carcinoma: results of a randomized phase III trial," *Journal of Clinical Oncology*, vol. 28, no. 6, pp. 1061–1068, 2010.

[29] B. Escudier, T. Eisen, W. M. Stadler et al., "Sorafenib in advanced clear-cell renal-cell carcinoma," *New England Journal of Medicine*, vol. 356, no. 2, pp. 125–134, 2007.

[30] R. J. Motzer, T. E. Hutson, P. Tomczak et al., "Overall survival and updated results for sunitinib compared with interferon alfa in patients with metastatic renal cell carcinoma," *Journal of Clinical Oncology*, vol. 27, no. 22, pp. 3584–3590, 2009.

[31] F. A. B. Schutz, T. K. Choueiri, and C. N. Sternberg, "Pazopanib: clinical development of a potent anti-angiogenic drug," *Critical Reviews in Oncology/Hematology*, vol. 77, no. 3, pp. 163–171, 2011.

[32] C. Robert, J. P. Arnault, and C. Mateus, "RAF inhibition and induction of cutaneous squamous cell carcinoma," *Current Opinion in Oncology*, vol. 23, no. 2, pp. 177–182, 2011.

[33] M. E. Lacouture, A. Desai, K. Soltani et al., "Inflammation of actinic keratoses subsequent to therapy with sorafenib, a multitargeted tyrosine-kinase inhibitor," *Clinical and Experimental Dermatology*, vol. 31, no. 6, pp. 783–785, 2006.

[34] D. S. Hong, S. B. Reddy, V. G. Prieto et al., "Multiple squamous cell carcinomas of the skin after therapy with sorafenib combined with tipifarnib," *Archives of Dermatology*, vol. 144, no. 6, pp. 779–782, 2008.

[35] J. P. Arnault, J. Wechsler, B. Escudier et al., "Keratoacanthomas and squamous cell carcinomas in patients receiving sorafenib," *Journal of Clinical Oncology*, vol. 27, no. 23, pp. e59–e61, 2009.

[36] T. Kamba and D. M. McDonald, "Mechanisms of adverse effects of anti-VEGF therapy for cancer," *British Journal of Cancer*, vol. 96, no. 12, pp. 1788–1795, 2007.

[37] C. F. Xu, B. H. Reck, Z. Xue et al., "Pazopanib-induced hyperbilirubinemia is associated with Gilbert's syndrome UGT1A1 polymorphism," *British Journal of Cancer*, vol. 102, no. 9, pp. 1371–1377, 2010.

[38] H. Minami, K. Kawada, H. Ebi et al., "Phase I and pharmacokinetic study of sorafenib, an oral multikinase inhibitor, in Japanese patients with advanced refractory solid tumors," *Cancer Science*, vol. 99, no. 7, pp. 1492–1498, 2008.

[39] J. L. Spivak, "Polycythemia vera: myths, mechanisms, and management," *Blood*, vol. 100, no. 13, pp. 4272–4290, 2002.

[40] B. Y. Y. Tam, K. Wei, J. S. Rudge et al., "VEGF modulates erythropoiesis through regulation of adult hepatic erythropoietin synthesis," *Nature Medicine*, vol. 12, no. 7, pp. 793–800, 2006.

[41] E. Wong, L. S. Rosen, M. Mulay et al., "Sunitinib induces hypothyroidism in advanced cancer patients and may inhibit thyroid peroxidase activity," *Thyroid*, vol. 17, no. 4, pp. 351–355, 2007.

[42] M. E. Cabanillas, S. G. Waguespack, Y. Bronstein et al., "Treatment with tyrosine kinase inhibitors for patients with differentiated thyroid cancer: the M. D. Anderson experience," *Journal of Clinical Endocrinology and Metabolism*, vol. 95, no. 6, pp. 2588–2595, 2010.

[43] E. R. Plimack, N. Tannir, E. Lin, B. N. Bekele, and E. Jonasch, "Patterns of disease progression in metastatic renal cell carcinoma patients treated with antivascular agents and interferon," *Cancer*, vol. 115, no. 9, pp. 1859–1866, 2009.

[44] K. Kim, K. Flaherty, P. Champman et al., "Pattern and outcome of disease progression in phase I study of vemurafenib in patients with metastatic melanoma (MM)," *Journal of Clinical Oncology*, vol. 29, supplement, 2011.

[45] J. A. Gottlieb and C. S. Hill Jr., "Chemotherapy of thyroid cancer with adriamycin. Experience with 30 patients," *New England Journal of Medicine*, vol. 290, no. 4, pp. 193–197, 1974.

[46] K. Zimmermann, A. Schmittel, U. Steiner et al., "Sunitinib treatment for patients with advanced clear-cell renal-cell carcinoma after progression on sorafenib," *Oncology*, vol. 76, no. 5, pp. 350–354, 2009.

[47] A. Fernández, A. Sanguino, Z. Peng et al., "An anticancer C-Kit kinase inhibitor is reengineered to make it more active and less cardiotoxic," *Journal of Clinical Investigation*, vol. 117, no. 12, pp. 4044–4054, 2007.

30

Incidental Papillary Thyroid Microcarcinoma in an Endemic Goiter Area

Emin Gürleyik,[1] Gunay Gurleyik,[2] Banu Karapolat,[1] and Ufuk Onsal[1]

[1]Department of Surgery, Duzce University Medical Faculty, 81650 Duzce, Turkey
[2]Haydarpasa Numune Hospital, Istanbul, Turkey

Correspondence should be addressed to Emin Gürleyik; egurleyik@yahoo.com

Academic Editor: Noriyuki Koibuchi

Clinical and pathological characteristics of incidental papillary thyroid microcancer cases, surgical, medical, and nuclear treatment methods, and patients' outcome were studied during follow-up period of 102 months. We studied 37 patients with incidental papillary thyroid microcancer (I-PTM). The surgical procedure was total thyroidectomy in 29 and hemithyroidectomy in 8 patients. Size, multifocality, and bilateralism of PTM foci, thyroid capsule invasion, and presence of lymphovascular invasion were histopathological parameters. We analysed adjuvant medical and nuclear treatment and patients' outcome during follow-up period of 102 (61–144) months. The prevalence rates of I-PTM were 9.4% in 395 thyroidectomy cases. Histopathological examination reported unifocal disease in 30 and multifocal disease in 7 (18%) patients. Multifocal disease was bilateral in 6 (20.1%) patients. The mean size of the PTM foci was 4.88 mm. The rate of thyroid capsule invasion was 5.4%. All patients received a suppressive dose of LT4 to achieve a low serum TSH level. Adjuvant surgical and nuclear treatment was not performed in our cases. We did not find any negative changes in blood chemistry and ultrasound imaging, and any unfavourable events as locoregional and systemic recurrence. In conclusion, diagnosis of I-PTM is common that multifocality and bilateralism appear as pathologic features. The prognosis is excellent after surgical treatment and TSH suppression. Routine adjuvant nuclear treatment is unnecessary in majority of patients.

1. Introduction

The incidence of well-differentiated thyroid carcinoma, particularly papillary cancer, has been increasing since the last 20–30 years. The Surveillance, Epidemiology and End Results (SEER) database shows more than a 2-fold increase in thyroid cancer since 1995 [1]. An important contributing factor for the increased incidence of such well-differentiated cancers is the increasing diagnostic rates of papillary thyroid microcarcinoma (PTM). Other factors such as iodination programmes in low iodine intake areas, detailed histopathological examination of the excised thyroid tissue, and the increase in bilateral total excision of the thyroid gland during thyroid surgery have also been attributed to the increasing rates of large (>10 mm) and micropapillary carcinoma [2–5]. A vast majority of PTM cases are incidentally determined on postoperative histopathological examination of the excised thyroid tissue for the surgical treatment of benign thyroid disorders.

PTM is defined as a tumour focus that is ≤10 mm in size. Incidental PTM (I-PTM) is a tumour focus that is clinically unsuspected before thyroid surgery and is identified in the final pathological examination of a thyroidectomy specimen. Therefore, several controversies regarding the need for completion surgery for excision of the remaining thyroid tissue and lymph nodes exist.

The objectives of this study were to describe the incidence and clinical/pathological characteristics of PTM and discuss our experience with I-PTM cases in an endemic goitre area.

2. Materials and Methods

2.1. Patients and Thyroid Surgery. Surgically treated patients between September 2003 and September 2010 were retrospectively analysed. The study involved 395 surgical patients with benign disease of the thyroid, without any diagnosis of preoperative malignancy. Total thyroidectomy or hemithyroidectomy was performed for the treatment of benign thyroid diseases. A total of 37 patients with PTM incidentally diagnosed on postoperative histopathological examination of the excised thyroid tissue were analysed for assessing the rate of incidental diagnosis of PTM and their demographic features and the surgical procedures used for their treatment.

2.2. Histopathology. Histopathological parameters were established by microscopic examination, including the size of PTM, location in the thyroid gland, multifocality and bilateralism in the thyroid lobes, thyroid capsule invasion, presence of lymphovascular invasion (LVI), lymph node metastasis, and tumour recurrence.

2.3. Adjuvant Treatment. As an adjuvant treatment, we analysed completion thyroidectomy for I-PTM cases with unilateral hemithyroidectomy, l-thyroxin (LT4) treatment for the suppression of thyroid stimulating hormone (TSH), and radioiodine (RAI) treatment.

2.4. Follow-Up. Patients with I-PTM were followed up for 12 years, mean 102 (61–144) months.

2.4.1. First and Third Month Postoperatively. Biochemical analyses for serum TSH and free thyroxin (FT4) were performed in order to determine the suppressive dose of LT4 (suppression of TSH at a level of <0.25 uIU/mL).

2.4.2. Sixth Month Postoperatively. Biochemical analyses for serum TSH, FT4, thyroglobulin (Tg), and anti-thyroglobulin antibody (anti-Tg Ab) were performed in total thyroidectomy cases. An ultrasound of the cervical lymph nodes in all patients and the remaining lobes in patients with hemithyroidectomy was also performed.

2.4.3. Yearly. An ultrasound of the cervical lymph nodes in all patients and the remaining lobes in patients with hemithyroidectomy was repeated. Biochemical analyses for serum TSH, FT4, Tg, and anti-Tg Ab were performed.

2.5. Outcome. Locoregional or distal recurrence of thyroid malignancy in the follow-up period and disease-free or overall survival of patients with I-PTM were the primary outcome parameters.

3. Results

During the study period, total thyroidectomy and right and left hemithyroidectomy were performed in 249, 75, and 71 patients, respectively, for the treatment of benign surgical diseases of the thyroid gland among the total 395 patients. The females consisted of 75% of the patients. I-PTM was diagnosed on histopathological examination in 37 (9.4%) of the 395 patients. Moreover, 47% of our thyroid papillary cancer cases were PTM, of which 78.7% were incidentally discovered. I-PTM was diagnosed in 10.8% and 5% of female and male patients, respectively (Table 1).

TABLE 1: Sex distribution of patients with surgical disease of the thyroid gland.

Patients	All	Female	Male
Thyroidectomy cases	395	295 (74.7%)	100 (25.3%)
Patients with I-PTM*	37	32 (86.5%)	5 (13.5%)
Rate of I-PTM	9.4%	10.8%	5%

*I-PTM: incidental papillary thyroid microcancer.

TABLE 2: Age distribution.

Age distribution	Patients with I-PTM*
0–20 years	1 (2.7%)
21–40 years	13 (35.1%)
41–60 years	21 (56.8%)
61–80 years	2 (5.4%)

*I-PTM: incidental papillary thyroid microcancer.

The mean age of the 37 patients with I-PTM was 44.1 (16–71) years. More than half of the patients (56.8%) were aged between 41 and 60 years (Table 2).

The prevalence rates of I-PTM were 11.6% (29/249) in the total thyroidectomy specimens and 5.5% (8/146) in the unilateral hemithyroidectomy specimens (Table 3).

3.1. Pathology. Histopathological examination revealed 45 foci of PTM in 37 patients. The disease was unifocal in 30 and multifocal in 7 (18%) patients (6 cases of two and 1 case of three foci). Of the 45 foci, 25 (55.6%) were located in the left lobe (Table 4). Bilateral location of the PTM foci was observed in 6 (20.1%) of the 29 total thyroidectomy cases (Table 3).

The mean size of the PTM foci was 4.88 (1–10) mm, and 42.2%, 64.4%, and 71% of the foci were ≤3 mm, 5 mm, and 6 mm, respectively (Tables 5(a) and 5(b)).

Microscopic examination revealed thyroid capsule invasion in 2 (5.4%) of the 37 patients and in 2 (4.4%) of the 45 foci. These two foci measured 3 and 6 mm in two female patients aged 41 and 57 years, respectively. LVI was not reported in the PTM cases.

3.2. Adjuvant Treatment. Based on the clinical and ultrasound findings of the cervical lymph nodes and thyroid gland, we did not perform completion thyroidectomy in eight PTM cases with unilateral hemithyroidectomy. Patients with I-PTM did not receive postoperative RAI treatment. All patients received a suppressive dose of LT4 to achieve a serum TSH level of <0.25 uIU/mL.

3.3. Follow-Up. During the follow-up period of 102 (61–144) months, we did not find any negative changes in blood chemistry and ultrasound imaging. We also did not find any unfavourable locoregional or distant events as recurrence in the remaining thyroid lobes, metastasis in the cervical nodes, and distant metastasis.

TABLE 3: Surgery of the thyroid gland and prevalence of I-PTM*.

| Surgery | Patients | Lobes | | I-PTM | Foci | Bilateral |
		Right	Left			
Total thyroidectomy	249 (63%)	249	249	29 (11.6%)	36	6 (20.1%)
Right hemithyroidectomy	75 (19%)	75	—	5 (6.7%)	6	—
Left hemithyroidectomy	71 (18%)	—	71	3 (4.2%)	3	—
Total	395	324	320	37 (9.4%)	45	—
		644				

*I-PTM: incidental papillary thyroid microcancer.

TABLE 4: Location of I-PTM* foci in thyroid lobes.

Surgery location	Total thyroidectomy	Right hemithyroidectomy	Left hemithyroidectomy	Total
Right lobe	14	6	—	20 (44.4%)
Left lobe	22	—	3	25 (55.6%)
Total	36	6	3	45 (100%)

*I-PTM: incidental papillary thyroid microcancer.

TABLE 5: (a) Size distribution of 45 I-PTM* foci. (b) Size distribution of 45 I-PTM* foci.

(a)

Size	Right lobe	Left lobe	Total
0–5 mm	11	18	29 (64.4%)
6–10 mm	9	7	16 (35.6%)
Total	20	25	45

*I-PTM: incidental papillary thyroid microcancer.

(b)

Size	Right lobe	Left lobe	Total
0–3 mm	8	11	19 (42.2%)
4–6 mm	4	9	13 (28.9%)
7–10 mm	8	5	13 (28.9%)
Total	20	25	45

*I-PTM: incidental papillary thyroid microcancer.

4. Discussion

PTM is an indolent neoplasia, often asymptomatic and discovered incidentally [4]. Papillary microcarcinoma is accordingly found more frequently and often incidentally upon histopathological examination of surgical specimens from presumed benign thyroid disease [5]. Our study region was formerly a low iodine intake (endemic goitre) area where preventive iodine supplementation programme has been ongoing since the last 30 years. Several changes have been observed in medical and surgical thyroid diseases. The significant increase in the diagnostic rates of PTM, particularly the incidental findings after thyroid surgery, raises an important issue. We observed the diagnostic rate of I-PTM to be 78.7% among all the PTM cases, which corroborates our previous results. In our endemic region, the increased frequency of PTM and higher diagnostic rates of I-PTM indicate the occurrence of papillary cancer after iodine supplementation.

The presence of incidental thyroid cancer is an important issue in patients with benign thyroid diseases who underwent thyroid surgery. Postoperatively, we discovered that the thyroid gland harboured PTM in approximately 1 (9.4%) out 10 of our patients with benign thyroid disease. Previous studies have also reported the prevalence of I-PTM to be between 7.1% and 16.3% [6–10]. Based on the present study and previous results of prevalence, we suggest that the presence of incidental cancer is not an uncommon situation. During our study period in the endemic area, the proportion of PTM was 47% among all papillary thyroid cancer cases, and a vast majority (78.7%) of them showed incidental diagnosis, which indicates the importance of this pathology in the increasing rates of differentiated thyroid cancers. Lombardi et al. [11] reported the proportion of I-PTM to be 42%, of which 75.5% were incidental in an area with a high prevalence of goitre. Rosa Pelizzo et al. [3] have also reported an increase in the proportion of PTM from 35% to 56%, of which 60% were incidental. In another study, the proportion of PTM in papillary thyroid cancer cases was determined to be 49%, of which 58% were incidental [8]. The proportion of incidental cases among all PTM cases was found to be between 49% and 75.5% [8, 11–15]. Londero et al. [5] recently reported that age-standardised rates increased from 0.35 per 100,000 per year in 1996 to 0.74 per 100,000 per year in 2008. About 59% of PTM cases were identified incidentally, and a significant rise in incidence was found only for the incidental cases.

The increasing number of total thyroidectomies appears to be an important factor for the higher rate of incidental PTM. In our study, the incidence (11.6%) of I-PTM among total thyroidectomy cases was more than twice the incidence (5.5%) after hemithyroidectomy. Rosa Pelizzo et al. [3] reported an increase in the proportion of total thyroidectomies (from 67% to 78%) and PTM (from 35% to 56%). The prevalence of PTM is higher in patients with bilateral surgery [10].

The important features of papillary thyroid cancer include multifocality and bilateralism. Our incidence rate of 18%

for the presence of two or more foci in the gland and the rate of 20% for the location of tumour foci in both lobes confirmed the pathological features of incidental PTM. Previous studies have also reported the multifocality rate of I-PTM to be between 13% and 44.1% [7–9, 15–19]. Some studies have reported multifocality as an independent risk factor for tumour recurrence [6, 8, 11, 14, 18, 20, 21]. On the other hand, the rate of recurrence is very low in patients with incidental PTM, which has been reported to range from 0% to 5% [6, 8, 11, 14, 15, 18, 19, 22]. Therefore, I-PTM cases with multifocality should be followed up more closely, despite the low risk of recurrence. Another pathological feature arising from our study was the rate of bilateralism (20%). Multiple foci were located in both lateral lobes in 20%–27.3% of patients with I-PTM [7, 9]. Based on the results of both the present and previous studies, the higher rate of bilateral tumour foci in both lobes draws our attention to the remaining lobes in patients with hemithyroidectomy. In such cases, sensitive imaging methods, such as ultrasound, should be used for the detection of nodules in the remaining lobes at both early postoperative and follow-up periods.

In general, incidental tumour foci are relatively smaller in size than nonincidental tumour foci. The average size of the tumour foci was <5 mm in patients with I-PTM [9, 15, 16, 18]. Our results confirmed the relatively small size (average 4.88 mm) of the tumour foci in the thyroid glands of patients with incidental PTM, of which 64% and 71% of foci were ≤5 mm and ≤6 mm, respectively. John et al. [15] reported that the tumour foci were ≤6 mm in 83% of such patients. Previous studies have reported tumour size as a risk factor for lymph node metastasis and recurrence. In general, tumour foci diameter >5 or 6 mm has appeared as an independent risk factor [6, 20, 21, 23, 24]. Therefore, patients with foci >6 mm in diameter should be followed up more closely. The recurrence rate of PTM is very low even among tumour foci > 6 mm, which has been reported to range from 0% to 5% [5, 6, 8, 14, 25–27].

Other important pathological features of thyroid malignancies are thyroid capsule invasion and LVI. The presence of LVI is a pathological feature showing the metastatic ability of malignancy. In our study, the absence of LVI in all our cases indicates the decreased ability of local and systemic spread of PTM. Previous studies have defined thyroid capsule invasion as extrathyroid or extracapsular spread, growth, extension, or invasion. Capsular invasion by PTM is an independent risk factor for tumour recurrence in the follow-up period [2, 6, 11, 12, 14, 20–23, 28]. Based on the rate of thyroid capsule invasion (5.4%) in the present study, we suggest that PTM with subcapsular localisation uncommonly invades the capsule of the thyroid gland. This rate has been reported to be 3.9% by John et al. [15] and 7.4% by Sakorafas et al. [9].

Locoregional and distant spread and recurrence of malignancy are the most important factors during the follow-up period. In our study, the absence of recurrence, lymph node, or distant metastasis indicates very low risk of tumour recurrence in patients with incidental PTM. The recurrence rate is 0% in some of the previous studies [12, 14, 19, 26]. In general, the overall recurrence rate was <2% in many case series [2, 5, 15, 22, 27]. Other studies have also reported a low recurrence rate between 2% and 5% [6, 8, 11, 13, 18, 25]. I-PTM is found in the thyroid tissue after surgical treatment of benign thyroid disease. Therefore, total thyroidectomy and unilateral hemithyroidectomy are usually performed in these cases. In this situation, is any adjuvant treatment required after the diagnosis of PTM? Completion thyroidectomy for hemithyroidectomy cases, RAI treatment, and suppression of TSH levels with LT4 treatment are the primary adjuvant procedures for patients with differentiated thyroid cancer. However, a very low rate of recurrence in a large series of I-PTM cases does not indicate the use of adjuvant treatment, except the suppression of TSH levels with LT4 treatment. After total excision of the gland, thyroidectomized patients receive L-thyroxin (LT4) replacement in order to maintain normal body function and TSH level in normal range [29]. On the other hand, well-differentiated malignant cells of papillary cancer have thyrotropin receptors in which the growth of differentiated malignant cells is controlled by TSH [30]. Therefore, inhibition of TSH secretion has beneficial effects on management of TSH-dependent tumour growth of well-differentiated malignancies that this secretion is inhibited by LT4 administration. Inhibition of TSH secretion should be provided by suppressive dose of LT4 in all patients with papillary cancer. The suppressive dose of LT4 is adjusted in individual basis by serum TSH level which is maintained between 0.1 and 0.25 uIU/mL according to patients' tolerability. In older patients, the dose of LT4 and suppression of TSH should be balanced with the cardiac risk [30]. After yearly follow-up the dose of LT4 can be decreased to maintain serum TSH levels between 0.5 and 1 uIU/mL in patients without unfavourable findings. In our study, surgical and nuclear adjuvant treatment was not attempted in any patients after a careful evaluation with imaging modalities and blood analysis. In our series of I-PTM cases, the absence of locoregional and distant recurrence during the follow-up period of 102 months confirmed the adequacy of the surgical treatment. Similarly, several previous studies have also reported no tumour recurrences after the surgical treatment of I-PTM [12, 14, 19, 26]. Based on our study and previous studies, we suggest that routine completion thyroidectomy after unilateral excision, lymph node dissection, and RAI application are unnecessary in most I-PTM cases.

In our endemic goitre area, diagnosis of I-PTM in thyroid tissue is not an uncommon situation after thyroid surgery for benign diseases. The prevalence of I-PTM increases parallel to the increase of total thyroidectomy rate for benign thyroid diseases. Multifocality and bilateralism are main pathologic features of PTM. Size of I-PTM foci in thyroid tissue is relatively small and the majority are smaller than 6 mm. Small foci of PTM create very low risk of lymph node metastasis and locoregional or distant recurrences in the follow-up period. The prognosis is excellent after surgical treatment and TSH suppression with LT4 administration. Routine adjuvant surgical and nuclear treatment as completion thyroidectomy, lymph node dissection, and RAI application is unnecessary in vast majority of patients due to low risk of recurrence. Such adjuvant procedures should be reserved for small number of recurrent cases discovered in the follow-up period.

References

[1] V. Bernet, "Approach to the patient with incidental papillary microcarcinoma," *Journal of Clinical Endocrinology and Metabolism*, vol. 95, no. 8, pp. 3586–3592, 2010.

[2] N. Neuhold, A. Schultheis, M. Hermann, G. Krotla, O. Koperek, and P. Birner, "Incidental papillary microcarcinoma of the thyroid—further evidence of a very low malignant potential: a retrospective clinicopathological study with up to 30 years of follow-up," *Annals of Surgical Oncology*, vol. 18, no. 12, pp. 3430–3436, 2011.

[3] M. Rosa Pelizzo, D. Rubello, C. Bernardi et al., "Thyroid surgical practices shaping thyroid cancer incidence in North-Eastern Italy," *Biomedicine and Pharmacotherapy*, vol. 68, no. 1, pp. 39–43, 2014.

[4] P. Malandrino, G. Pellegriti, M. Attard et al., "Papillary thyroid microcarcinomas: a comparative study of the characteristics and risk factors at presentation in two cancer registries," *Journal of Clinical Endocrinology and Metabolism*, vol. 98, no. 4, pp. 1427–1434, 2013.

[5] S. C. Londero, A. Krogdahl, L. Bastholt et al., "Papillary thyroid microcarcinoma in Denmark 1996–2008: a national study of epidemiology and clinical significance," *Thyroid*, vol. 23, no. 9, pp. 1159–1164, 2013.

[6] I. Vasileiadis, T. Karatzas, D. Vasileiadis et al., "Clinical and pathological characteristics of incidental and nonincidental papillary thyroid microcarcinoma in 339 patients," *Head and Neck*, vol. 36, no. 4, pp. 564–570, 2014.

[7] D. Costamagna, L. Pagano, M. Caputo, M. Leutner, F. Mercalli, and A. Alonzo, "Incidental cancer in patients surgically treated for benign thyroid disease: our experience at a single institution," *Giornale di Chirurgia*, vol. 34, no. 1-2, pp. 21–26, 2013.

[8] E. Dunki-Jacobs, K. Grannan, S. McDonough, and A. M. Engel, "Clinically unsuspected papillary microcarcinomas of the thyroid: a common finding with favorable biology?" *The American Journal of Surgery*, vol. 203, no. 2, pp. 140–144, 2012.

[9] G. Sakorafas, V. Stafyla, T. Kolettis, G. Tolumis, G. Kassaras, and G. Peros, "Microscopic papillary thyroid cancer as an incidental finding in patients treated surgically for presumably benign thyroid disease," *Journal of Postgraduate Medicine*, vol. 53, no. 1, pp. 23–26, 2007.

[10] N. Slijepcevic, V. Zivaljevic, J. Marinkovic, S. Sipetic, A. Diklic, and I. Paunovic, "Retrospective evaluation of the incidental finding of 403 papillary thyroid microcarcinomas in 2466 patients undergoing thyroid surgery for presumed benign thyroid disease," *BMC Cancer*, vol. 15, article 330, 2015.

[11] C. P. Lombardi, R. Bellantone, C. De Crea et al., "Papillary thyroid microcarcinoma: extrathyroidal extension, lymph node metastases, and risk factors for recurrence in a high prevalence of goiter area," *World Journal of Surgery*, vol. 34, no. 6, pp. 1214–1221, 2010.

[12] A. Pisanu, I. Reccia, O. Nardello, and A. Uccheddu, "Risk factors for nodal metastasis and recurrence among patients with papillary thyroid microcarcinoma: differences in clinical relevance between nonincidental and incidental tumors," *World Journal of Surgery*, vol. 33, no. 3, pp. 460–468, 2009.

[13] M. S. Elliott, K. Gao, R. Gupta, E. L. Chua, A. Gargya, and J. Clark, "Management of incidental and non-incidental papillary thyroid microcarcinoma," *The Journal of Laryngology and Otology*, vol. 127, supplement 2, pp. S17–S23, 2013.

[14] A. Antonaci, A. Anello, A. Aucello et al., "Microcarcinoma and incidental carcinoma of the thyroid in a clinical series: clinical behaviour and surgical management," *Clinica Terapeutica*, vol. 157, no. 3, pp. 225–229, 2006.

[15] A. M. John, P. M. Jacob, R. Oommen, S. Nair, A. Nair, and S. Rajaratnam, "Our experience with papillary thyroid microcancer," *Indian Journal of Endocrinology and Metabolism*, vol. 18, no. 3, pp. 410–413, 2014.

[16] S.-F. Wang, W.-H. Zhao, W.-B. Wang, X.-D. Teng, L.-S. Teng, and Z.-M. Ma, "Clinical features and prognosis of patients with benign thyroid disease accompanied by an incidental papillary carcinoma," *Asian Pacific Journal of Cancer Prevention*, vol. 14, no. 2, pp. 707–711, 2013.

[17] Y. K. So, M. W. Kim, and Y. I. Son, "Multifocality and bilaterality of papillary thyroid microcarcinoma," *Clinical and Experimental Otorhinolaryngology*, vol. 8, no. 2, pp. 174–178, 2015.

[18] B. Mantinan, A. Rego-Iraeta, A. Larrañaga, E. Fluiters, P. Sánchez-Sobrino, and R. V. Garcia-Mayor, "Factors influencing the outcome of patients with incidental papillary thyroid microcarcinoma," *Journal of Thyroid Research*, vol. 2012, Article ID 469397, 5 pages, 2012.

[19] D. Siassakos, S. Gourgiotis, P. Moustafellos, N. Dimopoulos, and E. Hadjiyannakis, "Thyroid microcarcinoma during thyroidectomy," *Singapore Medical Journal*, vol. 49, no. 1, pp. 23–25, 2008.

[20] N. Qu, L. Zhang, Q. H. Ji et al., "Risk factors for central compartment lymph node metastasis in papillary thyroid microcarcinoma: a meta-analysis," *World Journal of Surgery*, vol. 39, no. 10, pp. 2459–2470, 2015.

[21] Z. Z. Lu, Y. Zhang, S. F. Wei et al., "Outcome of papillary thyroid microcarcinoma: study of 1,990 cases," *Molecular and Clinical Oncology*, vol. 3, no. 3, pp. 672–676, 2015.

[22] E. Gschwandtner, T. Klatte, N. Swietek et al., "Increase of papillary thyroid microcarcinoma and a plea for restrictive treatment: a retrospective study of 1,391 prospective documented patients," *Surgery*, vol. 159, no. 2, pp. 503–511, 2016.

[23] L. Y. Zhang, Z. W. Liu, Y. W. Liu, W. S. Gao, and C. J. Zheng, "Risk factors for nodal metastasis in cN0 papillary thyroid microcarcinoma," *Asian Pacific Journal of Cancer Prevention*, vol. 16, no. 8, pp. 3361–3363, 2015.

[24] J. Y. Kim, E. J. Jung, T. Park et al., "Impact of tumor size on subclinical central lymph node metastasis in papillary thyroid microcarcinoma depends on age," *World Journal of Surgical Oncology*, vol. 13, article 88, 2015.

[25] Y. Ito, T. Higashiyama, Y. Takamura et al., "Prognosis of patients with benign thyroid diseases accompanied by incidental papillary carcinoma undetectable on preoperative imaging tests," *World Journal of Surgery*, vol. 31, no. 8, pp. 1672–1676, 2007.

[26] N. Besic, J. Zgajnar, M. Hocevar, and R. Petric, "Extent of thyroidectomy and lymphadenectomy in 254 patients with papillary thyroid microcarcinoma: a single-institution experience," *Annals of Surgical Oncology*, vol. 16, no. 4, pp. 920–928, 2009.

[27] Y. Ito and A. Miyauchi, "A therapeutic strategy for incidentally detected papillary microcarcinoma of the thyroid," *Nature Clinical Practice Endocrinology and Metabolism*, vol. 3, no. 3, pp. 240–248, 2007.

[28] L. Pedrazzini, A. Baroli, L. Marzoli, R. Guglielmi, and E. Papini, "Cancer recurrence in papillary thyroid microcarcinoma: a multivariate analysis on 231 patients with a 12-year follow-up," *Minerva Endocrinologica*, vol. 38, no. 3, pp. 269–279, 2013.

[29] V. Di Donna, M. G. Santoro, C. de Waure et al., "A new strategy to estimate levothyroxine requirement after total thyroidectomy for benign thyroid disease," *Thyroid*, vol. 24, no. 12, pp. 1759–1764, 2014.

31

Thyroid Hormone Receptor Mutations in Cancer and Resistance to Thyroid Hormone: Perspective and Prognosis

Meghan D. Rosen and Martin L. Privalsky

Department of Microbiology, University of California-Davis, Davis, CA 95616, USA

Correspondence should be addressed to Martin L. Privalsky, mlprivalsky@ucdavis.edu

Academic Editor: Michelina Plateroti

Thyroid hormone, operating through its receptors, plays crucial roles in the control of normal human physiology and development; deviations from the norm can give rise to disease. Clinical endocrinologists often must confront and correct the consequences of inappropriately high or low thyroid hormone synthesis. Although more rare, disruptions in thyroid hormone endocrinology due to aberrations in the receptor also have severe medical consequences. This review will focus on the afflictions that are caused by, or are closely associated with, mutated thyroid hormone receptors. These include Resistance to Thyroid Hormone Syndrome, erythroleukemia, hepatocellular carcinoma, renal clear cell carcinoma, and thyroid cancer. We will describe current views on the molecular bases of these diseases, and what distinguishes the neoplastic from the non-neoplastic. We will also touch on studies that implicate alterations in receptor expression, and thyroid hormone levels, in certain oncogenic processes.

1. Preface

More than two thousand years ago, Aristotle discovered a link between castration and disruption of male maturation. Through extensive experimentation on bird and beast, he hypothesized that the testes were vital to the development of secondary male sex characteristics [1]. Excision of these organs drastically altered body size and behavior, as well as hair, feather, and horn growth [2]. These experiments were the earliest seeds of what would eventually become our current understanding of endocrinology. And from these same beginnings arose the recognition that aberrant endocrine signaling, through intentional intervention, accident, or pathogenic processes, could lead to disease.

Comprehension of endocrine signaling grew slowly over the next two millennia until the mid-19th century, which oversaw a dramatic expansion of research into endocrine glands and their secretions. With these studies came the first hints of methods to clinically intervene when normal endocrine homeostasis was disturbed. In 1849, Berthold discovered how to undo the deed of Aristotle, showing that castrated roosters regained their comb and wattle if the testes were surgically transplanted back into the abdominal cavity;

Berthold correctly reasoned that the growth-enhancing compound in the testes must be soluble and blood-borne [3]. Similarly, the roles of the thyroid gland came to focus when Murray, in 1891, determined that a patient's symptoms (now known to be due to hypothyroidism) disappeared after grafting half of a sheep's thyroid beneath her skin. Because the patient's symptoms disappeared quickly after the operation, Murray surmised his patient's improvement could not be attributed to regained function of the sheep's gland but rather must be "due to the absorption of the juice of the healthy thyroid gland by the tissues of the patient" [4]. He later suggested that injections of thyroid gland extract would likely produce the same effect, a prediction subsequently confirmed by Baumann and Roos [5]. Graves reciprocally demonstrated that excessive thyroid gland activity leads to the pathological process now denoted hyperthyroidism [6]. In 1915, Kendall reported the successful isolation of thyroid hormone [7].

As more and more endocrine hormones were identified between the mid-19th to mid-20th centuries, interest turned toward understanding not only their synthesis and chemical structures, but also their mechanisms of action within their target tissues. In the 1960s, Jensen et al. demonstrated that radiolabeled estrogen injected into female rats localized, in part, to reproductive target tissues, hinting at the existence of a tissue-specific receptor for this hormone [8, 9]. In 1973, Jensen et al. demonstrated that the estrogen/estrogen receptor (ER) complex shuttled from the cytoplasm to the nucleus and enhanced RNA synthesis in uterine tissue (Jensen et al. referred to it as an "alleviation of a deficiency in RNA synthesis") [10]. This was one of the first indications that nuclear receptors could influence transcription, foreshadowing both the appellation of "nuclear" to the term "receptor" and the role of these receptors in gene regulation. Additional evidence for the participation of nuclear receptors in transcription control soon accumulated, extending this paradigm to glucocorticoids and thyroid hormones [11–19]. The molecular cloning of the cDNA for glucocorticoid receptor (GR) was reported in 1985, and, just a year later, the cDNAs for the human estrogen receptor and thyroid hormone receptors (TRs) were isolated and described [20–25]. Today, 48 members of the nuclear receptor family have been identified in humans, 49 in mice, 21 in flies, and 270 in worms [26–28].

This work ultimately led to the current model of endocrine signaling wherein minute amounts of potent compounds are carried from their site of synthesis through the blood to mediate distal physiological changes. In the cases of interest to us here, these compounds are small, lipophilic molecules derived from cholesterol (the androgens of Aristotle's observations), highly modified amino acids (the thyroid hormones), or a variety of other greasy compounds. Nuclear receptors within the target tissues are the regulatory ambassadors in this endocrine diplomacy: they receive extracellular information in the form of their cognate hormone, bind to specific target genes, collaborate with coregulatory partners, and initiate phenotypic change by altering the regulation of a broad array of gene targets [10, 29, 30]. We now know that nuclear receptors have a pervasive reach into nearly all aspects of animal biology and play key roles not only in endocrine signaling but also in metabolic and xenobiotic sensing [31–33]. In humans, frogs, flies, and likely every other form of metazoan life, nuclear receptors are key regulators of development, growth, metabolism, reproduction, homeostasis, and circadian rhythm. A recent hierarchical clustering analysis based on nuclear receptor expression, function, and physiology organized the known mouse nuclear receptors into six distinct clades that span steroidogenesis, reproduction, development, metabolism, and energy homeostasis [34].

Not surprisingly, departures from this normal pathway of endocrine signaling in humans have the potential to wreak developmental or physiological disorder and can require medical intervention. In the day-to-day routine of the clinical endocrinologist, these departures are most commonly the consequence of too little or too much hormone production. Although we will touch on these hormone deficiencies and excesses, the main topic of this paper lies on the other side of the equation: mutations in the nuclear receptors that receive the hormone signals, rather than defects in the hormone signals *per se*. This paper will introduce thyroid hormone

endocrinology and discuss how thyroid hormone receptors function as members of the larger nuclear receptor family. We will then discuss the role of TR signaling in human disease, with an emphasis on endocrine and neoplastic disorders.

2. Normal Thyroid Hormone Endocrinology

2.1. The Signal. In a healthy individual, thyroid hormone is produced in response to a cascade of signals originating in the hypothalamus, which synthesizes thyrotropin-releasing hormone (TRH) (Figure 1). TRH induces expression of thyroid-stimulating hormone (TSH) in the anterior pituitary, which induces, in turn, synthesis and release of T3/T4 thyronine by the follicular cells of the thyroid gland. T3 and T4 are the most abundant forms of thyroid hormone and are carried in the circulation chiefly as complexes with transthyretin, serum albumin, and thyroxine-binding globulin (TBG) [42, 43]. On arrival at a responsive cell, T3 and T4 are transported across the cell membrane primarily by monocarboxylate anion transporters 8 and 10 (MCT8 and MCT10) [44, 45] (Figure 1). T4 can be converted to T3 by deiodinase type 2 (DIO2) found in a variety of other responsive tissues [46]. Although both T3 and T4 can bind to, and modulate the activity of, intracellular TRs, T3 is considerably more active than T4, leading many to view the latter as a prohormone [46]. Deiodination of T3 or T4 on their inner ring by deiodinase type 3 (DIO3) leads to their inactivation. Interestingly, DIO1, a third deiodinase found primarily in the liver and kidney, can remove iodines from either the outer or inner ring and therefore can alternatively generate or inactivate T3 [46]. It should be noted that several metabolic derivatives of thyroid hormone can signal through membrane-associated G-protein coupled receptors such as TAAR1 [47]; however, the TRs appear to represent the key receptors for T3 and T4 and are the focus of the remainder of this paper.

2.2. The Receptor. Once in a target cell, T3 and T4 bind to the TR subfamily of nuclear receptors. In common with virtually all members of the nuclear receptor family, TRs are composed of a shared architecture consisting of an N-terminal (A/B) domain that contains binding sites for transcriptional coregulators, a central DNA binding domain C responsible for target gene recognition, an intervening "hinge" domain (D), and a C-terminal, hormone-binding domain (E/F) (Figure 2).

2.2.1. The "A/B" Domain. The "A/B" domains of the TRs recruit an assortment of coregulatory proteins that can participate in ligand-independent transcription regulation and/or modify the hormone-dependent transcriptional properties of the E/F domain (see below) [48–51]. This region is also a target of a variety of phosphorylation events that modulate TR function [52]. Interestingly, the (A/B) domain of many nuclear receptors appears to posses little inherent secondary or tertiary structure but is thought

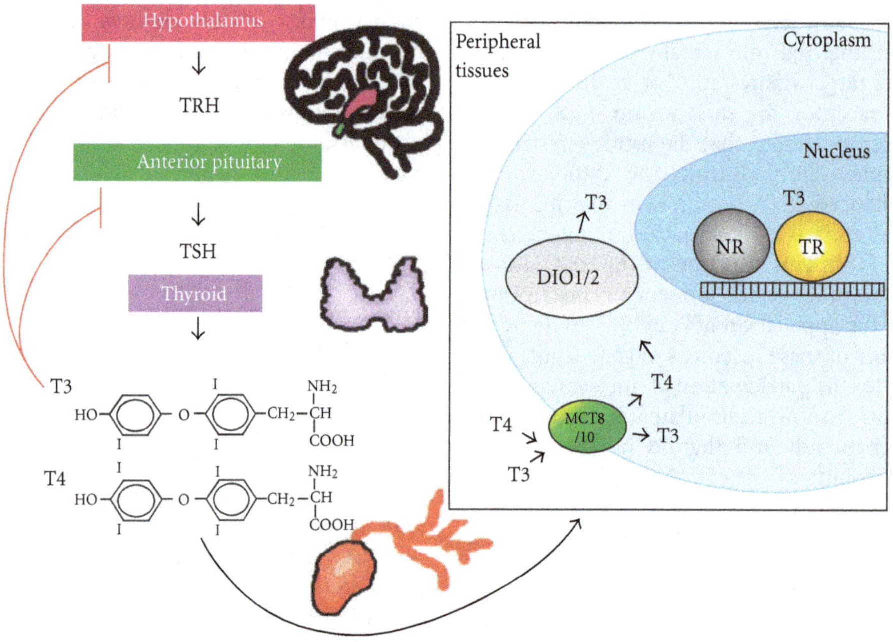

FIGURE 1: Regulation of thyroid hormone synthesis and activity. TRH is produced in the hypothalamus (shown in pink) and stimulates the anterior pituitary (shown in green) to create TSH, which stimulates the follicular cells of the thyroid gland (purple) to produce T3 and T4. T3 and T4 circulate through the blood to the peripheral tissues (see box at right), where they are transported across the cell membrane into the cytoplasm by MCT8/MCT10 (green oval). T4 can be converted to T3 by deiodinase type 1 and deiodinase type 2 (DIO1/2, gray sphere). Both T3 and T4 can enter the nucleus and regulate TR activity. TR is shown here as a yellow sphere bound to DNA. On most sites, TRs can dimerize, either as homodimers or as heterodimers, with another nuclear receptor partner (NR, dark gray sphere).

instead to assume more ordered conformations on interaction with other proteins; it has been suggested that this induced fit phenomenon allows the (A/B) domain to adapt to different coregulators and to different cellular environments [53–57].

2.2.2. The "C" Domain. The "C" domain in TRs, in common with virtually all other nuclear receptors, is comprised of two, highly conserved α-helical domains that are oriented and stabilized through interactions with coordinated zinc atoms [58–61]. The first α-helix tucks into the major groove of DNA and interacts intimately with a cognate hexanucleotide sequence on the DNA [62–64] (Figure 2). The most crucial base-specific contacts are made by the "P-box" amino acids within this first α-helix, and nuclear receptors with different P-box amino acids recognize different hexanucleotide sequences [65–67]. TRs possess an EGKG P-box and bind most tightly to consensus AGGTCA DNA sequences *in vitro* but can recognize a variety of variations on this theme; the presence of nonconsensus sequences in nature are likely to contribute to the specificity of target gene recognition by TRs *in vivo* [68].

The second α-helix in the "C" domain lies orthogonal to the first α-helix and stabilizes the receptor-DNA interaction through both direct and water-mediated contacts with the DNA phosphodiester backbone [60]. Amino acids within or flanking the second a-helix (the D-box) also can serve

as a receptor dimerization interface [60, 69]. In fact TRs can bind to DNA as receptor monomers, homodimers, or heterodimers with retinoid X receptors (RXRs) or other members of the nuclear receptor family [70–74]. The best characterized TR DNA binding sites ("thyroid hormone response elements" or TREs) consist of two hexanucleotide sequences (half-sites) and bind a TR-TR or TR-RXR receptor dimer. The sequence, orientation, and spacing of the half-sites all contribute to proper TR recognition. In TRs, the second α-helix is followed by a short, flexible loop of amino acids and a third α-helix; this "C-terminal extension" helix both makes additional dimerization contacts and can contact the minor groove of the DNA, permitting recognition of an extended DNA sequence that includes bases 5′ to the historically defined hexanucleotide half-site [61, 75]. In addition to its role in DNA binding, the "C" domain also represents a docking surface for several known coregulatory proteins [76].

2.2.3. The "D" Domain. The "D" domain is thought to act as a flexible linker joining together the more conformationally and evolutionarily constrained "C" and "E/F" domains. TRs can recognize a surprising variety of half-site orientations, and the receptor "D" domain has been proposed to provide the rotational flexibility to accommodate the necessary twists and turns [70–74]. Consistent with this concept, different crystal structures of TR reveal different structural options for

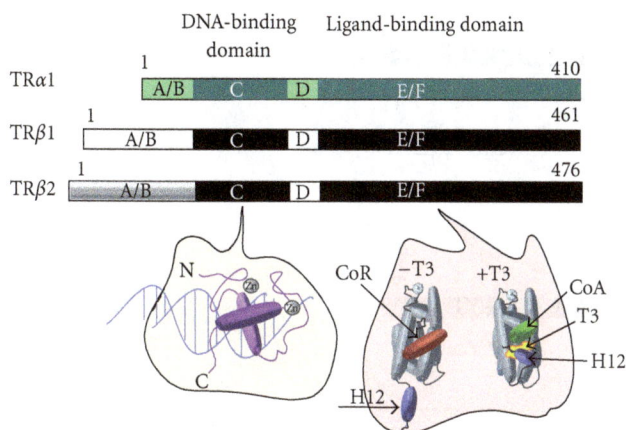

FIGURE 2: Domain comparison of different TR isoforms and schematic of DNA- and ligand-binding domain crystal structures. Each TR isoform is represented as a horizontal bar, from N to C termini. Total amino acid length is indicated at right [35, 36]. Within a given isoform, the location of each domain is lettered (A/B, C, D, and E/F). Identical domains of TRβ1 and TRβ2 are shown in matching colors. Note the unique A/B domain of TRβ2. Below left depicts the structure of the TR DNA-binding domain. α-helical domains are represented as purple cylinders and coordinating zinc atoms (Zn) as silver spheres. Below right depicts two conformations (−T3 and +T3) of the TR ligand-binding domain, which is composed of 12 α helices; the 12th helix (dark blue cylinder, labeled "H12") contains the ligand-dependent activation domain. In the −T3 conformation, helix 12 is in an extended position and the corepressor binding groove is filled with the CoRNR-box helical motifs found in SMRT and NCoR (red cylinder, labeled "CoR"). In the +T3 conformation, helix 12 has rotated to close around T3 hormone ligand (shown in yellow), and a novel docking surface for the LXXLL motifs of a transcriptional coactivator has formed (green cylinder, labeled "CoA").

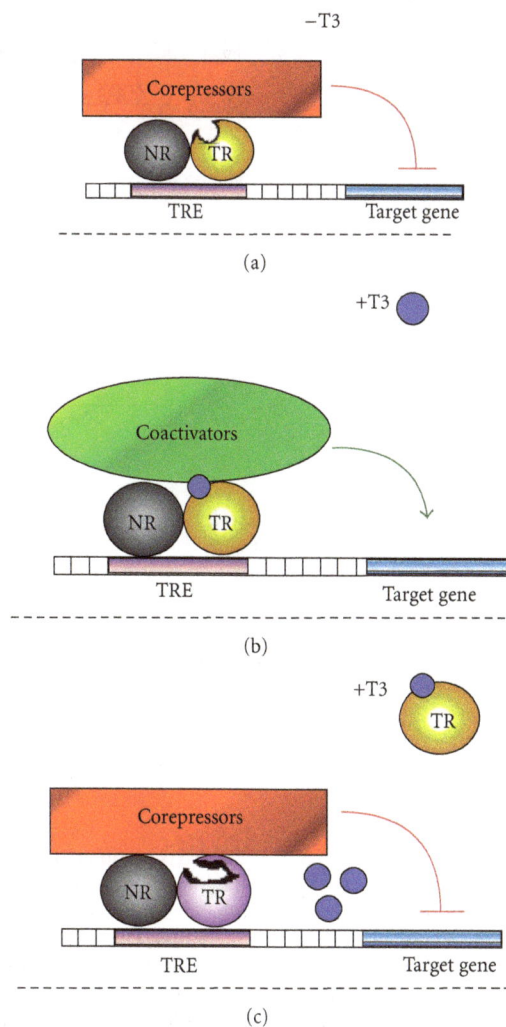

FIGURE 3: Transcriptional activity of wild-type and dominant-negative TRs. (a) In the absence of T3, wild-type TR (orange sphere plus a grey homo- or heterodimer partner) binds to thyroid hormone response elements (TREs-, shown as pink rectangle on DNA), recruits a cohort of corepressor proteins (shown as a red rectangle), and represses transcription of a given target gene (blue rectangle). (b) In the presence of T3 (dark blue sphere), wild-type TRs undergo a conformational change and exchange corepressor proteins for coactivators (green oval) to activate transcription of a target gene. (c) Dominant-negative TR mutants (shown here as a disfigured lavender sphere) have defects in hormone binding, corepressor release, or coactivator recruitment and consequently repress transcription even in the presence of hormone and other wild-type TRs.

the "D" domain, either a flexible loop or a short α-helix, as it exists from the "C" domain [77]. The "D" domain also possesses key nuclear localization motifs and can participate in recruitment of several regulatory proteins, either alone or in conjunction with the other nuclear receptor domains [77–80].

2.2.4. The "E/F" Domain. The "E/F" domain of TRs binds the thyroid hormone. It also forms a second receptor dimerization surface and is a major site of coregulator interaction (Figure 2). Although less than 35% sequence identity is conserved among the "E/F" domains of different nuclear receptors, structural analysis reveals a highly shared canonical architecture composed of a triple laminate of α-helices surrounding a variable-sized hollow pocket lined with hydrophobic residues (Figure 2) [81–88]. This pocket varies in size and shape for different nuclear receptors, thereby defining their ligand specificity. A C-terminal α-helix (denoted helix 12 or H12) exists from this triple helical stack and forms a short, pivoting structure that can adopt different conformations depending on presence and character of the hormone ligand. Binding to hormone induces a "mouse-trap mechanism" whereby portions of the "E/F" domain constrict

around the hormone, and H12 swings shut to close off the pocket [81, 89].

These hormone-driven conformational changes are the principal means by which ligand regulates TR-mediated transcriptional regulation (Figure 3). For example, the TR "E/F" domain possess a hydrophobic surface groove composed of portions of helices H3, H4, and H5 [90]. In the absence of hormone, this surface groove can interact with

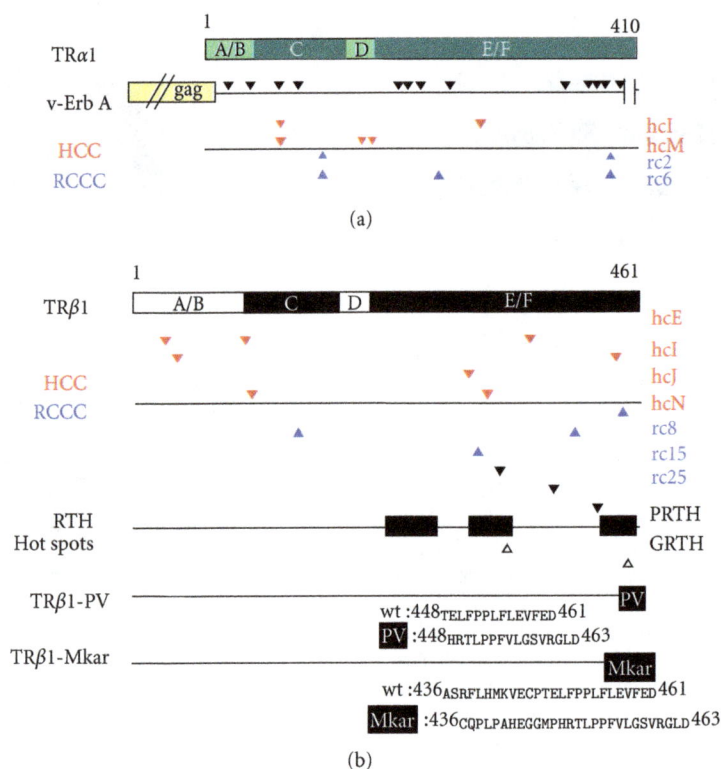

FIGURE 4: Oncogenic- and RTH-associated mutations in different TR isoforms. (a) A schematic of wild-type TRα1 is shown as a horizontal bar as in Figure 1; beneath, horizontal lines depict v-Erb A and several representative HCC/RCCC TRα1 mutants. As a result of fusion of retroviral gag-sequences, the N-terminus of v-erb A is 12 amino acids shorter than TRα1. V-erb A's 13 mutations are indicated by black arrowheads. From left to right, they are R24H, Y44C, G73S, K90T, K186R, P191L, P203L, K233N, T342S, P363S, T370A, C378Y, and F395S. A 9 amino-acid C-terminal deletion is indicated by vertical lines. All mutations and deletions are in relation to the avian TRα1 sequence [24]. Under the schematic for v-Erb A, red and blue arrowheads indicate mutations found in representative HCC and RCCC mutants, respectively, [37–39]. The nomenclature for each mutant is provided at the far right of the figure. For HCC, these mutants are hcI-TRα1 (K74E, A264V) and hcM-TRα1 (K74R, M150T, and E159K). For RCCC, these mutants are rc2-TRα1 (I116N and M388I) and rc6-TRα1 (I116N, A225T, and M388I). (b) A schematic of wild-type TRβ1 is shown as a horizontal bar as in Figure 1; beneath, horizontal lines depict several representative HCC/RCCC TRβ mutants, RTH hot spots, and the RTH mutant, TRβ1-PV. As above, red and blue arrowheads indicate representative mutations found in HCC and RCCC [37–39]. For HCC, these mutants are hcE-TRβ1 (M32I, C107R, and T368N), hcI-TRβ1 (S43L, C446R), hcJ-TRβ1 (M313I), and hcN-TRβ1 (K113N and T329P). For RCCC, these mutants are rc8-TRβ1 (F451S), rc15-TRβ1 (K155E, K411E), and rc25-TRβ1 (Y321H). Below the schematic for HCC/RCCC mutants, the locations of RTH hot spots are shown (amino acids 234–282, 310–353, and 429–460 [36]). Representative mutants for PRTH are: R338L, R383H, and R429Q. For GRTH, these mutations are G345S and P453S. The TRβ1-PV mutant has undergone a C-insertion at codon 448 that results in a frameshift at the C-terminus of the receptor [40]. The location of the 16 new PV-specific amino acids is indicated by a black box on the TRβ1-PV schematic, and the identities of these amino acids (and their wild-type TRβ1 counterparts) are shown below. The TRβ1-Mkar mutant has a T insertion at codon 436 that results in a frameshift at the C-terminus of the receptor. The locations of these new 28 amino acids are indicated by a black box on the TRβ1-Mkar schematic, and their identities are shown below. Note that Mkar shares with PV the amino acid sequence from codons 448 to 463 [41].

CoRNR-box helical motifs found in the SMRT and NCoR family of corepressors, resulting in recruitment of these corepressors. The corepressors, in turn, recruit deacetylases and additional histone modifiers that, by altering the chromatin template, lead to repression of transcription [91–94]. The reorientation of H12 that occurs in response to binding of hormone agonist occludes this corepressor docking surface, releasing corepressor and simultaneously forming a novel docking surface for the LXXLL motifs that are found in many transcriptional coactivators, such as SRC1 [90, 95–99]

(Figure 2). These coactivators typically possesess associated histone acetyl and methyl transferase activities that, by appropriately modifying the chromatin, enhance transcription. Other coactivators include the Mediator complex (which helps recruit the general transcriptional machinery) and ATP-dependent chromatin remodelers (which regulate nucleosomal packaging). Differences in the shape and size of the hormone ligand can operate the H12 conformational toggle switch in different fashions; hormone antagonists, for example, induce H12 conformations that further stabilize corepressor binding and/or destabilize coactivator binding [100–102].

Although this H12-driven mechanism by which TRs bind corepressors in the absence of hormone and release corepressors and bind coactivators on binding to T3 is the best worked out paradigm (Figure 3), a substantial number of genes are regulated by TRs in the inverse fashion (activated in the absence and repressed in the presence of T3) [103–105]. Additional genes appear to be constitutively regulated up or down by TRs in a hormone-independent manner [37]. The precise basis for this diversity in the transcriptional response is incompletely understood, but it presumably reflects mechanisms by which the nature of the DNA binding site, and/or the presence of additional transcription factors on the target gene, can alter coregulator recruitment or function. It should be noted that thyroid hormone receptors not only operate as transcription factors but also mediate nonnuclear effects by interacting with other proteins; although not the focus of this review, this aspect of TR function will arise again in our discussion of the TRβ-PV mutant (Figure 4) [106].

3. Diversification of Signal Reception: The TR Isoforms

TRs in humans are encoded by two distinct genetic loci: TRα on chromosome 17 and TRβ on chromosome 3. Alternative splicing and promoter usage produces additional diversity, leading to the synthesis of a series of TR "isoforms," the most studied of which are TRα1, TRβ1, and TRβ2 [35, 106] (Figure 2). All three bind T3 and can modulate expression of target genes in response to this hormone (not all splice variants do so; the TRα2 splice form, e.g., does not bind T3 and appears to mediate a hormone-independent mode of transcriptional regulation [35, 106]). Though virtually all cells express some form of TR, the ratios of the different isoforms vary in different tissue types and during development [106, 107]. TRα1 is expressed in the early stages of embryonic development, and is widely distributed, although particularly abundant in skeletal muscle and brown fat. TRβ1, in contrast, appears later in development and is present at the highest levels in the liver and kidney. TRβ2 is restricted to the pituitary, hypothalamus, sensory cells in the inner ear, and in the cone cells of the retina [35, 106–110].

TR knockout mice have helped delineate each isoform's role in thyroid hormone action. Mice missing the TRα1 isoform, for example, have cardiac abnormalities and lower body temperatures, whereas TR$\beta^{-/-}$ animals have hearing defects and a loss of negative feedback regulation of the hypothalamus/pituitary/thyroid axis (e.g., high T3/T4 and unsuppressed TSH and TRH levels) [111–114]. Of note, mice bearing genetic disruption of all TR isoforms also present with high circulating T3/T4 and unsuppressed TSH levels (apparently due to the loss of TRβ2 in the hypothalamus and pituitary) but otherwise display fewer systemic abnormalities than do the TRβ-specific isoform knockouts. Presumably the loss of the peripheral TRα1 and TRβ1 response in these combined knockout mice renders them resistant to the otherwise detrimental effects of their elevated T3/T4

levels [115, 116]. In fact, chemically or genetically induced hypothyroidism also presents as a much more severe syndrome than does the TRα/TRβ combined receptor knockout, indicating that the presence of unliganded TRs is more disruptive physiologically than is the complete lack of TR function. Taken as a whole, these genetic studies indicate that the different isoforms mediate both shared, and specific physiological and developmental functions and that TRs play major biological roles even in the absence of T3.

Although there appears to be significant overlap between the target genes regulated by the different TR isoforms, the detailed transcriptional response on a given gene can differ for each isoform [37, 117, 118]. For example, TRα1 can induce expression of certain genes more strongly than does TRβ1, whereas these isoforms confer nearly equal activity on other genes [37]. Similarly, TRβ2 fails to repress and instead activates certain genes under T3 conditions that confer repression by TRβ1 or TRα1 [50, 119–122]. These gene- and isoform-specific transcriptional responses are likely to reflect differences in the coregulatory factors that are recruited by each isoform once bound to a given target gene.

4. A Failed Response: TR Mutations and Resistance to Thyroid Hormone (RTH) Syndrome

Circulating T3/T4 levels are tightly controlled by a negative feedback loop wherein surges of thyroid hormone bind to TRs in the hypothalamus and pituitary, which then suppress TRH and TSH production and, as a consequence, repress further release of T3/T4 (Figure 1). Production of too much or too little thyroid hormone causes a number of clinically important endocrine disorders. In Graves' disease, for example, a hyperstimulated thyroid overproduces T3 leading to cardiac abnormalities, palpitations, fatigue, weight loss, dyspnea, myxedema, and muscle wasting [123, 124]. Conversely, insufficient T3 (hypothyroidism) produces depression, weight gain, edema, thickened speech, reduced cognition, cold intolerance, and, in a neonate, cretinism (a disorder marked by retarded physical and mental development) [124–126].

The consequences of over- or underproduction of circulating T3/T4 had been recognized for over a century when Refetoff et al., in 1967, reported an intriguing paradox in a study of two siblings with goiter, short stature, deafness, mutism, and bone deformations [127]. Although these symptoms shared several characteristics with hypothyroidism, both patients had high concentrations of thyroid hormone in the blood. Refetoff et al. suggested that the patients' tissues might be deficient in their ability to sense T3 and coined the phrase "Resistance to Thyroid Hormone (RTH) Syndrome: [127, 128]. This was soon confirmed and, since then, RTH syndrome has been recognized as an autosomal dominant genetic disease that affects approximately 1 in 40,000 people worldwide [36, 129].

The vast majority of RTH cases have been traced to mutations in the TRβ isoform (Figure 4) [130–134]. As of 2010, at least 137 different RTH-TRβ mutations have been identified, distributed among more than 300 families [36, 128, 135–138]. Despite this genetic diversity, virtually all of these RTH-TRβ mutations appear to share one key property: they encode mutant receptors that function as dominant-negative inhibitors of wild-type TR function [36] (Figure 3). RTH syndrome is, in fact, largely a disease of heterozygotes, and it is believed that RTH-TR mutant receptors interfere with normal T3 signaling by competing with the wild-type TRs expressed in the same cells from the unaffected TR alleles. Only two cases of patients homozygous/hemizygous for the TRβ mutation have been published: one was the product of a cousin marriage, and the other was born to a mother with goiter and a father of indeterminable genotype [139, 140].

RTH-TRβ mutants can interfere with both wt TRα1 and wt TRβ1 functions and are likely to mediate both isoform-specific and nonspecific effects *in vivo*, depending on the tissue and on the target gene. Interestingly, no RTH mutations have been mapped to TRα in humans, and, when TRβ RTH mutations are artificially targeted to TRα1 in mice, they do not produce RTH but generate instead a distinct slew of neoplastic and metabolic defects [141–145]. Although less frequently cataloged, and presenting with distinct symptoms, genetic defects in the MCT8 transporter, or in the incorporation of selenocysteines into the active sites of deiodinases, can also lead to defects in thyroid hormone signaling [36, 44]. This paper, however, will focus on RTH syndromes that arise due to lesions in the TRβ gene.

The genetic lesions responsible for RTH syndrome cluster in several "hot spots" mapping within the "D" and "E/F" domains of TRβ and result in defects in the hormone-driven release of corepressors and acquisition of coactivators (Figure 4) [79, 146–149]. In many cases, these mutations map to the hormone binding pocket and impair or eliminate the ability of the RTH-TRβ mutant to bind T3/T4 [36]. Although somewhat more rare, additional RTH mutants have been identified that retain a near wild-type affinity for T3/T4 but are defective in the conformational machinery that couples hormone binding to corepressor release and/or coactivator recruitment [150]. For example, proline 453 in TRβ1 is an important pivot on which H12 reorients in response to hormone agonist (Figure 4). Different amino acid substitutions at P453 have been identified in multiple human RTH syndrome kindreds; RTH-TR mutants bearing these substitutions retain significant T3 binding, but nonetheless exhibit defects in corepressor release, presumably due to a failure of H12 to properly reorient in response to bound hormone [151–155].

It is important to note that the symptoms of RTH syndrome are not identical to those of either a homozygous or heterozygous null mutation of TRβ. Instead it is the ability of the RTH syndrome TRβ mutants to function as dominant-negatives that plays a critical role in producing the disease phenotype. Is it the failure of the mutant TRβ to release corepressor, or to bind coactivator, that leads to this dominant-negative phenotype? In most RTH mutants tested, experimental inhibition of corepressor binding by biochemical or genetic manipulation reduces dominant-negative activity [150, 156]. Consistent with these findings,

RTH patients with TR mutants that interact weakly with corepressors generally have more minimal disease symptoms than those with a strong corepressor interaction [157]. Nonetheless, a defect in coactivator binding (rather than in corepressor release) represents the primary defect in at least one RTH-TR mutant [147] and appears to contribute to the dominant-negative phenotype exerted by several other RTH-TR mutants (see Pituitary Resistance, below). It is also important to note that there are multiple forms of corepressor, and RTH mutants can display alterations in corepressor selectivity, rather than global defects in corepressor release. For example, NCoR and SMRT are closely related corepressor paralogs found in many cells. Wild-type TRs preferentially interact with NCoR, whereas the Mkar RTH mutant of TRβ (representing a C-terminal frame shift mutation), significantly reduces NCoR binding, but results in an increase in the SMRT interaction (Figure 4) [41]. NCoR and SMRT also undergo alternative mRNA splicing, and several RTH-TRβ mutants differ from wtTRβs in their ability to bind to these different corepressor splice variants [38, 158, 159]. This point will be addressed again in our discussion of oncogenic versions of TR (below).

5. Different Paths to Resistance: Generalized versus Pituitary RTH Disease

RTH has been divided clinically into two main subtypes, generalized (GRTH) versus pituitary (PRTH) [118, 130, 160–164]. GRTH is characterized by a broad insensitivity to thyroid hormone; as a result GRTH patients display some characteristics suggestive of hypothyroidism (e.g., short stature, goiter, and hearing impairments, reflecting an impaired T3 hormone response in peripheral tissues) but also have inappropriately high circulating levels of T3 and T4 and nonsuppressed TSH (a consequence of a loss of negative feedback in the hypothalamus/pituitary/thyroid gland axis) [35]. In essence, GRTH patients make more T3 and T4 than normal, but "do not know it," and present in some fashion as if they make too little. In contrast, in PRTH patients, negative feedback sensing in the hypothalamus/pituitary/thyroid gland is selectively impaired (resulting in high levels of circulated T3/T4), whereas the peripheral tissue response remains relatively intact (resulting in symptoms of hyperthyroidism, such as cardiac palpitations, heat intolerance, and nervousness) [35, 165, 166]. Thus, PRTH patients make too much T3 and T4, and "do know it," often to the point of peripheral thyrotoxicity.

These subtypes are not completely discrete: a given mutation can manifest as either GRTH or PRTH in different individuals, or within a given individual at different times [36]. Nonetheless certain RTH mutations are more often associated with one or the other form of disease, an observation that has been recently confirmed in a mouse knock-in model of PRTH syndrome [167]. Notably, the mutations most often associated with GRTH typically map to amino acid substitutions in the hormone binding or pivot/H12 domains of TRβ and can be explained conceptually through their potential to interfere with hormone binding, corepressor release, or coactivator recruitment. In contrast, the most extensively characterized PRTH mutations map to a set of three arginines that form charged clusters on the surface of the TR "E" domain. In normal TRs, these arginines have been implicated in stabilizing the overall conformation of the "E/F" domain and also as important contacts in receptor homodimerization [168, 169].

Several explanations have been advanced for how PRTH mutations might impair T3 negative feedback in the hypothalamus/pituitary/thyroid axis while sparing the T3 response in the peripheral tissues. One proposal focuses on the observations that (a) TRβ1 forms homodimers more efficiently than does TRβ2, (b) TR homodimers recruit corepressors more efficiently than do TR/RXR heterodimers, and (c) many PRTH mutations impair homodimerization but retain the ability to form heterodimers with RXRs [94, 167, 170–177]. By this scenario, the diminished homodimerization properties of the PRTH mutants would favor TR-mediated activation over TR-mediated repression, resulting in a loss of repression of T3 synthesis in the hypothalamus and pituitary (producing increases in circulating T3 levels), yet enhancing T3-mediated positive gene regulation, resulting in the symptoms of peripheral thyrotoxicity characteristic of PRTH.

Alternatively, it is known that the hypothalamus and pituitary express primarily the TRβ2 splice form, whereas most peripheral tissues, such as liver, muscles, and kidneys, express primarily TRβ1 [35, 106, 178–183]. TRβ2 displays an enhanced ability to respond to T3 than does TRβ1, a phenomenon that may permit the hypothalamus and pituitary to sense, and suppress, surges of T3 before these elevated hormone levels saturate the more widely distributed TRβ1 isoforms [122, 184]. TRβ1 and TRβ2 share the same "C," "D," and "E/F" domains, and so RTH mutations are expressed as both splice forms. We have suggested that PRTH mutations have a more severe impact on the T3 response of TRβ2 compared to their impact on TRβ1, resulting in an increase in thyroid hormone levels (due to the impaired TRβ2-mediated negative feedback response in the hypothalamus/pituitary) while nonetheless conferring a thyrotoxic effect in peripheral tissues (mediated by the less-impaired TRβ1 splice form) [122]. As is most often the case with competing scientific theories, it is likely that both models play a role in the actual genesis of PRTH disease.

6. A Still Darker Side to Aberrant T3 Sensing: TRs and Their Mutations in Oncogenesis

In an ironic twist of history, TRs were linked to cancer before they were ever recognized as endocrine receptors. The avian erythroblastosis retrovirus (AEV) was first identified in 1935 as a retrovirus that could induce erythroleukemias and fibrosarcomas in infected chickens [185]. By the early 1980s it was realized that the oncogenic proclivities of AEV mapped to two viral oncogenes, v-Erb A and v-Erb B, that worked together to induce oncogenic transformation [186–188]. In 1986, v-Erb A was shown to be

a retrovirally acquired, mutated version of avian TRα1 (Figure 4) [24, 25], establishing the precedent that mutated versions of TR can participate in the initiation or progression of oncogenesis. Mutated versions of TRs have been subsequently linked to hepatocellular carcinoma (HCC), renal clear cell carcinoma (RCCC), pituitary adenomas, and thyroid malignancies (Figure 4) [189–192]. Conversely, wt TRs can function as tumor suppressors, and loss of wt TR expression has been associated with these and other tumors [193]. We will discuss these malignancies in turn.

6.1. V-Erb A. Acutely transforming retroviruses cause neoplasia by acquiring, mutating, and inappropriately expressing host cell genes involved in the control of normal cell proliferation or differentiation. AEV represents a model by which two virally acquired cell genes, v-Erb A and v-Erb B, cooperate to induce neoplasia [187, 194–196]. V-Erb B is a mutated version of the avian epidermal growth factor (EGF) receptor, a cell surface tyrosine kinase that induces a cascade of mitogenic signals in response to extracellular EGF [188, 197]. Through loss of its extracellular regulatory and C-terminal domain, compounded by internal point mutations, v-Erb B has acquired a constitutive kinase activity that can induce proliferation of immature erythroid cells and fibroblasts even in the absence of EGF. V-Erb A is, as noted above, a mutated version of chicken TRα1. However, in contrast to the constitutive activation seen for v-Erb B, the mutations in v-Erb A have turned the latter into a constitutive repressor [198–201]. V-Erb A cooperates with v-Erb B in oncogenesis by suppressing differentiation of AEV-infected erythroid cells and by promoting the growth and life span of AEV-infected fibroblasts.

The basis of the dominant-negative activity of v-Erb A is obvious on inspection: the H12 helix toggle switch critical for corepressor release and coactivator recruitment by the wt TRα1 is deleted from the v-Erb A coding region (Figure 4) [24, 25]. In addition to this C-terminal deletion, v-Erb A has sustained a fusion at its N-terminus with sequences derived from the retroviral "gag" protein and 13 internal amino acid substitutions (Figure 4) [24, 25]. Several of these substitutions map to the hormone binding pocket, virtually abolishing the ability to bind T3 and further favoring corepressor over coactivator binding, whereas others map to the "A/B" and "C" domains.

Thus, in many ways, one would expect v-Erb A to operate as a particularly virulent version of an RTH mutant. Why then does v-Erb A function in neoplasia, whereas the RTH mutants induce primarily endocrine disorders? Neither the avian origin nor the TRα1 isoform backbone of v-Erb A fully explains this phenomenon. Instead, the acquisition of oncogenesis by v-Erb A appears to result in large part from changes in its DNA recognition domains. V-Erb A has sustained two amino acid substitutions within the P- and D-boxes of the "C" domain that play crucial roles in DNA binding specificity, as well as two additional amino acid substitutions in the "A/B" domain that can modify

DNA recognition by the adjacent "C" domain [202]. As a consequence, v-Erb A possesses an altered specificity for artificial DNA response elements *in vitro* compared to wt TRα1 and an altered target gene specificity in transfected cells [196, 203–207]. It is likely that the oncogenic properties of v-Erb A reflect these changes in DNA recognition, permitting the viral protein to target a distinct set of "neoplastic" genes that differ from the "endocrine" genes normally targeted by TRα1. These novel v-Erb A targets may include those regulated by other nuclear receptors (such as retinoic acid receptor), or by other, nonreceptor transcription factors [194]. Consistent with this proposal, replacement of portions of the "C" domain of v-Erb A with the corresponding wt TRα1 sequences severely inhibits oncogenic transformation by AEV [208]. It should be noted that these DNA binding domain mutations probably work together with the other mutations in v-Erb A that favor repression by deleting H12, inhibiting T3 binding, enhancing homodimer formation, and widening the ability of v-Erb A to bind to both SMRT and NCoR forms of corepressor [205].

6.2. Hepatocellular Carcinoma.
The neoplastic properties of v-Erb A were viewed as an obscure tidbit of avian retrovirology exotica until eerily analogous TR mutants were discovered in a variety of human tumors. The first among these was human hepatocellular carcinoma (HCC). Worldwide, HCC ranks 5th out of all neoplasias for number of cases and third for number of deaths [209]. HCC can manifest as a medley of symptoms, including upper abdominal pain, weakness, weight loss, and jaundice [210]. Infection with hepatitis B or C virus is one of the major risk factors for HCC, along with cirrhosis, and exposure to aflatoxin, a highly mutagenic fungal compound often found in stores of contaminated grains or nuts [211].

Though the risk factors for HCC are known, the molecular mechanisms responsible for subsequent tumor initiation and progression are not fully understood. Alterations in a variety of tumor suppressors and oncogenes have been identified in HCC, as have a variety of chromosomal losses, gains, and translocations [212–216]. Most provocatively for the topic of this paper, however, is that TR mutants have been identified at high incidence in both HCC cell lines and in solid tumors [189, 217]. One study found that 65% of examined tumors had mutations in TRα and 76% had mutations in TRβ, with a significant subgroup of these tumors bearing mutations in both loci [189].

The HCC-TR mutants, when analyzed, resemble in many of their properties the RTH paradigm: they are impaired for transcriptional activation, many display defects in T3-driven corepressor release and/or coactivator binding, and the majority can function as dominant negative inhibitors of wild-type receptor activity in reporter gene assays (Figure 4) [39]. Unlike RTH syndrome, however, the TR mutations in HCC are not inherited, but instead arise *de novo* during the progression of the HCC tumors [189]. Also in stark contrast to RTH syndrome, the vast majority of HCC-TR mutants

analyzed had sustained two or more genetic lesions, with at least one lesion located so as to impact DNA recognition (i.e., in the "A/B" or "C" domains). Indeed, two of the HCC-TR mutants studied were able to bind *in vitro* to DNA sequences not recognized by the wild-type receptors [39].

This suite of molecular defects suggested a potential role for these HCC-TR mutants in the mismanagement of transcription of genes not normally under T3 regulation. Gene expression analysis of hepatoma cell lines expressing specific HCC-TR mutants confirmed this supposition by demonstrating that these mutants regulate a distinct set of genes from that regulated by the corresponding wild-type receptors [37]. Analysis of the HCC-TR target gene set revealed several provocative features. A subset of genes normally regulated by wt TRs were not targeted by the HCC-TR mutants tested; conversely, the HCC-TR mutants regulated a panel of novel genes that were not targets of wt TR regulation. Several genes were targeted by each of the HCC-TR mutants, such as AGR2, DKK1, CDC7AL, and SLC2A2 and were repressed in both the absence and presence of hormone compared to the wild-type receptors [37]. Interestingly, HCC-TR target genes included not only genes that were constitutively repressed by the mutant receptors, as expected from prior reporter gene assays, but also genes that were constitutively activated, including GNG12, GPC3, and KCNAB2 [37]. At least several of these aberrantly regulated genes have been previously implicated in cancer [37]. Therefore, although the TR mutations associated with HCC appear to impede the ability of the receptor to respond to T3, they do not necessarily prevent the receptor from mediating hormone-independent transcriptional effects, both down and up.

Although the role of many of the HCC target genes in oncogenesis remains to be determined, it was notable that the HCC-TR mutants gained the ability to activate several genes known to play proproliferative roles (CSF1, NRCAM, and CX3CR1) and to repress several genes known to function as tumor suppressors (DKK1, TIMP3). Conversely, several potential proproliferative genes repressed by wt TRs were not repressed by the HCC-TR mutant (e.g., GPC3, expression of which has been linked to cell proliferation in liver), and several potential tumor suppressor genes activated by wt TR were not activated by the HCC-TR mutant (e.g., TIMP3) [37].

These findings further extended the conceptual model first put forward for v-Erb A: TR mutants associated with disease act, at least in part, as dominant-negative inhibitors of normal TR action. In the absence of any additional changes, these TR mutants can cause endocrine disorders such as RTH syndrome. Acquisition of yet-additional lesions that impact the DNA recognition domains of the receptor, as observed for v-Erb A and for the HCC-TR mutants described above, appears to unleash a previously cryptic oncogenic function in the TRs, permitting the mutant receptors to extend their regulatory reach to genes capable of contributing to leukemogenesis and hepatocellular carcinogenesis. Drawing this conceptual link between v-Erb A and the HCC-TR mutants tantalizingly closer, systemic expression of v-Erb A in transgenic mice under a β-actin promoter results in a high incidence of HCC [218].

Given the evidence that multiply mutated TRs contribute to multiple neoplastic diseases, are there other forms of cancer in which TRs might play a role? To address this question, we next turn our discussion to renal clear cell carcinomas.

7. The Internist's Tumor: Renal Cell Carcinoma (RCCC)

RCC accounts for ~3% of all adult malignant diseases [219]. In men, it is the 7th most commonly occurring cancer; in women, it is the 9th [220]. Once known as "the internist's tumor" for its ability to produce an assortment of internal maladies and symptoms (flank pain, blood in the urine, fever, and palatable abdominal masses, to name a few), RCC actually encompasses a diverse assortment of tumor subtypes [221]. The most common of these subtypes (~75–80%) is of the clear cell variety and is abbreviated RCCC (or ccRCC) [219]. The name is derived from the appearance of the cytoplasm after histological prep of cancer tissue: high lipid content results in a clear solution [219]. Risk factors for RCC include tobacco use, high body mass index, and hypertension [219, 222–226]. Though methods of detecting renal tumors have improved in recent years, worldwide incidence and mortality rates are on the rise [220]. Metastatic RCC is highly resistant to conventional treatments (chemotherapy, radiation, and hormone therapy) and survival outcomes after diagnosis are typically less than one year [220, 227]. Though understanding the molecular basis of this disease has greatly advanced treatment options, therapy-refractory tumors typically develop 6–15 months after initial clinical intervention [228].

Approximately 80% of RCCCs bear inactivating mutations in the von Hippel Lindau gene (*VHL*) [229]. *VHL* encodes the targeting component of an E3 ubiquitin ligase complex, which marks the hypoxia inducible factor (HIF) for degradation. Normally, HIF functions as an oxygen-sensing transcription factor; under hypoxic conditions it activates an array of genes involved in the formation of new blood vessels [230–232]. When VHL is inactivated, HIF accumulates and proangiogenic factors are transcribed unchecked; this contributes to the highly vascular tumors characteristic of RCCC [233]. Additionally, VHL has been implicated in spindle misorientation and chromosome instability; a defective VHL protein may, therefore, drive formation of additional tumor-promoting mutations [234]. In RCCCs with this genetic root, one defective *VHL* allele is typically inherited, and the other is deleted or mutated somatically.

Although VHL inactivation is considered the predominant molecular change associated with development of RCCC, it alone is not sufficient to cause cancer in mice [235, 236]. It is likely that VHL inactivation serves as the first step towards tumorigenesis and that additional steps, or "hits," are required for tumor progression [237]. In fact, an intriguing diversity of TR mutations, deletions, and aberrant mRNA expression patterns have been observed in RCCC. For example, an analysis of 71 RCCC tumors found characteristic deletions at 3p26 and 3p24, which are home to *VHL* and *TRβ*, respectively [238]. Analysis of TR mRNA expression in RCCC tumor tissues revealed a significant reduction of TRβ mRNA in the majority of samples tested (although paradoxically, TRβ mRNA was overexpressed in several samples) [239]. Reduction of TRα mRNA was also observed in several RCCC tumors, although complete loss of the TRα locus on chromosome 17 was rare [238–240]. And, of greatest relevance to the topic of this paper, mutations in both TR isoforms have been identified in ~40% of RCCC tumors examined, in TRα, TRβ, or both [190]. It is therefore likely that defects in TR function can serve as a 2nd hit that triggers, or participates in, the transition from renal cyst to clear cell carcinoma.

Ten different RCCC-TR mutants have been studied in molecular detail [190]. In common with HCC, the majority of these RCCC mutants contain more than one genetic lesion each, with at least one or more of these lesions frequently mapping to the "A/B" or "C" domains; nonetheless, no two identical TR mutations have been isolated to date from the two different forms of neoplasia. The majority of the RCCC-TR mutants tested display hormone binding and coregulator release/acquisition defects *in vitro* and can function as dominant negatives in reporter gene assays (Figure 4) [38]. Several RCCC-TR mutants also display a gain in their specificity for certain splice forms of SMRT and NCoR compared to the wild-type receptor [38]. The multiple genetic lesions carried by a given mutant receptor can work together to contribute to the overall dominant-negative phenotype [38].

Do the mutations in the "A/B" and "C" domains of the RCCC-TR mutants alter their DNA specificity? Consistent with this idea, nuclear extracts from RCCC tumors were found to be impaired in their ability to bind to consensus TREs compared to extracts from wt tissues [190]. Expression array analyses of cells stably transfected with RCCC mutant receptors are in progress to determine if there are changes in target gene specificity (Rosen, Chan, and Privalsky unpublished observations).

8. Thyroid Neoplasia

A third example of an association of a human neoplasia with mutations in the TR loci was revealed by studies of papillary thyroid malignancies. Almost 63% of these malignancies were found to have mutations in TRα, and a remarkable 94% in TRβ; in contrast 22% and 11% of thyroid adenomas bore mutations in these isoforms, respectively, and no mutations were found in normal thyroid controls [191, 241]. This pattern is most consistent with a role of the TR mutants in cancer progression, rather than initiation. Further analysis demonstrated that the majority of these mutated TRs lost transcriptional activation function and displayed dominant-negative activity when coexpressed with their normal TR counterparts [191, 241]. Many, but not all, of these mutants contained multiple genetic lesions, with one tumor possessing 5 different lesions within a single TRβ1 allele and another possessing 6 in TRα1 and 2 in TRβ1 [191]. In many of these mutants, lesions included at least one mutation within the "A/B" or "C" domains. The effects of these mutations on DNA binding *in vitro*, or target gene specificity in cells, have not been reported.

9. Potential Cracks in the Wall Separating RTH Syndrome from HCC, RCC, and Thyroid Malignancy

The narrative to this point may have led the unwary reader to the conclusion that the absence or presence of DNA binding domain mutations determines if a given dominant-negative TR mutant induces endocrine or neoplastic disease. However, there is some evidence that this phenomenon may not be absolute. Although not associated with overt neoplasia, RTH-TR mutations in humans often lead to goiter, a nonneoplastic hyperplasia of the thyroid gland in response to the loss of T3/T4 feedback regulation. Further, a very strong dominant-negative RTH-TRβ mutant, denoted PV and representing a frameshift at the C-terminus of the receptor, causes not only severe disruption of the pituitary-thyroid axis and goiter, but also TSH-omas, and metastatic follicular thyroid carcinoma in homozygous-mutant mice [40, 242–245]. The "A/B" and "C" domains of the PV mutant are fully wild type in sequence (Figure 4), suggesting that strong, dominant-negative RTH-TR mutants may have an inherent oncogenic potential that is rarely displayed in humans (where homozygosity for the RTH mutation is very unusual) but can uncloak when presented with an appropriate opportunity.

Subsequent analysis of the PV/PV mutant mice revealed several mechanisms by which the mutant receptor appears to be mediating oncogenesis; significantly, none of these involved the classic mode of direct binding of the TR mutant receptors to DNA [163]. The PV mutant was found to heterodimerize with, and inhibit, another member of the nuclear receptor family, peroxisome proliferator-activated receptor-γ, removing an antiproliferative signal [246, 247]. Many nuclear receptors exert nongenomic functions outside of the nucleus, and the PV mutant also induced one of these: the phosphatidyl-inositol 3 kinase/AKT pathway [248, 249]. The PV mutant also makes protein-protein interactions with β-catenin and pituitary tumor transforming gene protein, increasing levels of these proteins by inhibiting their degradation [249–252]. Finally, through protein-protein interactions with the CREB transcription factor, the PV-TRβ mutant was able to induce cyclin D1 [245]. These PV-TR studies raise the possibility that similar TR signaling pathways, unrelated to DNA recognition *per se*, may also play a role in HCC-TR and RCCC-TR oncogenesis.

10. Ups and Downs of Wild-Type TR Expression in Oncogenesis

The impact of TRs on neoplasia is not restricted to scenarios involving receptor mutants. Wild-type TRs can act as tumor suppressors in many contexts, and losses in wild-type receptor expression appear to precipitate, or otherwise contribute to, several classes of neoplasia. For example, a double knockout of both TRα and TRβ in mice results in a higher incidence of follicular thyroid carcinoma and increased aggressiveness in a skin cancer model [253, 254]. Changes in TRα1 levels have been shown in 49% of human gastric cancers analyzed by immunoblotting [193]. Reduction in TRβ1 levels or changes in subcellular localization have been reported in colorectal cancers [255]. In several cases these changes in TR expression levels were associated with alterations in the restriction pattern of the TR gene, suggesting that loss of expression might reflect an underlying genetic event. In other cases, TR expression appears to be suppressed epigenetically by hypermethylation of the promoter region of the TR gene; for example, biallelic inactivation of TRβ expression by promoter methylation has been found in human breast cancers [192, 256]. Notably, reintroduction of wild-type TRβ into HCC or mammary carcinoma cell lines that have lost endogenous TR expression retards proliferation, results in partial mesenchymal to epithelial transitions, and suppresses invasiveness, extravasation, and metastasis in nude mice [253, 257].

11. Thyroid Hormone Status and Cancer

As noted above, changes in TR expression and function are associated with a wide variety of neoplastic events. Can changes in thyroid hormone levels exert similar effects? Answering this question has proven to be complex and somewhat contentious. In clinical studies, hypothyroidism has been reported to correlate with a lower risk of primary mammary carcinoma and a reduction in progression to invasive disease [258]. Pharmacologically induced hypothyroidism has similarly been reported to yield an improved survival in glioblastoma when used together with tamoxifen [259]. Consistent with hypothyroidism being beneficial, T3 has been reported to induce the proliferation and invasiveness of several types of tumor-derived cells in culture or in xenograft models, including HCC-derived cells [253].

In contrast, however, other studies indicate that low thyroid hormone levels increase the risk of HCC in humans, and high T3/T4 are therapeutic [260]. Dating back to the late 18th century, administration of thyroid extract was often used in conjunction with oophorectomy as a treatment for breast cancer [261–263] though its efficacy was not well established [264]. More recently, T3, operating through TRβ1, has been shown to retard the proliferation, anchorage-independent growth, and invasiveness of mammary cancer cells in culture [265]. Similarly, long-term hypothyroidism in women has been associated with an elevated risk of HCC [266], whereas T3 administration can reduce HCC progression in animal studies [267], and T4 has shown some success in reducing the risk of colorectal cancer [268].

Clearly "results may vary!" It is likely that the impact of thyroid hormone differs in different types of cancer and may control different aspects of the same cancer (proliferation, differentiation, invasion, metastasis, apoptosis, and senescence) differently. For example, the investigators that have shown T3 to be promitogenic in rodent liver have also shown that T3 suppresses formation of preneoplastic nodules in a diethylnitrosamine rat model of HCC; T3 is therefore likely to be exerting both proproliferative and prodifferentiation effects on liver [269]. It is worth noting that T3 also induces both differentiation and proliferation in several other contexts, such as the gut [270]. As is virtually always true in science, more studies will be required to fully reveal all of the intricate web of biological processes regulated by T3 and its receptors.

References

[1] J. D. Wilson and C. Roehrborn, "Long-term consequences of castration in men: lessons from the Skoptzy and the eunuchs of the Chinese and Ottoman courts," *Journal of Clinical Endocrinology and Metabolism*, vol. 84, no. 12, pp. 4324–4331, 1999.

[2] J. Barnes, Ed., *The Complete Works of Aristotle*, Princeton University Press, Princeton, NJ, USA, 1984.

[3] A. Berthold, "Transplantation der Hoden," *Archiv fur Anatomie, Physiologie und Wissenschaftliche*, vol. 16, pp. 42–46, 1849.

[4] G. R. Murray, "Note on the treatment of myxoedema by hypodermic injections of an extract of the thyroid gland of sheep," *British Medical Journal*, vol. 2, p. 796, 1891.

[5] E. Baumann and E. Z. Roos, "übernahm er mit Albrecht Kossel die Leitung von Hoppe-Seylers," *Zeitschrift für Physiologische Chemie*, vol. 21, p. 481, 1895.

[6] R. J. Graves, "Clinical lectures," *London Medical and Surgical Journal*, vol. 7, pp. 516–517, 1835.

[7] E. C. Kendall, "Landmark article, June 19, 1915. The isolation in crystalline form of the compound containing iodin, which occurs in the thyroid. Its chemical nature and physiologic activity. By E.C. Kendall," *Journal of the American Medical Association*, vol. 250, no. 15, pp. 2045–2046, 1983.

[8] E. V. Jensen, *Biological Activities of Steroids in Relation to Cancer*, Academic Press, New York, NY, USA, 1960.

[9] J. I. Macgregor and V. C. Jordan, "Basic guide to the mechanisms of antiestrogen action," *Pharmacological Reviews*, vol. 50, no. 2, pp. 151–196, 1998.

[10] E. V. Jensen, P. I. Brecher, M. Numata, S. Mohla, and E. R. De Sombre, "Transformed estrogen receptor in the regulation of RNA synthesis in uterine nuclei," *Advances in Enzyme Regulation*, vol. 11, pp. 1–16, 1973.

[11] J. R. Tata and C. C. Widnell, "Ribonucleic acid synthesis during the early action of thyroid hormones," *Biochemical Journal*, vol. 98, no. 2, pp. 604–620, 1966.

[12] G. M. Ringold, K. R. Yamamoto, and G. M. Tomkins, "Dexamethasone mediated induction of mouse mammary tumor virus RNA: a system for studying glucocorticoid action," *Cell*, vol. 6, no. 3, pp. 299–305, 1975.

[13] G. M. Ringold, K. R. Yamamoto, J. M. Bishop, and H. E. Varmus, "Glucocorticoid stimulated accumulation of mouse mammary tumor virus RNA: increased rate of synthesis of viral RNA," *Proceedings of the National Academy of Sciences of the United States of America*, vol. 74, no. 7, pp. 2879–2883, 1977.

[14] C. Scheidereit, S. Geisse, H. M. Westphal, and M. Beato, "The glucocorticoid receptor binds to defined nucleotide sequences near the promoter of mouse mammary tumour virus," *Nature*, vol. 304, no. 5928, pp. 749–752, 1983.

[15] F. Payvar, D. DeFranco, and G. L. Firestone, "Sequence-specific binding of glucocorticoid receptor to MTV DNA at sites within and upstream of the transcribed region," *Cell*, vol. 35, pp. 381–392, 1983.

[16] H. H. Samuels and L. E. Shapiro, "Thyroid hormone stimulates de novo growth hormone synthesis in cultured GH cells: evidence for the accumulation of a rate limiting RNA species in the induction process," *Proceedings of the National Academy of Sciences of the United States of America*, vol. 73, no. 10, pp. 3369–3373, 1976.

[17] B. J. Spindler, K. M. MacLeod, J. Ring, and J. D. Baxter, "Thyroid hormone receptors. Binding characteristics and lack of hormonal dependency for nuclear localization," *Journal of Biological Chemistry*, vol. 250, no. 11, pp. 4113–4119, 1975.

[18] S. R. Spindler, S. H. Mellon, and J. D. Baxter, "Growth hormone gene transcription is regulated by thyroid and glucocorticoid hormones in cultured rat pituitary tumor cells," *Journal of Biological Chemistry*, vol. 257, no. 19, pp. 11627–11632, 1982.

[19] A. Pascual, J. Casanova, and H. H. Samuels, "Photoaffinity labeling of thyroid hormone nuclear receptors in intact cells," *Journal of Biological Chemistry*, vol. 257, no. 16, pp. 9640–9647, 1982.

[20] S. M. Hollenberg, C. Weinberger, and E. S. Ong, "Primary structure and expression of a functional human glucocorticoid receptor cDNA," *Nature*, vol. 318, no. 6047, pp. 635–641, 1985.

[21] C. Weinberger, S. M. Hollenberg, and E. S. Ong, "Identification of human glucocorticoid receptor complementary DNA clones by epitope selection," *Science*, vol. 228, no. 4700, pp. 740–742, 1985.

[22] S. Green, P. Walter, and V. Kumar, "Human oestrogen receptor cDNA: Sequence, expression and homology to v-erb-A," *Nature*, vol. 320, no. 6058, pp. 134–139, 1986.

[23] G. L. Greene, P. Gilna, and M. Waterfield, "Sequence and expression of human estrogen receptor complementary DNA," *Science*, vol. 231, no. 4742, pp. 1150–1154, 1986.

[24] J. Sap, A. Munoz, and K. Damm, "The c-erb-A protein is a high-affinity receptor for thyroid hormone," *Nature*, vol. 324, no. 6098, pp. 635–640, 1986.

[25] C. Weinberger, C. C. Thompson, and E. S. Ong, "The c-erb-A gene encodes a thyroid hormone receptor," *Nature*, vol. 324, no. 6098, pp. 641–646, 1986.

[26] Z. Zhang, P. E. Burch, A. J. Cooney et al., "Genomic analysis of the nuclear receptor family: new insights into structure, regulation, and evolution from the rat genome," *Genome Research*, vol. 14, no. 4, pp. 580–590, 2004.

[27] A. M. Näär and J. K. Thakur, "Nuclear receptor-like transcription factors in fungi," *Genes and Development*, vol. 23, no. 4, pp. 419–432, 2009.

[28] A. E. Sluder and C. V. Maina, "Nuclear receptors in nematodes: themes and variations," *Trends in Genetics*, vol. 17, no. 4, pp. 206–213, 2001.

[29] R. M. Evans, "The nuclear receptor superfamily: a rosetta stone for physiology," *Molecular Endocrinology*, vol. 19, no. 6, pp. 1429–1438, 2005.

[30] P. Chambon, "The nuclear receptor superfamily: a personal retrospect on the first two decades," *Molecular Endocrinology*, vol. 19, no. 6, pp. 1418–1428, 2005.

[31] M. Lehrke and M. A. Lazar, "The many faces of PPARγ," *Cell*, vol. 123, no. 6, pp. 993–999, 2005.

[32] S. Mukherjee and S. Mani, "Orphan nuclear receptors as targets for drug development," *Pharmaceutical Research*, vol. 27, pp. 1439–1468, 2010.

[33] M. Schupp and M. A. Lazar, "Endogenous ligands for nuclear receptors: digging deeper," *Journal of Biological Chemistry*, vol. 285, no. 52, pp. 40409–40415, 2010.

[34] A. L. Bookout, Y. Jeong, M. Downes, R. T. Yu, R. M. Evans, and D. J. Mangelsdorf, "Anatomical profiling of nuclear receptor expression reveals a hierarchical transcriptional network," *Cell*, vol. 126, no. 4, pp. 789–799, 2006.

[35] P. M. Yen, "Physiological and molecular basis of Thyroid hormone action," *Physiological Reviews*, vol. 81, no. 3, pp. 1097–1142, 2001.

[36] S. Refetoff and A. M. Dumitrescu, "Syndromes of reduced sensitivity to thyroid hormone: genetic defects in hormone receptors, cell transporters and deiodination," *Best Practice and Research: Clinical Endocrinology and Metabolism*, vol. 21, no. 2, pp. 277–305, 2007.

[37] I. H. Chan and M. L. Privalsky, "Isoform-specific transcriptional activity of overlapping target genes that respond to thyroid hormone receptors α1 and β1," *Molecular Endocrinology*, vol. 23, no. 11, pp. 1758–1775, 2009.

[38] M. D. Rosen and M. L. Privalsky, "Thyroid hormone receptor mutations found in renal clear cell carcinomas alter corepressor release and reveal helix 12 as key determinant of corepressor specificity," *Molecular Endocrinology*, vol. 23, no. 8, pp. 1183–1192, 2009.

[39] I. H. Chan and M. L. Privalsky, "Thyroid hormone receptors mutated in liver cancer function as distorted antimorphs," *Oncogene*, vol. 25, no. 25, pp. 3576–3588, 2006.

[40] R. Parrilla, A. J. Mixson, J. A. McPherson, J. H. McClaskey, and B. D. Weintraub, "Characterization of seven novel mutations of the c-erbAβ gene in unrelated kindreds with generalized thyroid hormone resistance. Evidence for two "hot spot" regions of the ligand binding domain," *Journal of Clinical Investigation*, vol. 88, no. 6, pp. 2123–2130, 1991.

[41] S. Y. Wu, R. N. Cohen, E. Simsek et al., "A novel thyroid hormone receptor-β mutation that fails to bind nuclear receptor corepressor in a patient as an apparent cause of severe, predominantly pituitary resistance to thyroid hormone," *Journal of Clinical Endocrinology and Metabolism*, vol. 91, no. 5, pp. 1887–1895, 2006.

[42] G. C. Schussler, "The thyroxine-binding proteins," *Thyroid*, vol. 10, no. 2, pp. 141–149, 2000.

[43] J. A. Hamilton and M. D. Benson, "Transthyretin: a review from a structural perspective," *Cellular and Molecular Life Sciences*, vol. 58, no. 10, pp. 1491–1521, 2001.

[44] H. Heuer and T. J. Visser, "Minireview: pathophysiological importance of thyroid hormone transporters," *Endocrinology*, vol. 150, no. 3, pp. 1078–1083, 2009.

[45] W. M. Van Der Deure, R. P. Peeters, and T. J. Visser, "Molecular aspects of thyroid hormone transporters, including MCT8, MCT10, and OATPs, and the effects of genetic variation in these transporters," *Journal of Molecular Endocrinology*, vol. 44, no. 1, pp. 1–11, 2010.

[46] B. Gereben, A. Zeöld, M. Dentice, D. Salvatore, and A. C. Bianco, "Activation and inactivation of thyroid hormone by deiodinases: local action with general consequences," *Cellular and Molecular Life Sciences*, vol. 65, no. 4, pp. 570–590, 2008.

[47] R. Zucchi, G. Chiellini, T. S. Scanlan, and D. K. Grandy, "Trace amine-associated receptors and their ligands," *British Journal of Pharmacology*, vol. 149, no. 8, pp. 967–978, 2006.

[48] E. Hadzic, V. Desai-Yajnik, E. Helmer et al., "A 10-amino-acid sequence in the N-terminal A/B domain of thyroid hormone receptor α is essential for transcriptional activation and interaction with the general transcription factor TFIIB," *Molecular and Cellular Biology*, vol. 15, no. 8, pp. 4507–4517, 1995.

[49] C. Oberste-Berghaus, K. Zanger, K. Hashimoto, R. N. Cohen, A. N. Hollenberg, and F. E. Wondisford, "Thyroid hormone-independent interaction between the thyroid hormone receptor β2 amino terminus and coactivators," *Journal of Biological Chemistry*, vol. 275, no. 3, pp. 1787–1792, 2000.

[50] Z. Yang and M. L. Privalsky, "Isoform-specific transcriptional regulation by thyroid hormone receptors: hormone-independent activation operates through a steroid receptor mode of coactivator interaction," *Molecular Endocrinology*, vol. 15, no. 7, pp. 1170–1185, 2001.

[51] H. Tian, M. A. Mahajan, T. W. Chun, I. Habeos, and H. H. Samuels, "The N-terminal A/B domain of the thyroid hormone receptor-β2 isoform influences ligand-dependent recruitment of coactivators to the ligand-binding domain," *Molecular Endocrinology*, vol. 20, no. 9, pp. 2036–2051, 2006.

[52] N. L. Weigel, "Steroid hormone receptors and their regulation by phosphorylation," *Biochemical Journal*, vol. 319, no. 3, pp. 657–667, 1996.

[53] M. Adams, M. J. Reginato, D. Shao, M. A. Lazar, and V. K. Chatterjee, "Transcriptional activation by peroxisome proliferator-activated receptor γ is inhibited by phosphorylation at a consensus mitogen-activated protein kinase site," *Journal of Biological Chemistry*, vol. 272, no. 8, pp. 5128–5132, 1997.

[54] R. Kumar, J. C. Lee, D. W. Bolen, and E. B. Thompson, "The conformation of the glucocorticoid receptor af1/tau1 domain induced by osmolyte binds co-regulatory proteins," *Journal of Biological Chemistry*, vol. 276, no. 21, pp. 18146–18152, 2001.

[55] S. E. Wardell, S. C. Kwok, L. Sherman, R. S. Hodges, and D. P. Edwards, "Regulation of the amino-terminal transcription activation domain of progesterone receptor by a cofactor-induced protein folding mechanism," *Molecular and Cellular Biology*, vol. 25, no. 20, pp. 8792–8808, 2005.

[56] V. Chandra, P. Huang, Y. Hamuro et al., "Structure of the intact PPAR-γ-RXR-α nuclear receptor complex on DNA," *Nature*, vol. 456, no. 7220, pp. 350–356, 2008.

[57] R. Kumar and G. Litwack, "Structural and functional relationships of the steroid hormone receptors' N-terminal transactivation domain," *Steroids*, vol. 74, no. 12, pp. 877–883, 2009.

[58] L. P. Freedman, B. F. Luisi, Z. R. Korszun, R. Basavappa, P. B. Sigler, and K. R. Yamamoto, "The function and structure of the metal coordination sites within the glucocorticoid receptor DNA binding domain," *Nature*, vol. 334, no. 6182, pp. 543–546, 1988.

[59] B. F. Luisi, W. X. Xu, Z. Otwinowski, L. P. Freedman, K. R. Yamamoto, and P. B. Sigler, "Crystallographic analysis of the interaction of the glucocorticoid receptor with DNA," *Nature*, vol. 352, no. 6335, pp. 497–505, 1991.

[60] F. Rastinejad, T. Perlmann, R. M. Evans, and P. B. Sigler, "Structural determinants of nuclear receptor assembly on DNA direct repeats," *Nature*, vol. 375, no. 6528, pp. 203–211, 1995.

[61] P. L. Shaffer and D. T. Gewirth, "Structural basis of VDR-DNA interactions on direct repeat response elements," *EMBO Journal*, vol. 21, no. 9, pp. 2242–2252, 2002.

[62] Z. Smit-McBride and M. L. Privalsky, "DNA sequence specificity of the v-erb A oncoprotein/thyroid hormone receptor: role of the P-box and its interaction with more

N-terminal determinants of DNA recognition," *Molecular Endocrinology*, vol. 8, no. 7, pp. 819–828, 1994.

[63] C. C. Nelson, S. C. Hendy, J. S. Faris, and P. J. Romaniuk, "The effects of P-box substitutions in thyroid hormone receptor on DNA binding specificity," *Molecular Endocrinology*, vol. 8, no. 7, pp. 829–840, 1994.

[64] C. C. Nelson, S. C. Hendy, J. S. Faris, and P. J. Romaniuk, "Retinoid X receptor alters the determination of DNA binding specificity by the P-box amino acids of the thyroid hormone receptor," *Journal of Biological Chemistry*, vol. 271, no. 32, pp. 19464–19474, 1996.

[65] K. Umesono and R. M. Evans, "Determinants of target gene specificity for steroid/thyroid hormone receptors," *Cell*, vol. 57, no. 7, pp. 1139–1146, 1989.

[66] F. Claessens and D. T. Gewirth, "DNA recognition by nuclear receptors," *Essays in Biochemistry*, vol. 40, pp. 59–72, 2004.

[67] S. Khorasanizadeh and F. Rastinejad, "Nuclear-receptor interactions on DNA-response elements," *Trends in Biochemical Sciences*, vol. 26, no. 6, pp. 384–390, 2001.

[68] T. Q. Phan, M. M. Jow, and M. L. Privalsky, "DNA recognition by thyroid hormone and retinoic acid receptors: 3,4,5 rule modified," *Molecular and Cellular Endocrinology*, vol. 319, no. 1-2, pp. 88–98, 2010.

[69] H. Gronemeyer and D. Moras, "Nuclear receptors. How to finger DNA," *Nature*, vol. 375, no. 6528, pp. 190–191, 1995.

[70] R. Kurokawa, V. C. Yu, A. Naar et al., "Differential orientations of the DNA-binding domain and carboxy-terminal dimerization interface regulate binding site selection by nuclear receptor heterodimers," *Genes and Development*, vol. 7, no. 7 B, pp. 1423–1435, 1993.

[71] M. A. Lazar, T. J. Berrodin, and H. P. Harding, "Differential DNA binding by monomeric, homodimeric, and potentially heteromeric forms of the thyroid hormone receptor," *Molecular and Cellular Biology*, vol. 11, no. 10, pp. 5005–5015, 1991.

[72] A. M. Näär, J. M. Boutin, S. M. Lipkin et al., "The orientation and spacing of core DNA-binding motifs dictate selective transcriptional responses to three nuclear receptors," *Cell*, vol. 65, no. 7, pp. 1267–1279, 1991.

[73] G. M. Wahlstrom, M. Sjoberg, M. Andersson, K. Nordstrom, and B. Vennstrom, "Binding characteristics of the thyroid hormone receptor homo-and heterodimers to consensus AGGTCA repeat motifs," *Molecular Endocrinology*, vol. 6, no. 7, pp. 1013–1022, 1992.

[74] B. M. Forman, J. Casanova, B. M. Raaka, J. Ghysdael, and H. H. Samuels, "Half-site spacing and orientation determines whether thyroid hormone and retinoic acid receptors and related factors bind to DNA response elements as monomers, homodimers, or heterodimers," *Molecular Endocrinology*, vol. 6, no. 3, pp. 429–442, 1992.

[75] Y. Chen and M. A. Young, "Structure of a thyroid hormone receptor DNA-binding domain homodimer bound to an inverted palindrome DNA response element," *Molecular Endocrinology*, vol. 24, no. 8, pp. 1650–1664, 2010.

[76] M. Mathur, P. W. Tucker, and H. H. Samuels, "PSF is a novel corepressor that mediates its effect through Sin3A and the DNA binding domain of nuclear hormone receptors," *Molecular and Cellular Biology*, vol. 21, no. 7, pp. 2298–2311, 2001.

[77] A. S. Nascimento, S. M. G. Dias, F. M. Nunes et al., "Structural rearrangements in the thyroid hormone receptor hinge domain and their putative role in the receptor function," *Journal of Molecular Biology*, vol. 360, no. 3, pp. 586–598, 2006.

[78] K. Busch, B. Martin, A. Baniahmad, R. Renkawitz, and M. Muller, "At least three subdomains of v-erbA are involved in its silencing function," *Molecular Endocrinology*, vol. 11, no. 3, pp. 379–389, 1997.

[79] J. D. Safer, R. N. Cohen, A. N. Hollenberg, and F. E. Wondisford, "Defective release of corepressor by hinge mutants of the thyroid hormone receptor found in patients with resistance to thyroid hormone," *Journal of Biological Chemistry*, vol. 273, no. 46, pp. 30175–30182, 1998.

[80] A. Aranda and A. Pascual, "Nuclear hormone receptors and gene expression," *Physiological Reviews*, vol. 81, no. 3, pp. 1269–1304, 2001.

[81] J. P. Renaud, N. Rochel, M. Ruff et al., "Crystal structure of the RAR-γ ligand-binding domain bound to all-trans retinoic acid," *Nature*, vol. 378, no. 6558, pp. 681–689, 1995.

[82] R. L. Wagner, J. W. Apriletti, M. E. McGrath, B. L. West, J. D. Baxter, and R. J. Fletterick, "A structural role for hormone in the thyroid hormone receptor," *Nature*, vol. 378, no. 6558, pp. 690–697, 1995.

[83] W. Bourguet, M. Ruff, P. Chambon, H. Gronemeyer, and D. Moras, "Crystal structure of the ligand-binding domain of the human nuclear receptor RXR-α," *Nature*, vol. 375, no. 6530, pp. 377–382, 1995.

[84] J. M. Wurtz, W. Bourguet, J. P. Renaud et al., "A canonical structure for the ligandbinding domain of nuclear receptors," *Nature Structural Biology*, vol. 3, no. 1, pp. 87–94, 1996.

[85] J. Uppenberg, C. Svensson, M. Jaki, G. Bertilsson, L. Jendeberg, and A. Berkenstam, "Crystal structure of the ligand binding domain of the human nuclear receptor PPARγ," *Journal of Biological Chemistry*, vol. 273, no. 47, pp. 31108–31112, 1998.

[86] B. P. Klaholz, J. P. Renaud, A. Mitschler et al., "Conformational adaptation of agonists to the human nuclear receptor RARγ," *Nature Structural Biology*, vol. 5, no. 3, pp. 199–202, 1998.

[87] P. F. Egea, A. Mitschler, N. Rochel, M. Ruff, P. Chambon, and D. Moras, "Crystal structure of the human RXRα ligand-binding domain bound to its natural ligand: 9-cis retinoic acid," *EMBO Journal*, vol. 19, no. 11, pp. 2592–2601, 2000.

[88] N. Rochel, J. M. Wurtz, A. Mitschler, B. Klaholz, and D. Moras, "The crystal structure of the nuclear receptor for vitamin D bound to its natural ligand," *Molecular Cell*, vol. 5, no. 1, pp. 173–179, 2000.

[89] J. P. Renaud and D. Moras, "Structural studies on nuclear receptors," *Cellular and Molecular Life Sciences*, vol. 57, no. 12, pp. 1748–1769, 2000.

[90] M. L. Privalsky, "The role of corepressors in transcriptional regulation by nuclear hormone receptors," *Annual Review of Physiology*, vol. 66, pp. 315–360, 2004.

[91] J. D. Chen and R. M. Evans, "A transcriptional co-repressor that interacts with nuclear hormone receptors," *Nature*, vol. 377, no. 6548, pp. 454–457, 1995.

[92] A. J. Hörlein, A. M. Naar, T. Heinzel et al., "Ligand-independent repression by the thyroid hormone receptor mediated by a nuclear receptor co-repressor," *Nature*, vol. 377, no. 6548, pp. 397–404, 1995.

[93] A. Marimuthu, W. Feng, T. Tagami et al., "TR surfaces and conformations required to bind nuclear receptor corepressor," *Molecular Endocrinology*, vol. 16, no. 2, pp. 271–286, 2002.

[94] A. Makowski, S. Brzostek, R. N. Cohen, and A. N. Hollenberg, "Determination of nuclear receptor corepressor interactions with the thyroid hormone receptor," *Molecular Endocrinology*, vol. 17, no. 2, pp. 273–286, 2003.

[95] W. Feng, R. C. J. Ribeiro, R. L. Wagner et al., "Hormone-dependent coactivator binding to a hydrophobic cleft on nuclear receptors," *Science*, vol. 280, no. 5370, pp. 1747–1749, 1998.

[96] B. D. Darimont, R. L. Wagner, J. W. Apriletti et al., "Structure and specificity of nuclear receptor-coactivator interactions," *Genes and Development*, vol. 12, no. 21, pp. 3343–3356, 1998.

[97] M. A. Mahajan and H. H. Samuels, "Nuclear hormone receptor coregulator: role in hormone action, metabolism, growth, and development," *Endocrine Reviews*, vol. 26, no. 4, pp. 583–597, 2005.

[98] D. M. Lonard and B. W. O'Malley, "The expanding cosmos of nuclear receptor coactivators," *Cell*, vol. 125, no. 3, pp. 411–414, 2006.

[99] B. York and B. W. O'Malley, "Steroid Receptor Coactivator (SRC) family: masters of systems biology," *Journal of Biological Chemistry*, vol. 285, no. 50, pp. 38743–38750, 2010.

[100] P. Webb, N. H. Nguyen, G. Chiellini et al., "Design of thyroid hormone receptor antagonists from first principles," *Journal of Steroid Biochemistry and Molecular Biology*, vol. 83, no. 1–5, pp. 59–73, 2002.

[101] L. Nagy and J. W. R. Schwabe, "Mechanism of the nuclear receptor molecular switch," *Trends in Biochemical Sciences*, vol. 29, no. 6, pp. 317–324, 2004.

[102] A. C.M. Figueira, D. M. Saidemberg, P. C.T. Souza et al., "Analysis of agonist and antagonist effects on thyroid hormone receptor conformation by hydrogen/deuterium exchange," *Molecular Endocrinology*, vol. 25, no. 1, pp. 15–31, 2011.

[103] A. N. Hollenberg, T. Monden, T. R. Flynn, M. E. Boers, O. Cohen, and F. E. Wondisford, "The human thyrotropin-releasing hormone gene is regulated by thyroid hormone through two distinct classes of negative thyroid hormone response elements," *Molecular Endocrinology*, vol. 9, no. 5, pp. 540–550, 1995.

[104] M. Nygård, G. M. Wahlström, M. V. Gustafsson, Y. M. Tokumoto, and M. Bondesson, "Hormone-dependent repression of the E2F-1 gene by thyroid hormone receptors," *Molecular Endocrinology*, vol. 17, no. 1, pp. 79–92, 2003.

[105] S. Decherf, I. Seugnet, S. Kouidhi, A. Lopez-Juarez, M. S. Clerget-Froidevaux, and B. A. Demeneix, "Thyroid hormone exerts negative feedback on hypothalamic type 4 melanocortin receptor expression," *Proceedings of the National Academy of Sciences of the United States of America*, vol. 107, no. 9, pp. 4471–4476, 2010.

[106] S. Y. Cheng, J. L. Leonard, and P. J. Davis, "Molecular aspects of thyroid hormone actions," *Endocrine Reviews*, vol. 31, no. 2, pp. 139–170, 2010.

[107] D. J. Bradley, H. C. Towle, and W. S. Young III, "Spatial and temporal expression of α- and β-thyroid hormone receptor mRNAs, including the β2-subtype, in the developing mammalian nervous system," *Journal of Neuroscience*, vol. 12, no. 6, pp. 2288–2302, 1992.

[108] C. B. Cook, I. Kakucska, R. M. Lechan, and R. J. Koenig, "Expression of thyroid hormone receptor β2 in rat hypothalamus," *Endocrinology*, vol. 130, no. 2, pp. 1077–1079, 1992.

[109] M. Sjöberg, B. Vennstrom, and D. Forrest, "Thyroid hormone receptors in chick retinal development: differential expression of mRNAs for α and N-terminal variant β receptors," *Development*, vol. 114, no. 1, pp. 39–47, 1992.

[110] D. J. Bradley, H. C. Towle, and W. S. Young, "α And β thyroid hormone receptor (TR) gene expression during auditory neurogenesis: evidence for TR isoform-specific transcriptional regulation in vivo," *Proceedings of the National Academy of Sciences of the United States of America*, vol. 91, no. 2, pp. 439–443, 1994.

[111] D. Forrest, L. C. Erway, L. Ng, R. Altschuler, and T. Curran, "Thyroid hormone receptor β is essential for development of auditory function," *Nature Genetics*, vol. 13, no. 3, pp. 354–357, 1996.

[112] D. Forrest, E. Hanebuth, R. J. Smeyne et al., "Recessive resistance to thyroid hormone in mice lacking thyroid hormone receptor β: evidence for tissue-specific modulation of receptor function," *EMBO Journal*, vol. 15, no. 12, pp. 3006–3015, 1996.

[113] L. Wikström, C. Johansson, C. Saltó et al., "Abnormal heart rate and body temperature in mice lacking thyroid hormone receptor α1," *EMBO Journal*, vol. 17, no. 2, pp. 455–461, 1998.

[114] H. Marrif, A. Schifman, Z. Stepanyan et al., "Temperature homeostasis in transgenic mice lacking thyroid hormone receptor-α gene products," *Endocrinology*, vol. 146, no. 7, pp. 2872–2884, 2005.

[115] K. Gauthier, O. Chassande, M. Plateroti et al., "Different functions for the thyroid hormone receptors TRα and TRβ in the control of thyroid hormone production and post-natal development," *EMBO Journal*, vol. 18, no. 3, pp. 623–631, 1999.

[116] R. E. Weiss, O. Chassande, E. K. Koo et al., "Thyroid function and effect of aging in combined hetero/homozygous mice deficient in thyroid hormone receptors α and β genes," *Journal of Endocrinology*, vol. 172, no. 1, pp. 177–185, 2002.

[117] A. Flores-Morales, H. Gullberg, L. Fernandez et al., "Patterns of liver gene expression governed by TRβ," *Molecular Endocrinology*, vol. 16, no. 6, pp. 1257–1268, 2002.

[118] P. M. Yen, "Molecular basis of resistance to thyroid hormone," *Trends in Endocrinology and Metabolism*, vol. 14, no. 7, pp. 327–333, 2003.

[119] M.-F. Langlois, K. Zanger, T. Monden, J. D. Safer, A. N. Hollenberg, and F. E. Wondisford, "A unique role of the β-2 thyroid hormone receptor isoform in negative regulation by thyroid hormone: mapping of a novel amino-terminal domain important for ligand-independent activation," *Journal of Biological Chemistry*, vol. 272, no. 40, pp. 24927–24933, 1997.

[120] L. Ng, D. Forrest, B. R. Haugen, W. M. Wood, and T. Curran, "N-terminal variants of thyroid hormone receptor β: differential function and potential contribution to syndrome of resistance to thyroid hormone," *Molecular Endocrinology*, vol. 9, no. 9, pp. 1202–1213, 1995.

[121] M. Sjoberg and B. Vennstrom, "Ligand-dependent and -independent transactivation by thyroid hormone receptor β2 is determined by the structure of the hormone response element," *Molecular and Cellular Biology*, vol. 15, no. 9, pp. 4718–4726, 1995.

[122] W. Wan, B. Farboud, and M. L. Privalsky, "Pituitary resistance to thyroid hormone syndrome is associated with T3 receptor mutants that selectively impair β2 isoform function," *Molecular Endocrinology*, vol. 19, no. 6, pp. 1529–1542, 2005.

[123] M. Bettendorf, "Thyroid disorders in children from birth to adolescence," *European Journal of Nuclear Medicine*, vol. 29, supplement 2, pp. S439–S446, 2002.

[124] T. F. Davies and P. R. Larsen, "Thyrotoxicosis," in *Williams Textbook of Endocrinology*, P. R. Larsen, H. M. Kronenberg, S. Melmed, and K. S. Polonsky, Eds., pp. 374–421, 2003.

[125] J. S. Melish, "Thyroid disease," in *Clinical Methods: The History, Physical, and Laboratory Examinations*, H. K. Walker, W. D Hall, and J. W. Hurst, Eds., 1990.

[126] S. C. Boyages and J. P. Halpern, "Endemic cretinism: toward a unifying hypothesis," *Thyroid*, vol. 3, no. 1, pp. 59–69, 1993.

[127] S. Refetoff, L. T. DeWind, and L. J. DeGroot, "Familial syndrome combining deaf-mutism, stuppled epiphyses, goiter and abnormally high PBI: possible target organ refractoriness to thyroid hormone," *Journal of Clinical Endocrinology and Metabolism*, vol. 27, no. 2, pp. 279–294, 1967.

[128] T. O. Olateju and M. P. J. Vanderpump, "Thyroid hormone resistance," *Annals of Clinical Biochemistry*, vol. 43, no. 6, pp. 431–440, 2006.

[129] S. H. LaFranchi, D. B. Snyder, D. E. Sesser et al., "Follow-up of newborns with elevated screening T4 concentrations," *Journal of Pediatrics*, vol. 143, no. 3, pp. 296–301, 2003.

[130] J. L. Jameson, "Mechanisms by which thyroid hormone receptor mutations cause clinical syndromes of resistance to thyroid hormone," *Thyroid*, vol. 4, no. 4, pp. 485–492, 1994.

[131] D. Forrest, G. Golarai, J. Connor, and T. Curran, "Genetic analysis of thyroid hormone receptors in development and disease," *Recent Progress in Hormone Research*, vol. 51, pp. 1–22, 1996.

[132] R. T. Liu, S. Suzuki, T. Takeda, and L. J. DeGroot, "An artificial thyroid hormone receptor mutant without DNA binding can have dominant negative effect," *Molecular and Cellular Endocrinology*, vol. 120, no. 1, pp. 85–93, 1996.

[133] T. Nagaya, M. Fujieda, and H. Seo, "Requirement of corepressor binding of thyroid hormone receptor mutants for dominant negative inhibition," *Biochemical and Biophysical Research Communications*, vol. 247, no. 3, pp. 620–623, 1998.

[134] S. Refetoff, "Resistance to thyroid hormone with and without receptor gene mutations," *Annales d'Endocrinologie*, vol. 64, no. 1, pp. 23–25, 2003.

[135] H. Sato, Y. Koike, M. Honma, M. Yagame, and K. Ito, "Evaluation of thyroid hormone action in a case of generalized resistance to thyroid hormone with chronic thyroiditis: discovery of a novel heterozygous missense mutation (G347A)," *Endocrine Journal*, vol. 54, no. 5, pp. 727–732, 2007.

[136] M. F. Azevedo, G. B. Barra, L. D. De Medeiros, L. A. Simeoni, L. A. Naves, and F. De A. Rocha Neves, "A novel mutation of thyroid hormone receptor beta (I431V) impairs corepressor release, and induces thyroid hormone resistance syndrome," *Arquivos Brasileiros de Endocrinologia e Metabologia*, vol. 52, no. 8, pp. 1304–1312, 2008.

[137] B. A. Asadi, P. A. Torjesen, E. Haug, and J. P. Berg, "Biochemical characterization of four novel mutations in the thyroid hormone receptor β gene in patients with resistance to thyroid hormone," *Scandinavian Journal of Clinical and Laboratory Investigation*, vol. 68, no. 7, pp. 563–567, 2008.

[138] C. M. Rivolta, M. C. Olcese, F. S. Belforte et al., "Genotyping of resistance to thyroid hormone in South American population. Identification of seven novel missense mutations in the human thyroid hormone receptor β gene," *Molecular and Cellular Probes*, vol. 23, no. 3-4, pp. 148–153, 2009.

[139] S. Ono, I. D. Schwartz, O. T. Mueller, A. W. Root, S. J. Usala, and B. B. Bercu, "Homozygosity for a dominant negative thyroid hormone receptor gene responsible for generalized resistance to thyroid hormone," *Journal of Clinical Endocrinology and Metabolism*, vol. 73, no. 5, pp. 990–994, 1991.

[140] K. Frank-Raue, A. Lorenz, C. Haag et al., "Severe form of thyroid hormone resistance in a patient with homozygous/hemizygous mutation of T3 receptor gene," *European Journal of Endocrinology*, vol. 150, no. 6, pp. 819–823, 2004.

[141] M. Kaneshige, H. Suzuki, K. Kaneshige et al., "A targeted dominant negative mutation of the thyroid hormone α1 receptor causes increased mortality, infertility, and dwarfism in mice," *Proceedings of the National Academy of Sciences of the United States of America*, vol. 98, no. 26, pp. 15095–15100, 2001.

[142] A. Tinnikov, K. Nordström, P. Thorén et al., "Retardation of post-natal development caused by a negatively acting thyroid hormone receptor α1," *EMBO Journal*, vol. 21, no. 19, pp. 5079–5087, 2002.

[143] Y. Y. Liu, J. J. Schultz, and G. A. Brent, "A thyroid hormone receptor α gene mutation (P398H) is associated with visceral adiposity and impaired catecholamine-stimulated lipolysis in mice," *Journal of Biological Chemistry*, vol. 278, no. 40, pp. 38913–38920, 2003.

[144] M. Vujovic, K. Nordström, K. Gauthier et al., "Interference of a mutant thyroid hormone receptor α1 with hepatic glucose metabolism," *Endocrinology*, vol. 150, no. 6, pp. 2940–2947, 2009.

[145] S. Hadjab-Lallemend, K. Wallis, M. van Hogerlinden et al., "A mutant thyroid hormone receptor alpha1 alters hippocampal circuitry and reduces seizure susceptibility in mice," *Neuropharmacology*, vol. 58, no. 7, pp. 1130–1139, 2010.

[146] E. Macchia, M. Gurnell, M. Agostini et al., "Identification and characterization of a novel de novo mutation (L346V) in the thyroid hormone receptor β gene in a family with generalized thyroid hormone resistance," *European Journal of Endocrinology*, vol. 137, no. 4, pp. 370–376, 1997.

[147] T. N. Collingwood, R. Wagner, C. H. Matthews et al., "A role for helix 3 of the TRβ ligand-binding domain in coactivator recruitment identified by characterization of a third cluster of mutations in resistance to thyroid hormone," *EMBO Journal*, vol. 17, no. 16, pp. 4760–4770, 1998.

[148] R. J. Clifton-Bligh, F. De Zegher, R. L. Wagner et al., "A novel TRβ mutation (R383H) in resistance to thyroid hormone syndrome predominantly impairs corepressor release and negative transcriptional regulation," *Molecular Endocrinology*, vol. 12, no. 5, pp. 609–621, 1998.

[149] J. Lado-Abeal, A. M. Dumitrescu, X. H. Liao et al., "A de novo mutation in an already mutant nucleotide of the thyroid hormone receptor β gene perpetuates resistance to thyroid hormone," *Journal of Clinical Endocrinology and Metabolism*, vol. 90, no. 3, pp. 1760–1767, 2005.

[150] S. M. Yoh, V. K.K. Chatterjee, and M. L. Privalsky, "Thyroid hormone resistance syndrome manifests as an aberrant interaction between mutant T3 receptors and transcriptional corepressors," *Molecular Endocrinology*, vol. 11, no. 4, pp. 470–480, 1997.

[151] S. Refetoff, R. E. Weiss, J. R. Wing, D. Sarne, B. Chyna, and Y. Hayashi, "Resistance to thyroid hormone in subjects from two unrelated families is associated with a point mutation in the thyroid hormone receptor β gene resulting in the replacement of the normal proline 453 with serine," *Thyroid*, vol. 4, no. 3, pp. 249–254, 1994.

[152] A. M. Zavacki, J. W. Harney, G. A. Brent, and P. R. Larsen, "Structural features of thyroid hormone response elements that increase susceptibility to inhibition by an RTH mutant thyroid hormone receptor," *Endocrinology*, vol. 137, no. 7, pp. 2833–2841, 1996.

[153] M. L. Privalsky and S. M. Yoh, "Resistance to thyroid hormone (RTH) syndrome reveals novel determinants regulating interaction of T3 receptor with corepressor," *Molecular and Cellular Endocrinology*, vol. 159, no. 1-2, pp. 109–124, 2000.

[154] S. M. Yoh and M. L. Privalsky, "Molecular analysis of human resistance to thyroid hormone syndrome," *Methods in Molecular Biology*, vol. 202, pp. 129–152, 2002.

[155] T. Bayraktaroglu, J. Noel, F. Alagol, N. Colak, N. M. Mukaddes, and S. Refetoff, "Thyroid hormone receptor beta gene mutation (P453A) in a family producing resistance to thyroid hormone," *Experimental and Clinical Endocrinology and Diabetes*, vol. 117, no. 1, pp. 34–37, 2009.

[156] T. Tagami and J. Larry Jameson, "Nuclear corepressors enhance the dominant negative activity of mutant receptors that cause resistance to thyroid hormone," *Endocrinology*, vol. 139, no. 2, pp. 640–650, 1998.

[157] Y. Hayashi, R. E. Weiss, D. H. Sarne et al., "Do clinical manifestations of resistance to thyroid hormone correlate with the functional alteration of the corresponding mutant thyroid hormone-β receptors?" *Journal of Clinical Endocrinology and Metabolism*, vol. 80, no. 11, pp. 3246–3256, 1995.

[158] M. Malartre, S. Short, and C. Sharpe, "Alternative splicing generates multiple SMRT transcripts encoding conserved repressor domains linked to variable transcription factor interaction domains," *Nucleic Acids Research*, vol. 32, no. 15, pp. 4676–4686, 2004.

[159] M. L. Goodson, B. A. Jonas, and M. L. Privalsky, "Alternative mRNA splicing of SMRT creates functional diversity by generating corepressor isoforms with different affinities for different nuclear receptors," *Journal of Biological Chemistry*, vol. 280, no. 9, pp. 7493–7503, 2005.

[160] P. Beck-Peccoz and V. K. K. Chatterjee, "The variable clinical phenotype in thyroid hormone resistance syndrome," *Thyroid*, vol. 4, no. 2, pp. 225–232, 1994.

[161] J. D. Safer, M. F. Langlois, R. Cohen et al., "Isoform variable action among thyroid hormone receptor mutants provides insight into pituitary resistance to thyroid hormone," *Molecular Endocrinology*, vol. 11, no. 1, pp. 16–26, 1997.

[162] F. E. Wondisford, "Thyroid hormone action: insight from transgenic mouse models," *Journal of Investigative Medicine*, vol. 51, no. 4, pp. 215–220, 2003.

[163] S. Y. Cheng, "Thyroid hormone receptor mutations and disease: beyond thyroid hormone resistance," *Trends in Endocrinology and Metabolism*, vol. 16, no. 4, pp. 176–182, 2005.

[164] V. K.K. Chatterjee, "Nuclear receptors and human disease: resistance to thyroid hormone and lipodystrophic insulin resistance," *Annales d'Endocrinologie*, vol. 69, no. 2, pp. 103–106, 2008.

[165] H. Gharib and G. G. Klee, "Familial euthyroid hyperthyroxinemia secondary to pituitary and peripheral resistance to thyroid hormones," *Mayo Clinic Proceedings*, vol. 60, no. 1, pp. 9–15, 1985.

[166] P. Beck-Peccoz, F. Forloni, D. Cortelazzi et al., "Pituitary resistance to thyroid hormones," *Hormone Research*, vol. 38, no. 1-2, pp. 66–72, 1992.

[167] D. S. Machado, A. Sabet, L. A. Santiago et al., "A thyroid hormone receptor mutation that dissociates thyroid hormone regulation of gene expression in vivo," *Proceedings of the National Academy of Sciences of the United States of America*, vol. 106, no. 23, pp. 9441–9446, 2009.

[168] R. C.J. Ribeiro, J. W. Apriletti, R. L. Wagner et al., "Mechanisms of thyroid hormone action: insights from X-ray crystallographic and functional studies," *Recent Progress in Hormone Research*, vol. 53, pp. 351–392, 1998.

[169] M. Togashi, P. Nguyen, R. Fletterick, J. D. Baxter, and P. Webb, "Rearrangements in thyroid hormone receptor charge clusters that stabilize bound 3,5′,5-triiodo-L-thyronine and inhibit homodimer formation," *Journal of Biological Chemistry*, vol. 280, no. 27, pp. 25665–25673, 2005.

[170] T. R. Flynn, A. N. Hollenberg, O. Cohen et al., "A novel C-terminal domain in the thyroid hormone receptor selectively mediates thyroid hormone inhibition," *Journal of Biological Chemistry*, vol. 269, no. 52, pp. 32713–32716, 1994.

[171] S. Sasaki, H. Nakamura, T. Tagami, Y. Miyoshi, and K. Nakao, "Functional properties of a mutant T receptor β (R338W) identified in a subject with pituitary resistance to thyroid hormone," *Molecular and Cellular Endocrinology*, vol. 113, no. 1, pp. 109–117, 1995.

[172] S. Ando, H. Nakamura, S. Sasaki et al., "Introducing a point mutation identified in a patient with pituitary resistance to thyroid hormone (Arg 338 to Trp) into other mutant thyroid hormone receptors weakens their dominant negative activities," *Journal of Endocrinology*, vol. 151, no. 2, pp. 293–300, 1996.

[173] R. N. Cohen, F. E. Wondisford, and A. N. Hollenberg, "Two separate NCoR (nuclear receptor corepressor) interaction domains mediate corepressor action on thyroid hormone response elements," *Molecular Endocrinology*, vol. 12, no. 10, pp. 1567–1581, 1998.

[174] R. N. Cohen, A. Putney, F. E. Wondisford, and A. N. Hollenberg, "The nuclear corepressors recognize distinct nuclear receptor complexes," *Molecular Endocrinology*, vol. 14, no. 6, pp. 900–914, 2000.

[175] S. M. Yoh and M. L. Privalsky, "Transcriptional repression by thyroid hormone receptors. A role for receptor homodimers in the recruitment of SMRT corepressor," *Journal of Biological Chemistry*, vol. 276, no. 20, pp. 16857–16867, 2001.

[176] S. Lee and M. L. Privalsky, "Heterodimers of retinoic acid receptors and thyroid hormone receptors display unique combinatorial regulatory properties," *Molecular Endocrinology*, vol. 19, no. 4, pp. 863–878, 2005.

[177] I. Astapova, M. F. Dordek, and A. N. Hollenberg, "The thyroid hormone receptor recruits NCoR via widely spaced receptor-interacting domains," *Molecular and Cellular Endocrinology*, vol. 307, no. 1-2, pp. 83–88, 2009.

[178] M. A. Lazar, "Thyroid hormone receptors: multiple forms, multiple possibilities," *Endocrine Reviews*, vol. 14, no. 2, pp. 184–193, 1993.

[179] G. A. Brent, "Tissue-specific actions of thyroid hormone: insights from animal models," *Reviews in Endocrine and Metabolic Disorders*, vol. 1, no. 1-2, pp. 27–33, 2000.

[180] D. Forrest and B. Vennström, "Functions of thyroid hormone receptors in mice," *Thyroid*, vol. 10, no. 1, pp. 41–52, 2000.

[181] J. Zhang and M. A. Lazar, "The mechanism of action of thyroid hormones," *Annual Review of Physiology*, vol. 62, pp. 439–466, 2000.

[182] F. Flamant and J. Samarut, "Thyroid hormone receptors: lessons from knockout and knock-in mutant mice," *Trends in Endocrinology and Metabolism*, vol. 14, no. 2, pp. 85–90, 2003.

[183] A. Oetting and P. M. Yen, "New insights into thyroid hormone action," *Best Practice and Research in Clinical Endocrinology and Metabolism*, vol. 21, no. 2, pp. 193–208, 2007.

[184] M. L. Privalsky, S. Lee, J. B. Hahm, B. M. Young, R. N. G. Fong, and I. H. Chan, "The p160 coactivator PAS-B

motif stabilizes nuclear receptor binding and contributes to isoform-specific regulation by Thyroid hormone receptors," *Journal of Biological Chemistry*, vol. 284, no. 29, pp. 19554–19563, 2009.

[185] J. Engelbreth-Holm and A. Rothe Meyer, "On the connection between erythroblastosis (haemocytoblastosis), myelosis, and sarcoma in chicken," *Acta Pathologica Microbiologica Scandinavica*, vol. 12, pp. 352–377, 1935.

[186] B. Vennstrom, "Isolation and characterization of chicken DNA homologous to the two putative oncogenes of avian erythroblastosis virus," *Cell*, vol. 28, no. 1, pp. 135–143, 1982.

[187] T. Graf and H. Beug, "Role of the v-erbA and v-erbB oncogenes of avian erythroblastosis virus in erythroid cell transformation," *Cell*, vol. 34, no. 1, pp. 7–9, 1983.

[188] J. Downward, Y. Yarden, and E. Mayes, "Close similarity of epidermal growth factor receptor and v-erb-B oncogene protein sequences," *Nature*, vol. 307, no. 5951, pp. 521–527, 1984.

[189] K. H. Lin, H. Y. Shieh, S. L. Chen, and H. C. Hsu, "Expression of mutant thyroid hormone nuclear receptors in human hepatocellular carcinoma cells," *Molecular Carcinogenesis*, vol. 26, no. 1, pp. 53–61, 1999.

[190] Y. Kamiya, M. Puzianowska-Kuznicka, P. McPhie, J. Nauman, S. Y. Cheng, and A. Nauman, "Expression of mutant thyroid hormone nuclear receptors is associated with human renal clear cell carcinoma," *Carcinogenesis*, vol. 23, no. 1, pp. 25–33, 2002.

[191] M. Puzianowska-Kuznicka, A. Krystyniak, A. Madej, S. Y. Cheng, and J. Nauman, "Functionally impaired TR mutants are present in thyroid papillary cancer," *Journal of Clinical Endocrinology and Metabolism*, vol. 87, no. 3, pp. 1120–1128, 2002.

[192] S. Y. Cheng, "Thyroid hormone receptor mutations in cancer," *Molecular and Cellular Endocrinology*, vol. 213, no. 1, pp. 23–30, 2003.

[193] C. S. Wang, K. H. Lin, and Y. C. Hsu, "Alterations of thyroid hormone receptor alpha gene: frequency and association with Nm23 protein expression and metastasis in gastric cancer," *Cancer Letters*, vol. 175, pp. 121–127, 2002.

[194] M. L. Privalsky, "v-erb A, nuclear hormone receptors, and oncogenesis," *Biochimica et Biophysica Acta*, vol. 1114, no. 1, pp. 51–62, 1992.

[195] H. Beug, A. Bauer, H. Dolznig et al., "Avian erythropoiesis and erythroleukemia: towards understanding the role of the biomolecules involved," *Biochimica et Biophysica Acta*, vol. 1288, no. 3, pp. M35–M47, 1996.

[196] L. E. G. Rietveld, E. Caldenhoven, and H. G. Stunnenberg, "Avian erythroleukemia: a model for corepressor function in cancer," *Oncogene*, vol. 20, no. 24, pp. 3100–3109, 2001.

[197] A. Ullrich, L. Coussens, and J. S. Hayflick, "Human epidermal growth factor receptor cDNA sequence and aberrant expression of the amplified gene in A431 epidermoid carcinoma cells," *Nature*, vol. 309, no. 5967, pp. 418–425, 1984.

[198] A. Muñoz, M. Zenke, U. Gehring, J. Sap, H. Beug, and B. Vennström, "Characterization of the hormone-binding domain of the chicken c-erbA/thyroid hormone receptor protein," *EMBO Journal*, vol. 7, no. 1, pp. 155–159, 1988.

[199] M. Zenke, P. Kahn, C. Disela et al., "v-erbA specifically suppresses transcription of the avian erythrocyte anion transporter (band 3) gene," *Cell*, vol. 52, no. 1, pp. 107–119, 1988.

[200] K. Damm, C. C. Thompson, and R. M. Evans, "Protein encoded by v-erbA functions as a thyroid-hormone receptor antagonist," *Nature*, vol. 339, no. 6226, pp. 593–597, 1989.

[201] J. Sap, A. Munoz, J. Schmitt, H. Stunnenberg, and B. Vennstrom, "Repression of transcription mediated at a thyroid hormone response element by the v-erb-A oncogene product," *Nature*, vol. 340, no. 6230, pp. 242–244, 1989.

[202] H. Chen, Z. Smit-McBride, S. Lewis, M. Sharif, and M. L. Privalsky, "Nuclear hormone receptors involved in neoplasia: Erb A exhibits a novel DNA sequence specificity determined by amino acids outside of the zinc-finger domain," *Molecular and Cellular Biology*, vol. 13, no. 4, pp. 2366–2376, 1993.

[203] C. Judelson and M. L. Privalsky, "DNA recognition by normal and oncogenic thyroid hormone receptors: unexpected diversity in half-site specificity controlled by non-zinc-finger determinants," *Journal of Biological Chemistry*, vol. 271, no. 18, pp. 10800–10805, 1996.

[204] J. S. Subauste and R. J. Koenig, "Characterization of the DNA-binding and dominant negative activity of v-erbA homodimers," *Molecular Endocrinology*, vol. 12, no. 9, pp. 1380–1392, 1998.

[205] S. Lee and M. L. Privalsky, "Multiple mutations contribute to repression by the v-Erb A oncoprotein," *Oncogene*, vol. 24, no. 45, pp. 6737–6752, 2005.

[206] C. Bresson, C. Keime, C. Faure et al., "Large-scale analysis by SAGE reveals new mechanisms of v-erbA oncogene action," *BMC Genomics*, vol. 8, article 390, 2007.

[207] T. Ventura-Holman, A. Mamoon, M. C. Subauste, and J. S. Subauste, "The effect of oncoprotein v-erbA on thyroid hormone-regulated genes in hepatocytes and their potential role in hepatocellular carcinoma," *Molecular Biology Reports*, vol. 38, no. 2, pp. 1137–1144, 2011.

[208] M. Sharif and M. L. Privalsky, "v-erbA oncogene function in neoplasia correlates with its ability to repress retinoic acid receptor action," *Cell*, vol. 66, no. 5, pp. 885–893, 1991.

[209] D. Maxwell Parkin, F. Bray, J. Ferlay, and P. Pisani, "Estimating the world cancer burden: Globocan 2000," *International Journal of Cancer*, vol. 94, no. 2, pp. 153–156, 2001.

[210] M. Al Sarraf, T. S. Go, K. Kithier, and V. K. Vaitkevicius, "Primary liver cancer: a review of the clinical features, blood groups, serum enzymes, therapy, and survival of 65 cases," *Cancer*, vol. 33, no. 2, pp. 574–582, 1974.

[211] J. M. Llovet, A. Burroughs, and J. Bruix, "Hepatocellular carcinoma," *The Lancet*, vol. 362, no. 9399, pp. 1907–1917, 2003.

[212] Y. Murakami, K. Hayashi, S. Hirohashi, and T. Sekiya, "Aberrations of the tumor suppressor p53 and retinoblastoma genes in human hepatocellular carcinomas," *Cancer Research*, vol. 51, no. 20, pp. 5520–5525, 1991.

[213] S. Y. Peng, P. L. Lai, and H. C. Hsu, "Amplification of the c-myc gene in human hepatocellular carcinoma: biologic significance," *Journal of the Formosan Medical Association*, vol. 92, no. 10, pp. 866–870, 1993.

[214] N. Nishida, Y. Fukuda, T. Komeda et al., "Amplification and overexpression of the cyclin D1 gene in aggressive human hepatocellular carcinoma," *Cancer Research*, vol. 54, no. 12, pp. 3107–3110, 1994.

[215] H. B. El-Serag and K. L. Rudolph, "Hepatocellular carcinoma: epidemiology and molecular carcinogenesis," *Gastroenterology*, vol. 132, no. 7, pp. 2557–2576, 2007.

[216] Y. Hoshida, S. Toffanin, A. Lachenmayer, A. Villanueva, B. Minguez, and J. M. Llovet, "Molecular classification and novel targets in hepatocellular carcinoma: recent advancements," *Seminars in Liver Disease*, vol. 30, no. 1, pp. 35–51, 2010.

[217] K.-H. Lin, X.-G. Zhu, H.-Y. Shieh et al., "Identification of naturally occurring dominant negative mutants of thyroid

hormone $\alpha1$ and $\beta1$ receptors in a human hepatocellular carcinoma cell line," *Endocrinology*, vol. 137, no. 10, pp. 4073–4081, 1996.

[218] C. Barlow, B. Meister, M. Lardelli, U. Lendahl, and B. Vennstrom, "Thyroid abnormalities and hepatocellular carcinoma in mice transgenic for v-erbA," *EMBO Journal*, vol. 13, no. 18, pp. 4241–4250, 1994.

[219] B. I. Rini, S. C. Campbell, and B. Escudier, "Renal cell carcinoma," *The Lancet*, vol. 373, no. 9669, pp. 1119–1132, 2009.

[220] K. Gupta, J. D. Miller, J. Z. Li, M. W. Russell, and C. Charbonneau, "Epidemiologic and socioeconomic burden of metastatic renal cell carcinoma (mRCC): a literature review," *Cancer Treatment Reviews*, vol. 34, no. 3, pp. 193–205, 2008.

[221] J. M. Kiely, "Hypernephroma–the internist's tumor," *Medical Clinics of North America*, vol. 50, no. 4, pp. 1067–1083, 1966.

[222] J. D. Hunt, O. L. Van Der Hel, G. P. McMillan, P. Boffetta, and P. Brennan, "Renal cell carcinoma in relation to cigarette smoking: meta-analysis of 24 studies," *International Journal of Cancer*, vol. 114, no. 1, pp. 101–108, 2005.

[223] J. M. Yuan, J. E. Castelao, M. Gago-Dominguez, M. C. Yu, and R. K. Ross, "Tobacco use in relation to renal cell carcinoma," *Cancer Epidemiology Biomarkers and Prevention*, vol. 7, no. 5, pp. 429–433, 1998.

[224] T. Bjørge, S. Tretli, and A. Engeland, "Relation of height and body mass index to renal cell carcinoma in two million Norwegian men and women," *American Journal of Epidemiology*, vol. 160, no. 12, pp. 1168–1176, 2004.

[225] B. A.C. Van Dijk, L. J. Schouten, L. A.L.M. Kiemeney, R. A. Goldbohm, and P. A. Van Den Brandt, "Relation of height, body mass, energy intake, and physical activity to risk of renal cell carcinoma: results from the Netherlands Cohort Study," *American Journal of Epidemiology*, vol. 160, no. 12, pp. 1159–1167, 2004.

[226] J. K. McLaughlin, W. H. Chow, J. S. Mandel et al., "International renal-cell cancer study. VIII. Role of diuretics, other anti-hypertensive medications and hypertension," *International Journal of Cancer*, vol. 63, no. 2, pp. 216–221, 1995.

[227] C. Suárez, R. Morales, E. Muñoz, J. Muñoz, C. M. Valverde, and J. Carles, "Molecular basis for the treatment of renal cell carcinoma," *Clinical and Translational Oncology*, vol. 12, no. 1, pp. 15–21, 2010.

[228] B. I. Rini and M. B. Atkins, "Resistance to targeted therapy in renal-cell carcinoma," *The Lancet Oncology*, vol. 10, no. 10, pp. 992–1000, 2009.

[229] M. L. Nickerson, E. Jaeger, Y. Shi et al., "Improved identification of von Hippel-Lindau gene alterations in clear cell renal tumors," *Clinical Cancer Research*, vol. 14, no. 15, pp. 4726–4734, 2008.

[230] J. R. Gnarra, S. Zhou, M. J. Merrill et al., "Posttranscriptional regulation of vascular endothelial growth factor mRNA by the product of the VHL tumor suppressor gene," *Proceedings of the National Academy of Sciences of the United States of America*, vol. 93, no. 20, pp. 10589–10594, 1996.

[231] S. Kourembanas, R. L. Hannan, and D. V. Faller, "Oxygen tension regulates the expression of the platelet-derived growth factor-B chain gene in human endothelial cells," *Journal of Clinical Investigation*, vol. 86, no. 2, pp. 670–674, 1990.

[232] N. De Paulsen, A. Brychzy, M. C. Fournier et al., "Role of transforming growth factor-α in von Hippel-Lindau (VHL) clear cell renal carcinoma cell proliferation: a possible mechanism coupling VHL tumor suppressor inactivation and tumorigenesis," *Proceedings of the National Academy of*

Sciences of the United States of America, vol. 98, no. 4, pp. 1387–1392, 2001.

[233] R. R. Lonser, G. M. Glenn, M. Walther et al., "Von Hippel-Lindau disease," *The Lancet*, vol. 361, no. 9374, pp. 2059–2067, 2003.

[234] C. R. Thoma, A. Toso, K. L. Gutbrodt et al., "VHL loss causes spindle misorientation and chromosome instability," *Nature Cell Biology*, vol. 11, no. 8, pp. 994–1001, 2009.

[235] E. B. Rankin, J. E. Tomaszewski, and V. H. Haase, "Renal cyst development in mice with conditional inactivation of the von Hippel-Lindau tumor suppressor," *Cancer Research*, vol. 66, no. 5, pp. 2576–2583, 2006.

[236] W. Ma, L. Tessarollo, S. B. Hong et al., "Hepatic vascular tumors, angiectasis in multiple organs, and impaired spermatogenesis in mice with conditional inactivation of the VHL gene," *Cancer Research*, vol. 63, no. 17, pp. 5320–5328, 2003.

[237] A. G. Knudson, "Genetics of human cancer.," *Annual Review of Genetics*, vol. 20, pp. 231–251, 1986.

[238] Z. Zhang, B. Wondergem, and K. Dykema, "A comprehensive study of progressive cytogenetic alterations in clear cell renal cell carcinoma and a new model for ccRCC tumorigenesis and progression," *Advances in Bioinformatics*, vol. 2010, Article ID 428325, 2010.

[239] M. Puzianowska-Kuznicka, A. Nauman, A. Madej, Z. Tanski, S. Y. Cheng, and J. Nauman, "Expression of thyroid hormone receptors is disturbed in human renal clear cell carcinoma," *Cancer Letters*, vol. 155, no. 2, pp. 145–152, 2000.

[240] J. C. Presti, V. E. Reuter, C. Cordon-Cardo, M. Mazumdar, W. R. Fair, and S. C. Jhanwar, "Allelic deletions in renal tumors: histopathological correlations," *Cancer Research*, vol. 53, no. 23, pp. 5780–5783, 1993.

[241] J. M. González-Sancho, V. García, F. Bonilla, and A. Muñoz, "Thyroid hormone receptors/THR genes in human cancer," *Cancer Letters*, vol. 192, no. 2, pp. 121–132, 2003.

[242] M. Kaneshige, K. Kaneshige, X. U. G. Zhu et al., "Mice with a targeted mutation in the thyroid hormone β receptor gene exhibit impaired growth and resistance to thyroid hormone," *Proceedings of the National Academy of Sciences of the United States of America*, vol. 97, no. 24, pp. 13209–13214, 2000.

[243] H. Suzuki, M. C. Willingham, and S. Y. Cheng, "Mice with a mutation in the thyroid hormone receptor β gene spontaneously develop thyroid carcinoma: a mouse model of thyroid carcinogenesis," *Thyroid*, vol. 12, no. 11, pp. 963–969, 2002.

[244] Y. Kato, H. Ying, M. C. Willingham, and S. Y. Cheng, "A tumor suppressor role for thyroid hormone β receptor in a mouse model of thyroid carcinogenesis," *Endocrinology*, vol. 145, no. 10, pp. 4430–4438, 2004.

[245] H. Furumoto, H. Ying, G. V. R. Chandramouli et al., "An unliganded thyroid hormone β receptor activates the cyclin D1/cyclin-dependent kinase/retinoblastoma/E2F pathway and induces pituitary tumorigenesis," *Molecular and Cellular Biology*, vol. 25, no. 1, pp. 124–135, 2005.

[246] H. Ying, O. Araki, F. Furuya, Y. Kato, and S.-Y. Cheng, "Impaired adipogenesis caused by a mutated thyroid hormone $\alpha1$ receptor," *Molecular and Cellular Biology*, vol. 27, no. 6, pp. 2359–2371, 2007.

[247] C. Lu and S. Y. Cheng, "Thyroid hormone receptors regulate adipogenesis and carcinogenesis via crosstalk signaling with peroxisome proliferator-activated receptors," *Journal of Molecular Endocrinology*, vol. 44, no. 3, pp. 143–154, 2010.

[248] F. Furuya, J. A. Hanover, and S. Y. Cheng, "Activation of phosphatidylinositol 3-kinase signaling by a mutant thyroid

hormone β receptor," *Proceedings of the National Academy of Sciences of the United States of America*, vol. 103, no. 6, pp. 1780–1785, 2006.

[249] C. J. Guigon and S. Y. Cheng, "Novel oncogenic actions of TRβ mutants in tumorigenesis," *IUBMB Life*, vol. 61, no. 5, pp. 528–536, 2009.

[250] H. Ying, H. Suzuki, H. Furumoto et al., "Alterations in genomic profiles during tumor progression in a mouse model of follicular thyroid carcinoma," *Carcinogenesis*, vol. 24, no. 9, pp. 1467–1479, 2003.

[251] H. Ying, F. Furuya, LI. Zhao et al., "Aberrant accumulation of PTTG1 induced by a mutated thyroid hormone β receptor inhibits mitotic progression," *Journal of Clinical Investigation*, vol. 116, no. 11, pp. 2972–2984, 2006.

[252] C. J. Guigon, LI. Zhao, C. Lu, M. C. Willingham, and S. Y. Cheng, "Regulation of β-catenin by a novel nongenomic action of thyroid hormone β receptor," *Molecular and Cellular Biology*, vol. 28, no. 14, pp. 4598–4608, 2008.

[253] O. Martínez-Iglesias, S. García-Silva, J. Regadera, and A. Aranda, "Hypothyroidism enhances tumor invasiveness and metastasis development," *PLoS ONE*, vol. 4, no. 7, Article ID e6428, 2009.

[254] X. G. Zhu, L. Zhao, M. C. Willingham, and S. Y. Cheng, "Thyroid hormone receptors are tumor suppressors in a mouse model of metastatic follicular thyroid carcinoma," *Oncogene*, vol. 29, no. 13, pp. 1909–1919, 2010.

[255] T. T. Hörkkö, K. Tuppurainen, S. M. George, P. Jernvall, T. J. Karttunen, and M. J. Mäkinen, "Thyroid hormone receptor β1 in normal colon and colorectal cancer-association with differentiation, polypoid growth type and K-ras mutations," *International Journal of Cancer*, vol. 118, no. 7, pp. 1653–1659, 2006.

[256] Z. Li, Z. H. Meng, R. Chandrasekaran et al., "Biallelic inactivation of the thyroid hormone receptor β1 gene in early stage breast cancer," *Cancer Research*, vol. 62, no. 7, pp. 1939–1943, 2002.

[257] S. García-Silva and A. Aranda, "The thyroid hormone receptor is a suppressor of ras-mediated transcription, proliferation, and transformation," *Molecular and Cellular Biology*, vol. 24, no. 17, pp. 7514–7523, 2004.

[258] M. Cristofanilli, Y. Yamamura, S. W. Kau et al., "Thyroid hormone and breast carcinoma: primary hypothyroidism is associated with a reduced incidence of primary breast carcinoma," *Cancer*, vol. 103, no. 6, pp. 1122–1128, 2005.

[259] A. A. Hercbergs, L. K. Goyal, J. H. Suh et al., "Propyl-thiouracil-induced chemical hypothyroidism with high-dose tamoxifen prolongs survival in recurrent high grade glioma: a phase I/II study," *Anticancer Research*, vol. 23, no. 1 B, pp. 617–626, 2003.

[260] A. Reddy, C. Dash, A. Leerapun et al., "Hypothyroidism: a possible risk factor for liver cancer in patients with no known underlying cause of liver disease," *Clinical Gastroenterology and Hepatology*, vol. 5, no. 1, pp. 118–123, 2007.

[261] G. Beatson, "On treatment of inoperable cases of carcinoma of the mamma: suggestions for a new method of treatment with illustrative cases," *The Lancet*, vol. 148, no. 3802, pp. 104–107, 1896.

[262] F. Page, "Recurrent carcinoma of the breast entirely disappearing under persistent use of thyorid extract continued for 18 months," *The Lancet*, vol. 151, no. 3900, pp. 1460–1461, 1898.

[263] R. R. Love and J. Philips, "Oophorectomy for breast cancer: history revisited," *Journal of the National Cancer Institute*, vol. 94, no. 19, pp. 1433–1434, 2002.

[264] A. Thomson, "Analysis of cases in which oophorectomy was performed for inoperable carcinoma of the breast," *British Medical Journal*, vol. 2, pp. 1538–1541, 1902.

[265] O. Martínez-Iglesias, S. Garcia-Silva, S. P. Tenbaum et al., "Thyroid hormone receptor β1 acts as a potent suppressor of tumor invasiveness and metastasis," *Cancer Research*, vol. 69, no. 2, pp. 501–509, 2009.

[266] M. M. Hassan, A. Kaseb, D. Li et al., "Association between hypothyroidism and hepatocellular carcinoma: a case-control study in the United States," *Hepatology*, vol. 49, no. 5, pp. 1563–1570, 2009.

[267] G. M. Ledda-Columbano, A. Perra, R. Loi, H. Shinozuka, and A. Columbano, "Cell proliferation induced by triiodothyronine in rat liver is associated with nodule regression and reduction of hepatocellular carcinomas," *Cancer Research*, vol. 60, no. 3, pp. 603–609, 2000.

[268] G. Rennert, H. S. Rennert, M. Pinchev, and S. B. Gruber, "A case-control study of levothyroxine and the risk of colorectal cancer," *Journal of the National Cancer Institute*, vol. 102, no. 8, pp. 568–572, 2010.

[269] A. Perra, M. A. Kowalik, M. Pibiri, G. M. Ledda-Columbano, and A. Columbano, "Thyroid hormone receptor ligands induce regression of rat preneoplastic liver lesions causing their reversion to a differentiated phenotype," *Hepatology*, vol. 49, no. 4, pp. 1287–1296, 2009.

[270] E. Kress, J. Samarut, and M. Plateroti, "Thyroid hormones and the control of cell proliferation or cell differentiation: paradox or duality?" *Molecular and Cellular Endocrinology*, vol. 313, no. 1-2, pp. 36–49, 2009.

32

Thyroid Hormone and the Neuroglia: Both Source and Target

Petra Mohácsik,[1] Anikó Zeöld,[1] Antonio C. Bianco,[2] and Balázs Gereben[1]

[1] Laboratory of Endocrine Neurobiology, Institute of Experimental Medicine, Hungarian Academy of Sciences, Budapest, H-1083, Hungary
[2] Division of Endocrinology, Diabetes, and Metabolism, University of Miami Miller School of Medicine, Miami, FL 33136, USA

Correspondence should be addressed to Balázs Gereben, gereben@koki.hu

Academic Editor: Juan Bernal

Thyroid hormone plays a crucial role in the development and function of the nervous system. In order to bind to its nuclear receptor and regulate gene transcription thyroxine needs to be activated in the brain. This activation occurs via conversion of thyroxine to T3, which is catalyzed by the type 2 iodothyronine deiodinase (D2) in glial cells, in astrocytes, and tanycytes in the mediobasal hypothalamus. We discuss how thyroid hormone affects glial cell function followed by an overview on the fine-tuned regulation of T3 generation by D2 in different glial subtypes. Recent evidence on the direct paracrine impact of glial D2 on neuronal gene expression underlines the importance of glial-neuronal interaction in thyroid hormone regulation as a major regulatory pathway in the brain in health and disease.

1. Introduction

Thyroid hormone is a fundamental regulator of biological processes, including cell proliferation, differentiation, and metabolic balance [1]. Thyroid hormone plays a crucial role in brain development, which is illustrated by the dramatic neurologic impairment observed in untreated neonatal hypothyroidism, a condition leading to cretinism [2–4]. The adult brain is also sensitive to thyroid hormone in view of mood disorders, depression, memory, cognitive and motoric impairments frequently observed in hypothyroid patients [5].

The major secretory product of the human thyroid gland is thyroxine (T4), a prohormone that does not efficiently bind thyroid hormone receptor (TR). T4 has to be converted to 3,5,3′-triiodothyronine (T3) in order to bind to TR and initiate thyroid hormone-mediated changes in gene expression profiles. Notably, a significant amount of brain T3 is derived from the local activation of prohormone T4 to T3 (80% in the cortex), suggesting that most T3 acting in the brain is generated *in situ* from T4 deiodination [6]. Plasma T3 was also shown to enter the brain [7], and studies on the monocarboxylate transporter 8 (MCT8) knock-out mice indicate that MCT8 plays an important role

in this process, but other transporters might also be involved [8, 9]. However, only supraphysiological doses of T3 were sufficient to suppress pro-TRH mRNA in the hypothalamic paraventricular nucleus of hypothyroid rats [10] indicating that T4 uptake into the brain is important for normal function of T3-mediated processes in this tissue. Further studies are required to better understand the transport of different thyroid hormone derivatives across the blood-brain and CSF-brain barrier, the consequences of this mechanism, and the factors affecting this process (see also Section 3.3).

Local T3 generation in the brain is catalyzed by the type 2 deiodinase (D2), a tightly controlled selenoenzyme [11–14]. D2 is the only known protein capable of producing T3 in the human brain [15]. Beyond D2-mediated T3 generation, type 3 deiodinase (D3) is also similarly important for thyroid hormone economy in the brain [16, 17]. D3 inactivates T3 and converts T4 to reverse-T3 that cannot bind to TR. Thus, in contrast to D2, D3 catalyzes the inactivation pathway of thyroid hormone metabolism.

D2 is expressed in glial cells, including astrocytes in different brain regions and tanycytes, the specialized glial cells in the walls and floor of the third ventricle of the mediobasal hypothalamus [18–20]. In contrast to the glial D2, D3 expression in the brain is restricted to neurons [21].

While historically glial elements of the brain were viewed as a type of connective tissue of the CNS without any real function, this view was overturned by the abundant data on the complex role of glial cells in brain metabolism [22]. According to this more recent hypothesis, glial D2 provides T3 for neighboring neurons that express TR but lack T3 generating capacity [4, 19, 20, 23–25].

Thyroid hormone exerts its biological effects predominantly via binding to its nuclear TR, but specific nongenomic effects have also been suggested [26–29]. Two TR isoforms, α and β, act as ligand-regulated transcription factor and have a central role in transducing the hormonal signal into a cellular response in the brain (reviewed in [30, 31]). Despite accumulating evidence demonstrating that thyroid hormone alters astrocytes function (see Section 2), the presence of TR in astrocytes remains controversial.

The presence of TR in astrocytes has been suggested by in vitro studies [32–34], but lower receptor concentrations have been detected compared to oligodendrocytes or neurons [34]. The presence of TR could also be detected in purified glial nuclei from postnatal rat brain [35]. In contrast, in vivo data suggested that thyroid hormone would mediate astrocyte function indirectly, based on the lack of immunofluorescence staining of TR receptor isoforms $\alpha 1$, $\beta 1$, and $\beta 2$ in GFAP positive astrocytes of the adult rat brain [36]. Interestingly the same group used immunofluorescent to locate TR in cultured astrocytes [37], in line with other in vitro data. Astrocytes from distinct developing brain regions are differently responsive to thyroid hormone, with the highest sensitivity in the hemispheres [38]. Thyroid hormone has been shown to be essential for maturation of rat cerebellar astrocytes [39], and TR$\alpha 1$ knock-out mice display astrocyte maturation defects suggesting the role of this TR isoform to mediate a direct effect of thyroid hormone action in astrocytes [40]. Presently, most studies agree with the presence of TR$\alpha 1$ isoform in astrocytes; discrepancies remain in the case of TRβ receptor subtypes. Expression of different TR isoforms has been reported in human astrocytomas [41]. Thyroid hormone action occurs within limited time windows, a spatially and timely controlled phenomenon. Cultured cells and most astrocytomas are devoid of the same control conditions, which normally act on cells in the brain, and this could be a background of the different experimental results obtained between in vitro and in vivo data. In addition, cultured astrocytes are most likely reactive astrocytes, and the heterogeneity of the in vitro experimental results regarding TR expression in these cells may reflect the different experimental conditions, such as the brain region and the age of the animals used for cultivation or the different culture conditions.

Active transport of thyroid hormone into brain cells adds to the complexity of thyroid hormone economy in the central nervous system [42, 43]. The MCT8 (SLC16A2) and organic anion transporter 1C1 (OATP1C1) are the best studied thyroid hormone transporters [44, 45]. MCT8 seems to be the predominant neuronal T3 transporter, and its mutations are associated with the Allan-Herndon-Dudley syndrome characterized by congenital hypotonia that progresses to spasticity with severe psychomotor delays [44, 46, 47].

OATP1C1 has high affinity to T4 and is expressed in brain endothelial cells and also in vascular end-feet of astrocytes [48]. Interestingly, tanycytes seem to coexpress MCT8 and OATP1C1 [48]. Other thyroid hormone transporters have also been identified including MCT10, which seems to transport T3 more effectively than MCT8 [49] and the L-type amino acid transporters (LATs) [50]. MCT10 expression was demonstrated in microglia while LAT1 and LAT2 expression was found both in astrocytes and neurons; LAT2 was also present in microglia [51]. Studies on the MCT8 deficient mouse revealed that in the absence of functional MCT8, alternative thyroid hormone transporters play an important complementary role in neuronal T3 transport. In contrast, the lack of alternative pathways, for example, LAT2 in developing human neurons, might be involved in the devastating neurodevelopmental phenotype seen in MCT8-deficient patients with Allan-Herndon-Dudley syndrome [8, 52].

Studies on transgenic mice with targeted inactivation of different members of the deiodinase enzyme family, MCT8, or their combined deletion provided important information on the complex nature of functional interactions between factors regulating thyroid hormone metabolism and transport in the brain and other tissues [8, 9, 53–58]. Despite the relatively mild brain phenotype of D2KO or MCT8KO mice, their combined inactivation led to aggravated manifestation of thyroid hormone deprivation and resulted in similar effects as observed in hypothyroidism [9, 59]. These data confirmed the crucial role of D2 in local T3 generation in the brain and suggested that changes in D2 expression could compensate for defects in MCT8 function in the rodent brain.

Numerous aspects of deiodinase-mediated changes of thyroid hormone metabolism have been carefully reviewed and provide a comprehensive view on the molecular and biochemical properties, structure, regulation, and biological functions of these enzymes in the brain and different tissues [24, 60–69]. In the present paper we will focus on the role and regulation of thyroid hormone in neuroglia, representing an exciting aspect of emerging significance for thyroid hormone economy. We provide a concise overview on the most important effects of thyroid hormone on glial cells, followed by the discussion of novel data on D2-mediated glial T3 generation and its role under specific physiological and pathophysiological conditions.

2. Thyroid Hormone-Mediated Changes in Neuroglial Cells

Brain development provides the best studied model of thyroid hormone action in the brain. It has been known for decades that hypothyroidism can result in numerous brain defects, including decreased dendritic arborization of Purkinje cells, diminished axonal outgrow and myelinization, and insufficient cortical layer organization [70]. Although thyroid hormone also impacts the adult brain, the underlying cellular and molecular events are less understood [71, 72]. Various aspects of thyroid hormone-mediated brain function were extensively reviewed (see Section 1).

Available data on thyroid-hormone-regulated gene networks are yet limited, but accumulating evidence indicates that various sets of genes are regulated along this pathway. In a recent study, thyroid hormone action on adult rat striatum was monitored using gene expression profiling [73]. The numerous up or down regulated sets of genes involved various pathways affecting for example, circadian regulation, oxidative stress response, phenylethylamine degradation, MAPK pathway, phosphate metabolism, signal transduction, and cell structure. These findings revealed novel aspects of brain related thyroid hormone action that need to be studied in details. Numerous examples of thyroid hormone-dependent gene expression in the brain are related to neurons, which could be a result of direct neuronal effect or an indirect glia-mediated signal [74]. Neuroglial cells are heavily involved in the regulation of neuronal metabolism and activity, glucose supply, cerebral blood flow, and neurotransmitter levels in mature brain [22]. The detailed description of mechanisms how glial cells are involved in this process is an ongoing effort and requires further studies. We will briefly summarize below how thyroid hormone targets glial cells and mediates their function that has also consequence on glia-mediated neuronal activities.

2.1. Differentiation, Maturation.

Thyroid hormone affects the differentiation and maturation of different glial subtypes including astrocytes, oligodendrocytes, and microglia [75–77]. Although many aspects of glial linages are yet controversial, evidence has been obtained *in vitro* that oligodendrocytes and astrocytes are derived from a common precursor, the glial restricted precursor cells (GRP) [78]. GRPs are tripotential cells, owning the ability to divide into myelin producing oligodendrocyte or two types of astrocytes, depending on the factors contained in growth medium. *In vitro* studies demonstrated that mature oligodendrocytes were developed from precursor cells in the presence of thyroid hormone and platelet-derived growth factor (PDGF) [79]. The concept that these two glial cell types originate from a common lineage was also supported by findings that show reciprocal changes in oligodendrocyte/astrocyte cell density in the rat white matter upon changes in serum T4 level [80]. Furthermore, the number of matured oligodendrocytes and astrocytes was reduced in the brain of hypothyroid animals within white matter tracts [81, 82]. Morphological differentiation of astrocytes from progenitors to mature cells has been explained by thyroid hormone-mediated actions affecting cytoskeletal proteins (F-actin, GFAP) [40, 83]. In hypothyroid neonatal rats, there was reduced GFAP content in hippocampus and basal forebrain [84]. In cell cultures, T3 upregulates GFAP production and reorganizes GFAP filaments and transforms the flat polygonal astrocytes into process-bearing cells [85, 86]. Not only T3, but T3-mediated growth factor secretion can enhance GFAP expression, thanks to several growth factor binding domains in its promoter region [87, 88].

Microglial cell development is also affected by thyroid hormone. In the cortical forebrain of hypothyroid neonatal rat there is diminished amount of cell bodies and less abundant microglial process density. T3 favored survival of microglias *in vitro* and have triggered their process extension [77, 89].

The mechanisms by which thyroid hormone promotes differentiation were not yet fully revealed, but there are several candidates for this process, for example, cell-cycle modulators like E2F-1, cyclin D1, and p27 [90]. E2F1 is a key transcription factor, that controls G1 to S phase transition and has an impact on cyclin D1 [91]. E2F-1 and cyclin D1 expression is down regulated via TR-mediated transcriptional repression [92, 93]. Another candidate of this pathway, p27 cyclin-dependent kinase inhibitor was upregulated in response to T3 [94, 95]. Decreased amount of E2F-1 and cyclin D1 protein and increased levels of the p27 cell-cycle inhibitor may shift cell fate towards differentiation.

2.2. Myelination.

Myelination represents the best characterized T3-dependent glial action in the brain [96–98]. Thyroid hormone regulates oligodendrocyte differentiation and myelin production via TR-mediated transcriptional effects [34, 99]. Thyroid hormone depletion resulted in delayed expression of oligodendrocyte-specific markers [100] and decreased the number of oligodendrocyte cell bodies in the main white matter tracts [81]. Hypothyroidism delayed the expression of genes encoding structural proteins of myelin, for example, myelin basic protein (MBP), proteolipid protein (PLP), and myelin-associated glycoprotein (MAG) [101] and resulted in reduced numbers of myelinated axons and lower myelin content [102]. Sensitivity period of these genes for thyroid hormone extends from the end of the first postnatal week up to the end of the first month in rat [76, 103].

2.3. Extracellular Matrix Formation and Cytoskeleton Organization.

Thyroid hormone action on astrocytes during brain development is illustrated by enhanced secretion of extracellular matrix proteins and growth factors. Astrocytes were previously shown to produce laminin and fibronectin [104, 105]. Subsequent studies demonstrated T3-induced expression of laminin and fibronectin in cultured cerebellar astrocytes and revealed that both laminin and fibronectin were organized in fibrillar pattern on the cell surface, while hypothyroid conditions changed this distribution for a disorganized extracellular matrix of punctuate pattern [106]. As an underlying mechanism it was suggested that astrocytes modulate extracellular matrix composition via T3-mediated growth factor secretion [104, 107].

Basic fibroblast growth factor (bFGF) and epidermal growth factor (EGF) are secreted by cerebellar astrocytes in response to T3 and seem to promote extracellular matrix protein secretion and organization in an autocrine manner [106]. EGF was suggested to exert its effect on extracellular matrix protein secretion through MAPK/phosphatidylinositol 3-kinase pathway [108]. Astrocytes also secrete nerve growth factor (NGF) in a T3-dependent manner, which allows potent control of neurite growth and survival [109–111].

Beyond T3, the effect of T4 on astrocytes was also demonstrated suggesting that thyroid hormone could also impact astrocytes via a nongenomic pathway. T4 exerts its effect on the microfilament network of astrocytes by dynamically organizing F-actin filaments, facilitating integrin clustering, and focal contact formation [112, 113]. Polymerized actin filament network was observed in cultured astrocytes after treatment with T4 and reverse T3 while T3 did not affect the polimerization rate [114, 115].

Adhesive interactions among the extracellular matrix protein laminin, integrins, and the microfilament network play a fundamental role in the regulation of neural cell migration during brain development. *In vitro* studies on neurite development demonstrated that neurons, cocultured with astrocytes under thyroid hormone-depleted conditions, showed reduced total neurite length and decreased neurite numbers [108]. As a consequence, these data suggest that thyroid hormone-mediated actions on astrocytes are important events in neuron migration and axon formation.

3. Thyroid Hormone Activation in Neuroglia

3.1. Regulation of Type 2 Deiodinase in Glial Cells. While thyroid hormone impacts glial function in various manner (see above), neuroglia is not only target but also the predominant source of T3 in the brain. As mentioned above, astrocytes and tanycytes express type 2 deiodinase (D2), the enzyme catalyzing thyroid hormone activation. Below, we will discuss factors and conditions affecting D2 regulation in glial cells, since they can contribute to the better understanding of thyroid hormone signaling in the brain.

3.1.1. Thyroid Hormone. D2 is negatively regulated by thyroid hormone, through a mechanism that involves product (T3-) mediated transcriptional downregulation of the *Dio2* gene and substrate (T4-) induced posttranslational decrease of D2 protein levels (reviewed in [66], see Section 3.2). The negative regulation of D2 activity suggests a homeostatic regulation of T3 generation [116–118]. However, region-specific differences within the brain regarding the response to hyper- or hypothyroidism are reflected by changes in D2 regulation. D2 is reciprocally regulated by thyroid hormone in various brain regions but shows only modest response in the hypothalamus [19, 119–121]. The fact that D2 activity in the hypothalamus is concentrated in tanycytes [19] suggests marked differences between astrocytes and tanycytes regarding thyroid hormone response and balance. While in astrocytes T3 production seems to serve homeostatic purposes, the relative insensitivity of D2 to T3 in tanycytes would indicate that other signals act more importantly on D2 expression, thus controlling local T3 production [25]. The mechanisms responsible for this difference between astrocytes and tanycytes remain to be determined. However, a link has been suggested between the developmental state of astrocytes and their responsiveness to thyroid hormone [38]. Although tanycytes are still considered as terminally differentiated cells, data have been accumulating that at least a subpopulation of this inhomogeneous cell layer might behave as progenitor cells. This is supported by observations that the tanycyte layer in the wall of the third ventricle regenerates in two weeks following alloxan-induced destruction

[122], and tanycytes could be considered a neurogenic niche in response to IGF-I [123]. This is presently unclear whether differences in differentiation stages or a more specific factor is responsible for the different responsiveness to thyroid hormone of the two cell types.

3.1.2. Infection, Nonthyroidal Illness. It has been suggested that D2-generated T3 in tanycytes of the mediobasal hypothalamus could play a role in the pathogenesis of nonthyroidal illness during infection [63, 66, 67, 124]. Nonthyroidal illness syndrome (euthyroid sick syndrome or low T3 syndrome) is accompanied by low T3 and sometimes low T4 serum levels and associated with nonelevated or inappropriately elevated TSH levels during infection, sepsis, starvation, malignancy, life-threatening trauma, and other critical illness [125–128]. Although the syndrome has been known for decades, it is still a matter of debate whether the changes of thyroid hormone profile provide physiologic compensation for illness or it represents pathological conditions [129–131]. Systemic administration of bacterial lipopolysaccharide (LPS) increased D2 mRNA expression in tanycytes and D2 activity in the rat mediobasal hypothalamus (Figure 1) accompanied by falling serum thyroid hormone and TSH levels [132]. This phenomenon was also observed in mice, immediately followed by decreased expression of thyroid receptor β2, TSHβ in the pituitary and decreased type 1 deiodinase mRNA in the pituitary and liver [133].

LPS induced suppression of TRH expression in the hypothalamic paraventricular nucleus of wild type but the effect was abolished in the D2 knock-out mice (Figure 2) (see Section 3.3) [23]. Although this model is not suitable to dissect the role of specific glial subtypes in this mechanism, it clearly demonstrated the fundamental role of D2 activity in TRH suppression during infection and supported the hypothesis of a close interaction between neurons and glial cells and their role in regulating brain functions via T3 availability. Importantly, while the continuous increase in D2 activity of cortical astrocytes seemed to be the consequence of falling T4 levels, D2 activation in tanycytes followed kinetics that was independent of thyroid hormone levels [132, 134]. It was also demonstrated that LPS-induced D2 expression on the mediobasal hypothalamus was not dependent on circulating corticosterone, either [135]. Unexpectedly, cultured astrocytes of the rat cerebral hemispheres increased their D2 activity in response to LPS, and glucocorticoids enhanced this effect [136]. It is presently not clear why this effect is not reflected *in vivo* by the kinetics of cortical D2 induction. Importantly NF-κB, a potent effector of LPS-induced signaling, transcriptionally activated the D2 encoding *Dio2* gene, and a functional NF-κB binding site was identified and characterized in the human *Dio2* 5′ flanking region [132, 137]. NF-κB was also involved in the LPS-induced increase in D2 activity in cultured astrocytes [136].

Further studies on the kinetics of LPS-induced activation of the NF-κB pathway in the rat mediobasal hypothalamus indicated that NF-κB activation contributes to sustaining the LPS-induced D2 response in a subset of α tanycytes [138]. However, this is not the initiating mechanism of LPS-induced D2 response in tanycytes. The same study suggested

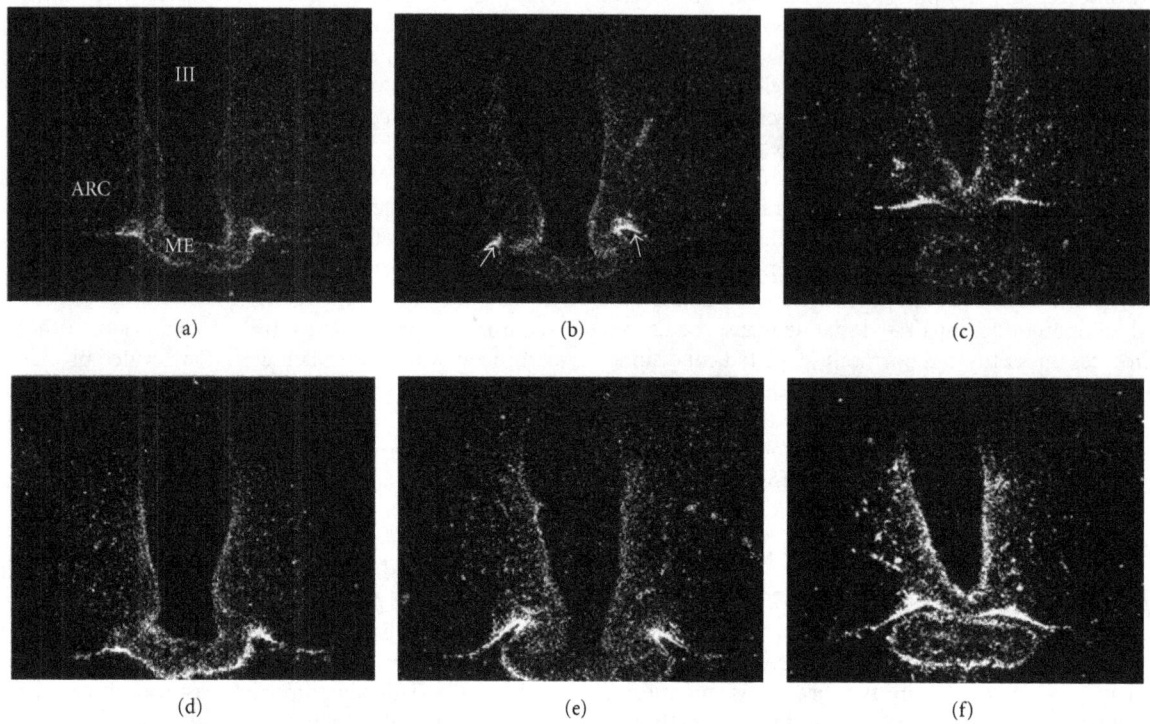

FIGURE 1: Infection upregulates D2 expression in tanycytes of the rat mediobasal hypothalamus. Dark-field micrographs from three different rostrocaudal levels of the median eminence (ME) showing the effect of *i.p.* LPS treatment on D2 mRNA expression. (a)–(c), Controls; (d)-(f), LPS-treatment. Note: D2 *in situ* hybridization signal is increased in the tanycytes lining the wall of the third ventricle (III), and in the tanycyte processes in the tuberoinfundibular sulci (arrows), in the external zone of the ME. ARC, arcuate nucleus. Reprinted with permission from Fekete et al. [132], The Endocrine Society.

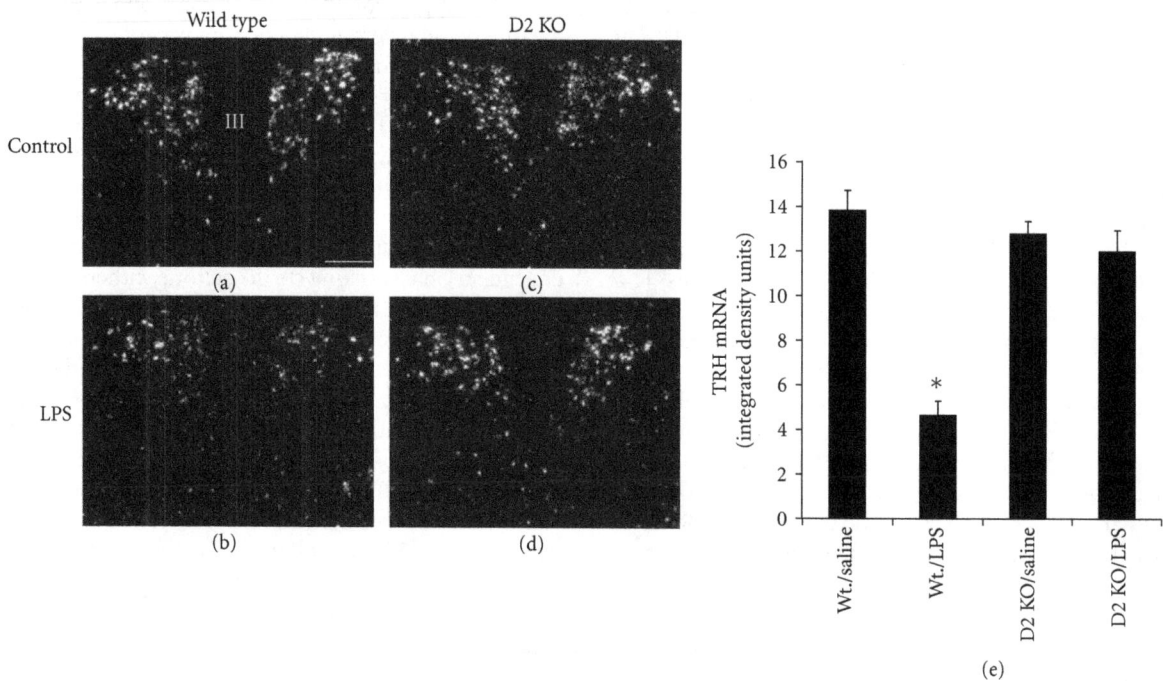

FIGURE 2: LPS-induced infection downregulates TRH mRNA expression in the hypothalamic paraventricular nucleus of wildtype but in D2 knock-out mice. (a,b), wild-type; (c,d), D2 KO mice; (a,c), control; (b,d), *i.p.* LPS-treated animals; (e), quantification of the TRH mRNA signal by densitometry. Printed from Freitas et al. American Society for Clinical Investigation [23].

that TSH of the part tuberalis could also play a role in this process [138]. The factor(s) that initiate tanycytal D2 induction in the starting phase of LPS-evoked infection are presently not known. However, taking into account the highly active nature of D2-catalyzed T3 generation even a subpopulation of tanycytes could provide a significant amount of T3 for the modulation of TRH expression. To asses this appropriately, it would be important to understand in details the pathways that allow tanycyte-generated T3 to reach hypophysiotropic TRH neurons in the paraventricular nucleus.

3.1.3. Iodine.

Iodine availability is critically important to maintain proper thyroid hormone levels. During moderate iodine deficiency most thyroid hormone target tissues are only mildly affected, due to rapid physiological adaptations of the hypothalamo-hypophyseal-thyroid axis, which maintains plasma T3 at the normal range [139, 140]. Via glial D2 and neuronal D3, the brain is capable of adapting to iodine deficiency in a complex manner. A moderately severe iodine deficiency resulted in increased D2 mRNA and activity in different brain regions [140]. D2 sensitivity to iodine deficiency was region specific, the hippocampus and cerebral cortex represented the most responsive regions. D2 induction in this regions indicated that astrocytes increase their T3-generating activity under iodine deficiency. Tanycytes of the mediobasal hypothalamus also increased their D2 expression and activity although their response was lower compared to astrocytes in the cortex and hippocampus. Since increase of D2 activity was higher than that of mRNA expression, it could be speculated that not only pretranslational events are involved here in D2 regulation but also prolonged D2 half-life due to decreased D2 ubiquitination (see Section 3.2) could contribute to this effect. Increased glial D2 in iodine deficiency was paralleled with reduced neuronal D3 [140]. Thus mitigating the effects of iodine deficiency by both increased T3 generation and reduced T3 degradation reflected the particular importance of adaptation of the brain to iodine deficiency. Various aspects of iodine deficiency modulated alterations of thyroid hormone deiodination were extensively reviewed elsewhere [141].

3.1.4. Fasting.

D2 expression in tanycytes is modulated by food restriction. Fasting resulted in twofold increase in D2 mRNA expression and activity in rat mediobasal hypothalamus, and it was straightforward to suggest that this could suppress TRH expression in the hypothalamic paraventricular nucleus and downregulate this way the hypothalamo-hypophyseal-thyroid axis. [121]. However, fasting-mediated decrease of TRH expression in the paraventricular nucleus of the TRβ2-null transgenic mice remained unaffected although TRβ2 represents the key TR isoform involved in T3-mediated negative regulation of TRH expression in transgenic mice [142]. This finding demonstrated that tanycyte-generated T3 during fasting should not have major direct effects on TRH expression in the paraventricular nucleus. As an alternative pathway, the hypothalamic ventromedial nucleus was also suggested as a target translating changing

hypothalamic T3 levels into the modulation of food intake [143]. The role of glial D2-mediated hypothalamic T3 in fasting is not yet resolved, and related data are reviewed elsewhere [25, 61, 63, 66].

3.1.5. Light.

D2 expression in the mediobasal hypothalamus is controlled by light, and this has consequences on reproductive function. Light exposure-induced D2 expression in the mediobasal hypothalamus of the Japanese quail (Coturnix japonica) represents a crucial event in the signal transduction pathway ensuring photoperiodic response of gonads. Intracerebroventricular administration of T3 mimicked the photoperiodic response, whereas the D2 inhibitor iopanoic acid prevented gonadal growth [144]. Interestingly, beyond median eminence and infundibular nucleus D2 induction was also observed in the dorsal and lateral hypothalamus. Based on this finding it cannot be excluded that not only tanycytes but other cell types, for example, hypothalamic astrocytes could be also involved in this mechanism, but this aspect was not studied in details. A mechanism for light-induced D2 expression in the mediobasal hypothalamus was also revealed in quail showing a preceding peak of TSHβ-subunit expression in the pars tuberalis via a cAMP-dependent mechanism. It was demonstrated that intracerebroventricular administration of TSH to short-day quail stimulated gonadal growth and D2 expression and proved that TSH in the pars tuberalis therefore seems to trigger long-day photoinduced seasonal breeding [145].

A homology between avian and mammalian photoperiodic regulation of reproduction has been observed since D2 expression was also increased in Djungarian (Siberian) hamsters (Phodopus sungorus) under long days; the signal was weaker under short days while melatonin injection decreased D2 expression under long days [146]. These results indicate that D2 expression in tanycytes may be involved in the regulation of seasonal reproduction both in mammals and birds. Regulation of seasonal reproduction by photoperiodic regulation of hypothalamic thyroid hormone levels also involves reciprocal changes of D2 and D3 expression that is reviewed elsewhere along with data on other models of seasonal reproduction [66, 147, 148].

3.1.6. Trauma.

After traumatic brain injury D2 mRNA was upregulated in reactive astrocytes in rat. In the cerebral cortex near the contusion D2 mRNA was upregulated on the first day after injury; in the following days the signal was shown to have expanded to the hippocampus, where the astrocytic localization of upregulated D2 mRNA was obvious and bordered the neuronal granule cell layer [149]. Furthermore, different stressors including relatively mild ones (e.g., handling) increased D2 activity in a stressor- and brain-region dependent manner [150]. The frontal cortex showed the highest D2 response, and motor stress was the most dominant stressor in this region while no effect was seen in the cerebellum. A stressor-dependent decrease of T4 tissue concentration was also observed but stressor-dependent deviations were also found since, for example, gently handling resulted in elevated T4 in the frontal cortex.

A strict correlation between D2 activity and tissue T4 levels could not be found suggesting the role of specific factors and not simply the falling T4 level in stress-related D2 increase [150].

3.1.7. Development. Deiodinases are tightly regulated during various developmental processes (reviewed in [4, 151]). It was shown that the human fetal brain is already sensitive to thyroid hormones before the onset of the fetal thyroid [152, 153]. The presence of high-affinity T3 binding sites with a specificity that resembles that of the nuclear T3 receptors was also demonstrated in the human fetal brain and its concentration increased by tenfold from ten to sixteen weeks [154]. D2 expression and activity was detected in the human fetal cortex already from seven to eight weeks of gestation [155]. It has been also demonstrated that during the second trimester T3 increases in the cortex due to D2 activity, while it remains very low in cerebellum because of D3-mediated thyroid hormone inactivation [156]. Although deiodinase activities were also studied in the developing rat brain, [157], data are limited on ontogenic aspects of D2 expression in different glial subtypes. Increasing D2 expression was detected in the developing chicken brain in perivascular localizations probably localized to glial cells [158]. It was also demonstrated that D2 was expressed in chicken tanycytes before the onset of thyroid hormone-dependent negative feedback. Furthermore, D2 and Nkx2.1 were coexpressed at E13 and P2 in tanycytes but not in the perivascular glia indicating a glial-subtype-specific regulation of D2 expression [159].

3.1.8. Other Factors. It has been demonstrated that D2 expression in glial cells is under the control of multiple factors. These include the increase of D2 activity upon cAMP induction [160, 161] that is in line with the finding of an evolutionary conserved CRE site in the *Dio2* promoter [61, 162–164]. Selenium dependence [165], phorbol esters and glucocorticoids [166], acidic fibroblast growth factor [167] also impact D2 activity.

3.2. Posttranslational Regulation of Glial D2 Activity. It has been demonstrated that D2 activity in the brain undergoes rapid and substrate-induce changes [116, 117]. The underlying mechanism was later identified demonstrating that D2 undergoes substrate-induced ubiquitination followed by its degradation in the proteasome [168–170]. This was a unique example of substrate-induced selective proteolysis that involves ubiquitination of an endoplasmic reticulum resident enzyme and represented the first demonstration that such a regulatory pathway controls activation of a hormone [170]. The pathway works also in primary cultures of astrocytes, since MG132 a proteasome uptake inhibitor could block substrate-induced D2 inactivation [171]. Interestingly, D2 inactivation via ubiquitination does not necessarily involve proteasomal proteolysis. It has been revealed that D2 forms homodimers that undergo ubiquitination-mediated transient and reversible conformation changes. Since dimerization of D2 monomers is crucial to maintain the proper conformation of the active center of the enzyme,

ubiquitination-mediated changes result in the rapid loss of D2 activity [172].

Since D2 ubiquitination represents a rapid way for the regulation of T3 generation its mechanism was studied in detail in the past several years. UBC6 and 7 were identified as the ubiquitin conjugases (E2) involved in the ubiquitination of D2 [173, 174], while USP-33 and USP-20 (VDU1 and 2) deubiquitinate D2 and prolong its half-life [175]. A novel type of ubiquitination motif containing a 18-aa-loop structure of the D2 protein was identified and characterized [176, 177]. WSB1 (Swip1) was recognized as a sonic hedgehog-induced SOCS-box containing protein of unknown function [178, 179]. Importantly, it could be shown that WSB1 serves as the ubiquitin ligase (E3) that links D2 to the Elongin BC-Cul5-Rbx1 ubiquitinating catalytic core complex [176]. Later, Teb4 has been also identified as a D2 E3 ligase [180].

Data are accumulating on how crucial elements of the D2 ubiquitination machinery are expressed in D2-expressing glial subtypes. The available data revealed cell-type-specific differences in the expression of crucial elements of the D2 ubiquitinating/deubiquitinating machinery in the rodent brain. WSB1, the D2 E3 ligase, is expressed both in GFAP-expressing astrocytes in different brain regions and in tanycytes in the mediobasal hypothalamus (Figure 3) [181]. This suggested that the WSB1-D2 interaction, a process required for D2 ubiquitination, could be functional in these cells. In contrast to WSB1, the TEB4 E3 ligase could not be detected in GFAP-expressing astrocytes, only in the cerebellum, but it was expressed in tanycytes [180]. Furthermore, the USP33 (VDUI) D2 deubiquitinase is co-expressed with D2 only in tanycytes but not in astrocytes (Figure 3) [181]. WSB1 and USP33 expression in the brain was not affected by thyroid hormone status indicating that these genes are not involved in the homeostatic response to hypo- or hyperthyroidism [181].

The available data suggested that kinetics of D2 ubiquitination and consequent selective proteolysis in the proteasome could be different among different subtypes of glial cells. Among D2-expressing cell types of the brain, tanycytes express the most comprehensive set of genes involved in ubiquitination-mediated D2 regulation, that ensures both WSB1- and TEB4-mediated ubiquitination ligation to D2- and also USP33 deubiquitinase-mediated D2 reactivation. In astrocytes D2 deubiquitinaton is either not possible, or it works via USP20 or other unidentified D2 deubiquitinases.

3.3. Neuroglial Thyroid Hormone Metabolism Affects Neuronal Gene Expression. Astrocytes and tanycytes of the neuroglial compartment are the predominant source of T3 present in the brain while TR in neurons represents a major target of thyroid hormone. As discussed above, neurons cannot generate T3 but express type 3 deiodinase (D3), the T3 degrading enzyme. While numerous observations suggested that glial thyroid hormone metabolism could affect neuronal function (see Section 3.1), until recently no direct evidence could be obtained to prove the existence of deiodinase-mediated transcriptional T3 footprints in neurons. Recently a two-dimensional coculture was used based on the D2-expressing

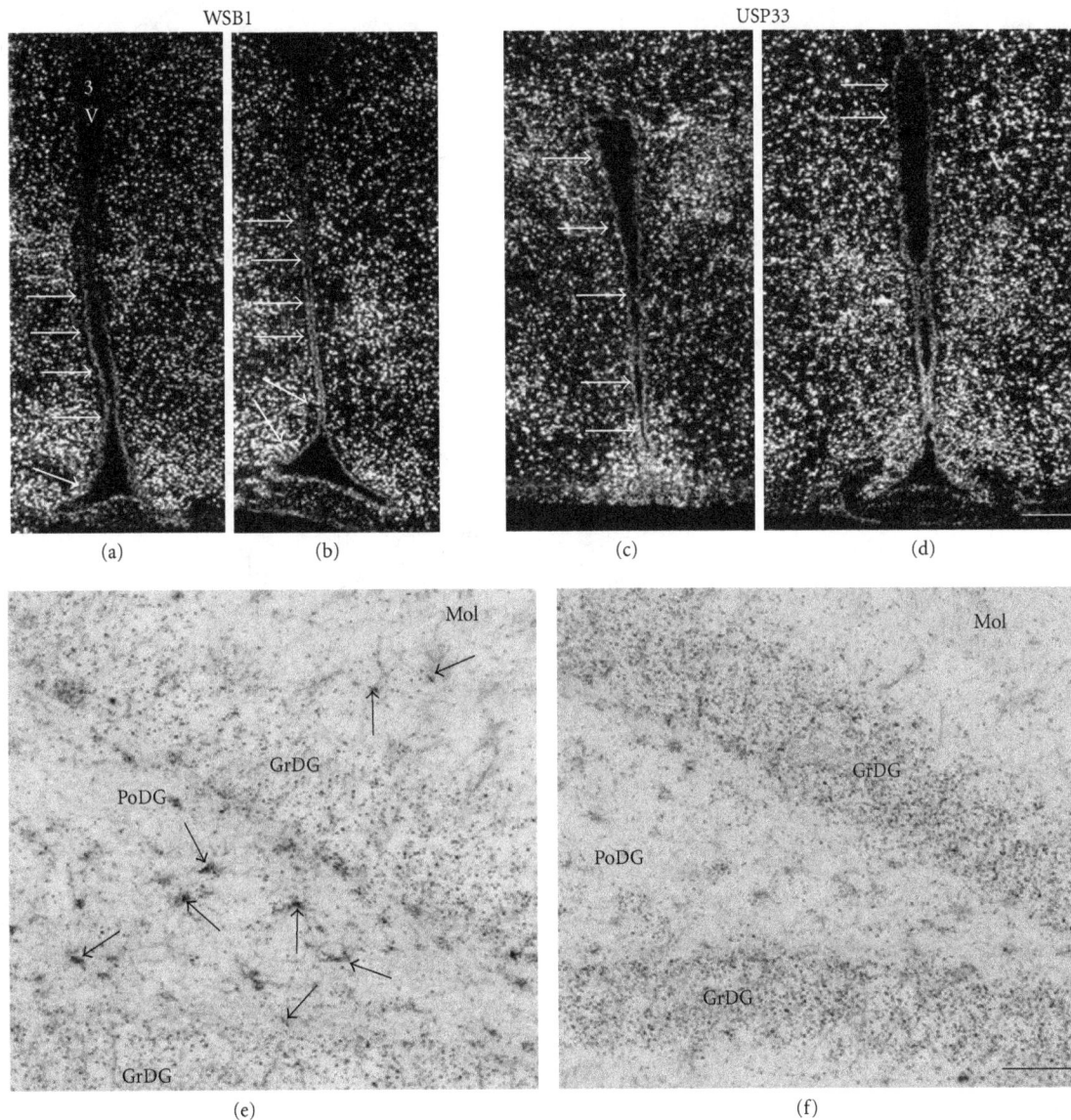

FIGURE 3: Expression of crucial elements of the D2 ubiquitination machinery in glial cells in the rat brain. (a,b) mRNA of WSB1, the D2 ubiquitin ligase is expressed in tanycytes lining the wall of the third ventricle (3V). WSB1 expression *(arrows)* extended from the anterior lower part (not shown) to the lower two thirds of the wall of the third ventricle in more caudal regions. Neuronal cells also express WSB1. (c,d) Hybridization signal of the USP33 D2 deubiquitinase was also detected over tanycytes and ependymal cells lining all regions of the wall of the third ventricle *(arrows)*. Neuronal cells also express USP33. (e) WSB1 *in situ* hybridization signal (arrows) is observed over the majority of GFAP-expressing astrocytes (brown immunoreactivity) demonstrated here in the hippocampal dentate gyrus. (f) The mRNA of USP33 was absent from GFAP-expressing astrocytes (brown) in the hippocampus, but it was expressed in granular neurons. The sense probes for WSB1 or USP33 did not produce any signal (not shown). Mol, molecular layers of the dentate gyrus; GrDG, granular layer of the dentate gyrus; PoDG, polymorph layer of the dentate gyrus. Reprinted with permission from Fekete et al. [181] The Endocrine Society.

H4 glioma cells and the D3-expressing SK-N-AS neuronal cell line. It has been shown that T4 could activate the endogenously expressed T3-sensitive ENPP2 gene of the neuronal compartment only if the glial compartment was present. This model led to the demonstration that D2-mediated glial T3 generation from physiological amount of T4 can directly affect thyroid hormone-dependent gene expression in a paracrine fashion [23]. A different approach using expression profiling-based assessment of thyroid-hormone-regulated gene expression in the cerebral cortex of the MCT8,

D2, and MCT8/D2 knock-out mice suggested that negative regulation required D2-generated T3, while peripheral T3 entering the brain should be sufficient to maintain normal expression of positively regulated genes [59].

Specific signals as hedgehog proteins [176, 182], bacterial lipopolysaccharide (LPS) [132, 133, 137, 183], and hypoxia [184] have been established as regulators of deiodinase activities. It was also studied how these specific signals impact neuroglial thyroid hormone metabolism in the coculture system. The sonic hedgehog morphogene decreases glial thyroid

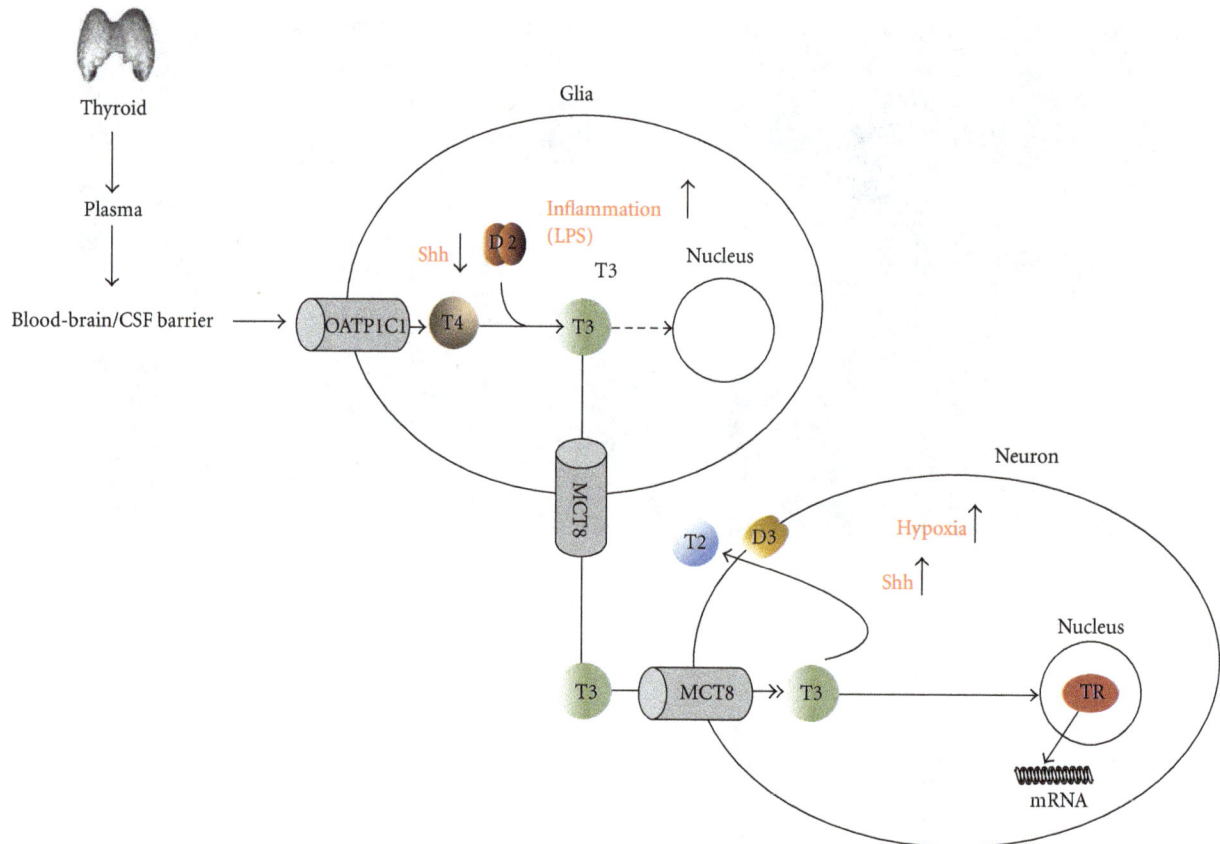

FIGURE 4: Proposed model of neuroglia-neuron interaction of thyroid hormone signaling in the brain. D2 activates the prohormone T4 in glial cells (astrocytes and tanycytes); the generated T3 exits the glial compartment and enters adjacent neurons, where it establishes a transcriptional footprint via liganding TR. Only the two best-characterized thyroid hormone transporters, OATP1C1 and MCT8, are indicated, but data are also accumulating on the role of LAT1 and LAT2 in the thyroid hormone transport both in neurons and astrocytes (discussed in Section 1). In the glial compartment LPS activates D2 transcription while sonic hedgehog (Shh) promotes D2 inactivation via WSB1—mediated ubiquitination; both hypoxia and Shh activate D3 gene transcription in neurons. Figure modified from Freitas et al. American Society for Clinical Investigation [23].

hormone activation via WSB1-mediated posttranslational downregulation of D2 (see Section 3.2) and increases neuronal D3 expression [23]. This demonstrates the existence of a mechanism ensuring a fine-tuned balance between sonic hedgehog-mediated proliferation and T3-evoked differentiation. This is interesting since astrocytes are targets of sonic hedgehog signaling [185]. It has been also demonstrated that in the brain T3 upregulates crucial elements of the sonic hedgehog signaling pathway that could represent a compensatory feedback loop for sonic hedgehog-mediated T3 regulation [186].

The effect of LPS on D2 expression and its relation to nonthyroidal illness were discussed in Section 3.1. In contrast to sonic hedgehog, LPS-induced glial D2 activity and decreased neuronal D3 in the H4-SK-N-AS system and as a consequence resulted in a decreased T3-mediated gene expression in the neuronal compartment [23]. These data were complemented with in vivo observation on the LPS evoked model of nonthyroidal illness. LPS could not induce TRH suppression on the paraventricular nucleus of the D2 knock-out mice only in wild types (Figure 2) (see also

Section 3.1). This indicated that glial (highly probably tany-cytal) D2-generated T3 in the hypothalamus could play an important role in T3-mediated suppression of the hypophys-iotropic TRH neurons and consequently in the decreased activity of the hypothalamo-hypophyseal-thyroid axis during the infection-evoked subtype of nonthyroidal illness [23].

In contrast, hypoxia affected predominantly neuronal D3 activity in the H4- SK-N-AS system. This effect could be also demonstrated in a rat in vivo hypoxia/ischemia model showing D3 induction in cortical neurons and in the hippocampal pyramidal and granular cell layers [23]. This suggested that lowered local T3 levels improve neuronal survival under hypoxic challenge. The glial aspect of this phenomenon requires further studies since an independent study on primary cultures of astrocytes demonstrated hypoxia-induced increase of D2 activity [171]. These data established deiodinase enzymes as glial and neuronal control points for the regulation of thyroid hormone action in the brain during health and disease (Figure 4) [23].

Abbreviations

D2:   type 2 deiodinase
D3:   type 3 deiodinase
GFAP: glial fibrillary acidic protein
T4:   thyroxine
T3:   3,5,3'-triiodothyronine
TR: thyroid hormone receptor
LPS: bacterial lipopolysaccharide
TSH: thyrotropin
TRH: thyrotropin-releasing hormone.

Acknowledgments

This work was supported by the Hungarian Scientific Research Fund Grant OTKA K81226 and the János Bolyai Research Scholarship of the Hungarian Academy of Sciences. Petra Mohácsik, Anikó Zeöld contributed equally to this work.

References

[1] P. R. Larsen, T. F. Davies, and I. D. Hay, "The thyroid gland," in *Williams Textbook of Endocrinology*, J. D. Wilson, D. W. Foster, H. M. Kronenberg, and P. R. Larsen, Eds., pp. 389–515, W.B. Saunders Co., Philadelphia, Pa, USA, 9th edition, 1998.

[2] W. M. Ord, "Report of the committee of the clinical society of london nominated December 14, 1883, to investigate the subject of myxoedema," *Transactions of the Clinical Society of London*, vol. 21, supplement, pp. 1–215, 1888.

[3] J. H. Oppenheimer and H. L. Schwartz, "Molecular basis of thyroid hormone-dependent brain development," *Endocrine Reviews*, vol. 18, no. 4, pp. 462–475, 1997.

[4] J. Bernal, A. Guadaño-Ferraz, and B. Morte, "Perspectives in the Study of Thyroid hormone action on brain development and function," *Thyroid*, vol. 13, no. 11, pp. 1005–1012, 2003.

[5] G. R. Williams, "Neurodevelopmental and neurophysiological actions of thyroid hormone," *Journal of Neuroendocrinology*, vol. 20, no. 6, pp. 784–794, 2008.

[6] F. R. Crantz, J. E. Silva, and P. R. Larsen, "An analysis of the sources and quantity of 3,5,3'-triiodothyronine specifically bound to nuclear receptors in rat cerebral cortex and cerebellum," *Endocrinology*, vol. 110, no. 2, pp. 367–375, 1982.

[7] J. H. Greenberg, M. Reivich, J. T. Gordon, M. B. Schoenhoff, C. S. Patlak, and M. B. Dratman, "Imaging triiodothyronine binding kinetics in rat brain: a model for studies in human subjects," *Synapse*, vol. 60, no. 3, pp. 212–222, 2006.

[8] A. Ceballos, M. M. Belinchon, E. Sanchez-Mendoza et al., "Importance of monocarboxylate transporter 8 for the blood-brain barrier-dependent availability of 3,5,3'-triiodo-L-thyronine," *Endocrinology*, vol. 150, no. 5, pp. 2491–2496, 2009.

[9] X.-H. Liao, C. Di Cosmo, A. M. Dumitrescu et al., "Distinct roles of deiodinases on the phenotype of Mct8 defect: a comparison of eight different mouse genotypes," *Endocrinology*, vol. 152, no. 3, pp. 1180–1191, 2011.

[10] I. Kakucska, W. Rand, and R. M. Lechan, "Thyrotropin-releasing hormone gene expression in the hypothalamic paraventricular nucleus is dependent upon feedback regulation by both triiodothyronine and thyroxine," *Endocrinology*, vol. 130, no. 5, pp. 2845–2850, 1992.

[11] J. C. Davey, K. B. Becker, M. J. Schneider, D. L. S. Germain, and V. A. Galton, "Cloning of a cDNA for the type II iodothyronine deiodinase," *Journal of Biological Chemistry*, vol. 270, no. 45, pp. 26786–26789, 1995.

[12] D. Salvatore, T. Bartha, J. W. Harney, and P. R. Larsen, "Molecular biological and biochemical characterization of the human type 2 selenodeiodinase," *Endocrinology*, vol. 137, no. 8, pp. 3308–3315, 1996.

[13] W. Croteau, J. C. Davey, V. A. Galton, and D. L. S. Germain, "Cloning of the mammalian type II iodothyronine deiodinase. A selenoprotein differentially expressed and regulated in human and rat brain and other tissues," *Journal of Clinical Investigation*, vol. 98, no. 2, pp. 405–417, 1996.

[14] B. Gereben, T. Bartha, H. M. Tu, J. W. Harney, P. Rudas, and P. R. Larsen, "Cloning and expression of the chicken type 2 iodothyronine 5'—deiodinase," *Journal of Biological Chemistry*, vol. 274, no. 20, pp. 13768–13776, 1999.

[15] A. Campos-barros, T. Hoell, A. Musa et al., "Phenolic and tyrosyl ring iodothyronine deiodination and thyroid hormone concentrations in the human central nervous system," *Journal of Clinical Endocrinology and Metabolism*, vol. 81, no. 6, pp. 2179–2185, 1996.

[16] D. L. S. Germain, R. A. Schwartzman, W. Croteau et al., "A thyroid hormone-regulated gene in Xenopus laevis encodes a type III iodothyronine 5-deiodinase," *Proceedings of the National Academy of Sciences of the United States of America*, vol. 91, no. 16, pp. 7767–7771, 1994.

[17] W. Croteau, S. L. Whittemore, M. J. Schneider, and D. L. S. Germain, "Cloning and expression of a cDNA for a mammalian type III iodothyronine deiodinase," *Journal of Biological Chemistry*, vol. 270, no. 28, pp. 16569–16575, 1995.

[18] P. N. Riskind, J. M. Kolodny, and P. R. Larsen, "The regional hypothalamic distribution of type II 5'-monodeiodinase in euthyroid and hypothyroid rats," *Brain Research*, vol. 420, no. 1, pp. 194–198, 1987.

[19] H. M. Tu, S. W. Kim, D. Salvatore et al., "Regional distribution of type 2 thyroxine deiodinase messenger ribonucleic acid in rat hypothalamus and pituitary and its regulation by thyroid hormone," *Endocrinology*, vol. 138, no. 8, pp. 3359–3368, 1997.

[20] A. Guadaño-Ferraz, M. J. Obregón, D. L. S. Germain, and J. Bernal, "The type 2 iodothyronine deiodinase is expressed primarily in glial cells in the neonatal rat brain," *Proceedings of the National Academy of Sciences of the United States of America*, vol. 94, no. 19, pp. 10391–10396, 1997.

[21] H. M. Tu, G. Legradi, T. Bartha, D. Salvatore, R. M. Lechan, and P. R. Larsen, "Regional expression of the type 3 iodothyronine deiodinase messenger ribonucleic acid in the rat central nervous system and its regulation by thyroid hormone," *Endocrinology*, vol. 140, no. 2, pp. 784–790, 1999.

[22] H. Kettenmann and B. R. Ransom, *Neuroglia*, Oxford University Press, New York, NY, USA, 1995.

[23] B. C. G. Freitas, B. Gereben, M. Castillo et al., "Paracrine signaling by glial cell-derived triiodothyronine activates neuronal gene expression in the rodent brain and human cells," *Journal of Clinical Investigation*, vol. 120, no. 6, pp. 2206–2217, 2010.

[24] A. C. Bianco, D. Salvatore, B. Gereben, M. J. Berry, and P. R. Larsen, "Biochemistry, cellular and molecular biology, and physiological roles of the iodothyronine selenodeiodinases," *Endocrine Reviews*, vol. 23, no. 1, pp. 38–89, 2002.

[25] R. M. Lechan and C. Fekete, "Role of thyroid hormone deiodination in the hypothalamus," *Thyroid*, vol. 15, no. 8, pp. 883–897, 2005.

[26] Y. Wu and R. J. Koenig, "Gene regulation by thyroid hormone," *Trends in Endocrinology and Metabolism*, vol. 11, no. 6, pp. 207–211, 2000.

[27] J. Zhang and M. A. Lazar, "The mechanism of action of thyroid hormones," *Annual Review of Physiology*, vol. 62, pp. 439–466, 2000.

[28] P. M. Yen, S. Ando, X. Feng, Y. Liu, P. Maruvada, and X. Xia, "Thyroid hormone action at the cellular, genomic and target gene levels," *Molecular and Cellular Endocrinology*, vol. 246, no. 1-2, pp. 121–127, 2006.

[29] S. Y. Cheng, J. L. Leonard, and P. J. Davis, "Molecular aspects of thyroid hormone actions," *Endocrine Reviews*, vol. 31, no. 2, pp. 139–170, 2010.

[30] J. Nunez, F. S. Celi, L. Ng, and D. Forrest, "Multigenic control of thyroid hormone functions in the nervous system," *Molecular and Cellular Endocrinology*, vol. 287, no. 1-2, pp. 1–12, 2008.

[31] J. Bernal, "Thyroid hormone receptors in brain development and function," *Nature Clinical Practice Endocrinology and Metabolism*, vol. 3, no. 3, pp. 249–259, 2007.

[32] J. Ortiz-Caro, B. Yusta, and F. Montiel, "Identification and characterization of L-triiodothyronine receptors in cells of glial and neuronal origin," *Endocrinology*, vol. 119, no. 5, pp. 2163–2167, 1986.

[33] J. Puymirat, "Thyroid receptors in the rat brain," *Progress in Neurobiology*, vol. 39, no. 3, pp. 281–294, 1992.

[34] B. Yusta, F. Besnard, J. Ortiz-Caro, A. Pascual, A. Aranda, and L. Sarlieve, "Evidence for the presence of nuclear 3,5,3'-triiodothyronine receptors in secondary cultures of pure rat oligodendrocytes," *Endocrinology*, vol. 122, no. 5, pp. 2278–2284, 1988.

[35] M. Hubank, A. K. Sinha, D. Gullo, and R. P. Ekins, "Nuclear tri-iodothyronine (T3) binding in neonatal rat brain suggests a direct glial requirement for T3 during development," *Journal of Endocrinology*, vol. 126, no. 3, pp. 409–415, 1990.

[36] D. J. Carlson, K. A. Strait, H. L. Schwartz, and J. H. Oppenheimer, "Immunofluorescent localization of thyroid hormone receptor isoforms in glial cells of rat brain," *Endocrinology*, vol. 135, no. 5, pp. 1831–1836, 1994.

[37] D. J. Carlson, K. A. Strait, H. L. Schwartz, and J. H. Oppenheimer, "Thyroid hormone receptor isoform content in cultured type 1 and type 2 astrocytes," *Endocrinology*, vol. 137, no. 3, pp. 911–917, 1996.

[38] F. R. S. Lima, N. Gonçalves, F. Carvalho, A. Gomes, M. S. De Freitas, and V. M. Neto, "Thyroid hormone action on astroglial cells from distinct brain regions during development," *International Journal of Developmental Neuroscience*, vol. 16, no. 1, pp. 19–27, 1998.

[39] J. Manzano, J. Bernal, and B. Morte, "Influence of thyroid hormones on maturation of rat cerebellar astrocytes," *International Journal of Developmental Neuroscience*, vol. 25, no. 3, pp. 171–179, 2007.

[40] B. Morte, J. Manzano, T. S. Scanlan, B. Vennström, and J. Bernal, "Aberrant maturation of Astrocytes in Thyroid hormone receptor α1 knockout mice reveals an interplay between Thyroid hormone receptor isoforms," *Endocrinology*, vol. 145, no. 3, pp. 1386–1391, 2004.

[41] S.-L. Hwang, C.-L. Lin, A.-S. Lieu et al., "The expression of thyroid hormone receptor isoforms in human astrocytomas," *Surgical Neurology*, vol. 70, supplement 1, pp. S1–S8, 2008.

[42] J. Bernal, "The significance of thyroid hormone transporters in the brain," *Endocrinology*, vol. 146, no. 4, pp. 1698–1700, 2005.

[43] D. Braun, E. K. Wirth, and U. Schweizer, "Thyroid hormone transporters in the brain," *Reviews in the Neurosciences*, vol. 21, no. 3, pp. 173–186, 2010.

[44] E. C. H. Friesema, P. A. Grueters, H. Biebermann et al., "Association between mutations in a thyroid hormone transporter and severe X-linked psychomotor retardation," *Lancet*, vol. 364, no. 9443, pp. 1435–1437, 2004.

[45] W. E. Visser, E. C. H. Friesema, J. Jansen, and T. J. Visser, "Thyroid hormone transport in and out of cells," *Trends in Endocrinology and Metabolism*, vol. 19, no. 2, pp. 50–56, 2008.

[46] A. M. Dumitrescu, X. H. Liao, T. B. Best, K. Brockmann, and S. Refetoff, "A Novel syndrome combining thyroid and neurological abnormalities is associated with mutations in a monocarboxylate transporter gene," *American Journal of Human Genetics*, vol. 74, no. 1, pp. 168–175, 2004.

[47] C. E. Schwartz, M. M. May, N. J. Carpenter et al., "Allan-Herndon-Dudley syndrome and the monocarboxylate transporter 8 (MCT8) gene," *American Journal of Human Genetics*, vol. 77, no. 1, pp. 41–53, 2005.

[48] L. M. Roberts, K. Woodford, M. Zhou et al., "Expression of the thyroid hormone transporters monocarboxylate transporter-8 (SLC16A2) and organic ion transporter-14 (SLCO1C1) at the blood-brain barrier," *Endocrinology*, vol. 149, no. 12, pp. 6251–6261, 2008.

[49] E. C. H. Friesema, J. Jansen, J. W. Jachtenberg, W. E. Visser, M. H. A. Kester, and T. J. Visser, "Effective cellular uptake and efflux of thyroid hormone by human monocarboxylate transporter 10," *Molecular Endocrinology*, vol. 22, no. 6, pp. 1357–1369, 2008.

[50] J. Jansen, E. C. H. Friesema, C. Milici, and T. J. Visser, "Thyroid hormone transporters in health and disease," *Thyroid*, vol. 15, no. 8, pp. 757–768, 2005.

[51] D. Braun, A. Kinne, A. U. Brauer et al., "Developmental and cell type-specific expression of thyroid hormone transporters in the mouse brain and in primary brain cells," *GLIA*, vol. 59, no. 3, pp. 463–471, 2011.

[52] E. K. Wirth, S. Roth, C. Blechschmidt et al., "Neuronal 3',3,5-triiodothyronine (T3) uptake and behavioral phenotype of mice deficient in Mct8, the neuronal T3 transporter mutated in Allan-Herndon-Dudley syndrome," *Journal of Neuroscience*, vol. 29, no. 30, pp. 9439–9449, 2009.

[53] D. L. S. Germain, A. Hernandez, M. J. Schneider, and V. A. Galton, "Insights into the role of deiodinases from studies of genetically modified animals," *Thyroid*, vol. 15, no. 8, pp. 905–916, 2005.

[54] M. J. Schneider, S. N. Fiering, S. E. Pallud, A. F. Parlow, D. L. St Germain, and A. V. Galton, "Targeted disruption of the type 2 selenodeiodinase gene (*DIO2*) results in a phenotype of pituitary resistance to T4," *Molecular Endocrinology*, vol. 15, no. 12, pp. 2137–2148, 2001.

[55] M. J. Schneider, S. N. Fiering, B. Thai et al., "Targeted disruption of the type 1 selenodeiodinase gene (Dio1) results in marked changes in thyroid hormone economy in mice," *Endocrinology*, vol. 147, no. 1, pp. 580–589, 2006.

[56] A. Hernandez, M. E. Martinez, S. Fiering, V. A. Galton, and D. S. Germain, "Type 3 deiodinase is critical for the maturation and function of the thyroid axis," *Journal of Clinical Investigation*, vol. 116, no. 2, pp. 476–484, 2006.

[57] V. A. Galton, E. T. Wood, E. A. S. Germain et al., "Thyroid hormone homeostasis and action in the type 2 deiodinase-deficient rodent brain during development," *Endocrinology*, vol. 148, no. 7, pp. 3080–3088, 2007.

[58] V. A. Galton, M. J. Schneider, A. S. Clark, and D. L. S. Germain, "Life without thyroxine to 3,5,3'-triiodothyronine conversion: studies in mice devoid of the 5'-deiodinases," *Endocrinology*, vol. 150, no. 6, pp. 2957–2963, 2009.

[59] B. Morte, A. Ceballos, D. Diez et al., "Thyroid hormone-regulated mouse cerebral cortex genes are differentially dependent on the source of the hormone: a study in monocarboxylate transporter-8- and deiodinase-2-deficient mice," *Endocrinology*, vol. 151, no. 5, pp. 2381–2387, 2010.

[60] D. L. S. Germain and V. A. Galton, "The deiodinase family of selenoproteins," *Thyroid*, vol. 7, no. 4, pp. 655–668, 1997.

[61] B. Gereben and D. Salvatore, "Pretranslational regulation of type 2 deiodinase," *Thyroid*, vol. 15, no. 8, pp. 855–864, 2005.

[62] F. Courtin, H. Zrouri, A. Lamirand et al., "Thyroid hormone deiodinases in the central and peripheral nervous system," *Thyroid*, vol. 15, no. 8, pp. 931–942, 2005.

[63] C. Fekete and R. M. Lechan, "Negative feedback regulation of hypophysiotropic thyrotropin-releasing hormone (TRH) synthesizing neurons: role of neuronal afferents and type 2 deiodinase," *Frontiers in Neuroendocrinology*, vol. 28, no. 2-3, pp. 97–114, 2007.

[64] A. C. Bianco and B. W. Kim, "Deiodinases: implications of the local control of thyroid hormone action," *Journal of Clinical Investigation*, vol. 116, no. 10, pp. 2571–2579, 2006.

[65] J. Kohrle, "Thyroid hormone transporters in health and disease: advances in thyroid hormone deiodination," *Best Practice and Research in Clinical Endocrinology and Metabolism*, vol. 21, no. 2, pp. 173–191, 2007.

[66] B. Gereben, A. M. Zavacki, S. Ribich et al., "Cellular and molecular basis of deiodinase-regulated thyroid hormone signaling," *Endocrine Reviews*, vol. 29, no. 7, pp. 898–938, 2008.

[67] B. Gereben, A. Zeöld, M. Dentice, D. Salvatore, and A. C. Bianco, "Activation and inactivation of thyroid hormone by deiodinases: local action with general consequences," *Cellular and Molecular Life Sciences*, vol. 65, no. 4, pp. 570–590, 2008.

[68] D. L. St Germain, V. A. Galton, and A. Hernandez, "Minireview: defining the roles of the Iodothyronine deiodinases: current concepts and challenges," *Endocrinology*, vol. 150, no. 3, pp. 1097–1107, 2009.

[69] G. R. Williams and J. H. Bassett, "Local control of thyroid hormone action: role of type 2 deiodinase: deiodinases: the balance of thyroid hormone," *Journal of Endocrinology*, vol. 209, no. 3, pp. 261–272, 2011.

[70] J. Legrand, "Thyroid hormone effects on growth and development," in *Thyroid Hormone Metabolism*, G. Hennemann, Ed., pp. 503–534, Marcel Dekker, New York, NY, USA, 1986.

[71] M. Bauer and P. C. Whybrow, "Thyroid hormone, neural tissue and mood modulation," *The world Journal of Biological Psychiatry*, vol. 2, no. 2, pp. 59–69, 2001.

[72] R. T. Joffe and S. T. H. Sokolov, "Thyroid hormones, the brain, and affective disorders," *Critical Reviews in Neurobiology*, vol. 8, no. 1-2, pp. 45–63, 1994.

[73] D. Diez, C. Grijota-Martinez, P. Agretti et al., "Thyroid hormone action in the adult brain: gene expression profiling of the effects of single and multiple doses of triiodo-L-thyronine in the rat striatum," *Endocrinology*, vol. 149, no. 8, pp. 3989–4000, 2008.

[74] F. C. A. Gomes, C. G. Maia, J. R. L. De Menezes, and V. Moura Neto, "Cerebellar astrocytes treated by thyroid hormone modulate neuronal proliferation," *GLIA*, vol. 25, no. 3, pp. 247–255, 1999.

[75] A. G. Trentin, "Thyroid hormone and astrocyte morphogenesis," *Journal of Endocrinology*, vol. 189, no. 2, pp. 189–197, 2006.

[76] G. Almazan, P. Honegger, and J. M. Matthieu, "Triiodothyronine stimulation of oligodendroglial differentiation and myelination. A developmental study," *Developmental Neuroscience*, vol. 7, no. 1, pp. 45–54, 1985.

[77] F. R. S. Lima, A. Gervais, C. Colin, M. Izembart, V. M. Neto, and M. Mallat, "Regulation of microglial development: a novel role for thyroid hormone," *Journal of Neuroscience*, vol. 21, no. 6, pp. 2028–2038, 2001.

[78] M. Noble, C. Pröschel, and M. Mayer-Pröschel, "Getting a GR(i)P on oligodendrocyte development," *Developmental Biology*, vol. 265, no. 1, pp. 33–52, 2004.

[79] J. C. Lee, M. Mayer-Proschel, and M. S. Rao, "Gliogenesis in the central nervous system," *GLIA*, vol. 30, no. 2, pp. 105–121, 2000.

[80] D. S. Sharlin, D. Tighe, M. E. Gilbert, and R. T. Zoeller, "The balance between oligodendrocyte and astrocyte production in major white matter tracts is linearly related to serum total thyroxine," *Endocrinology*, vol. 149, no. 5, pp. 2527–2536, 2008.

[81] C. M. Schoonover, M. M. Seibel, D. M. Jolson et al., "Thyroid hormone regulates oligodendrocyte accumulation in developing rat brain white matter tracts," *Endocrinology*, vol. 145, no. 11, pp. 5013–5020, 2004.

[82] J. R. Martínez-Galán, P. Pedraza, M. Santacana, F. E. Del Rey, G. M. De Escobar, and A. Ruiz-Marcos, "Early effects of iodine deficiency on radial glial cells of the hippocampus of the rat fetus. A model of neurological cretinism," *Journal of Clinical Investigation*, vol. 99, no. 11, pp. 2701–2709, 1997.

[83] S. Paul, R. Poddar, and P. K. Sarkar, "Role of thyroid hormone in the morphological differentiation and maturation of astrocytes: temporal correlation with synthesis and organization of actin," *European Journal of Neuroscience*, vol. 8, no. 11, pp. 2361–2370, 1996.

[84] C. Faivre-Sarrailh, A. Rami, C. Fages, and M. Tardy, "Effect of thyroid deficiency on glial fibrillary acidic protein (GFAP) and GFAP-mRNA in the cerebellum and hippocampal formation of the developing rat," *Glia*, vol. 4, no. 3, pp. 276–284, 1991.

[85] F. R. S. Lima, A. G. Trentin, D. Rosenthal, C. Chagas, and V. Moura Neto, "Thyroid hormone induces protein secretion and morphological changes in astroglial cells with an increase in expression of glial fibrillary acidic protein," *Journal of Endocrinology*, vol. 154, no. 1, pp. 167–175, 1997.

[86] A. G. Trentin and V. M. Neto, "T3 affects cerebellar astrocyte proliferation, GFAP and fibronectin organization," *NeuroReport*, vol. 6, no. 2, pp. 293–296, 1995.

[87] F. C. A. Gomes, D. Paulin, and V. M. Neto, "Glial fibrillary acidic protein (GFAP): modulation by growth factors and its implication in astrocyte differentiation," *Brazilian Journal of Medical and Biological Research*, vol. 32, no. 5, pp. 619–631, 1999.

[88] N. J. Laping, B. Teter, N. R. Nichols, I. Rozovsky, and C. E. Finch, "Glial fibrillary acidic protein: regulation by hormones, cytokines, and growth factors," *Brain Pathology*, vol. 4, no. 3, pp. 259–275, 1994.

[89] M. Mallat, F. R. S. Lima, A. Gervais, C. Colin, and V. Moura Neto, "New insights into the role of thyroid hormone in the CNS: the microglial track," *Molecular Psychiatry*, vol. 7, no. 1, pp. 7–8, 2002.

[90] S. Garcia-Silva, G. Perez-Juste, and A. Aranda, "Cell cycle control by the thyroid hormone in neuroblastoma cells," *Toxicology*, vol. 181-182, pp. 179–182, 2002.

[91] J. R. Nevins, "Transcriptional regulation. A closer look at E2F," *Nature*, vol. 358, no. 6385, pp. 375–376, 1992.

[92] M. Nygírd, G. M. Wahlström, M. V. Gustafsson, Y. M. Tokumoto, and M. Bondesson, "Hormone-dependent repression of the E2F-1 gene by thyroid hormone receptors," *Molecular Endocrinology*, vol. 17, no. 1, pp. 79–92, 2003.

[93] H. Furumoto, H. Ying, G. V. R. Chandramouli et al., "An unliganded thyroid hormone β receptor activates the cyclin D1/cyclin-dependent kinase/retinoblastoma/E2F pathway and induces pituitary tumorigenesis," *Molecular and Cellular Biology*, vol. 25, no. 1, pp. 124–135, 2005.

[94] B. Durand, F. B. Gao, and M. Raff, "Accumulation of the cyclin-dependent kinase inhibitor p27/Kip1 and the timing of oligodendrocyte differentiation," *EMBO Journal*, vol. 16, no. 2, pp. 306–317, 1997.

[95] G. Perez-Juste and A. Aranda, "The cyclin-dependent kinase inhibitor p27(Kip1) is involved in thyroid hormone-mediated neuronal differentiation," *Journal of Biological Chemistry*, vol. 274, no. 8, pp. 5026–5031, 1999.

[96] T. Valcana, E. R. Einstein, and J. Csejtey, "Influence of thyroid hormones on myelin proteins in the developing rat brain," *Journal of the Neurological Sciences*, vol. 25, no. 1, pp. 19–27, 1975.

[97] A. Compston, J. Zajicek, J. Sussman et al., "Glial lineages and myelination in the central nervous system," *Journal of Anatomy*, vol. 190, part 2, pp. 161–200, 1997.

[98] B. Emery, "Regulation of oligodendrocyte differentiation and myelination," *Science*, vol. 330, no. 6005, pp. 779–782, 2010.

[99] K. A. Strait, D. J. Carlson, H. L. Schwartz, and J. H. Oppenheimer, "Transient stimulation of myelin basic protein gene expression in differentiating cultured oligodendrocytes: a model for 3,5,3'- triiodothyronine-induced brain development," *Endocrinology*, vol. 138, no. 2, pp. 635–641, 1997.

[100] A. Rodríguez-Peña, "Oligodendrocyte development and thyroid hormone," *Journal of Neurobiology*, vol. 40, no. 4, pp. 497–512, 1999.

[101] N. Ibarrola and A. Rodríguez-Peña, "Hypothyroidism coordinately and transiently affects myelin protein gene expression in most rat brain regions during postnatal development," *Brain Research*, vol. 752, no. 1-2, pp. 285–293, 1997.

[102] P. Berbel, A. Guadano-Ferraz, A. Angulo, and J. R. Cerezo, "Role of thyroid hormones in the maturation of interhemispheric connections of rats," *Behavioural Brain Research*, vol. 64, no. 1-2, pp. 9–14, 1994.

[103] A. Rodriguez-Pena, N. Ibarrola, M. A. Iniguez, A. Munoz, and J. Bernal, "Neonatal hypothyroidism affects the timely expression of myelin- associated glycoprotein in the rat brain," *Journal of Clinical Investigation*, vol. 91, no. 3, pp. 812–818, 1993.

[104] A. G. Trentin, D. Rosenthal, and V. M. Neto, "Thyroid hormone and conditioned medium effects on astroglial cells from hypothyroid and normal rat brain: factor secretion, cell differentiation, and proliferation," *Journal of Neuroscience Research*, vol. 41, no. 3, pp. 409–417, 1995.

[105] A. P. Farwell and S. A. Dubord-Tomasetti, "Thyroid hormone regulates the expression of laminin in the developing rat cerebellum," *Endocrinology*, vol. 140, no. 9, pp. 4221–4227, 1999.

[106] A. Gonçalves Trentin, C. B. Nedel Mendes De Aguiar, R. Castilho Garcez, and M. Alvarez-Silva, "Thyroid hormone modulates the extracellular matrix organization and expression in cerebellar astrocyte: effects on astrocyte adhesion," *GLIA*, vol. 42, no. 4, pp. 359–369, 2003.

[107] A. G. Trentin, V. Alvarez-Silva, and Moura Neto, "Thyroid hormone induces cerebellar astrocytes and C6 glioma cells to secrete mitogenic growth factors," *American Journal of Physiology , Endocrinology and Metabolism*, vol. 281, no. 5 44-5, pp. E1088–E1094, 2001.

[108] R. Martinez and F. C. A. Gomes, "Neuritogenesis induced by thyroid hormone-treated astrocytes is mediated by epidermal growth factor/mitogen-activated protein kinase-phosphatidylinositol 3-kinase pathways and involves modulation of extracellular matrix proteins," *Journal of Biological Chemistry*, vol. 277, no. 51, pp. 49311–49318, 2002.

[109] R. M. Lindsay, "Adult rat brain astrocytes support survival of both NGF-dependent and NGF-insensitive neurones," *Nature*, vol. 282, no. 5734, pp. 80–82, 1979.

[110] M. Alvarez-Dolado, T. Iglesias, A. Rodríguez-Peña, J. Bernal, and A. Muñoz, "Expression of neurotrophins and the trk family of neurotrophin receptors in normal and hypothyroid rat brain," *Molecular Brain Research*, vol. 27, no. 2, pp. 249–257, 1994.

[111] Y. Hashimoto, S. Furukawa, F. Omae, Y. Miyama, and K. Hayashi, "Correlative regulation of nerve growth factor level and choline acetyltransferase activity by thyroxine in particular regions of infant rat brain," *Journal of Neurochemistry*, vol. 63, no. 1, pp. 326–332, 1994.

[112] J. L. Leonard and A. P. Farwell, "Thyroid hormone-regulated actin polymerization in brain," *Thyroid*, vol. 7, no. 1, pp. 147–151, 1997.

[113] C. A. Siegrist-Kaiser, C. Juge-Aubry, M. P. Tranter, D. M. Ekenbarger, and J. L. Leonard, "Thyroxine-dependent modulation of actin polymerization in cultured astrocytes. A novel, extranuclear action of thyroid hormone," *Journal of Biological Chemistry*, vol. 265, no. 9, pp. 5296–5302, 1990.

[114] J. L. Leonard, "Non-genomic actions of thyroid hormone in brain development," *Steroids*, vol. 73, no. 9-10, pp. 1008–1012, 2008.

[115] A. P. Farwell, M. P. Tranter, and J. L. Leonard, "Thyroxine-dependent regulation of integrin-laminin interactions in astrocytes," *Endocrinology*, vol. 136, no. 9, pp. 3909–3915, 1995.

[116] J. L. Leonard, M. M. Kaplan, and T. J. Visser, "Cerebral cortex responds rapidly to thyroid hormones," *Science*, vol. 214, no. 4520, pp. 571–573, 1981.

[117] L. A. Burmeister, J. Pachucki, and D. L. S. Germain, "Thyroid hormones inhibit type 2 iodothyronine deiodinase in the rat cerebral cortex by both pre- and posttranslational mechanisms," *Endocrinology*, vol. 138, no. 12, pp. 5231–5237, 1997.

[118] A. Guadaño-Ferraz, M. J. Escámez, E. Rausell, and J. Bernal, "Expression of type 2 iodothyronine deiodinase in hypothyroid rat brain indicates an important role of thyroid hormone in the development of specific primary sensory systems," *Journal of Neuroscience*, vol. 19, no. 9, pp. 3430–3439, 1999.

[119] O. Broedel, M. Eravci, S. Fuxius et al., "Effects of hyper- and hypothyroidism on thyroid hormone concentrations in regions of the rat brain," *American Journal of Physiology, Endocrinology and Metabolism*, vol. 285, no. 3 48-3, pp. E470–E480, 2003.

[120] B. Anguiano, A. Quintanar, M. Luna et al., "Neuroendocrine regulation of adrenal gland and hypothalamus 5'deiodinase activity. II. Effects of splanchnicotomy and hypophysectomy," *Endocrinology*, vol. 136, no. 8, pp. 3346–3352, 1995.

[121] S. Diano, F. Naftolin, F. Goglia, and T. L. Horvath, "Fasting-induced increase in type II iodothyronine deiodinase activity and messenger ribonucleic acid levels is not reversed by thyroxine in the rat hypothalamus," *Endocrinology*, vol. 139, no. 6, pp. 2879–2884, 1998.

[122] N. M. Sanders, A. A. Dunn-Meynell, and B. E. Levin, "Third ventricular alloxan reversibly impairs glucose counterregulatory responses," *Diabetes*, vol. 53, no. 5, pp. 1230–1236, 2004.

[123] M. Pérez-Martín, M. Cifuentes, J. M. Grondona et al., "IGF-I stimulates neurogenesis in the hypothalamus of adult rats," *European Journal of Neuroscience*, vol. 31, no. 9, pp. 1533–1548, 2010.

[124] R. M. Lechan and C. Fekete, "Feedback regulation of thyrotropin-releasing hormone (TRH): mechanisms for the non-thyroidal illness syndrome," *Journal of Endocrinological Investigation*, vol. 27 Suppl, no. 6, pp. 105–119, 2004.

[125] J. Faber and K. Siersbæk-Nielsen, "Serum free 3,5,3'-triiodothyronine (T3) in non-thyroidal somatic illness, as measured by ultrafiltration and immunoextraction," *Clinica Chimica Acta*, vol. 256, no. 2, pp. 115–123, 1996.

[126] I. J. Chopra, "Simultaneous measurement of free thyroxine and free 3,5,3'- triiodothyronine in undiluted serum by direct equilibrium dialysis/radioimmunoassay: evidence that free triiodothyronine and free thyroxine are normal in many patients with the low triiodothyronine syndrome," *Thyroid*, vol. 8, no. 3, pp. 249–257, 1998.

[127] M. M. Kaplan, P. R. Larsen, and F. R. Crantz, "Prevalence of abnormal thyroid function test results in patients with acute medical illnesses," *American Journal of Medicine*, vol. 72, no. 1, pp. 9–16, 1982.

[128] P. R. Larsen, T. F. Davies, M.-J Schlumberger, and I. D. Hay, "hyroid Physiology and Diagnostic Evaluation of Patients with Thyroid Disorders," in *Williams Textbook of Endocrinology*, P. R. Larsen, H. M. Kronenberg, S. Melmed, and K. S. Polonsky, Eds., pp. 331–373, W.B. Saunders Co., Philadelphia, Pa, USA, 10th edition, 2003.

[129] R. D. Utiger, "Decreased extrathyroidal triiododthyronine production in nonthyroidal illness: benefit or harm?" *American Journal of Medicine*, vol. 69, no. 6, pp. 807–810, 1980.

[130] L. J. de Groot, "Dangerous dogmas in medicine: the non-thyroidal illness syndrome," *Journal of Clinical Endocrinology and Metabolism*, vol. 84, no. 1, pp. 151–164, 1999.

[131] B. McIver and C. A. Gorman, "Euthyroid sick syndrome: an overview," *Thyroid*, vol. 7, no. 1, pp. 125–132, 1997.

[132] C. Fekete, B. Gereben, M. Doleschall et al., "Lipopolysaccharide induces type 2 iodothyronine deiodinase in the mediobasal hypothalamus: implications for the nonthyroidal illness syndrome," *Endocrinology*, vol. 145, no. 4, pp. 1649–1655, 2004.

[133] A. Boelen, J. Kwakkel, D. C. Thijssen-Timmer, A. Alkemade, E. Fliers, and W. M. Wiersinga, "Simultaneous changes in central and peripheral components of the hypothalamus-pituitary-thyroid axis in lipopolysaccharide-induced acute illness in mice," *Journal of Endocrinology*, vol. 182, no. 2, pp. 315–323, 2004.

[134] C. Fekete, S. Sarkar, M. A. Christoffolete, C. H. Emerson, A. C. Bianco, and R. M. Lechan, "Bacterial lipopolysaccharide (LPS)-induced type 2 iodothyronine deiodinase (D2) activation in the mediobasal hypothalamus (MBH) is independent of the LPS-induced fall in serum thyroid hormone levels," *Brain Research*, vol. 1056, no. 1, pp. 97–99, 2005.

[135] E. Sánchez, P. S. Singru, C. Fekete, and R. M. Lechan, "Induction of type 2 iodothyronine deiodinase in the mediobasal hypothalamus by bacterial lipopolysaccharide: role of corticosterone," *Endocrinology*, vol. 149, no. 5, pp. 2484–2493, 2008.

[136] A. Lamirand, M. Ramaugé, M. Pierre, and F. Courtin, "Bacterial lipopolysaccharide induces type 2 deiodinase in cultured rat astrocytes," *Journal of Endocrinology*, vol. 208, no. 2, pp. 183–192, 2011.

[137] A. Zeold, M. Doleschall, M. C. Haffner et al., "Characterization of the nuclear factor-κB responsiveness of the human dio2 gene," *Endocrinology*, vol. 147, no. 9, pp. 4419–4429, 2006.

[138] E. Sánchez, P. S. Singru, G. Wittmann et al., "Contribution of TNF-α and nuclear factor-κB signaling to type 2 iodothyronine deiodinase activation in the mediobasal hypothalamus after lipopolysaccharide administration," *Endocrinology*, vol. 151, no. 8, pp. 3827–3835, 2010.

[139] M. A. Greer and Y. Grimm, "Changes in thyroid secretion produced by inhibition of iodotyrosine deiodinase," *Endocrinology*, vol. 83, no. 3, pp. 405–410, 1968.

[140] R. Peeters, C. Fekete, C. Goncalves et al., "Regional physiological adaptation of the central nervous system deiodinases to iodine deficiency," *American Journal of Physiology, Endocrinology and Metabolism*, vol. 281, no. 1 44-1, pp. E54–E61, 2001.

[141] M. J. Obregon, F. Escobar del Rey, and G. Morreale de Escobar, "The effects of iodine deficiency on thyroid hormone deiodination," *Thyroid*, vol. 15, no. 8, pp. 917–929, 2005.

[142] E. D. Abel, R. S. Ahima, M. -E. Boers, J. K. Elmquist, and F. E. Wondisford, "Critical role for thyroid hormone receptor β2 in the regulation of paraventricular thyrotropin-releasing hormone neurons," *Journal of Clinical Investigation*, vol. 107, no. 8, pp. 1017–1023, 2001.

[143] W. M. Kong, N. M. Martin, K. L. Smith et al., "Triiodothyronine stimulates food intake via the hypothalamic ventromedial nucleus independent of changes in energy expenditure," *Endocrinology*, vol. 145, no. 11, pp. 5252–5258, 2004.

[144] T. Yoshimura, S. Yasuo, M. Watanabe et al., "Light-induced hormone conversion of T4 to T3 regulates photoperiodic response of gonads in birds," *Nature*, vol. 426, no. 6963, pp. 178–181, 2003.

[145] N. Nakao, H. Ono, T. Yamamura et al., "Thyrotrophin in the pars tuberalis triggers photoperiodic response," *Nature*, vol. 452, no. 7185, pp. 317–322, 2008.

[146] M. Watanabe, S. Yasuo, T. Watanabe et al., "Photoperiodic regulation of type 2 deiodinase gene in djungarian hamster: possible homologies between avian and mammalian photoperiodic regulation of reproduction," *Endocrinology*, vol. 145, no. 4, pp. 1546–1549, 2004.

[147] S. Yasuo, N. Nakao, S. Ohkura et al., "Long-day suppressed expression of type 2 deiodinase gene in the mediobasal hypothalamus of the Saanen goat, a short-day breeder: implication for seasonal window of thyroid hormone action on reproductive neuroendocrine axis," *Endocrinology*, vol. 147, no. 1, pp. 432–440, 2006.

[148] P. Barrett, F. J. P. Ebling, S. Schuhler et al., "Hypothalamic thyroid hormone catabolism acts as a gatekeeper for the seasonal control of body weight and reproduction," *Endocrinology*, vol. 148, no. 8, pp. 3608–3617, 2007.

[149] L. Zou, L. A. Burmeister, S. D. Styren, P. M. Kochanek, and S. T. DeKosky, "Up-regulation of type 2 iodothyronine deiodinase mRNA in reactive astrocytes following traumatic brain injury in the rat," *Journal of Neurochemistry*, vol. 71, no. 2, pp. 887–890, 1998.

[150] A. Baumgartner, L. Hiedra, G. Pinna, M. Eravci, H. Prengel, and H. Meinhold, "Rat brain type II 5'-iodothyronine deiodinase activity is extremely sensitive to stress," *Journal of Neurochemistry*, vol. 71, no. 2, pp. 817–826, 1998.

[151] V. A. Galton, "The roles of the iodothyronine deiodinases in mammalian development," *Thyroid*, vol. 15, no. 8, pp. 823–834, 2005.

[152] V. J. Pop, J. L. Kuijpens, A. L. van Baar et al., "Low maternal free thyroxine concentrations during early pregnancy are associated with impaired psychomotor development in infancy," *Clinical Endocrinology*, vol. 50, no. 2, pp. 147–155, 1999.

[153] J. E. Haddow, G. E. Palomaki, W. C. Allan et al., "Maternal thyroid deficiency during pregnancy and subsequent neuropsychological development of the child," *New England Journal of Medicine*, vol. 341, no. 8, pp. 549–555, 1999.

[154] J. Bernal and F. Pekonen, "Ontogenesis of the nuclear 3,5,3'-triiodothyronine receptor in the human fetal brain," *Endocrinology*, vol. 114, no. 2, pp. 677–679, 1984.

[155] S. Chan, S. Kachilele, C. J. McCabe et al., "Early expression of thyroid hormone deiodinases and receptors in human fetal cerebral cortex," *Developmental Brain Research*, vol. 138, no. 2, pp. 109–116, 2002.

[156] M. H.A. Kester, R. Martinez De Mena, M. J. Obregon et al., "Iodothyronine levels in the human developing brain: major regulatory roles of iodothyronine deiodinases in different areas," *Journal of Clinical Endocrinology and Metabolism*, vol. 89, no. 7, pp. 3117–3128, 2004.

[157] J. M. Bates, D. L. S. Germain, and V. A. Galton, "Expression profiles of the three iodothyronine deiodinases, D1, D2, and D3, in the developing rat," *Endocrinology*, vol. 140, no. 2, pp. 844–851, 1999.

[158] B. Gereben, J. Pachucki, A Kollár, Z. Liposits, and C. Fekete, "Expression of type 2 deiodinase in the developing chicken brain," *Thyroid*, vol. 13, p. 724, 2003.

[159] T. É. H. Füzesi, E. Szabó, M. Doleschall et al., "Developmental co-expression of type 2 deiodinase (D2) and Nkx-2.1 in chicken tanycytes," in *Proceedings of the 14th International Thyroid Congress*, Paris, France, 2010.

[160] F. Courtin, F. Chantoux, M. Pierre, and J. Francon, "Induction of type II 5'-deiodinase activity by cyclic adenosine 3',5'-monophosphate in cultured rat astroglial cells," *Endocrinology*, vol. 123, no. 3, pp. 1577–1581, 1988.

[161] J. L. Leonard, "Dibutyryl cAMP induction of type II 5'deiodinase activity in rat brain astrocytes in culture," *Biochemical and Biophysical Research Communications*, vol. 151, no. 3, pp. 1164–1172, 1988.

[162] T. Bartha, S. W. Kim, D. Salvatore et al., "Characterization of the 5'-flanking and 5'-untranslated regions of the cyclic adenosine 3',5'-monophosphate-responsive human type 2 iodothyronine deiodinase gene," *Endocrinology*, vol. 141, no. 1, pp. 229–237, 2000.

[163] G. Canettieri, F. S. Celi, G. Baccheschi, L. Salvatori, M. Andreoli, and M. Centanni, "Isolation of human type 2 deiodinase gene promoter and characterization of a functional cyclic adenosine monophosphate response element," *Endocrinology*, vol. 141, no. 5, pp. 1804–1813, 2000.

[164] B. Gereben, D. Salvatore, J. W. Harney, H. M. Tu, and P. R. Larsen, "The human, but not rat, dio2 gene is stimulated by thyroid transcription factor-1 (TTF-1)," *Molecular Endocrinology*, vol. 15, no. 1, pp. 112–124, 2001.

[165] S. Pallud, A. M. Lennon, M. Ramauge et al., "Expression of the type II iodothyronine deiodinase in cultured rat astrocytes is selenium-dependent," *Journal of Biological Chemistry*, vol. 272, no. 29, pp. 18104–18110, 1997.

[166] F. Courtin, F. Chantoux, J. M. Gavaret, D. Toru-Delbauffe, C. Jacquemin, and M. Pierre, "Induction of type II 5'-deio-dinase activity in cultured rat astroglial cells by 12-O-tetra-decanoylphorbol-13-acetate: dependence on glucocorticoids," *Endocrinology*, vol. 125, no. 3, pp. 1277–1281, 1989.

[167] F. Courtin, J. M. Gavaret, D. Toru-Delbauffe, and M. Pierre, "Induction of 5'-deiodinase activity in rat astroglial cells by acidic fibroblast growth factor," *Developmental Brain Research*, vol. 53, no. 2, pp. 237–242, 1990.

[168] J. Steinsapir, J. Harney, and P. R. Larsen, "Type 2 iodo-thyronine deiodinase in rat pituitary tumor cells is inactivated in proteasomes," *Journal of Clinical Investigation*, vol. 102, no. 11, pp. 1895–1899, 1998.

[169] J. Steinsapir, A. C. Bianco, C. Buettner, J. Harney, and P. R. Larsen, "Substrate-induced down-regulation of human type 2 deiodinase (hD2) is mediated through proteasomal degradation and requires interaction with the enzyme's active center," *Endocrinology*, vol. 141, no. 3, pp. 1127–1135, 2000.

[170] B. Gereben, C. Goncalves, J. W. Harney, P. R. Larsen, and A. C. Bianco, "Selective proteolysis of human type 2 deiodinase: a novel ubiquitin-proteasomal mediated mechanism for regulation of hormone activation," *Molecular Endocrinology*, vol. 14, no. 11, pp. 1697–1708, 2000.

[171] A. Lamirand, G. Mercier, M. Ramaugé, M. Pierre, and F. Courtin, "Hypoxia stabilizes type 2 deiodinase activity in rat astrocytes," *Endocrinology*, vol. 148, no. 10, pp. 4745–4753, 2007.

[172] G. D. V. Sagar, B. Gereben, I. Callebaut et al., "Ubiquitina-tion-induced conformational change within the deiodinase dimer is a switch regulating enzyme activity," *Molecular and Cellular Biology*, vol. 27, no. 13, pp. 4774–4783, 2007.

[173] D. Botero, B. Gereben, C. Goncalves, L. A. De Jesus, J. W. Harney, and A. C. Bianco, "Ubc6p and Ubc7p are required for normal and substrate-induced endoplasmic reticulum-associated degradation of the human selenoprotein type 2 iodothyronine monodeiodinase," *Molecular Endocrinology*, vol. 16, no. 9, pp. 1999–2007, 2002.

[174] B. W. Kim, A. M. Zavacki, C. Curcio-Morelli et al., "Endo-plasmic reticulum-associated degradation of the human Type 2 iodothyronine deiodinase (D2) is mediated via an association between mammalian UBC7 and the carboxyl region of D2," *Molecular Endocrinology*, vol. 17, no. 12, pp. 2603–2612, 2003.

[175] C. Curcio-Morelli, A. M. Zavacki, M. Christofollete et al., "Deubiquitination of type 2 iodothyronine deiodinase by von Hippel-Lindau protein-interacting deubiquitinating enzymes regulates thyroid hormone activation," *Journal of Clinical Investigation*, vol. 112, no. 2, pp. 189–196, 2003.

[176] M. Dentice, A. Bandyopadhyay, B. Gereben et al., "The Hedgehog-inducible ubiquitin ligase subunit WSB-1 modulates thyroid hormone activation and PTHrP secretion in the developing growth plate," *Nature Cell Biology*, vol. 7, no. 7, pp. 698–705, 2005.

[177] A. Zeöld, L. Pormüller, M. Dentice et al., "Metabolic instability of type 2 deiodinase is transferable to stable proteins independently of subcellular localization," *Journal of Biological Chemistry*, vol. 281, no. 42, pp. 31538–31543, 2006.

[178] D. Vasiliauskas, S. Hancock, and C. D. Stern, "SWiP-1: novel SOCS box containing WD-protein regulated by signalling centres and by Shh during development," *Mechanisms of Development*, vol. 82, no. 1-2, pp. 79–94, 1999.

[179] D. J. Hilton, R. T. Richardson, W. S. Alexander et al., "Twenty proteins containing a C-terminal SOCS box form five structural classes," *Proceedings of the National Academy of Sciences of the United States of America*, vol. 95, no. 1, pp. 114–119, 1998.

[180] A. M. Zavacki, R. A. E Drigo, B. C. G. Freitas et al., "The E3 ubiquitin ligase TEB4 mediates degradation of type 2 iodothyronine deiodinase," *Molecular and Cellular Biology*, vol. 29, no. 19, pp. 5339–5347, 2009.

[181] C. Fekete, B. C.G. Freitas, A. Zeöld et al., "Expression patterns of WSB-1 and USP-33 underlie cell-specific posttranslational control of type 2 deiodinase in the rat brain," *Endocrinology*, vol. 148, no. 10, pp. 4865–4874, 2007.

[182] M. Dentice, C. Luongo, S. Huang et al., "Sonic hedgehog-induced type 3 deiodinase blocks thyroid hormone action enhancing proliferation of normal and malignant keratinocytes," *Proceedings of the National Academy of Sciences of the United States of America*, vol. 104, no. 36, pp. 14466–14471, 2007.

[183] A. Boelen, J. Kwakkel, W. M. Wiersinga, and E. Fliers, "Chronic local inflammation in mice results in decreased TRH and type 3 deiodinase mRNA expression in the hypothalamic paraventricular nucleus independently of diminished food intake," *Journal of Endocrinology*, vol. 191, no. 3, pp. 707–714, 2006.

[184] W. S. Simonides, M. A. Mulcahey, E. M. Redout et al., "Hypoxia-inducible factor induces local thyroid hormone inactivation during hypoxic-ischemic disease in rats," *Journal of Clinical Investigation*, vol. 118, no. 3, pp. 975–983, 2008.

[185] J. D. Cahoy, B. Emery, A. Kaushal et al., "A transcriptome database for astrocytes, neurons, and oligodendrocytes: a new resource for understanding brain development and function," *Journal of Neuroscience*, vol. 28, no. 1, pp. 264–278, 2008.

[186] L. A. Desouza, M. Sathanoori, R. Kapoor et al., "Thyroid hormone regulates the expression of the sonic hedgehog signaling pathway in the embryonic and adult mammalian brain," *Endocrinology*, vol. 152, no. 5, pp. 1989–2000, 2011.

33

Biological Behavior of Papillary Carcinoma of the Thyroid Including Squamous Cell Carcinoma Components and Prognosis of Patients Who Underwent Locally Curative Surgery

Yasuhiro Ito,[1] Mitsuyoshi Hirokawa,[2] Takuya Higashiyama,[1] Minoru Kihara,[1] Chisato Tomoda,[1] Yuuki Takamura,[1] Kaoru Kobayashi,[1] Akihiro Miya,[1] and Akira Miyauchi[1]

[1] *Department of Surgery, Kuma Hospital, Shimoyamate-Dori, Chuo-Ku, Kobe 650-0011, Japan*
[2] *Department of Pathology, Kuma Hospital, Kobe 650-0011, Japan*

Correspondence should be addressed to Yasuhiro Ito, ito01@kuma-h.or.jp

Academic Editor: Nikola Bešič

Thyroid carcinoma showing squamous differentiation throughout the entire lesion is diagnosed as squamous cell carcinoma of the thyroid (SCCT) in the WHO classification. This entity is a rare disease and shows a dire prognosis; however, squamous differentiation is more frequently detected in only a portion of papillary thyroid carcinoma. In this paper, we present our experience of 10 patients (8 primary lesions and 2 with recurrence in the lymph nodes) with papillary thyroid carcinoma having an SCC component (PTC-SCC). Only 3 of 8 primary lesions (38%) and none of the 2 recurrent nodes were preoperatively diagnosed as or suspected of having SCC components. All 10 patients underwent locally curative surgery. To date, 3 patients have died of carcinoma, and 2 had distant metastasis at diagnosis or had an undifferentiated carcinoma component. The other 7 are currently alive 5 to 43 months after diagnosis. Systemic adjuvant therapy after the detection of recurrence was effective for 2 patients. It is possible that some PTC-SCC patients without distant metastasis who undergo locally curative surgery can survive for a prolonged period and adjuvant therapies can be effective for local and distant recurrences.

1. Introduction

Squamous cell carcinoma of the thyroid (SCCT) is known to show very aggressive characteristics and a dire prognosis. In the WHO classification [1], SCCT is defined as "squamous cell carcinoma of the thyroid should be composed entirely of tumour cells with squamous differentiation." According to this definition, SCCT is an extremely rare disease [2–5]. However, squamous differentiation can be more frequently observed as a SCC component in a portion of the papillary carcinoma (PTC) lesion, especially in the tall cell variant [6]. Most previous studies investigating a comparably large number of patients investigated SCCT and PTC with an SCC component (PTC-SCC) as a single group, and our knowledge regarding the biological characteristics of PTC-SCC remains poor because of its rarity. To date, we have encountered 10 patients who were diagnosed as having PTC-SCC on

postoperative pathological examination. In this study, we present their clinicopathological features, therapies, and clinical outcomes to elucidate the biological behavior of this disease.

2. Patients and Methods

We reviewed the surgical and pathological records of patients who underwent surgery for thyroid carcinoma between 2006 and 2010. In this period, 5749 patients underwent surgery for primary or recurred PTC. Of these, 10 patients (0.2%) were diagnosed as PTC-SCC and were enrolled in this study. In this period, no patients were diagnosed as SCCT. These diagnoses were rereviewed by a thyroid pathologist (M.H.) based on the WHO classification [1]. PTC-SCC was diagnosed in 8 primary lesions obtained at initial surgery and

2 recurrent lymph nodes obtained at second surgery. Patients who had SCC sites other than the thyroid were excluded from the series. Patients who were diagnosed as having PTC with squamous cell metaplasia (squamous lesions appear benign) or squamoid subtype in undifferentiated carcinoma (UC) were excluded from the study. In this period, 3 patients were suspected as having PTC-SCC (1 primary lesion and 2 recurring lesions) but underwent biopsy only. One patient died of carcinoma one month after detection, and two patients were referred to other hospitals, and their prognoses are unknown. These patients were also excluded from the study. In our department, all patients with PTC undergo thyroid ultrasonography, and neck CT scan is also performed for those who have clinical lymph node metastasis and whose primary lesions are suspected of having extension to adjacent organs. All patients in our series also underwent ultrasonography. Neck CT scan (plain and enhanced) was performed for 9 patients. Furthermore, all patients underwent chest CT scan to screen for lung metastasis and 3 patients who were cytologically suspected of having SCC or UC also underwent abdominal CT scan also. None of these patients underwent PET-CT preoperatively, although two underwent PET-CT after surgery. All patients underwent ultrasound-guided fine needle aspiration biopsy (FNAB) for diagnosis. Furthermore, 3 patients who were suspected of SCC or UC on cytology underwent also ultrasound-guided core needle biopsy (CNB) to confirm the diagnosis. None of these patients showed any complications of CNB, such as hemorrhage, hematoma, and recurrent laryngeal nerve paralysis. On pathological examination, UC lesion was also detected in 2 patients (one primary lesion and one recurrent lymph node). One patient also had primary lung carcinoma, which was detected on CT scan before thyroid surgery. After thyroid surgery, this patient was referred to another hospital and underwent surgery and chemotherapy for lung carcinoma. The histology of lung carcinoma was adenocarcinoma.

3. Results

We analyzed the backgrounds and preoperative findings on imaging studies of 10 PTC-SCC (Table 1). Patients consisted of 7 females and 3 males, and patient ages ranged from 68 to 83 years. Of 8 patients who underwent initial surgery, only 3 (38%) (patient nos. 1, 4, and 8) were preoperatively diagnosed as or suspected of having an SCC component on FNAB or CNB. Tumors of these 3 patients were suspected to significantly extend to adjacent organs. Therefore, these patients underwent chemotherapy using paclitaxel [7] before surgery, considering the possibility of UC with Stage IVB [8], to promote tumor shrinkage and make locally curative surgery easier. There was no evidence of carcinoma progression during preoperative chemotherapy, *although no patients were judged as complete response* (manuscript in preparation). The remaining 5 primary lesions were diagnosed as PTC on cytology. Tumor size ranged from 3.5 to 5.6 cm, and 7 of these patients also had lymph node metastasis detected on preoperative imaging studies. Three patients (patient nos. 6, 7, and 8) also underwent FNAB for metastatic nodes and

were diagnosed as or suspected of having PTC. Two patients (patients nos. 2 and 3) had previously undergone initial surgery for PTC, and recurrence was detected in the lymph nodes, which measured 0.9 cm and 3.9 cm, respectively. The cytological results of these nodes were PTC and UC, respectively. Two patients (patient nos. 1 and 3) had lung metastasis at surgery, and one (patient no. 10) had primary lung carcinoma that was treated after surgery for thyroid carcinoma at another hospital, as indicated above.

Table 2 summarizes the intraoperative and postoperative findings and clinical courses of these 10 patients. All 8 primary lesions showed significant extrathyroid extension corresponding to T4a in the UICC TNM classification [8], but all these patients could undergo locally curative surgery. Of 8 patients, 2 (patient nos. 4 and 5) were SCC dominant, and the remaining 6 (patient nos. 1, 6–10) were PTC dominant on pathological examination for primary lesions. PTC lesion was dominant in 2 patients who underwent surgery for lymph node recurrence (patient nos. 2 and 3). The range of the portion of SCC component was less than 10% in 2 patients (patient nos. 2 and 6), 10–20% in 5 patients (patient nos. 1, 7–10), and 40% or more in 3 patients (patient nos. 3–5). The PTC lesions of 4 patients (50%) were tall cell variant. Two patients (patient nos. 3 and 4) also demonstrated UC lesion.

None of these 10 patients underwent radioactive iodine (RAI) therapy after surgery. The 3 patients who underwent preoperative chemotherapy continued to receive it after surgery. Chemotherapy was initiated after surgery for patient nos. 3 and 5. Patient no. 3 underwent chemotherapy immediately after initial surgery because of lung metastasis and involvement of a UC component and patient no. 5 underwent chemotherapy after the detection of local recurrence. Patient no. 9 showed recurrence in the lung 3 months after surgery and underwent immunotherapy using dendritic cells pulsed with WT1 peptide at the patient's request [9]. Three patients (patients nos. 5, 7, and 8) underwent external beam radiotherapy (EBRT) of the whole neck at 50–60 Gy immediately after surgery. However, 2 local recurrences were detected during EBRT in patient no. 5. One was located in front of the common carotid artery and was diagnosed as SCC on CNB, and another was found in the skin, for which neither FNAB nor CNB was performed. The former disappeared by postoperative chemotherapy, and the latter was resected by second surgery. The histology of the second surgical specimen was SCC.

During followup, patient no. 1, who had lung metastasis at surgery, developed recurrence in the bone and died of carcinoma 18 months after diagnosis because of the enlargement of lung metastasis. Patient no. 3 is currently alive despite the development of lung metastasis that had been present before surgery. Patient no. 4, who had a UC component, developed recurrence in the larynx and underwent a second surgery at another hospital. The recurrent tumor was pathologically diagnosed as UC, and this patient died of UC progression 23 months after diagnosis. In patient no. 5, there has been no further evidence of carcinoma recurrence to date after chemotherapy and second surgery.

TABLE 1: Backgrounds and preoperative evaluation of 10 patients with PTC-SCC.

Patient no.	Gender	Age	Initial surgery?	Rapid growth	*Preoperative diagnosis (primary)	*Preoperative diagnosis (LN meta)	Tumor size (cm)	LN meta size (cm)	Distant metastasis at surgery
1	Female	71	Yes	Yes?	SCC	x	5.6	1.6	Lung
2	Female	71	No	No	x	PTC	x	0.9	No
3	Female	69	No	Yes	x	UC	x	3.9	Lung
4	Female	67	Yes	No	UC or SCC	x	4.9	x	No
5	Female	83	Yes	No	PTC or PDC	x	5.2	1.7	No
6	Male	76	Yes	No	PTC	PTC	4.0	1.4	No
7	Male	71	Yes	No	PTC	PTC	3.5	0.9	No
8	Female	68	Yes	No	PTC or SCC	PTC?	4.4	2.7	No
9	Male	70	Yes	No	PTC	x	4.4	3.6	No
^10	Female	71	Yes	No	PTC	x	4.7	2.7	No

PTC: papillary thyroid carcinoma, UC: undifferentiated carcinoma; PDC: poorly differentiated carcinoma, SCC: squamous cell carcinoma.
*Based on FNAB or CNB.
^Also had lung carcinoma.

TABLE 2: Intraoperative and pathological findings and prognosis of 10 patients with PTC-SCC.

Patient no.	Surgical designs	Resection	Extrathyroid extension	Pathology (primary)	Pathology (LN meta)	Adjuvant therapies	Carcinoma recurrence	Outcome after diagnosis
1	TT + MND	R0?	Yes	**PTC > SCC (10%)	PTC	*chemo	Bone	18 m DOC
2	CT + MND	R0	x	x	PTC > SCC (<10%)	x	x	43 m ANEC
3	MND	R0	x	x	PTC > SCC (40%) > UC	Chemo	x	33 m AWC
4	TT + CND	R0	Yes	SCC (40%) > UC > PTC	PTC	*chemo	^Laryn, Bone	23 m DOC
5	TT + MND	R0	Yes	SCC (80%) > PTC (tall)	PTC	Chemo + EBRT	Skin, local	18 m ANEC
6	TT + MND	R0?	Yes	PTC > SCC (<10%)	PTC	x	x	14 m ANEC
7	TT + MND	R0	Yes	PTC (tall) > SCC (40%)	PTC	EBRT	x	13 m ANEC
8	LI + MND	R0	Yes	PTC (tall) > SCC (10%)	PTC	*chemo + EBRT	x	9 m ANEC
9	TT + MND	R0	Yes	PTC (tall) > SCC (20%)	PTC	Immunotherapy	Lung	9 m DOC
10	TT + MMD	R1	Yes	PTC > SCC (20%)	PTC	Chemo for lung carcinoma	x	5 m ANEC

*Preoperative chemotherapy was also performed. ^Recurrence of UC. **A > B indicates A occupied a larger portion than B.
TT: total thyroidectomy, CT: completion total thyroidectomy, LI: lobectomy with isthymectomy, CND: central node dissection, MND: modified radical neck dissection, EBRT; external beam radiotherapy.
DOC; Died of carcinoma.
ANEC: Alive with no evidence of Carcinoma.
AWC: Alive with carcinoma.

Lung metastasis was stable in patient no. 9 for 6 months after the initiation of immunotherapy, but he died of sudden respiratory tract hemorrhage 9 months after surgery. The remaining 5 (patients nos. 2, 6–8, 10) are currently alive with no evidence of carcinoma recurrence, although patient no. 10 is currently undergoing chemotherapy for lung carcinoma.

4. Discussion

In this study, we demonstrated that it is difficult to diagnose PTC-SCC on preoperative FNAB or CNB. Only 3 of 8 patients (38%) having primary lesions were preoperatively diagnosed as or suspected of having SCC components. This is partially because of the difficulty in differential diagnosis between SCC and UC on cytology. Furthermore, SCC cells may not be aspirated or biopsied if the needle does not appropriately hit SCC components. In our series, all patients were older, 7 patients had carcinoma larger than 4 cm, clinical node metastasis was detected in 7 patients, all had significant extrathyroid extension, and the PTC lesions of 4 patients were diagnosed as tall cell variant. These clinicopathological features were recognized as predicting poor prognosis, indicating that squamous differentiation occurs in PTC with biologically aggressive behavior [10–13].

Previous studies investigated SCCT and PTC-SCC as a single group and demonstrated that most of these patients showed a poor prognosis. Booya et al. showed that the median survival period was only 8.6 months for 10 patients [2]. According to a review by Syed et al. in 2010 [14], median survival periods in reports published between 1985 and 2009 ranged from 3 to 24 months but mostly 12 months or even shorter. Furthermore, Cook et al. demonstrated that all patients with SCCT or PTC-SCC who underwent incomplete resection or biopsy died within a short period despite adjuvant therapies [3], which was similar to the results of UC, as we previously demonstrated [15].

In this study, we investigated 10 patients with PTC-SCC who underwent locally curative resection, indicating that they were potential long-term survivors. In our series, 7 patients have survived for 8 months to 43 months to date. Two patients (patients nos. 2 and 6) with only focal SCC lesions who did not show distant metastasis at diagnosis have survived without any further recurrence for 14 and 43 months after diagnosis, respectively, although they underwent no adjuvant therapies. The remaining 5 with larger lesions of SCC components, who underwent either or both chemotherapy and EBRT, have also survived with or without recurrence. Of the 3 patients who died of carcinoma, 2 had distant metastasis at diagnosis or had a UC component. These findings suggest that long-term survival can be expected for some PTC-SCC patients if they undergo locally curative surgery and do not have distant metastasis at diagnosis or a UC component.

Previous studies demonstrated controversial results of adjuvant chemotherapy [16–18]. In our series, 3 patients who were cytologically diagnosed as or suspected of having SCC underwent preoperative adjuvant chemotherapy. These tumors were large and were suspected of extending to adjacent organs. In order to make locally curative surgery easier, we performed preoperative chemotherapy based on the protocol for UC [7]. If a tumor is small without the suspicion of extrathyroid extension and locally curative surgery is expected to be easy, immediate surgery may be preferred to avoid losing time. Postoperative chemotherapy should be performed for patients having distant metastasis at surgery or those who have undergone only palliative surgery. It remains unclear whether chemotherapy immediately after locally curative surgery for patients without distant metastasis is effective to prolong the survival of PTC-SCC patients, because we did not perform a comparative study. However, it may be an alternative in order to control minute carcinoma lesions that remained unresected in local lesions

and micrometastases in distant organs. Another strategy is to initiate chemotherapy when recurrence is clinically detected. Since one of the local recurrences disappeared in patient no. 5, this may also promise a certain level of effect.

EBRT is another adjuvant therapy for local control. However, previous studies of SCCT and PTC-SCC showed controversial findings of its effectiveness [2, 3, 18, 19]. In our series, 3 patients underwent EBRT immediately after surgery. Two patients showed no evidence of local recurrence, but in 1 patient, local recurrences became apparent during EBRT. Therefore, we cannot conclude that EBRT has a significant effect on the local control of PTC-SCC. However, it may be better to perform postoperative EBRT, especially for cases with significant extension to adjacent organs, because multimodality therapy should be considered for aggressive diseases such as PTC-SCC.

In summary, we have presented our experience of treating 10 patients with PTC-SCC, which is difficult to diagnose preoperatively. Long-term survival can be expected for PTC-SCC patients if locally curative resection can be performed and distant metastasis at surgery is not detected. Adjuvant chemotherapy and EBRT may contribute to the control of carcinoma recurrence, but further studies of a large number of patients are necessary to establish therapeutic protocols for PTC-SCC patients.

References

[1] K. Y. Lam and A. Sakamoto, "Squamous cell carcinoma," in *Pathology and Genetics of Tumours of Endocrine Organs*, R. A. Delellis, R. V. Lloyd, P. U. Heitz et al., Eds., p. 81, International Agency for Research on Cancer, Lyon, France, 2004.

[2] F. Booya, T. J. Sebo, J. L. Kasperbauer, and V. Fatourechi, "Primary squamous cell carcinoma of the thyroid: report of ten cases," *Thyroid*, vol. 16, no. 1, pp. 89–93, 2006.

[3] A. M. Cook, L. Vini, and C. Harmer, "Squamous cell carcinoma of the thyroid: outcome of treatment in 16 patients," *European Journal of Surgical Oncology*, vol. 25, no. 6, pp. 606–609, 1999.

[4] W. J. Simpson and J. Carruthers, "Squamous cell carcinoma of the thyroid gland," *The American Journal of Surgery*, vol. 156, no. 1, pp. 44–46, 1988.

[5] A. K. Sarda, S. Bal, Arunabh, M. K. Singh, and M. M. Kapur, "Squamous cell carcinoma of the thyroid," *Journal of Surgical Oncology*, vol. 39, no. 3, pp. 175–178, 1988.

[6] C. G. Kleer, T. J. Giordano, and M. J. Merino, "Squamous cell carcinoma of the thyroid: an aggressive tumor associated with tall cell variant of papillary thyroid carcinoma," *Modern Pathology*, vol. 13, no. 7, pp. 742–746, 2000.

[7] T. Higashiyama, Y. Ito, M. Hirokawa et al., "Induction chemotherapy with weekly paclitaxel administration for anaplastic thyroid carcinoma," *Thyroid*, vol. 20, no. 1, pp. 4–14, 2010.

[8] L. H. Sobin and C. H. Wittekindeds, *UICC; TNM Classification of Malignant Tumors*, Wiley-Liss, New York, NY, USA, 6th edition, 2002.

[9] M. Okamoto, S. Furuichi, Y. Nishioka et al., "Expression of toll-like receptor 4 on dendritic cells is significant for anticancer effect of dendritic cell-based immunotherapy in combination with an active component of OK-432, a streptococcal preparation," *Cancer Research*, vol. 64, no. 15, pp. 5461–5470, 2004.

[10] Y. Ito, C. Tomoda, T. Uruno et al., "Ultrasonographically and anatomopathologically detectable node metastases in the lateral compartment as indicators of worse relapse-free survival in patients with papillary thyroid carcinoma," *World Journal of Surgery*, vol. 29, no. 7, pp. 917–920, 2005.

[11] Y. Ito, C. Tomoda, T. Uruno et al., "Prognostic significance of extrathyroid extension of papillary thyroid carcinoma: massive but not minimal extension affects the relapse-free survival," *World Journal of Surgery*, vol. 30, no. 5, pp. 780–786, 2006.

[12] Y. Ito, M. Hirokawa, M. Fukushima et al., "Prevalence and prognostic significance of poor differentiation and tall cell variant in papillary carcinoma in Japan," *World Journal of Surgery*, vol. 32, no. 7, pp. 1535–1543, 2008.

[13] Y. Ito and A. Miyauchi, "Prognostic factors and therapeutic strategies for differentiated carcinomas of the thyroid," *Endocrine Journal*, vol. 56, no. 2, pp. 177–192, 2009.

[14] M. I. Syed, M. Stewart, S. Syed et al., "Squamous cell carcinoma of the thyroid gland: primary or secondary disease?" *The Journal of Laryngology and Otology*, vol. 125, no. 1, pp. 3–9, 2010.

[15] Y. Ito, T. Higashiyama, M. Hirokawa et al., "Investigation of the validity of UICC stage grouping of anaplastic carcinoma of the thyroid," *Asian Journal of Surgery*, vol. 32, no. 1, pp. 47–50, 2009.

[16] K. Shimaoka and Y. Tsukada, "Squamous cell carcinomas and adenosquamous carcinomas originating from the thyroid gland," *Cancer*, vol. 46, no. 8, pp. 1833–1842, 1980.

[17] T. Harada, K. Shimaoka, K. Yakumaru, and K. Ito, "Squamous cell carcinoma of the thyroid gland—transition from adenocarcinoma," *Journal of Surgical Oncology*, vol. 19, no. 1, pp. 36–43, 1982.

[18] T. Y. Huang and D. Assor, "Primary squamous cell carcinoma of the thyroid gland: a report of four cases," *American Journal of Clinical Pathology*, vol. 55, no. 1, pp. 93–98, 1971.

[19] X. H. Zhou, "Primary squamous cell carcinoma of the thyroid," *European Journal of Surgical Oncology*, vol. 28, no. 1, pp. 42–45, 2002.

34

Ameliorative Effect of Vitamin C on Alterations in Thyroid Hormones Concentrations Induced by Subchronic Coadministration of Chlorpyrifos and Lead in Wistar Rats

Suleiman F. Ambali, Chinedu Orieji, Woziri O. Abubakar, Muftau Shittu, and Mohammed U. Kawu

Department of Veterinary Physiology and Pharmacology, Ahmadu Bello University, Zaria 800007, Nigeria

Correspondence should be addressed to Suleiman F. Ambali, fambali2001@yahoo.com

Academic Editor: Duncan Topliss

The present study evaluated the ameliorative effect of vitamin C on alteration in thyroid hormones induced by low-dose subchronic coadministration of chlorpyrifos (CPF) and lead (Pb). Forty Wistar rats were divided into 4 groups of 10 animals each. Groups I and II were administered soya oil (2 mL/kg) and vitamin C (100 mg/kg), respectively. Group III was coadministered CPF (4.25 mg/kg $\sim$1/20th LD_{50}) and Pb (250 mg/kg $\sim$1/20th LD_{50}), respectively. Group IV was pretreated with vitamin C (100 mg/kg) and then coadministered with CPF (4.25 mg/kg) and Pb (250 mg/kg), 30 min later. The regimens were administered by gavage for a period of 9 weeks. The marginal decrease in serum triiodothyronine and thyroxine and the significant increase in the concentrations of thyroid stimulating hormone and malonaldehyde in the group coadministered with CPF and Pb were ameliorated by vitamin C partly due to its antioxidant properties.

1. Introduction

Man and animals are exposed to a "soup" of chemical contaminants in the environment, which directly or indirectly affect their health and well-being. Pesticides and heavy metals are the most common environmental contaminants because of their respective widespread use in agriculture and industries. Hitherto, most studies on these chemical contaminants have centered on the examination of one single agent and therefore, current understanding of the toxicity of many environmental toxicants/pollutants is based primarily on toxicity studies performed on laboratory animals exposed to a single toxic agent [1, 2]. However, the environment is heavily contaminated with many chemicals, which interact with each other in such a way that modify their toxic response in humans and animals.

Organophosphate (OP) compounds are the most widely used insecticides accounting for 50% of global insecticidal use [3] while Pb is the most widespread heavy metal contaminants with wide applications [4]. Occupational and environmental Pb exposure continues to be among the most significant public health problems [4–7]. Due to their persistent nature in the environment and their toxicodynamics, CPF and Pb have resulted in deleterious effects in man and animals [8].

The toxicity of Pb remains a matter of public health concern [9] due to its pervasiveness in the environment and the awareness about its toxic effects [10] at exposure levels lower than what was previously considered harmful [11]. Reproductive consequences of Pb exposure are widespread [12], affecting almost all aspects of reproduction [13]. Pb induces decreased sperm count and motility and increased morphological abnormalities in animals [14, 15]. CPF is one of the most common insecticidal environmental contaminants [16, 17]. Despite restrictions placed on some of its domestic uses by United States Environmental Protection Agency (USEPA) in 2000, CPF is still widely used as residues have been detected in citrus fruits in some parts of the world [18]. Adverse reproductive outcomes have been observed following CPF poisoning [16, 17, 19–21]. The adverse reproductive health outcomes even as a result of environmental exposure to CPF have been partly linked to hypothyroidism [17]. Furthermore, other studies have found hypothyroidism in both CPF [17, 22–24] and Pb [25–28] poisonings. Since adequate thyroidal function is essential for effective and optimal reproductive performance, therefore, measures aimed at mitigating the thyroid dysfunction instigated by exposure to low-dose environmental contaminants are pertinent.

Although the mechanisms of toxicity of the two agents differ, oxidative stress is a common feature in CPF [29–33] and Pb [34–36] poisoning. However, ascorbic acid has shown tremendous promise in mitigating toxicity evoked by CPF [31, 33, 37, 38] and Pb [28, 39]. Therefore, the present paper was aimed at evaluating the effect of low dose subchronic exposure to CPF and Pb on thyroid functions, the role of thyroidal lipoperoxidation, and ameliorative effect of vitamin C in Wistar rats.

2. Material and Methods

2.1. Experimental Animals. Forty 6-week-old adult male Wistar rats were obtained from the Animal House of the Department of Veterinary Physiology and Pharmacology, Ahmadu Bello University, Zaria, Nigeria. The rats were fed on standard rat pellets, and water was provided *ad libitum*. The experiment was performed in compliance with the National Institutes of Health Guide for Care and Use of Laboratory Animals [40].

2.2. Chemicals. Commercial grade CPF (Termicot 20% EC, Sabero Organics, Gujarat, India) was reconstituted in soya oil to 10% solution, which was subsequently used for the experiment. Analytical grade lead acetate (Kiran Light Laboratories, Mumbai, India) used for the study was reconstituted into a 20% solution using distilled water. Commercial grade vitamin C tablets (100 mg/tablet; Emzor Pharmaceutical Ltd, Nigeria, BN : 618 N) were dissolved in distilled water to 10% solution just before daily administration.

2.3. Animal Treatments. Forty adult male Wistar rats were divided into 4 groups of 10 animals per group. The rats in group I (C/oil) were administered corn oil (2 mL/kg), while those in group II (VC) were administered vitamin C (100 mg/kg). Rats in group III (CPF) were coadministered CPF 4.25 mg/kg, ~1/20th LD$_{50}$ [24] and lead acetate 225 mg/kg, ~1/20th LD$_{50}$ [28], respectively. Rats in group IV (VC + CPF + Pb) were pretreated with vitamin C, and then coadministered with CPF (4.25 mg/kg) and Pb (225 mg/kg), 30 min later. These regimens were administered orally by gavage once daily for a period of 9 weeks. At the end of the dosing period, the rats were sacrificed by jugular venisection after light chloroform anesthesia. Serum obtained from each blood sample was used to evaluate for the concentrations of triodothyronine (T3), thyroxine (T4), and thyroid stimulating hormone (TSH), while the thyroid gland was weighed and then evaluated for the malonaldehyde (MDA) concentration as an index of lipoperoxidation.

2.4. Evaluation of Concentrations of Triodothyronine—Thyroid Stimulating Hormone and Thyroxine. The concentrations of T$_3$, T$_4$, and TSH were assayed using enzyme-linked immunosorbent assay (ELISA) kits (Microwell TSH, T$_3$,T$_4$ kits; Synthron Bioresearch, Inc, USA).

2.5. Effect of Treatments on Thyroid Gland Lipoperoxidation. The level of thiobarbituric acid reactive substance, malonaldehyde (MDA) as an index of lipid peroxidation was evaluated in the thyroid gland using the double heating method of Draper and Hadley [41]. The principle of the method was based on spectrophotometric measurement of the color developed during reaction of thiobarbituric acid (TBA) with malonaldehyde. The thyroid glands from each animal in all the groups were weighed and then homogenized in a known volume of ice-cold phosphate buffer to obtain a 10% homogenate, which was centrifuged at 2000 g for 10 min to obtain the supernatant. The supernatant was then used to assess the level of protein and MDA in the sample. The assessment of MDA concentration in the supernatant of thyroid gland homogenate was performed thus; 2.5 mL of 100 g/L trichloroacetic acid solution was added to 0.5 mL of the thyroid gland homogenate in a centrifuge tube and placed in a boiling water bath for 15 min. After cooling under tap water for 5 min, the mixtures were then centrifuged at 1000 g for 10 min. 2 mL of the supernatant was added to 1 mL of 6.7 g/L (0.67%) thiobarbituric acid (TBA) solution in a test tube and placed in a boiling water (100°C) bath for 15 min. The solution was cooled under tap water and the absorbance was thereafter measured at 532 nm using a UV spectrophotometer (T80$^+$UV/VIS Spectrometer PG Instruments Ltd, UK). The concentration of MDA calculated by the absorbance coefficient of MDA-TBA complex (1.56 × 10^5 cm^{-1}) and expressed as nmol/mg of tissue protein. The protein concentration was determined using the method described by Lowry et al. [42].

2.6. Statistical Analysis. Data obtained were expressed as mean + SEM and then subjected to one-way analysis of variance followed by Tukey's post hoc test using Graphpad prism version 4.0. Values of $P < .05$ were considered significant.

3. Results

3.1. Effect of Treatments on Serum Triiodothyronine Concentration. The effect of treatments on serum T$_3$ level is shown in Figure 1. There was no significant difference in the serum T$_3$ level between the groups. However, the CPF + Pb group had the lowest T$_3$ concentration with its level decreasing by 14.3%, 29%, and 14.3%, respectively, relative to the S/oil, VC, and VC + CPF + Pb groups.

3.2. Effect of Treatments on Serum Thyroxine Concentration. There was no significant ($P > .05$) difference in the serum T$_4$ level between the groups. However, the lowest T$_4$ level was recorded in the CPF + Pb group as its level decreased by 0.6%, 32%, and 26% compared to S/oil, VC, and VC + CPF + Pb groups, respectively (Figure 2).

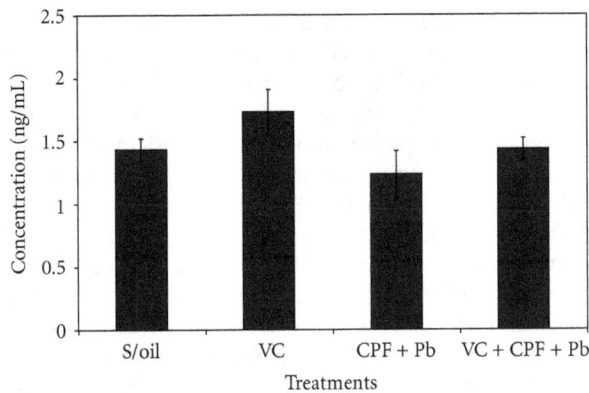

FIGURE 1: Effect of subchronic coexposure of soya oil (S/oil) and vitamin C (VC) and/or combination of chlorpyrifos (CPF) and lead (Pb) on triodothyronine concentration in Wistar rats.

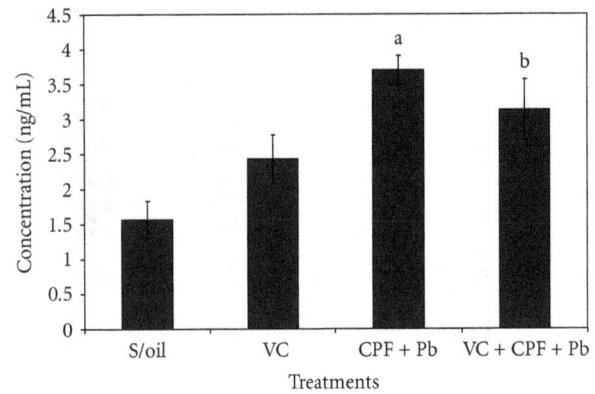

FIGURE 2: Effect of subchronic coexposure of soya oil (S/oil) and vitamin C (VC) and/or combination of chlorpyrifos (CPF) and lead (Pb) on serum thyroxine concentration in Wistar rats.

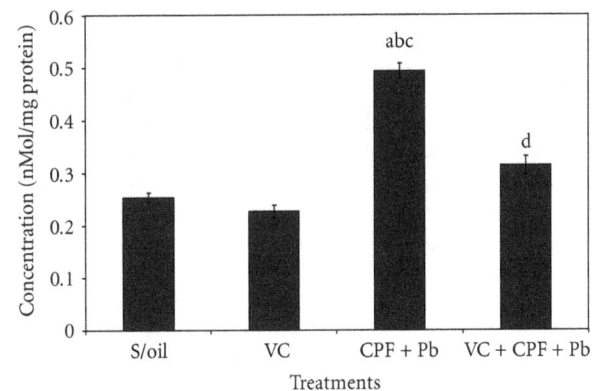

FIGURE 3: Effect of subchronic coexposure of soya oil (S/oil) and vitamin C (VC) and/or combination of chlorpyrifos (CPF) and lead (Pb) on thyroid stimulating hormone concentration in Wistar rats. [a]$P < .01$ versus S/oil group, [b]$P < .05$ versus S/oil group.

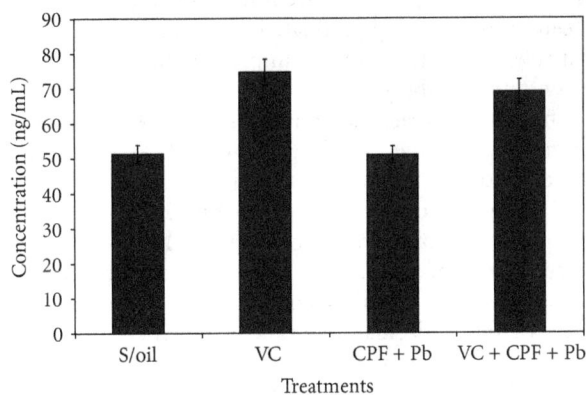

FIGURE 4: Effect of subchronic coexposure of soya oil (S/oil) and vitamin C (VC) and/or combination of chlorpyrifos (CPF) and lead (Pb) on thyroid malonaldehyde concentration in Wistar rats. [abc]$P < .01$ versus S/oil, VC and VC + CPF + Pb groups, respectively; [d]$P < .01$ versus VC.

3.3. Effect of Treatments on Serum Thyroid Stimulating Hormone Concentration. The effect of treatments on TSH concentration is shown in Figure 3. There was a significant ($P < .01$) increase in the TSH concentration in CPF + Pb group compared to S/oil group. The TSH concentration in the VC + CPF + Pb group significantly ($P < .05$) increased compared to S/oil group. There was no significant ($P > .05$) change in the TSH concentration in the VC group compared to S/oil, CPF + Pb, or VC + CPF + Pb group.

3.4. Effect of Treatments on Thyroid Malondialdehyde Concentration. The effect of treatments on thyroidal MDA concentration of various groups is shown in Figure 4. There was a significant ($P < .01$) increase in the MDA concentration in the CPF + Pb group when compared to S/oil, VC, or VC + CPF group. The MDA concentration significantly ($P < .01$) increased in the VC + CPF + Pb group compared to VC group.

3.5. Effect of Treatments on the Weight of Thyroid Gland. The effect of treatments on the weight of thyroid gland is shown in Figure 5. There was no significant change ($P > .05$) in the

weight of the thyroid gland in between the groups. However, the thyroid weight was higher in the CPF group by 11.4%, 8%, and 7.2% relative to C/oil, VC, and VC + CPF groups, respectively.

4. Discussion

Low-dose subchronic coadministration of CPF and Pb mimicking environmental exposure, which did not cause any apparent systemic toxicity, has been shown to cause a nonsignificant decrease in the serum level of T_3 and T_4 in the present study. Although, the alteration in the concentration of thyroid hormone was not significant, the fact that these very low doses of CPF and Pb did cause some level of hormonal changes should not be ignored as it may indicate ongoing subclinical metabolic alterations within the system. CPF has been shown to induce hypothyroidism in ewes [22] and rats [23, 24, 43]. Zaidi et al. [44] recorded hypothyroidism in the serum of some pesticide formulators. Similarly, Meeker et al. [17] demonstrated an

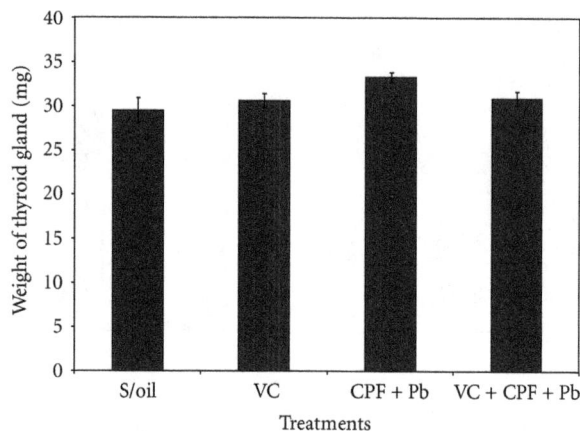

FIGURE 5: Effect of subchronic coexposure of soya oil (S/oil) and vitamin C (VC), and/or combination of chlorpyrifos (CPF) and lead (Pb) on the weight of thyroid gland in Wistar rats.

inverse association between urinary concentration of CPF metabolites, 3,5,6-trichloro-2-pyridinol and T_4 level and a positive association with TSH. In the same vein, hypothyroidism has been associated with Pb [45, 46] poisoning. Perhaps the reason why the coadministration of CPF and Pb did not result in significant alteration in thyroid hormone concentrations may be due to the very low doses of the two chemicals used.

Although T_3 is a poor indicator of subclinical or overt hypothyroidism, the marginal decrease in serum T_3 level observed in the group subchronically coadministered with CPF and Pb may be due to the low T_4 level observed in the group rather than a decrease synthesis. This is because T_4 have to be converted to T_3 for the biological effect of the hormone to be manifested. In addition, the relative low T_3 level may also be due to deficiency in the synthesis of 5'-deiodionase, an enzyme responsible for the conversion of T_4 to the more metabolically active T_3. Indeed, Pb has been shown to inhibit the activity of type-I iodothyronine 5'-monodeiodinase (5'-D) activity [45]. CPF has been suggested to differentially affect peripheral deiodination [23]. The low 5'-deioodinase activity may have been due to pathological changes in the organs responsible for its synthesis by both CPF and Pb.

The marginal decrease in the level of T_4 observed in the group coadministered with CPF and Pb may be due to some level of damage to the thyroid acinar probably due to oxidative stress induction by both CPF [23, 24, 43, 44] and Pb [47, 48]. Although, the present study did not evaluate histological changes in the thyroid glands, Pb on its own has been shown to cause hypothyroidism either by inhibiting iodine uptake [25, 26] and to cause functional impairment of the pituitary—thyroid axis [27].

Some level of improvement in the concentration of T_3 and T_4 in group pretreated with vitamin C probably underscores the role of oxidative stress in thyroid dysfunction evoked by coadministration of CPF and Pb as indicated by low lipoperoxidative changes in the VC + CPF + Pb group. The vitamin C having protected the thyroid acinar

from oxidative damage may have aided in restoring thyroid hormones' synthetic function. Apart from its antioxidant properties, some other nonantioxidant activity of vitamin C may have complemented the restoration of thyroidal function. For example, vitamin C has been demonstrated to aid the synthesis of paraoxonase, an important esterase that aids in the detoxification of OPs [49].

The significant increase in the TSH concentration in the group coadministered with CPF and Pb may be due to the attempt by the body to stimulate the thyroid gland to increase the synthesis and elaboration of T_4 in order to compensate for the apparent deficit in the system. CPF-induced increase in TSH concentration has been recorded in humans [17, 44] and laboratory animal models [23, 24]. The low T_4 concentration in the CPF + Pb group may have stimulated the hypothalamic neurons to secrete thyrotrophin releasing hormone (TRH) leading to increased stimulation of TSH synthesis [50]. The apparent normalization of the TSH concentration in group pretreated with vitamin C correlates positively with the marginal improvement in T_4 and T_3 concentration in the group.

The study revealed a significant increase in the MDA concentration in the thyroid gland of CPF + Pb group as compared to other groups. This increased MDA concentration is indicative of oxidative damage to the thyroid gland. This may be attributed to the high metabolic rate, high level of free radicals accumulation, and low level of endogenous antioxidant in the thyroid gland. Oxidative stress induction is one of the molecular mechanism of CPF [31–33] and Pb [28, 34] poisoning. Oxidative stress, characterized by an elevation in the steady-state concentration of reactive oxygen species (ROS), has been implicated in a wide range of biological and pathological conditions [51]. Thyroid hormones are associated with the oxidative and antioxidative status of the organism [52]. Because of its role in oxidative metabolism, increase concentration of ROS is formed in the thyroid glands. However, the combination of CPF and Pb was shown to have exacerbated the ROS induction perhaps due to their direct interaction with the thyroid acinar. Lipid peroxidation inactivates cell constituents by oxidation or causes oxidative stress by undergoing radical chain reaction, ultimately leading to loss of membrane integrity [53]. Similarly, the increased MDA concentration may have been exacerbated due to impairment of antioxidant enzymes that have been reported in hypothyroidism [54]. Pb on its own induces lipoperoxidation by inhibiting the activity of δ-aminolevulinic acid dehydrase leading to accumulation of its substrate δ-aminolevulinic acid, which rapidly oxidize to generate free radicals as superoxide ion, hydroxyl radical, and hydrogen peroxide [7].

Pretreatment with vitamin C has been shown by the present study to ameliorate the lipoperoxidative changes induced by subchronic administration of coadministration of CPF and Pb. This was apparently due to antioxidant property of the vitamin. The antioxidant properties of vitamin C have been demonstrated in numerous studies involving CPF-induced lipoperoxidation [31, 33, 37, 38].

The weight of the thyroid was marginally higher in the CPF + Pb group than any of the other three groups. The reason for the relatively higher weight in the CPF + Pb group may be related to the significantly higher TSH concentration, which may have partly stimulated the proliferation of the thyroid follicular cell [55], apparently to compensate for the marginal decrease in thyroid hormones. Although, the weight of the thyroid gland was marginally higher in the group pretreated with vitamin C than those of C/oil and VC groups, the fact that it was lower compared to CPF + Pb group demonstrates apparent restoration of the weight of the thyroid gland by vitamin C.

5. Conclusion

Subchronic coadministration of CPF and Pb has been shown by the present study to marginally decrease thyroid hormones concentration, increase TSH concentration and thyroid lipoperoxidation, and marginally increase the weight of the thyroid gland. The alterations in these thyroid gland parameters were ameliorated by pretreatment with vitamin C apparently due to its antioxidant properties.

References

[1] A. Brouwer, D. C. Morse, M. C. Lans et al., "Interactions of persistent environmental organohalogens with the thyroid hormone system: mechanisms and possible consequences for animal and human health," *Toxicology and Industrial Health*, vol. 14, no. 1-2, pp. 59–84, 1998.

[2] M. G. Wade, G. K. Warren, V. Y. Edwards et al., "Effects of subchronic exposure to a complex mixture of persistent contaminants in male rats: systemic, immune and reproductive effects," *Toxicological Sciences*, vol. 67, pp. 131–143, 2002.

[3] J. E. Casida and G. B. Quistad, "Organophosphate toxicity: safety aspects of non acetylcholinesterase secondary targets," *Chemical Research in Toxicology*, vol. 17, no. 8, pp. 983–998, 2004.

[4] S. M. Levin and M. Goldberg, "Clinical evaluation and management of lead-exposed construction workers," *American Journal of Industrial Medicine*, vol. 37, no. 1, pp. 23–43, 2000.

[5] Y. Lolin and P. O'Gorman, "δ-Aminolaevulinic acid dehydratase as an index of the presence and severity of lead poisoning in acute and chronic lead exposure," *Annals of Clinical Biochemistry*, vol. 23, no. 5, pp. 521–528, 1986.

[6] L. M. Fels, M. Wünsch, J. Baranowski et al., "Adverse effects of chronic low level lead exposure on kidney function—a risk group study in children," *Nephrology Dialysis Transplantation*, vol. 13, no. 9, pp. 2248–2256, 1998.

[7] H. Gurer-Orhan, H. U. Sabir, and H. Ozgüneş, "Correlation between clinical indicators of lead poisoning and oxidative stress parameters in controls and lead-exposed workers," *Toxicology*, vol. 195, no. 2-3, pp. 147–154, 2004.

[8] H. Krishna and A. V. Ramachandran, "Biochemical alterations induced by the acute exposure to combination of chlorpyrifos and lead in Wistar rats," *Biology and Medicine*, vol. 1, no. 2, pp. 1–6, 2009.

[9] N. S. Duzgoren-Aydin, "Sources and characteristics of lead pollution in the urban environment of Guangzhou," *Science of the Total Environment*, vol. 385, no. 1–3, pp. 182–195, 2007.

[10] A. M. Saleh, C. Vijayasarathy, L. Masoud, L. Kumar, A. Shahin, and A. Kambal, "Paraoxon induces apoptosis in EL4 cells via activation of mitochondrial pathways," *Toxicology and Applied Pharmacology*, vol. 190, no. 1, pp. 47–57, 2003.

[11] R. Sandhir, D. Julka, and K. D. Gill, "Lipoperoxidative damage on lead exposure in rat brain and its implications on membrane bound enzymes," *Pharmacology and Toxicology*, vol. 74, no. 2, pp. 66–71, 1994.

[12] L. Patrick, "Lead toxicity part II: the role of free radical damage and the use of antioxidants in the pathology and treatment of lead toxicity," *Alternative Medicine Review*, vol. 11, no. 2, pp. 114–127, 2006.

[13] W. Zheng, M. Aschner, and J. F. Ghersi-Egea, "Brain barrier systems: a new frontier in metal neurotoxicological research," *Toxicology and Applied Pharmacology*, vol. 192, no. 1, pp. 1–11, 2003.

[14] P. C. Hsu, M. Y. Liu, C. C. Hsu, L. Y. Chen, and Y. Leon Guo, "Lead exposure causes generation of reactive oxygen species and functional impairment in rat sperm," *Toxicology*, vol. 122, no. 1-2, pp. 133–143, 1997.

[15] P. C. Hsu, C. C. Hsu, M. Y. Liu, L. Y. Chen, and Y. L. Guo, "Lead-induced changes in spermatozoa function and metabolism," *Journal of Toxicology and Environmental Health Part A*, vol. 55, no. 1, pp. 45–64, 1998.

[16] J. D. Meeker, L. Ryan, D. B. Barr et al., "The relationship of urinary metabolites of carbaryl/naphthalene and chlorpyrifos with human semen quality," *Environmental Health Perspectives*, vol. 112, no. 17, pp. 1665–1670, 2004.

[17] J. D. Meeker, L. Ryan, D. B. Barr, and R. Hauser, "Exposure to nonpersistent insecticides and male reproductive hormones," *Epidemiology*, vol. 17, no. 1, pp. 61–68, 2006.

[18] M. Iwasaki, I. Sato, Y. Jin, N. Saito, and S. Tsuda, "Problems of positive list system revealed by survey of pesticide residue in food," *Journal of Toxicological Sciences*, vol. 32, no. 2, pp. 179–184, 2007.

[19] S. C. Joshi, R. Mathur, and N. Gulati, "Testicular toxicity of chlorpyrifos (an organophosphate pesticide) in albino rat," *Toxicology and Industrial Health*, vol. 23, no. 7, pp. 439–444, 2007.

[20] S. F. Ambali, S. O. Abbas, M. Shittu et al., "Effects of gestational exposure to chlorpyrifos on implantation and neonatal mice," *Journal of Cell and Animal Biology*, vol. 3, no. 4, pp. 050–057, 2009.

[21] S. F. Ambali, H. O. Imana, M. Shittu, M. U. Kawu, S. O. Salami, and J. O. Ayo, "Effect of chlorpyrifos on pre-implantation loss in Swiss Albino mice," *Journal of Agriculture and Biology of North America*, vol. 1, no. 2, pp. 152–155, 2010.

[22] N. C. Rawlings, S. J. Cook, and D. Waldbillig, "Effects of the pesticides carbofuran, chlorpyrifos, dimethoate, lindane, triallate, trifluralin, 2,4-D, and pentachlorophenol on the metabolic endocrine and reproductive endocrine system in ewes," *Journal of Toxicology and Environmental Health Part A*, vol. 54, no. 1, pp. 21–36, 1998.

[23] S. De Angelis, R. Tassinari, F. Maranghi et al., "Developmental exposure to chlorpyrifos induces alterations in thyroid and thyroid hormone levels without other toxicity signs in CD-1 mice," *Toxicological Sciences*, vol. 108, no. 2, pp. 311–319, 2009.

[24] S. F. Ambali, *Ameliorative Effect of Vitamins C and E on Neurotoxicological, Hematological and Biochemical Changes Induced by Chronic Chlorpyrifos in Wistar Rats*, Ph.D. thesis, Ahmadu Bello University, Zaria, Nigeria, 2009.

[25] D. W. Slingerland, "The influence of various factors on the uptake of iodine by the thyroid," *Journal of Clinical Endocrinology and Metabolism*, vol. 15, pp. 131–141, 1955.

[26] H. H. Sandstead, E. G. Stant, A. B. Brill, L. I. Arias, and R. T. Terry, "Lead intoxication and the thyroid," *Archives of Internal Medicine*, vol. 123, no. 6, pp. 632–635, 1969.

[27] B. Singh, V. Chandran, H. K. Bandhu et al., "Impact of lead exposure on pituitary-thyroid axis in humans," *Biometals*, vol. 13, no. 2, pp. 187–192, 2000.

[28] O. O. Oladipo, *Ameliorative Effects of Ascorbic Acid on Neurobehavioural, Haematological and Biochemical Changes Induced by Subchronic Lead Exposure in Wistar Rats*, M.S. thesis, Ahmadu Bello University, Zaria, Nigeria, 2010.

[29] B. D. Banerje, V. Seth, A. Bhattacharya, S. T. Pasha, and A. K. Chakraborty, "Biochemical effects of some pesticides on lipid peroxidation and free radical scavengers," *Toxicology Letters*, vol. 107, pp. 33–47, 1999.

[30] F. Gultekin, N. Delibas, S. Yasar, and I. Kilinc, "*In vivo* changes in antioxidant systems and protective role of melatonin and a combination of vitamin C and vitamin E on oxidative damage in erythrocytes induced by chlorpyrifos-ethyl in rats," *Archives of Toxicology*, vol. 75, no. 2, pp. 88–96, 2001.

[31] S. F. Ambali, S. B. Idris, C. Onukak, M. Shittu, and J. O. Ayo, "Ameliorative effects of vitamin C on short-term sensorimotor and cognitive changes induced by acute chlorpyrifos exposure in Wistar rats," *Toxicology and Industrial Health*, vol. 26, no. 9, pp. 547–558, 2010.

[32] S. F. Ambali, J. O. Ayo, S. A. Ojo, and K. A. N. Esievo, "Vitamin E protects rats from chlorpyrifos-induced increased erythrocyte osmotic fragility in Wistar rats," *Food and Chemical Toxicology*, vol. 48, pp. 3477–3480, 2010.

[33] S. F. Ambali, J. O. Ayo, S. A. Ojo, and K. A. N. Esievo, "Ameliorative effect of vitamin C on chlorpyrifos-induced increased erythrocyte fragility in Wistar rats," *Human and Experimental Toxicology*, vol. 30, no. 1, pp. 19–24, 2011.

[34] E. G. Moreira, I. Vassilieff, and V. S. Vassilieff, "Developmental lead exposure: behavioral alterations in the short and long term," *Neurotoxicology and Teratology*, vol. 23, no. 5, pp. 489–495, 2001.

[35] M. K. Nihei, J. L. McGlothan, C. D. Toscano, and T. R. Guilarte, "Low level Pb^{2+} exposure affects hippocampal protein kinase Cαf gene and protein expression in rats," *Neuroscience Letters*, vol. 298, no. 3, pp. 212–216, 2001.

[36] K. Slawomir, K. Aleksandra, S. Horakb et al., "Activity of SOD and catalase in people protractedly exposed to lead compounds," *Annals of Agricultural and Environmental Medicine*, vol. 11, pp. 291–296, 2004.

[37] S. Ambali, D. Akanbi, N. Igbokwe, M. Shittu, M. Kawu, and J. Ayo, "Evaluation of subchronic chlorpyrifos poisoning on hematological and serum biochemical changes in mice and protective effect of vitamin C," *Journal of Toxicological Sciences*, vol. 32, no. 2, pp. 111–120, 2007.

[38] G. G. El-Hossary, S. M. Mansour, and A. S. Mohamed, "Neurotoxic effects of chlorpyrifos and the possible protective role of antioxidant supplements: an experimental study," *Journal of Applied Sciences Research*, vol. 5, no. 9, pp. 1218–1222, 2009.

[39] R. C. Patra, D. Swarup, and S. K. Dwivedi, "Antioxidant effects of α tocopherol, ascorbic acid and L-methionine on lead induced oxidative stress to the liver, kidney and brain in rats," *Toxicology*, vol. 162, no. 2, pp. 81–88, 2001.

[40] "Guide for the care and use of laboratory animals," DHEW Publication No. (NIH) 85-23, Office of Science and Health Reports, DRR/NIH, Bethesda, Md, USA, 1985.

[41] H. H. Draper and M. Hadley, "Malondialdehyde determination as index of lipid peroxidation," *Methods in Enzymology*, vol. 186, pp. 421–431, 1990.

[42] O. H. Lowry, N. J. Rosebrough, A. L. Farr, and R. J. Randall, "Protein measurement with the Folin phenol reagent," *The Journal of Biological Chemistry*, vol. 193, no. 1, pp. 265–275, 1951.

[43] S. H. Jeong, B. Y. Kim, H. G. Kang, H. O. Ku, and J. H. Cho, "Effect of chlorpyrifos-methyl on steroid and thyroid hormones in rat F0- and F1-generations," *Toxicology*, vol. 220, no. 2-3, pp. 189–202, 2006.

[44] S. S. A. Zaidi, V. K. Bhatnagar, S. J. Gandhi, M. P. Shah, P. K. Kulkarni, and H. N. Saiyed, "Assessment of thyroid function in pesticide formulators," *Human and Experimental Toxicology*, vol. 19, no. 9, pp. 497–501, 2000.

[45] S. S. Chaurasia, S. Panda, and A. Kar, "Lead inhibit type-1 iodothyronine 5'-monodeinodinase in the Indian rock pigeon *Columba livia*: a possible involvement of essential thiol groups," *Journal of Biosciences*, vol. 22, no. 2, pp. 247–254, 1997.

[46] K. Badiei, P. Nikghadam, K. Mostaghni, and M. Zariti, "Effect of lead on thyroid function in sheep," *Iranian Journal of Veterinary Research Shiraz University*, vol. 10, no. 3, Ser. no. 28, pp. 223–227, 2009.

[47] M. K. Kale, S. N. Umathe, and K. P. Bhusari, "Oxidative Stress and the Thyroid," Positive Health, http://www.encognitive.com/files/Oxidative%20Stress%20and%20the%20Thyroid_0.pdf, 2006.

[48] M. Ahamed and M. K. J. Siddiqui, "Low level lead exposure and oxidative stress: current opinions," *Clinica Chimica Acta*, vol. 383, no. 1-2, pp. 57–64, 2007.

[49] G. P. Jarvik, N. T. Tsai, L. A. McKinstry et al., "Vitamin C and E intake is associated with increased paraoxonase activity," *Arteriosclerosis, Thrombosis, and Vascular Biology*, vol. 22, no. 8, pp. 1329–1333, 2002.

[50] S. Nussey and S. A. Whitehead, *Endocrinology: An Integrated Approach*, Bios Scientific Publishers, Oxford, UK, 2001.

[51] Z. E. Suntres and E. M. K. Lui, "Antioxidant effect of zinc and zinc-metallothionein in the acute cytotoxicity of hydrogen peroxide in Ehrlich ascites tumour cells," *Chemico-Biological Interactions*, vol. 162, no. 1, pp. 11–23, 2006.

[52] A. A. Alturfan, E. Zengin, N. Dariyerli et al., "Investigation of zinc and copper levels in methimazole-induced hypothyroidism: relation with the oxidant-antioxidant status," *Folia Biologica*, vol. 53, no. 5, pp. 183–188, 2007.

[53] M. A. Abdel-Wahhab and S. E. Aly, "Antioxidant property of *Nigella sativa* (black cumin) and *Syzygium aromaticum* (clove) in rats during aflatoxicosis," *Journal of Applied Toxicology*, vol. 25, no. 3, pp. 218–223, 2005.

[54] D. K. Sahoo, A. Roy, S. Bhanja, and G. B. N. Chainy, "Hypothyroidism impairs antioxidant defence system and testicular physiology during development and maturation," *General and Comparative Endocrinology*, vol. 156, no. 1, pp. 63–70, 2008.

[55] A. Hood, Y. P. Liu, V. H. Gattone, and C. D. Klaassen, "Sensitivity of thyroid gland growth to thyroid stimulating hormone (TSH) in rats treated with antithyroid drugs," *Toxicological Sciences*, vol. 49, no. 2, pp. 263–271, 1999.

Permissions

Contributors

Shannon R. Bales and Inder J. Chopra
Division of Endocrinology, Diabetes, and Hypertension, University of California, Los Angeles, CA 90095, USA

Navin Rudolph, Claudia Dominguez, Anthony Beaulieu, Pierre De Wailly and Jean-Louis Kraimps
Department of Endocrine Surgery, University Hospital of Poitiers, 86021 Poitiers, France

Hatixhe Latifi-Pupovci, Besa Gacaferri-Lumezi and Violeta Lokaj-Berisha
Department of Physiology and Immunology, Faculty of Medicine, University of Prishtina, Deshmoret e Kombit Street, 10000 Prishtina, Kosovo

Ugur Deveci, Mahmut Sertan Kapakli, Manuk Norayk Manukyan and Abut Kebudi
General Surgery Department, School of Medicine, Maltepe University, 34843 Istanbul, Turkey

Fatih Altintoprak
General Surgery Department, School of Medicine, Sakarya University, 54100 Sakarya, Turkey

Rahmi Cubuk
Radiology Department, School of Medicine, Maltepe University, 34843 Istanbul, Turkey

Nese Yener
Pathology Department, School of Medicine, Maltepe University, 34843 Istanbul, Turkey

Anjali Amin, Waljit S. Dhillo and Kevin G.Murphy
Section of Investigative Medicine, Faculty of Medicine, Imperial College London, 6th Floor, Commonwealth Building, Hammersmith Hospital, Du Cane Road, London W12 0NN, UK

Ceren Eke Koyuncu, Sembol Turkmen Yildirmak and Yüksel Gülen Ozbanazi
Department of Clinical Biochemistry, Ministry of Health Okmeydani Educational and Research Hospital, Okmeydani, Istanbul 34384, Turkey

Mustafa Temizel
Department of Internal Medicine, Ministry of Health Okmeydani Educational and Research Hospital, Okmeydani, Istanbul 34384, Turkey

Tevfik Ozpacaci
Department of Nuclear Medicine, Ministry of Health Okmeydani Educational and Research Hospital, Okmeydani, Istanbul 34384, Turkey

Pinar Gunel
Department of Biostatistics, Uludag University Medical Faculty, Bursa 16059, Turkey

Mustafa Cakmak
Department of Clinical Chemistry, Gulkent State Hospital, Isparta 32100, Turkey

Iordanis Mourouzis, Efstathia Politi and Constantinos Pantos
Department of Pharmacology, University of Athens, 75 Mikras Asias Avenue, Goudi, 11527 Athens, Greece

R. L.Margraf, J. D. Durtschi, J. E. Stephens and M. Perez
Research and Development, ARUP Institute for Clinical and Experimental Pathology, 500 Chipeta Way, Salt Lake City, UT 84108, USA

K. V. Voelkerding
Research and Development, ARUP Institute for Clinical and Experimental Pathology, 500 Chipeta Way, Salt Lake City, UT 84108, USA
Department of Pathology, University of Utah School of Medicine, Salt Lake City, UT 84112, USA

F. Brucker-Davis, P. Fenichel and S. Hieronimus
Department of Endocrinology, Diabetology and Reproductive Medicine, l'Archet Hospital, CHU de Nice, 151 route de Saint-Antoine, 06200 Nice, France

P. Ferrari
Department of Biochemistry, CHU de Nice, 151 route de Saint-Antoine, 06200 Nice, France

J. Gal and F. Berthier
Department of Biostatistics, CHU de Nice, 151 route de Saint-Antoine, 06200 Nice, France

Rabia Cherqaoui
Howard University Hospital, 2041 Georgia Avenue NW, Washington, DC 20060, USA

K. M. Mohamed Shakir
Department of Endocrinology, National Naval Medical Center, 8901Wisconsin Avenue, Bethesda, MD 20889, USA

Babak Shokrani
Department of Pathology, 2041 Georgia Avenue NW,Washington, DC 20060, USA

SujayMadduri
Division of Endocrinology and Metabolism, 2041 Georgia Avenue NW,Washington, DC 20060, USA

Faria Farhat and Vinod Mody
Division of Infectious Disease, Department of Internal Medicine, Howard University Hospital, 2041 Georgia Avenue NW, Washington, DC 20060, USA

VeerleM. Darras, Stijn L. J. Van Herck and Marjolein Heijlen
1Division Animal Physiology and Neurobiology, Biology Department, Laboratory of Comparative Endocrinology, K.U.Leuven, 3000 Leuven, Belgium

Bert De Groef
Division Animal Physiology and Neurobiology, Biology Department, Laboratory of Comparative Endocrinology, K.U.Leuven, 3000 Leuven, Belgium
Department of Agricultural Sciences, Centre for Agribiosciences, La Trobe University, Bundoora, VIC 3086, Australia

Francesca Marini, Ettore Luzi and Maria Luisa Brandi
Unit of Metabolic Bone Diseases, Department of Internal Medicine, University of Florence, Viale Pieraccini 6, 50139 Florence, Italy

Maria Carmela Di Marcantonio and Chiara Tarantelli
Department of Oncology and Experimental Medicine, University "G. d'Annunzio" Chieti-Pescara, 66013 Chieti, Italy

GabriellaMincione
Department of Oncology and Experimental Medicine, University "G. d'Annunzio" Chieti-Pescara, 66013 Chieti, Italy

Center of Excellence on Aging, Ce.S.I., "G. d'Annunzio" University Foundation, 66013 Chieti, Italy

Sonia D'Inzeo, Arianna Nicolussi, Francesco Nardi, Caterina Francesca Donini and Anna Coppa
Department of Experimental Medicine and Department of Radiological Sciences Oncology and Anatomical Pathology, Sapienza University of Rome, Viale Regina Elena, 324, 00161 Rome, Italy

Hala Ahmadieh and Sami T. Azar
Division of Endocrinology, Department of Internal Medicine, American University of Beirut Medical Center, 3 Dag Hammarskjold Plaza, New York, NY 10017, USA

Carles Zafon, Gabriel Obiols, Belen Dalama and JordiMesa
Department of Endocrinology, Hospital General Universitari Vall d'Hebron, Pg. Vall d'Hebron 119-129, 08035 Barcelona, Spain

Juan Antonio Baena
Department of Surgery, Unit of Endocrinological Surgery, Hospital General Universitari Vall d'Hebron, 08035 Barcelona, Spain

Josep Castellví
Department of Pathology, Hospital General Universitari Vall d'Hebron, 08035 Barcelona, Spain

Maureen Groer
University of South Florida College of Nursing, 12910 Bruce B. Downs Boulevard, Tampa, FL 33612, USA

Cecilia Jevitt
Yale University School of Nursing, P.O. Box 27399,West Haven, CT 06515-7399, USA

Syed Ali Imran
Division of Endocrinology and Metabolism, Dalhousie University, Halifax, NS, Canada B3H 2Y9

Murali Rajaraman
Department of Radiation Oncology, Dalhousie University, Halifax, NS, Canada B3H 2Y9

Naifa Lamki Busaidy and Maria E. Cabanillas
Department of Endocrine Neoplasia and Hormonal Disorders, University of Texas MD Anderson Cancer Center, 1515 Holcombe Boulevard, Unit 1461, Houston, TX 77030, USA

Luca Ceriani and Sergio Suriano
Department of Nuclear Medicine and Thyroid Unit, Oncology Institute of Southern Switzerland, Street Ospedale 12, 6500 Bellinzona, Switzerland

Luca Giovanella
Department of Nuclear Medicine and Thyroid Unit, Oncology Institute of Southern Switzerland, Street Ospedale 12, 6500 Bellinzona, Switzerland
Department of Clinical Chemistry and Laboratory Medicine, Ente Ospedaliero Cantonale, 6500 Bellinzona, Switzerland

Leonidas H. Duntas
Endocrine Unit, Evgenidion Hospital, University of Athens, 20 Papadiamantopoulou Street, 11528 Athens, Greece

Mohamed Osama Hegazi and Sherif Ahmed
Medical Department, Al Adan Hospital, P.O. Box 262, Hadiya 52853, Kuwait

Norman Blumenthal
Department of Obstetrics and Gynaecology, Blacktown Hospital and Norwest Private Hospital, 9 Norbrik Drive, Bella Vista 2153, Sydney, NSW, Australia

Karen Byth
NHMRC Clinical Trials Centre, Faculty of Medicine, 92 Parramatta Road, Camperdown, Sydney, NSW 2050, Australia

Creswell J. Eastman
International Council for Control of Iodine Deficiency Disorders, Sydney Medical School, University of Sydney, Sydney, NSW, Australia

Sydney Thyroid Clinic, Westmead Specialist Centre, Suite 8, 16-18 Mons Road Westmead, NSW 2145, Australia

Yoshiyuki Ban, Michiya Takada and Tsutomu Hirano
Division of Diabetes, Metabolism and Endocrinology, Department of Medicine, Showa University School of Medicine, 1-5-8 Hatanodai, Shinagawa-ku, Tokyo 142-8666, Japan

Gou Yamamoto and Shigeo Hayashi
Department of Oral Pathology and Diagnosis, School of Dentistry, Showa University, 1-5-8 Hatanodai, Shinagawa-ku, Tokyo 142-8555, Japan

Tetsuhiko Tachikawa
Department of Oral Pathology and Diagnosis, School of Dentistry, Showa University, 1-5-8 Hatanodai, Shinagawa-ku, Tokyo 142-8555, Japan Comprehensive Research Center of Oral Cancer, Showa University, 1-5-8 Hatanodai, Shinagawa-ku, Tokyo 142-8555, Japan

Yoshio Ban
Ban Thyroid Clinic, 2-11-16 Jiyugaoka, Megro-ku, Tokyo 152-0035, Japan

Kazuo Shimizu, Haruki Akasu and Takehito Igarashi
Division of Endocrine Surgery, Department of Surgery, Nippon Medical School, 1-1-5 Sendagi, Bunkyo-ku, Tokyo 113-8602, Japan

Yasuhiko Bando
Biosys Technologies, Inc., 2-13-18 Nakane, Meguro-ku, Tokyo 152-0031, Japan

Karen Gómez
Department of Endocrinology, Hospital San Juan de Dios, Avenida 14, Calles 6 Y 7 Paseo Colon, 1475-1000 San José, Costa Rica

Jeena Varghese and Camilo Jiménez
Department of Endocrine Neoplasia and Hormonal Disorders, Unit 1461, The University of Texas MD Anderson Cancer Center, 1515 Holcombe Boulevard, Houston, TX 77030, USA

Alex Stagnaro-Green
GeorgeWashington University School of Medicine and Health Sciences, 2300 Eye Street, Ross Hall, Suite 712, Washington, DC 20037, USA

Enrique Grande
Department of Medical Oncology, Ram´on y Cajal University Hospital, 28034 Madrid, Spain

Juan José Díez
Department of Endocrinology, Ram´on y Cajal University Hospital, 28034 Madrid, Spain

Carles Zafon
Department of Endocrinology, Vall d'Hebron University Hospital, 08035 Barcelona, Spain

Jaume Capdevila
Department of Medical Oncology, Vall d'Hebron University Hospital, 08035 Barcelona, Spain

Mourouzis Iordanis, Zisakis Athanasios, Economou Konstantinos and Pantos Constantinos
Department of Pharmacology, University of Athens, 75 Mikras Asias Avenue,11527 Goudi, Athens, Greece

Liappas Alexandros
Department of Pharmacology, University of Athens, 75 Mikras Asias Avenue,11527 Goudi, Athens, Greece
School of Pharmacy and Biomedical Sciences, University of Central Lancashire, Preston PR1 2HE, Lancashire, UK

Lea Robert-William
School of Pharmacy and Biomedical Sciences, University of Central Lancashire, Preston PR1 2HE, Lancashire, UK

Yaniv S. Ovadia and Dov Gefel
Department of Internal Medicine "C", Barzilai Medical Center Ashkelon, Hahistadrout Street 2, 7830604 Ashkelon, Israel

Nutrition and Brain Health Laboratory, School of Nutritional Sciences, Institute of Biochemistry, Food Science and Nutrition, Robert H. Smith Faculty of Agriculture, Food and Environment,The Hebrew University of Jerusalem, P.O. Box 12, 76100 Rehovot, Israel

AronM. Troen
Nutrition and Brain Health Laboratory, School of Nutritional Sciences, Institute of Biochemistry, Food Science and Nutrition, Robert H. Smith Faculty of Agriculture, Food and Environment,The Hebrew University of Jerusalem, P.O. Box 12, 76100 Rehovot, Israel

Svetlana Turkot
Endocrinology Clinic, Barzilai Medical Center Ashkelon, Hahistadrout Street 2, 7830604 Ashkelon, Israel

Dorit Aharoni and Shlomo Fytlovich
Laboratory of Clinical Biochemistry, Barzilai Medical Center Ashkelon, Hahistadrout Street 2, 7830604 Ashkelon, Israel

Maria E. Cabanillas, Mimi I. Hu and Naifa L. Busaidy
Department of Endocrine Neoplasia and Hormonal Disorders, The University of Texas MD Anderson Cancer Center, Houston, TX 77030, USA

Jean-Bernard Durand
Department of Cardiology, The University of Texas MD Anderson Cancer Center, Houston, TX 77030, USA

Emin Gürleyik, Banu Karapolat and Ufuk Onsal
Department of Surgery, Duzce University Medical Faculty, 81650 Duzce, Turkey

Gunay Gurleyik
Haydarpasa Numune Hospital, Istanbul, Turkey

Meghan D. Rosen and Martin L. Privalsky
Department of Microbiology, University of California-Davis, Davis, CA 95616, USA

PetraMohácsik, Anikó Zeöld and Balázs Gereben
Laboratory of Endocrine Neurobiology, Institute of Experimental Medicine, Hungarian Academy of Sciences, Budapest, H-1083, Hungary

Antonio C. Bianco
Division of Endocrinology, Diabetes, and Metabolism, University of Miami Miller School of Medicine, Miami, FL 33136, USA

Yasuhiro Ito, Takuya Higashiyama, Minoru Kihara, Chisato Tomoda, Yuuki Takamura, Kaoru Kobayashi, AkihiroMiya and AkiraMiyauchi
Department of Surgery, Kuma Hospital, Shimoyamate-Dori, Chuo-Ku, Kobe 650-0011, Japan

Mitsuyoshi Hirokawa
Department of Pathology, Kuma Hospital, Kobe 650-0011, Japan

Suleiman F. Ambali, Chinedu Orieji, Woziri O. Abubakar, Muftau Shittu, and Mohammed U. Kawu
Department of Veterinary Physiology and Pharmacology, Ahmadu Bello University, Zaria 800007, Nigeria

Index